A TEXTBOOK FOR NURSING ASSISTANTS

A TEXTBOOK FOR NURSING ASSISTANTS

GERTRUDE D. CHERESCAVICH, R.N., B.S., M.S.

Director of Nursing Services, Community General Hospital; Assistant Professor, Syracuse University School of Nursing, Syracuse, New York; Project Director, Regional Medical Program Supported Project to Expand the Health Care Delivery System Through the Use of Nurse Clinicians

THIRD EDITION

with 179 illustrations

THE C. V. MOSBY COMPANY
Saint Louis 1973

THIRD EDITION

Copyright © 1973 by The C. V. Mosby Company

All rights reserved. No part of this book may be reproduced in any manner without written permission of the publisher.

Previous editions copyrighted 1964, 1968

Printed in the United States of America

Distributed in Great Britain by Henry Kimpton, London

Library of Congress Cataloging in Publication Data

Cherescavich, Gertrude D
  A textbook for nursing assistants.

    1. Nurses and nursing. 2. Nurses' aides.
I. Title. [DNLM: 1. Nurses' aides. WY 193 C521t 1973]
RT41.C56 1973   610.73   72-12852
ISBN 0-8016-0957-7

To those corpsmen in World War II,
nursing assistants at the New York Veterans Administration Hospital,
and orderlies in the Neurological Department at Philadelphia General Hospital
who taught me how effectively a well-trained nonprofessional nursing assistant
can care for patients.

Foreword

If safe, efficient, therapeutic nursing care is the objective of departments of nursing service, then priority must be placed upon preparation of *all* nursing service personnel for their changing role and functions. At the same time we are expanding and planning for further expansion of services to individuals and families in a community, the department of nursing service is employing and assigning more auxiliary personnel for the provision of these services. The responsibilities involved in the selection, training, and assignment of these personnel are serious, and the author has established guidelines and goals as well as the techniques to be employed.

Currently, more than 400,000 aides, orderlies, and attendants are employed in hospitals, but there is a wide diversity of potential within this group based primarily on selection policies and training programs. The important contribution of the supportive assistance rendered by the auxiliary worker in nursing services is in the performance of tasks that assist the nurse in direct patient care. But major problems in a significant proportion of institutions and agencies are the result of dilution of the nursing service program of care through ineffective utilization of nursing service personnel and through assignment for tasks for which the worker is not prepared.

The auxiliary worker, working under the direction of a professional nurse or licensed practical nurse, performs tasks delegated by the nurse responsible for the nursing service of the unit. Two practices which appear to be prevalent need to be modified —one is that which tends to limit the tasks of auxiliary workers so that they cannot make the contribution to patient care which they should and the other is that which allows them to take on more and more responsibility for nursing care with little or no preparation.

The Statement on Auxiliary Personnel in Nursing Service of the American Nurses' Association clearly identifies examples of tasks which demonstrate the potentiality of auxiliary workers in nursing services. These examples were presented with the acknowledgement that the choice and diversity of tasks assigned to the worker depend upon many variables, including but not limited to the nature of the supporting service, the type of patient, the size and kind of institution or agency, the potentiality of the auxiliary worker, and the currently accepted principles of good patient care.

In a dynamic social order, continuous change is evident in occupational patterns, resulting in inevitable changes in the role and activities of personnel. Advances in technology and in research in the fundamental and applied sciences have augmented the body of knowledge available to special interest vocational groups. A set of skills, accepted as professional when first developed, may become so routine that they can be taught to or "caught" by other individuals through the use of concise directional statements. Knowledge has a similar filtering process. One has only to be aware of the reporting on all matters concerning the health field in the daily press and magazines for the general public. Other evidences of the shifting emphasis and availability of knowledge are developments in the elementary and secondary school systems of the nation. Observations of auxiliary workers in the work situation, the types of questions they ask, and the comments they make clearly indicate a need for understanding the "why" as well as the "how" with respect to assignments for patient care services. Since we expect the general public to be informed about matters of health and illness, it is imperative that personnel employed in health agencies are informed so as to guide those to whom service is being rendered.

The on-the-job training program projected in this text is based upon the assumption that auxiliary personnel must be informed workers if they are to function effectively as members of the nursing team, for observations are misconstrued unless the basic elements for understanding are provided. There is no intent to extend the scope of tasks beyond those which are supportive and complimentary to nursing practice. Auxiliary personnel must be properly instructed and properly supervised. This is a primary responsibility of the professional nurse if nursing assistants are to contribute to the patient's comfort and welfare.

Eleanor C. Lambertsen
Dean, Cornell University-
New York Hospital
School of Nursing,
New York, N. Y.

Preface

This era of the expanding responsibilities of the nurse will have many implications for the role of the nursing assistant, a role that has traditionally expanded when nursing personnel was scarce and contracted when nurses were plentiful. But now as nursing matures into a truly clinical and therapeutic profession, the role of the nursing assistant as a deliverer of personal care may finally be clearly established, and accepted. However, since notably definitive changes in the role of the nurse and, therefore, in the role of the nursing assistant are yet to come, this revision has not attempted to identify the new practice patterns or the skills they require. Instead, this book has continued to focus on the nursing assistant as a team member in the health care delivery system.

The major portion of the book is concerned with the patient and his needs: why he needs a particular care, how to provide that care, and what results can be expected. To assist the nonprofessional team members to understand the specific disease mechanisms and nursing care techniques, 179 illustrations are included.

In this revision, techniques are simplified, disposable equipment is emphasized, and the discussions of reusable types are deleted. The section on isolation has been completely revised in accord with the latest thinking on the subject.

Although this book cannot provide any one existing health care delivery facility with the precise job description and training program for its nursing assistants, it should meet the needs of most with a moderate amount of exclusion and addition.

Throughout the book, study questions are included at the beginning of each chapter, and discussion questions, along with a glossary of terms and sources of additional information, where deemed desirable, are included at the end of each chapter. These self-help aids should prove extremely valuable to students.

A teaching guide is available for instructors in in-service programs who use this book as a text in their training programs. This guide includes a plan for developing a job description for nursing assistants, a method of teaching, and a list of recommended teaching aids.

Gertrude D. Cherescavich

Contents

SECTION I Introduction

    1 The hospital and the extended care facility, 3
    2 Your job as assistant, 6
    3 The patient care team, 9
    4 The patient needs you to care, 15
    5 The patient is a person, 17
    6 The patient's home in the hospital, 20

SECTION II The nursing assistant meets the patient's basic daily needs in the health care facility

    7 Meeting the patient's need for a comfortable bed, 27
    8 Meeting the patient's need for food, 40
    9 Meeting the patient's need for water, 57
    10 Meeting the patient's need for cleanliness and movement—complete, partial, and out-of-bed baths, 65
    11 Caring for the patient's toilet needs, 80
    12 Caring for the patient's need to move, 91
    13 Caring for the patient's need to get out of bed, 107
    14 Meeting the patient's need for sleep, 122

SECTION III The nursing assistant meets the patient's particular needs in the hospital and extended care facility

    15 Receiving the patient on the ward, 131
    16 Caring for the patient's emotional environment, 142
    17 Maintaining a safe physical environment for the patient, 147
    18 Identifying, recording, and reporting the patient's needs, 159
    19 The vital signs, 165

- 20 Taking the patient's temperature, 167
- 21 Taking the patient's pulse, 176
- 22 Counting the patient's respirations, 181
- 23 Taking the patient's blood pressure, 186
- 24 Observing the patient's level of consciousness, 194
- 25 Charting temperature, pulse, and respiration, 198
- 26 Collecting specimens from the patient, 201
- 27 Giving the patient an enema, 209
- 28 Caring for the patient with a colostomy, 226
- 29 Caring for the patient with an ileostomy, a "wet" ileostomy, or ureterostomies, 248
- 30 Applying heat to the patient's body in the presence of infection, 260
- 31 Reducing the patient's temperature, 271
- 32 Internal and external urinary drainage, 284

SECTION IV The nursing assistant meets the needs of special patients in the hospital

- 33 Caring for the patient with a communicable disease, 303
- 34 Caring for the patient in reverse isolation, 324
- 35 Caring for the patient who is unable to cope with the problems in living, 329
- 36 Caring for the preoperative patient, 339
- 37 Caring for the postoperative patient, 351
- 38 Caring for the patient who is breathless, 371
- 39 Care of the aged person with problems in living, 395
- 40 Meeting the first-aid needs of the patient, 404
- 41 Caring for the dying patient, 413
- 42 Meeting the patient's need for comfort and safety on an off-ward trip, 423
- 43 Assisting the patient to get ready to go home, 428

INTRODUCTION

SECTION I

Chapter 1   The hospital and the extended care facility
         2   Your job as assistant
         3   The patient care team
         4   The patient needs you to care
         5   The patient is a person
         6   The patient's home in the hospital

1/The hospital and the extended care facility

STUDY QUESTIONS

1. Why does a hospital exist?
2. How does the law control the operation of the hospital?
3. What does the law require from us in caring for patients?
4. How do hospitals differ?
5. How are hospitals alike?
6. What does the hospital do for those patients who cannot be cured?

PURPOSE OF THE HOSPITAL

The purpose of every hospital is patient care. The patient is the primary reason for the hospital's existence. Without patients, we would not need hospitals, doctors, nurses, or nursing assistants.

TYPES OF HOSPITALS

There are many different types of hospitals. There are general hospitals that care for patients with all types of illness, and there are specialty hospitals that specifically care for patients with one particular kind of illness. Some examples of specialty hospitals are (1) mental disease hospitals and (2) cancer hospitals.

Hospitals may differ also in their ownership. Some examples are (1) the university hospital, (2) the city hospital, (3) the state hospital, (4) the church-supported hospital, and (5) the private hospital.

In one way, however, all hospitals are the same—they are all concerned with patient care.

HOSPITAL PROGRAMS

In looking around most hospitals, we see doctors, nurses, and nursing assistants caring for patients, groups of students (medical, nursing, psychology, social work, etc.), and groups of research workers. In fact, some patients might complain of being a guinea pig. All of these groups take part in the three programs conducted by the hospital: (1) patient care, (2) teaching, and (3) research. All three groups contribute to the basic purpose of the hospital—patient care. Each group makes its contribution as follows:

1. The doctors, nurses, and nursing assistants giving patient care contribute by caring for the patient now.
2. The students are learning patient care now so that they will be able to care for patients next year or even 5 years from now.
3. The research workers are looking for cures for incurable diseases and for improved methods of treating patients.

It is our responsibility to be helpful to students and to research workers whenever we can because they are a vital part of our hospital patient care team.

RESPONSIBILITY OF THE HOSPITAL

We have said that the purpose of the hospital is to care for patients, and the law expects us to do this well. The law expects us to give the patient the care he needs. It expects us to carry out this care in such a way that the patient is safe and free from any harm. In fact, the patient has a right to sue us in the courts if we fail to give him the care he needs, or if we carry out this care in an unsafe manner and he receives bodily harm. Examples of this might be as follows:

1. Burning the patient with a hot-water bottle that is too hot
2. Amputating the leg of a patient who went to the operating room to have his eye removed
3. Removing the eye of a patient who went to the operating room to have his leg amputated
4. Permitting an unconscious patient to roll out of bed because the crib side was left down
5. Permitting the patient to slip in the bath water we spilled and to fall and break his leg

Not one of us wants to hurt a patient in any way. We all want to help him get well, but we can hurt the patient unless we learn to work carefully at all times. The more rushed we are, the more likely we are to make mistakes. However, regardless of how busy we are, we must always check our work and take the time to give the patient the very best nursing care we know how to give. The temperature of the water must be exactly the right temperature before we pour the water into the hot-water bottle. The patient's bed tag and name tag on his wrist must be checked carefully before we place the patient on a stretcher to go to the operating room. Spilled water must be mopped up quickly before the patient slips. We can never afford to be so busy that our careless work causes a patient to be injured. Not only do we want it this way, but the law says it **must** be this way.

PATIENT CARE

The hospital gives health care to the acutely ill patient. This acute-type care is both intensive and expensive. Because of this, the patient is usually discharged to his family for his convalescent care. Sometimes, however, this convalescent care is really extensive rehabilitative training in activities of living such as talking, walking, and toileting. When this is so, the patient is not discharged to family care but is, instead, transferred to an extended care facility or a nursing home. In this type of facility patient care consists of a minimum amount of diagnostic and therapeutic services and a maximum amount of retraining in living.

The hospital gives the patient the best care it can, the best it knows how to give. The doctor uses all the newest advances in science to diagnose and treat the patient. The nurse uses all of her skill to alleviate the patient's discomfort and pain. You, the nursing assistant, help the patient carry out all the daily living activities that he cannot do for himself or by himself because of his illness. The hospital cures many, many patients, but not all of them.

The cure for some diseases is still not known, but the hospital finds ways to help patients with incurable diseases to live as painlessly, as comfortably, and as enjoyably as possible for as long as possible. Once these ways are found—the medicines, the treatments, and the exercises to keep him comfortable—the patient no longer needs the hospital but he does need living assistance. Now he needs help with all the living activities he once did for himself—getting a drink of water, taking a bath, going to the toilet, finding a friend—and so he is ready to go back home and live with this help and caring. The Visiting Nurse Service and their Home Health Aides will assist the family in caring for the incurably ill family member. However, if the patient has no family or if the family is unable to give the care the patient requires (for example, an old and feeble mate), the hospital can arrange to transfer the patient to an extended care facility. In the extended care facility a patient is given living assistance from a foster family (nurses and nursing assistants), when his own family cannot give it.

SUMMARY

The hospital exists for the care of patients. Although hospitals may differ in their ownership or in the types of disease they treat, all hospitals are the same in their desire to help patients get well when possible or to find ways to help incurably ill patients live comfortably for as long as possible. Making the patient's life comfortable can be done at home with the help of a family member or in a nursing home, when the family cannot give the help the patient needs. The hospital provides diagnosis and treatment and the nursing home gives living assistance.

Health care personnel (hospital and extended care facility personnel) are required by law to carry out these purposes by giving the best patient care they can. Health care facilities may be sued by the patient if he receives bodily harm from the care given him or from the lack of care that he needs.

DISCUSSION QUESTIONS

1 What kind of hospital is the one in which you work?
2 What does the law in your state say about your care of patients?
3 How does the hospital help you keep your nursing care safe?
4 What would you say to a patient who complained to you that he was a guinea pig?
5 Discuss the error in this statement: You are taught one way in the classroom, but when you get on the ward, you forget that and do it your own way.
6 When is the incurably ill patient discharged from the hospital? Why?

VOCABULARY

extended care facility An intensive rehabilitative setting for the patient who has recovered from the acute phase of illness but who has not as yet attained his maximum recovery potential.
health care facility Any setting in which health care is delivered. Examples of newer type settings might be extended care units, day hospitals, and neighborhood health centers. The goal of these settings is to provide the essential health care and/or periodic foster parent–type supervision (day hospital) to enable a person, even with living skill deficiencies, to live effectively at home.

2/Your job as assistant

STUDY QUESTIONS

1 Why do you feel so strange in your new hospital job?
2 What will you be required to do?
3 What is involved in caring for patients?
4 How will you know what to do and when to do it?
5 Why are health care facilities kept so clean?

As you begin your new job, you may feel a little strange and quite worried. Perhaps you have never worked with patients before. Perhaps you have been a patient at one time, and now you remember all the pain you had then and the great relief you felt when you were discharged. Perhaps you walk a little more slowly as you ask yourself the following questions: What am I doing here now? What can I possibly do to help patients? How can I ever do this job?

THE NURSE'S JOB

The job of the nurse in the hospital and extended care facility may be outlined as follows:
1. Give the patient nursing care.
   a. Help the patient get as well as possible.
   b. Help the incurable patient to live as comfortably and as enjoyably as possible.
   c. Teach the patient who is getting ready to go home how to stay as well as possible.
2. Provide the patient with the facilities for living.
   a. Give the patient the kind of home he needs (patient's unit—bed, overbed table, wheelchair, etc.).
   b. Keep the patient's home clean.
3. Assist the doctor in caring for the pa-

tient; help him diagnose and treat the patient.
  a. Give the doctor clues to the patient's condition (observing the signs and symptoms he presents).
  b. Assist the doctor with diagnostic and therapeutic procedures for the patient (giving intravenous injections, taking blood specimens, etc.).
  c. Give the patient the treatments and medications the doctor orders.

THE NURSING ASSISTANT'S JOB

The nurse has a big job, too big for her to do alone, and so you have been employed to assist her. The way in which you can assist her has been drawn up into a list of duties that you will be able to do after your training program is completed. These duties are the ones that the nurses in this hospital or extended care facility need you to do to help them take care of their patients and not those you performed in any previous health care facility.

Your new job will not consist of a great many new and strange duties. You have been taking care of yourself for a long time. Now you are going to do the same things you do for yourself, but you are going to do them for the patient.

Patient care

The patient is a person who has lost his ability to take care of himself because of his illness. So you take over—you become his arms, his legs, and his muscles. The patient may be unconscious and not aware of what he needs, but you know that he needs all the same things you do. You are able to care for him by thinking about your own needs.

You know how unpleasant your mouth feels in the morning until you brush your teeth, so you brush his teeth and clean his mouth. You know how good it feels to take a bath, so you give him a bath. The patient cannot get out of bed, so you take a pan of water to the bedside and bathe him in bed. You know how tired you get sitting in one position for a long time (think of your last long trip), so you move the patient frequently, shifting his position and relieving the pressures on his body. The patient cannot swallow, but the doctor will feed him by intravenous injections or by passing a tube so that you can feed him. The patient cannot tell you of his pains and aches, so you watch him carefully for clues to his condition—clues that he is getting better or that he is getting worse.

Remember, you do not have the full responsibility for patient care. You are the nurse's assistant, and the nurse will tell you what patients you are to care for and what care you are to give them. Now you do not know how to give this care, but you will after your training is completed.

Care of the patient's hospital home

Some, and maybe all, of the care of the patient's unit will be the unit housekeeper's job. However, it must be stressed that daily damp dusting of the unit and daily mopping of the floor are essential to keep the patient safe from germs and infections. Dust is a vehicle on which germs ride. With the help of air currents, germs can ride across hallways and through ventilating systems from floor to floor. Dust, therefore, is the companion of germs and the enemy of safe patient care.

Assisting the doctor

Assisting the doctor in the only aspect of your job that will be new to you. You may learn how to get clues to the patient's condition by taking vital signs (temperature, pulse, respiration, blood pressure) and by learning the signs and symptoms of illness and how to observe the patient for these. You will also learn how to collect specimens from the patient and how to prepare them for the laboratory.

You may learn how to help the doctor examine the patient and how to help him do diagnostic tests and perform treatments.

You may learn how to give the patient enemas, colostomy irrigations, bladder irrigations, how to apply wet dressings, etc.

• • •

You will like your job. You will like the many new things you learn every day, and you will become more and more skilled in caring for patients. The feeling of warmth and satisfaction you get from easing the pain or soothing the fears of a patient will more than make up for all the little problems encountered on the job.

SUMMARY

The job of the nursing assistant is helping the nurse and the doctor care for the patients in the health care facility. Most of this work is already familiar to the nursing assistant, since it involves doing those daily activities of living that one does for himself but that will now be done for the patient. Some aspects of the job will be entirely new. This is the part that deals with taking vital signs, giving treatments, and helping the doctor. The nurse determines the patients' nursing care and assigns the nursing assistant to that part of the care he is able to do.

A good rule to follow in caring for the patient is to care for him as you would want him to care for you if you were the patient and he were the nursing assistant.

DISCUSSION QUESTIONS

1 What are the duties and responsibilities of the nursing assistant in your health care facility?
2 How does the nurse make out the assignments on your unit?
3 Who does unit housekeeping activities?
4 Which unit housekeeping activities are the nursing assistant's responsibility?
5 Observe the patients and note how closely their needs resemble yours.
6 How do your duties differ from those you had in a previous health care facility?

3/The patient care team

STUDY QUESTIONS

1 What is a nursing care team?
2 Who is the team leader?
3 What is the value of a nursing care team?
4 Who are the team members?
5 How does the team leader lead?
6 What is the role of the team members?
7 How good is a nursing care team?

THE NURSING CARE TEAM

The patient care team is comprised of a nurse team leader and nursing assistant team members. This team works together in caring for a group of patients.

The nurse is responsible to the patient, to the doctor, and to the health care facility for providing the patient with the specialized nursing care that he needs. She has been prepared through an extensive educational program to diagnose the patient's nursing needs and to give the skilled care to meet these needs. She understands that each patient is different and, because of this difference, requires an individualized type of nursing care. Therefore the nurse guides her team members (nursing assistants) in doing an intensive study of each patient so that his physical and emotional needs can be identified. She guides her team members in this study through an assignment plan in which she focuses their attention on the kind of patient observations they are to make.

After the team members have studied the patient they meet with the team leader for a patient care planning conference. In this conference, the nurse and the nursing assistants pool their patient information and observations and determine the nursing care approach required to meet the specific physical and emotional needs of that particular patient. The nurse then decides how the nursing care can best be given. She considers the patient's need and the education or training of her team members. She then develops a patient care assignment. In this assignment, each team member is delegated that part of the patient's nursing care that he is able to do and that he has been trained to do.

The patient's needs change as his condition changes. Therefore the nursing care plan will require constant revision if it is to meet the patient's changing needs. These revisions are determined each day in the evaluation conference when the team comes together to evaluate the patient care they have given. In these conferences the team members discuss how they have carried out their patient care assignment and how effective their care has been in meeting the patient's needs, and then they identify new patient needs and plan new nursing approaches to meet them.

The nurse gives patient care that requires nursing skill and clinical judgment, and the nursing assistants give patient care that requires nursing assistant skill and observational ability. For example, the nurse carefully evaluates the patient's condition when he returns from the operating room. Then, after she has determined that he is breathing properly, that his secretions are not blocking his airway, and that his vital signs are within normal limits, she delegates such duties as checking the blood pressure, the pulse, and the respirations at 15-minute intervals to the nursing assistant. When the nurse delegates this part of the patient's care to the nursing assistant, she specifically tells the nursing assistant what vital signs to take, how often to take them, what patient observations to make, what vital sign changes indicate, and at what vital sign change she wishes to be notified.

The nurse does not leave the recovery room. She remains there. The nursing assistant takes the patient's vital signs every 15 minutes, and this frees the nurse to suction the patient's airway, to irrigate any tubes, to give medication, to start oxygen, and to encourage the patient to breathe deeply and to cough. The nurse also assists the doctor in giving blood transfusions and in doing emergency treatments. At least once each hour, the nurse carefully evaluates each patient's condition with the nursing assistant. At this time, the nurse identifies changes in the patient's condition and revises her patient care plan and her patient care directions to the nursing assistant in order to meet the patient's changing physical and emotional needs.

The nurse does not have the time or the physical capacity to care for a group of postoperative patients alone, and the nursing assistant does not have sufficient nursing knowledge and skill to safely care for the postoperative patient alone. However, when the nurse and the nursing assistants work together as a team and share the patient care work load, they can give a group of postoperative patients the specialized nursing care they need. In the team relationship the nurse is able to care for a group of patients when she can delegate part of their care to well-trained nursing assistants. The nursing assistant team members can give this care safely and effectively when the nurse team leader assigns them patient care activities that they have been taught to do and when she works with them in giving, planning, and evaluating this care.

PREPARATION OF THE NURSING ASSISTANT FOR TEAM NURSING

Since the nurse assigns patient care activities to members of the nursing team, the nursing assistant must be adequately trained to give this care before he can accept an assignment and function as a full-fledged team member. This training must prepare him to do all the patient care activities that the nurse may assign him to do. The nursing assistant's patient care activities will differ from one health care facility to another and will depend upon the following:

1. The availability of professional nurses
2. The degree of the patient's illness
3. The preemployment qualifications for nursing assistants
4. The type of training program provided for nursing assistants
5. The turnover rates in the nursing assistant group
6. The opportunities for advancement in the nursing assistant role

Therefore each nursing service will develop a job description for the nursing assistant team members and will institute a training program to prepare them to meet these job requirements. This job description is usually developed as a result of the head nurses' identifying those patient care activities that they believe an assistant could be trained to do. They also identify the qualifications the assistant must have in order to be able to learn the skills taught in the training program.

After the job description is prepared and approved by the director of nursing, it is given to the in-service education and training staff, who use it as a guide in developing a training program for the nursing assistant team members. Then a group of nursing assistants are employed and trained with this program. Constant evaluations are made throughout the training program, and many revisions are made until it finally becomes the exact training program the nursing assistant needs to assist him in developing the patient care skills he will be required to do in the health care facility.

As the trained nursing assistant functions on the team and becomes more skilled in patient care, he may be rewarded with salary increases. Perhaps, he may even receive advanced training in additional patient care skills, with promotions to new patient care activities and higher salary scales.

The nursing assistant team member always works under the direction and guidance of the professional nurse team leader, just as the team leader always works under the direction and guidance of the head nurse or supervisor.

HOW THE TEAM LEADER LEADS THE TEAM

The nurse team leader will lead her patient care team in the following ways:

1. *The team leader will make a team assignment.* Each day, near the end of the tour of duty, she will get her team together to plan the coming day's work. Patient care activities for the coming day will be discussed, and plans will be made for carrying out these activities. Each team member will be assigned a share of the work to be done, and he will be given specific directions on how to do it and where to get help if he needs it. At the end of the conference, the team leader will post the written assignment on the personnel bulletin board. This assignment will give each team member specific directions as to:

   a. What patients he is to care for
   b. What care he is to give the patients
   c. How this care is to be given
   d. What care the team leader will give the patients
   e. How he can locate his team leader
   f. Patient observations he is to make
   g. Patient observations that are to be reported to the team leader immediately

2. *The team leader will conduct a planning conference soon after the tour of duty begins.* After she receives a report on the condition of her patients from the nurse on the previous tour of duty, she will meet with her team. At this meeting, she will acquaint her team with any significant changes in the patients' conditions that necessitate revisions in the patient care plans and the assignment. Together, the team will make these revisions.

3. *The team leader will conduct evaluation rounds.* She will visit her team members and evaluate their progress in the

assignment. She will identify areas of difficulty and will assist the team members in avoiding or overcoming these difficulties. At the completion of the patient care assignment, the entire team will make evaluation rounds to determine the quality of care they have given. One member of the team carries the Kardex and serves as team secretary.

Before the team enters the patient's room, the team member who gave most of the patient's care discusses the care that he gave, the problems he had in giving the care, and any new patient needs that he identified. Then all of the team members enter the patient's room. The nurse talks with the patient in such a way as to get information about problem areas or changing needs. She also observes the quality of care given to the patient. Then the team members leave the patient's room. In the hall they identify patient problems and new needs, and the secretary jots these down on the Kardex.

After the rounds, the team members discuss the quality of care they have given and identify ways in which they can improve this care.

4. *The team leader will determine what skills should be included in a teaching program* (Fig. 3-1). During evaluation rounds, she will identify the training needs of her team. These may include identifying patient's problems, giving patient care, or making patient observations. The leader will discuss the training needs of her team members with the head nurse, and together they will decide what skills should be taught in a ward teaching program to meet the team's needs.

5. *The team leader will conduct a teaching program for the team* (Fig. 3-2). She will work with individual team members in a buddy system. She will teach them good patient care by actually helping them give this care. She will also teach them that the patient is a person of dignity and worth by her attitude toward and manner of dealing with the patients and by her concern for their wants as well as their needs.

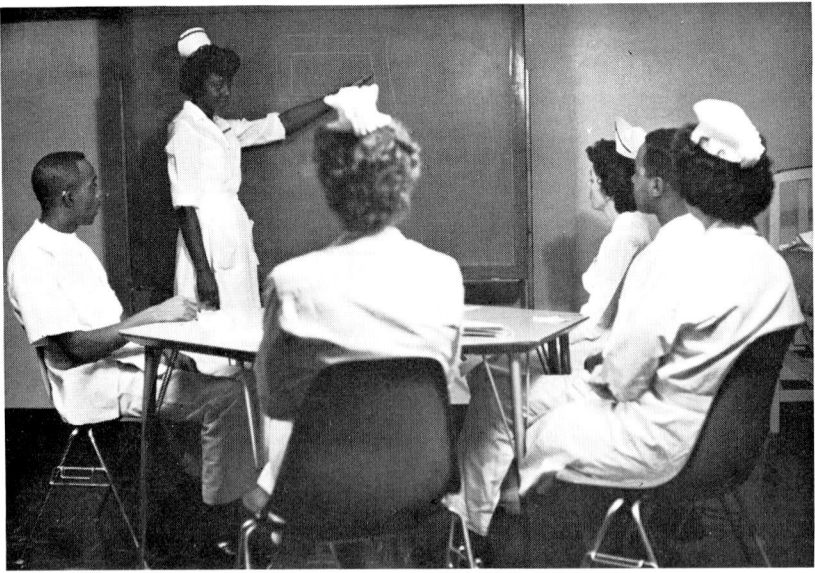

Fig. 3-1. The head nurse conducts a ward teaching program.

6. The team leader will give patient care that will serve as a model to the team. She will give individualized care to the patient who needs her attention. She will give this care in such a way as to satisfy the patient's needs and wants. The team members will be aware of their leader's skill and ability and will seek her assistance when they are unable to cope with the patient's nursing needs. They will strive to give patient care the way their leader does and the way their leader expects them to.

HOW THE TEAM MEMBER WORKS ON THE TEAM

The nursing team means togetherness. The team is only a team when the leader and members plan together, work together, learn together, and evaluate their work together. Therefore the nursing assistant team member must accept and carry out the assignment the leader gives to him. He knows that she has more nursing knowledge and skill than he has, so he seeks her help and assistance whenever he has a problem. Since he knows that she is vitally concerned with helping him learn to do his patient care job better, he asks her questions about things he does not understand, and he asks her to demonstrate new procedures and to discuss the implications they have on the care he gives.

The team member participates in the patient care rounds, and he likes to have the care he gave evaluated by the team. He knows the team does this evaluation so that he can learn what aspects of his job he is doing well and what additional training he needs in order to do it even better. He knows that these evaluations will result in a team or ward teaching program that will help him learn more about patient care.

The team leader is aware of the nursing assistant's importance and will convey this to the head nurse. The head nurse will evaluate his skills, and his salary will increase in relationship to his increasing patient care skills and his increasing worth as a member of the patient care team.

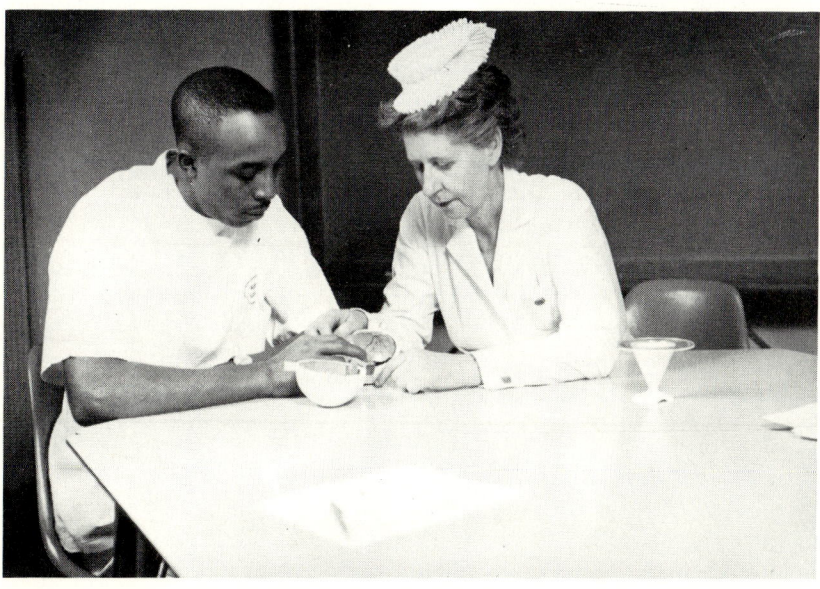

Fig. 3-2. The team leader teaches a team member the "why" of eye care.

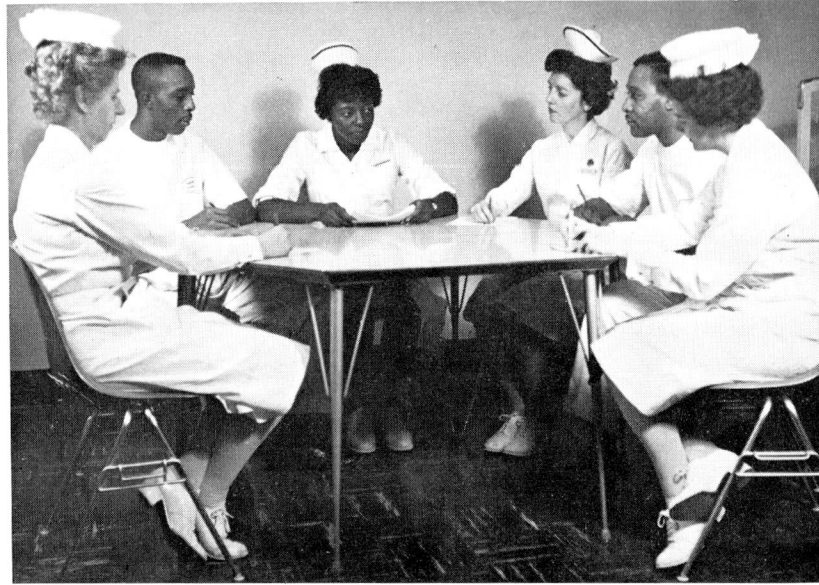

Fig. 3-3. The head nurse assists two teams develop the nursing care plans to meet the patients' needs.

SUMMARY

The quality of care the team gives is determined by that which the leader has prepared the members to give through her direction and guidance. The team is only as effective as the leader. The team members reflect her skills and her weaknesses, her attitudes and her problems, her concerns and her unconcern.

The nurse and the nursing assistants work together as a team to care for a group of patients (Fig. 3-3). The effectiveness of this nursing care team depends on the direction, guidance, evaluation, instruction, and skill of the leader. A team member cannot do what he does not know how to do.

DISCUSSION QUESTIONS

1 Do you receive a written assignment?
2 Do you participate in making this assignment?
3 Do you feel it is important for the entire team to participate in making the assignment? Why?
4 Do you have a team leader?
5 When do you seek assistance from the team leader?
6 Do you have a ward teaching program?
7 What patient care activities would you like the team leader to discuss at your next team teaching program?
8 How does your team leader evaluate the patient care that you give?
9 What kind of patient care does your team leader give?
10 What part of the team's assignment did your leader give you today?
11 How often did you see your team leader today? Did you need to see her more often? Less often? Why?

4/The patient needs you to care

STUDY QUESTIONS

1. Does a worried mind go with a sick body?
2. How can the patient's worry, fear, and apprehension be lessened?
3. What is friendship therapy, and when can the nursing assistant find time to do this?
4. What does the patient have to worry about?
5. What kind of answers should you give to patients?

EMOTIONAL ASPECTS OF ILLNESS

The patient comes to the hospital because he has some disease or discomfort. He also comes with worry about himself (whether or not he will get well and whether or not the treatment will cause him even more pain) and worry about his family and his job. He also comes with fear—fear that he might die, fear that he might have cancer, or fear that he will be left paralyzed and helpless.

The patient comes to an extended care facility because he is helpless. He can not do his own living activities anymore. He needs help with everything, even his most personal and private living functions such as going to the toilet. He hates this depending on others for everything, but he hates even more the fact that he is not home with his family. He worries about his helplessness and he longs for the good old days when he was strong and healthy and the head of his family. These daydreams only make him angry with his today in the nursing home. Angry with his helplessness, angry with the nursing assistant who is not the family, angry with his own feebleness, and yet angry with his helpers. He is frightened, lonely, helpless, and angry.

We must be aware of this worry, fear, and anger. We must recognize that the patient has a sick body and a worried mind. Taking care of the patient then means that we must take care of both the sick body and the worried mind.

THE WORRIED MIND

When we give the patient physical care such as a bath we must observe him closely for clues to determine whether he is getting better or worse. Does he move his painful arm better today? Are his lips as blue as they were yesterday? Are his legs more or less edematous today? In addition, we must listen closely to his conversation for clues on how his worried mind is today. What did he talk about? Did he talk at all? Was he discouraged? Did he say that he would be better off dead? Is he anxious to go home? Did he say that his boss would not hold the job for him? In every contact with the patient, we must be aware of both the physical and mental aspects of illness and look for clues as to how his sick body is today and for clues as to how his worried mind is today. These clues must be reported to the nurse and the doctor after the patient's care is finished. In Chapter 18 we will learn how to chart these clues on the patient's chart.

Care of the worried mind

Care for his worried mind consists of being the patient's friend. Listen to his conversation carefully and with sincere interest. Visit with him while you are caring for him. Let him set the tone of the visit. Give him a chance to talk over his problems, his fears, and his worries with you. Talking about them will release some of his tension. So listen carefully and answer as a friend who cares. Do not worry about giving him answers to medical problems. He really does not want medical information from you. He can get that from the doctor or nurse.

When the nurse gives you your nursing care assignment, she will give you confidential medical information about the patient and his family that will help you to understand how and why care is required by the patient. In your conversations with the patient, you are not to share this confidential medical and family information with him. If you have any doubts about how to answer your patient or how to care for his worried mind, ask the nurse.

The hospital day is long and lonely for the patient. He needs your friendship, your visits, your concern for him. Go to see the patient frequently throughout the day—even when you *do not have something* to do for him. All the personnel go in when they must; a friend goes to see the patient because he cares.

Remember how you felt when you started this job, your very first day. Remember how ill at ease you felt because no one knew you or went out of his way to help you. Remember how frightened you were making the first bed or giving the first bath alone.

The patient feels all this aloneness too, but he feels much worse because he also has pain and worry. Remember how your feelings of strangeness and your uncertainty disappeared when you made friends among the staff. So will they disappear for your patient. The patient needs you not only to take care of him but also to care about him.

SUMMARY

The patient has two kinds of needs; needs of the body and needs of the mind. When you take care of the patient, you must take care of his worried mind as well as his sick body in order to help him get well as quickly as possible.

DISCUSSION QUESTIONS

1 What subjects do we discuss with our friends?
2 Do we seek answers from friends, or do we seek sympathy and understanding?
3 What kind of information must we keep confidential?
4 If the patient's chart pertains to the patient, why should we not let him read it?
5 If you were going to die soon, would you like to know it?
6 If you had cancer, would you like to know it? Why? Why not?
7 If you were incurably ill, would you like your nursing assistant to share with you information about your incurable illness, or would you like him to protect you from it?

5/The patient is a person

STUDY QUESTIONS

1 What are the bodily needs of the patients?
2 What are the emotional needs of the patient or the needs of the patient's mind?
3 What is a patient?
4 How is the health care facility similar to a hotel? How dissimilar?
5 How can we show the patient who is being admitted that we are going to help him?

THE PATIENT IS OUR GUEST

As mentioned previously, the patient is a person who has come to the hospital because he is sick or to the extended care facility because he is helpless. Therefore he is really a guest, and we should treat him in the same way a guest in a hotel is treated. Just as a hotel does everything possible for a guest's comfort, health care facilities, too, do everything possible for the patient's comfort.

RECEIVING THE PATIENT IN THE HOSPITAL AND EXTENDED CARE FACILITY

In order to understand your job of caring for the patient and observing his progress, you must think about what he needs to live comfortably in the health care facility. Let us first consider your needs when you go to a hotel and see how the hotel meets them.

As you approach the hotel, loaded down with luggage, the doorman steps forth, tips his hat, takes your bag, helps you into the hotel, and takes you to the hotel desk. The desk clerk courteously listens to your request for room accommodations, helps you register, and then summons a bellboy to carry your bag and take you to your room. Upon entering the room, the bellboy makes the room comfortable for you. In summer, he opens the windows or turns up the air-conditioning. In winter, he turns up the heat. He shows you where the bathroom is and where the heat-regulating or cooling-regulating apparatus is located; then he gives you a brochure explaining all the hotel services available. The entire hotel staff makes you feel wanted because they seem to be glad that you came.

The patient needs this same kind of help when he comes into the hospital or health care facility. It may be a new experience for him. He does not know where to go or what to do next, and unlike the hotel guest, he is sick and worried. He is also filled with fear of what his illness might be and of what is going to be done to him. He is torn with doubts about leaving his job, his wife, and his family. He is not too sure that he wants to come to the hospital and he is very sure that he does not want to come to the extended care facility. Therefore you must let the patient see by the way you receive him in the admitting department, by the way you help him to the ward, by the way you receive him on the ward, and by the way you orient him to his health care home that you really want him here and that you have the knowledge, the ability, and the desire to help him get well or to care for him in his helplessness. Do this by receiving him just as you would want your mother received in a health care facility.

The nursing assistant in the admitting area should be on the lookout for new patients. When a new patient enters, assist him as he needs to be assisted. If he appears to be walking with great difficulty, get a wheelchair for him. If he has a suitcase, carry it for him and take him to the admission desk. Be friendly and show concern. Do not joke. Answer the patient's questions and tell him where you are taking him and what he can expect there.

If the patient is to be examined in the admitting department, wait for him at the business desk until he completes the application. Then take him to the examining room. Help him to undress, and help him onto the examining table. Inform the examining doctor when the patient is ready. Remain with the examining physician and assist him during the examination. Expose only the body area the doctor is examining. Keep the rest of the patient's body covered. Explain each step of the examination to the patient to reduce his fear and apprehension.

After the examination is completed, assist the patient into hospital dress or his own clothing, as indicated, in preparation for his trip to the ward. Find out from the nurse or doctor the floor or ward to which the patient is assigned and whether he is to walk there or be taken on a stretcher or in a wheelchair. Then take the patient and his family and the admission slip or chart to his room or ward. Answer any questions asked by the patient or his family in a friendly, truthful, courteous manner, but do not disclose any confidential information you may have about the patient's medical condition. Do not show the patient his chart or admission slip.

When you arrive on the assigned ward, proceed to the nurse's station and introduce the new patient to the head nurse. The nurse will take the chart and admission slip and escort you to the patient's room or bed area. Help the ward nurse get the new patient into bed, and then return to the admitting area (taking with you any equipment you may have brought to the ward) to await the next new patient.

NEEDS OF THE PATIENT

Now let us think about the daily needs of a patient. Supplying these needs will be a large part of your job. Patient needs are the same as any person's needs, the same as your needs. These needs of the body and mind for comfortable living are as follows:
1. Needs of the body
    a. The need to *eat* (adequate food)
    b. The need to *drink* (adequate fluids)
    c. The need to *sleep* (adequate body rest)

d. The need to *eliminate* waste (feces and urine)
   e. The need to *breathe* (adequate air)
   f. The need to *move* (shift weight to relieve pressure)
   g. The need to be free of pain or disability
   h. The need to do these things for oneself (be independent)
   i. The need to be clean (feel refreshed; be free of odors)
2. Needs of the mind
   a. The need to feel cared about and worthwhile (self-worth)
   b. The need to know what is being done, why it is being done, etc. (minimize threats)
   c. The need to know that there is relief or cure for your illness (hope)
   d. The need to feel that members of the hospital staff are skilled, competent people who will help you (security)
   e. The need to know that one's family is getting along well (fulfill obligations)
   f. The need to know what the future means in relation to this illness and how to live in this future (self-control, independence)
   g. The need to live (self-preservation)
   h. The need to have a friend (purpose for being—belonging; this is especially true of the nursing home patient who has no family)

The signs and symptoms of illness, which will be discussed in Chapter 18, are really signs that the patient is unable to meet his needs comfortably by himself and therefore comes to the hospital. Your job of caring for the patient, then, consists of doing those activities that will enable him to meet both the needs of his body and the needs of his mind.

SUMMARY

The patient is a person who has the same needs you have. Disease has interrupted the patient's ability to meet these needs, and so he has come to the health care facility for help.

DISCUSSION QUESTIONS

1 Why would a newly admitted patient ask to see his chart?
2 Why should a patient not see his chart?
3 What needs (other than those listed) do you have?
4 Think about the last time you were ill. What needs (body or mind) did you have difficulty in meeting?
5 Discuss the statement: Signs of illness are really signs that the body or mind is not meeting a need of living.
6 Talk to a patient on your ward. What are his physical (body) needs? What are his emotional (mind) needs?
7 Discuss your patient care assignment in terms of what needs you are helping the patient meet with your care.

6/The patient's home in the hospital

STUDY QUESTIONS

1. What are the furnishings of the patient's hospital home?
2. Why do some patients have a private room while other have ward living facilities?
3. What is the difference between the medical and nursing care for a private room patient and that of a ward patient?
4. Why does a patient move from one type of hospital home to another?
5. What is an intensive care unit?
6. How can you know the names of all the patients?

THE PATIENT'S HOSPITAL HOME

In the hospital, the patient's home contains a bed, a bedside stand, a chair, and toilet facilities. Just as you and I rent or buy the most comfortable living quarters we can afford, the patient rents the hospital living facilities that he can afford. Therefore some patients have a private room, some have a semiprivate room, and some are in wards. The private room patient may have more comfortable living quarters and more privacy than the ward patient, but here the difference ceases. All patients get the medical and nursing care they need to get as well as possible. Each patient's unit is prepared in such a way as to help the patient attain the maximum degree of health possible for him regardless of his ability to pay. The patient is seeking health, and giving the patient care so that he can achieve this aim is the primary role of the hospital regardless of where the patient lives in the hospital.

Certain hospital floors or wards are designated for the care of certain kinds of patients, (for example, medical, orthopedic, surgical, or psychiatric). This is a matter of convenience for the hospital. The physicians, nurses, and nursing assistants skilled in a particular type of patient care can remain on that floor or in that ward. This saves their time (avoids the need for them to travel from floor to floor), and it ensures the patient of proper care.

NEED DETERMINES CONDITIONS IN THE HOSPITAL HOME

Just as we make our home fit our needs, the patient's hospital home is made to fit his needs.

If the patient had a coronary thrombosis and needs to be quiet, to conserve his energy, and to be away from noise and excitement, the nurse will place him in a quiet section of the ward if he is a ward patient or in a single room at the end of the corridor if he is a private patient. In both cases (ward or private patient) visitors would be limited or excluded and nursing care would be spaced throughout the day. On the other hand, if a patient who does not need a quiet atmosphere is bored or depressed, the nurse would assign him to a cheerful section of the ward if he is a ward patient or to a private room nearer the nurses' station where there is activity if he is a private patient.

If the nurse is caring for several dangerously ill patients whose breathing should be observed constantly so that any choking on saliva can be prevented by suctioning, she will move these patients as close to the nurses' desk as possible. The ward patients are moved to the front of the ward, and the private patients are moved to the rooms just across from the nurses' station.

THE PATIENT'S HOME CHANGES AS HIS CONDITION CHANGES
Recovery room

Because the patient's condition changes, his living facilities in the hospital change. The patient may spend his preoperative period in the ward or in a single room. However, after he has been operated on, he is sent from the operating room to the recovery room. Since the recovery room is close to the operating room, the patient just operated upon has only a short distance to travel through well-protected (draft-free) areas for his postoperative care. He remains close to his doctor and the operating room. This means that the doctor can visit him frequently throughout the immediate postoperative period and that he can easily be returned to the operating room should postoperative complications occur.

In the recovery room skilled nurses and nursing assistants watch the patient's vital signs (signs of life) to see how effectively he is living, and they assist him in carrying out the body functions essential to living when he needs such assistance. If the unconscious patient just operated upon becomes blue and needs oxygen, the nurse gives him oxygen; if he chokes or gurgles on his own saliva, the nurse suctions out his trachea (air tube to the lungs), thus enabling him to breathe easily again.

Intensive care unit

When the hospital staff members believe that the patient is in need of skilled medical and nursing care because his condition is constantly changing, he may be moved to the intensive care unit. Here there is an intensive concentration of skilled doctors and nurses, an intensive concentration of emergency equipment and drugs, and an intensive concentration of medical supplies. In this unit, the patient will receive maximum hospital services to assist him in getting well.

It is interesting to point out here that the recovery room and the intensive care unit have no private room or ward facilities. Instead, they have an intensive concentration of medical and nursing services for the patient who needs them. Both the ward patient and the private patient have the same living facilities and get the exact care they need. Any patient whose life is being threatened by hemorrhage or by the inability to breathe needs hospital health services fast, and the intensive care unit is where emergency services are the routine of the day.

PATIENTS MOVE ABOUT THE HOSPITAL

We see, then, that patients may move about the floor or the ward or even about the hospital. It is extremely dangerous to assume that the patient who was in room 1, or bed 1 yesterday is the same one who is there today. Even if the patient looks like the patient who was there yesterday, he may not be the same one. It is much easier and safer to check the patient's name tag on his wrist (or his bed tag if he does not have a wrist tag) before taking him to the operating room or before giving him a treatment than it is to rectify the wrong we might do to him by giving him the treatment intended for another patient or by sending him to the operating room for an operation intended for another.

Begin immediately to learn the names of your patients. Each time you enter a patient's room to give him care, address the patient by name and explain what you are going to do and why you are going to do it. If you address the patient by a name other than his, he will correct you immediately and thus help you avoid making errors. If you are in doubt about the patient's identity, check his name on the tag on his wrist. Always check the patient's name on his wrist tag before giving any treatment or care to a patient who is unconscious and unable to answer to his name. Checking takes only a minute, but careless errors cannot be undone in a lifetime.

THE PATIENT'S NAME TAG ON HIS WRIST

At home we have our name on the mailbox or on our door, but in his hospital home the patient has his name on his wrist. One reason for this, as already mentioned, is that the patient's hospital home changes as frequently as his condition changes. Another reason is that the patient travels extensively throughout the hospital to diagnostic and therapeutic services, such as x-ray, operating room, physical therapy, or electrocardiogram laboratory. Most of his need to be identified occurs away from his room or ward. The third reason is that the patient receives diagnostic tests and treatments from a variety of hospital personnel who do not know who he is except for the name tag on his wrist.

Since the patient moves about the hospital among hospital services where he is unknown, the only way we can be sure that the right patient gets the right test or treatment is to check his name tag each time we care for him, each time we assist the doctor or nurse treat him, and each time we prepare him for an off-ward trip for a diagnostic study.

SUMMARY

The patient's hospital home contains the essentials for living in the hospital: a bed, a bedside stand, a chair, and toilet facilities. All patients have the same type of furniture in their hospital home. However, the amount of privacy they have in their hospital living depends on their ability or willingness to pay for private, semiprivate, or ward accommodations. Regardless of where the patient lives in the hospital, the medical and nursing care is the same. In fact, even the hospital home (the recovery room and intensive care unit) is the same for all acutely ill or newly operated upon patients in the hospital.

The patient moves about the hospital, changing his hospital home as his needs for health care change. Therefore it is important that each patient wear his name tag on his wrist so that nursing personnel (as well as all hospital personnel) giving patient care can identify the patient correctly, thus ensuring that the right patient gets the right care.

DISCUSSION QUESTIONS

1 What are the differences in the living facilities for private room patients and ward patients?
2 What differences are there in your nursing care of patients living in private rooms and that of patients living in the ward?
3 Visit the recovery room and intensive care unit. What differences are there in these units for private and for ward patients? Why?
4 Are there two types of nursing care, private and ward? Discuss.

5 Why is it necessary to be sure that the patient is wearing a wrist name tag when he goes to the operating room?
6 What could you do to avoid hospital accidents if you had two patients on your ward with the same first and last names?

VOCABULARY

coronary arteries Arteries that take blood to the heart muscles.

intensive care unit A special hospital unit prepared with equipment and staff to care for the acutely ill patient who needs constant medical and nursing observation and care. The surgical intensive care unit might receive acutely ill surgical patients from the recovery room after they have recovered from the immediate effects of anesthesia and surgery. However, it might also receive those preoperative patients who need intensive observation (possibility of bleeding) or intensive care (replacement of blood loss in preparation for surgery).

orthopedics A medical specialty concerned with the diagnosis and treatment of patients with diseases of the bones, muscles, tendons, and joints.

postoperative After an operation.

preoperative Before an operation.

psychiatry A medical specialty concerned with the diagnosis and treatment of patients with mental illness.

recovery room A special hospital unit prepared with equipment and staff to care for the patient immediately after his operation. The patient goes directly from the operating room to the recovery room. He remains here until he recovers from the effects of anesthesia and from the immediate effects of surgery.

suctioning Sucking out body secretions with a vacuum and a tube.

surgery A medical specialty concerned with the diagnosis and treatment of patients requiring operative procedures to remove disease that is obstructing a body part or to remove or bypass the diseased body part itself.

thrombosis Blood clot.

trachea Windpipe.

THE NURSING ASSISTANT MEETS THE PATIENT'S BASIC DAILY NEEDS IN THE HEALTH CARE FACILITY

SECTION II

Chapter
- 7   Meeting the patient's need for a comfortable bed
- 8   Meeting the patient's need for food
- 9   Meeting the patient's need for water
- 10 Meeting the patient's need for cleanliness and movement—complete, partial, and out-of-bed baths
- 11 Caring for the patient's toilet needs
- 12 Caring for the patient's need to move
- 13 Caring for the patient's need to get out of bed
- 14 Meeting the patient's need for sleep

7/Meeting the patient's need for a comfortable bed

STUDY QUESTIONS

1. What are the two principles of bedmaking?
2. How is the patient's bed similar to your shoes?
3. How is a blister on your foot similar to the patient's bedsore?
4. How does the way the patient's bed is made help you to know something about the patient?
5. Since the patient may live in his bed 24 hours a day, how can the bed be adjusted to help the patient eat, sleep, eliminate waste, etc.?

THE PATIENT'S BED

The patient spends most of his time in the hospital in bed. You and I spend most of our time in the hospital on our feet. Therefore the patient's bed is to him what our shoes are to us. You and I do not wear the same kind of shoes. So, too, patients' beds differ. Each patient has the kind of bed that he needs.

One patient may have a painful back, so a bedboard is placed under the mattress to keep his back straight. Another patient may be confused and cannot understand where he is and what is being said to him, so crib sides are placed on his bed. Another one may have difficulty moving and turning and, because of this, is very likely to develop pressure sores on his back, so an alternating pressure mattress is placed on his bed. Still another patient may have one side of his body paralyzed, which creates a problem for him in getting in and out of bed, so his bed is lower than that of other patients. Still another patient may have painful legs, so a cradle (frame) is placed over his feet to keep the bedclothes off his legs.

The bed, then, is not made in any routine, set way. It is made for one particular patient and is made exactly as that patient needs it. There is a routine way beds are made at home or in hotels for well people, and this serves as the basic hospital bed.

BEDMAKING

Basic bedmaking

The basic hospital bed is prepared in the following way (Figs. 7-1 to 7-7):

1. Clean the bed first by damp dusting it thoroughly; also clean the bedside stand.
2. Cover the mattress with a mattress cover. This may be a muslin, plastic, or rubberized mattress cover.
3. Place a mattress pad on the bed. This is usually made of thick cotton, quilted material.
4. Put a sheet on the bed, even with the bottom of the bed, fold the excess under the head of the mattress, and miter the corner on one side to hold it in place.
5. Put another sheet on the bed, even with the top of the bed. Fold the excess under the bottom of the mattress and miter the corner to hold it in place.
6. Place a blanket over the sheet (about 6 inches from the top of the bed). Fold the excess under the mattress at the bottom of the bed, and miter the corner to hold it in place.
7. Finish making the side of the bed as follows: put a spread on even with the top of the bed. Fold in the excess under the mattress at the bottom of the bed, and miter the corner to hold it in place.
8. Go to the opposite side of the bed and repeat steps 4 to 7, thus making up the second side of the bed.
9. Fold the spread in and over the blanket at the head of the bed. Then fold the sheet over this fold to make a 4-inch to 6-inch fold at the top of the bed. Then fanfold the top covers halfway down to the foot of the bed.
10. Put pillowcases on a firm pillow and a soft pillow and place the pillows at the head of the bed.

Modifications of basic bedmaking

The basic bed just described may be modified to meet various patient needs as shown in Table 7-1.

Text continued on p. 34.

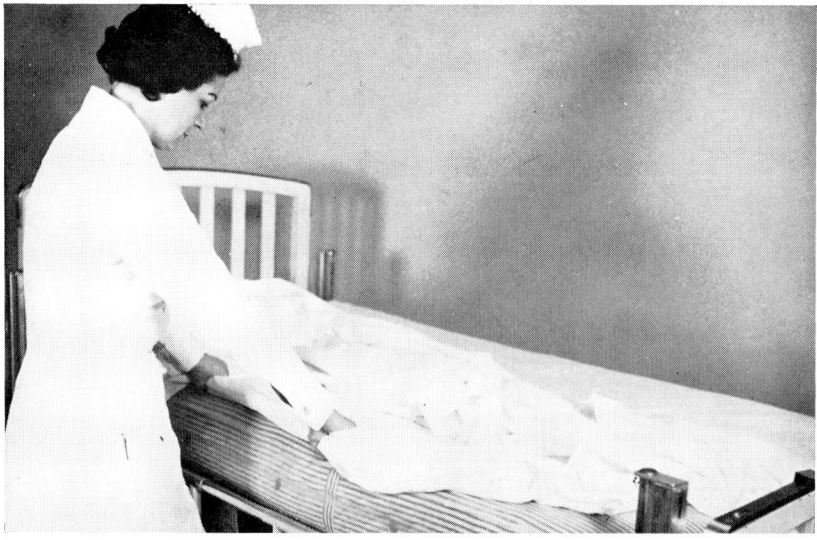

Fig. 7-1. The nurse demonstrating how to pull the mattress pad over to begin making up the second side of an unoccupied bed. Note that the first side is completely made.

Meeting the patient's need for a comfortable bed   29

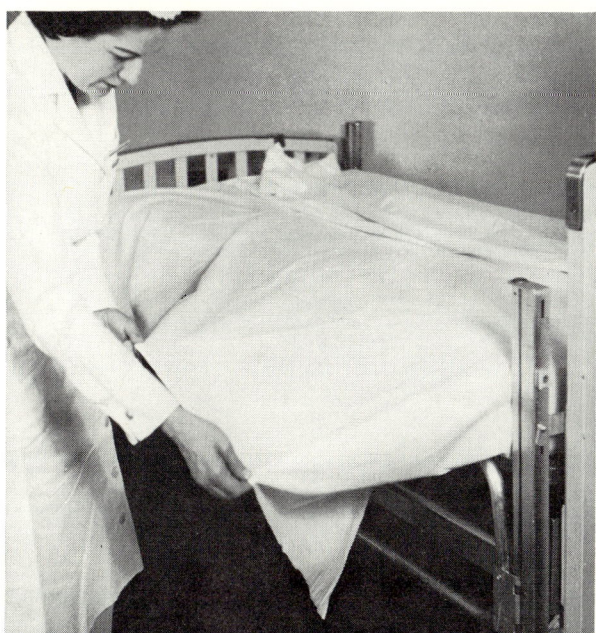

Fig. 7-2. Making a mitered corner in the bottom sheet on the second side of the bed. Note how the nurse's left hand measures off a distance equal to that of the distance from the bed to her right hand. She actually measures off a square.

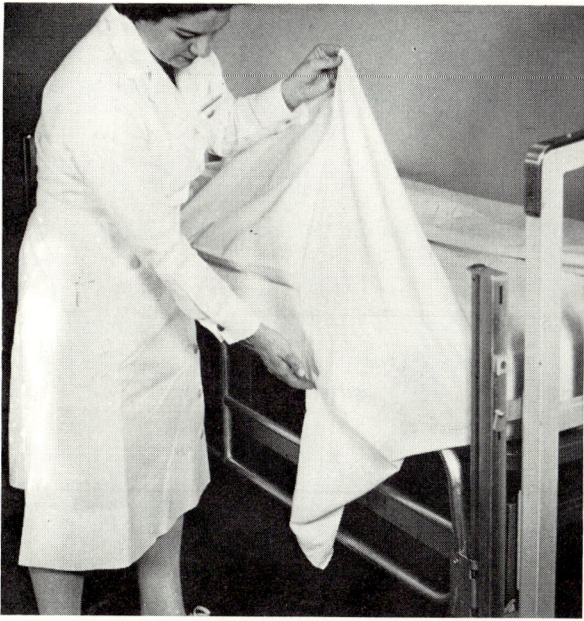

Fig. 7-3. The sheet is picked up by the left hand while it is dropped by the right hand, and the square becomes two right angles.

30 Nursing assistant meets patient's basic daily needs in health care facility

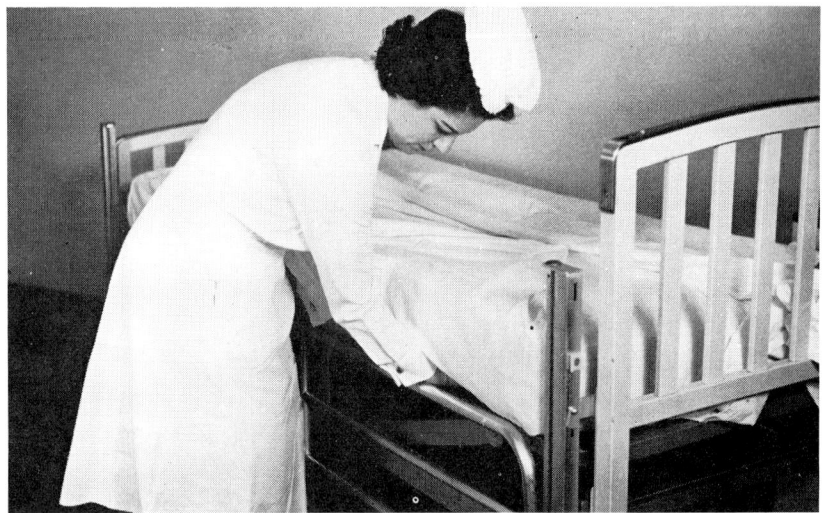

Fig. 7-4. The bottom angle is tucked under the mattress while the top one rests on the bed.

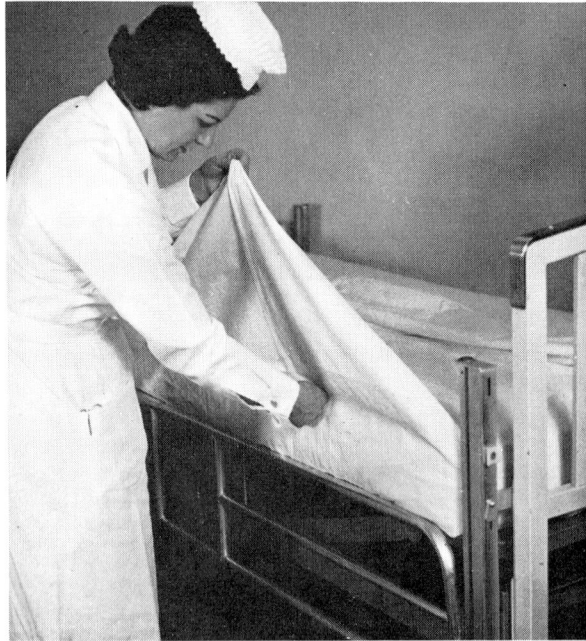

Fig. 7-5. The sheet is held in position on the mattress with the right hand while the top angle is brought down over it.

Meeting the patient's need for a comfortable bed 31

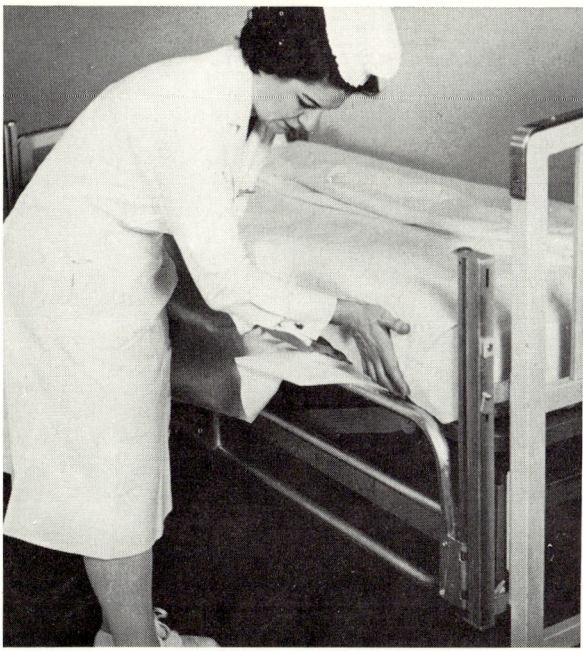

Fig. 7-6. Then the top angle is tucked under the mattress to form a mitered corner.

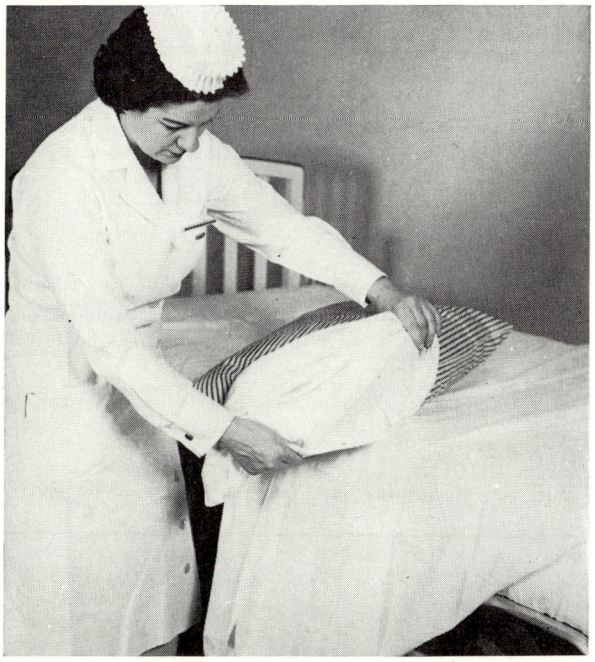

Fig. 7-7. The pillow is grasped through the closed end of the pillowcase and is held firmly while the sides of the pillowcase are pulled up and over the pillow.

Table 7-1. Modifications of the basic bed and the needs they meet

Modification	Need

1. Rubber drawsheet covered with a linen sheet (Figs. 7-8 and 7-9)
   a. Placed so that it will be under the lower half of the patient's body if the patient is incontinent
   b. Placed so that it will be under any area of the patient's body that is draining profusely, such as a draining ulcer
	1. To protect the mattress

2. Trapezelike apparatus suspended over the head of the bed	2. To assist the patient in lifting and moving himself about in bed when he has no legs or when one or both of his legs are paralyzed.
3. Board perpendicular to the mattress at the foot of the bed (Fig. 7-10)	3. To hold the patient's feet in a standing position when the patient has a paralyzed foot that tends to drop or when, as a result of being in bed for a long time, he has weakened muscles of the foot and the weight of the bedclothes tends to pull his feet down, causing footdrop
4. Bed with board under mattress (Fig. 7-11)	4. To keep the patient's back straight
5. Bed with crib sides (Fig. 7-12)	5. To keep the patient from rolling or falling out of bed when he is confused, unconscious, or unaware of his surroundings
6. Bed with alternating pressure pad (Fig. 7-13)	6. To alternate the areas of the patient's body that are pressing against the bed, thus relieving the pressure points on the patient's body and enabling recirculation of the blood in these areas to avoid the ulcers caused by poor circulation (decubitus ulcers)

7. High-low bed
   a. Placed at regular height when the patient is receiving care
   b. Lowered so that the feet reach the floor when the patient sits on the side of the bed
	7. To help the patient who has difficulty in shifting his balance and in standing (due to old age, paralysis, or amputations) to get in and out of bed easily

8. Bed with lifting sheet—sheet placed under the patient (from the shoulders to the hips) (Fig. 7-9)	8. To enable the nursing personnel to lift and move the helpless patient by lifting and moving him on the sheet

9. Postoperative bed
   a. Top covers folded to one side of the bed
   b. A rubber sheet covered with a linen sheet placed under the head
   c. A rubber sheet covered with a linen sheet placed under the operative area
	9. a. To receive an unconscious patient
	
	   b. To facilitate cleaning of the bed if the patient vomits
	
	   c. To protect the bed from drainage or blood

10. Bed with cradle—frame over an area of the patient's body and fixed under the mattress	10. To support bed clothing and keep them off a painful or oozing (burned) body part

Meeting the patient's need for a comfortable bed   33

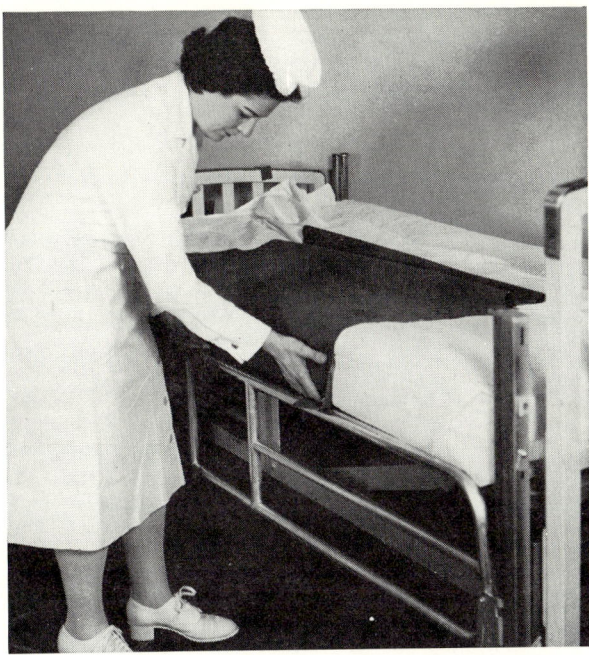

Fig. 7-8. Tucking the rubber drawsheet into position under the mattress on the second side of the bed.

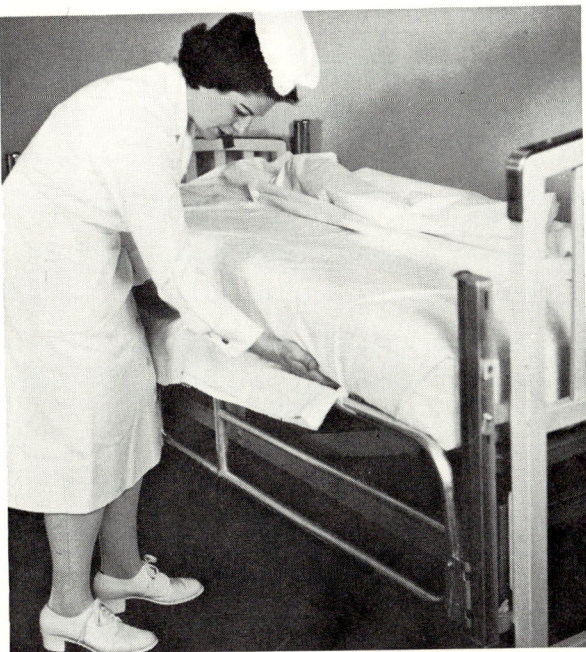

Fig. 7-9. The linen drawsheet is placed over the rubber drawsheet and tucked into position under the mattress.

First principle of bedmaking

The bed, then, is made in such a way as to meet the needs of the individual patient. However, there are a few principles that do apply to the making of all beds. Remember, the patient's bed is to the patient what our shoes are to us.

Let us take a look at our shoes. Suppose there is a little wrinkle in the lining. What happens as we stand—as the weight of our

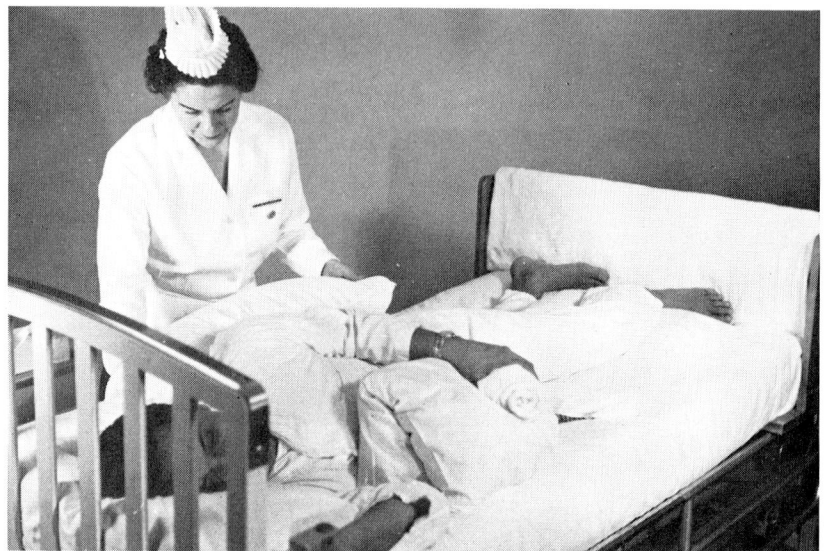

Fig. 7-10. A footboard in place to maintain the feet of the unconscious patient in correct position.

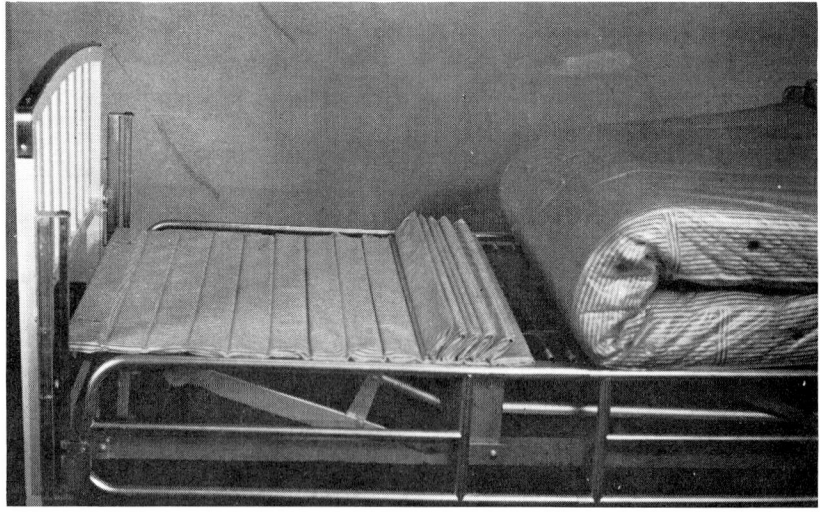

Fig. 7-11. A bed board being placed in position under the mattress to prevent it from sagging.

Meeting the patient's need for a comfortable bed 35

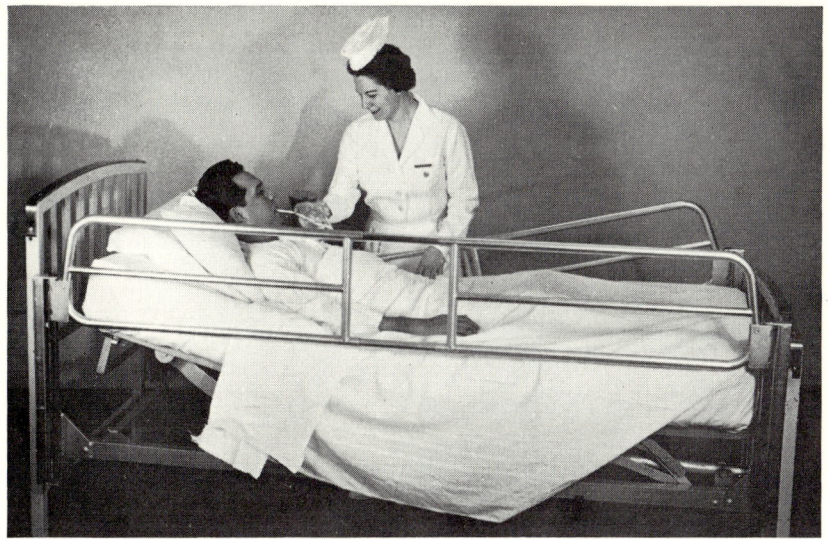

Fig. 7-12. Crib sides in position on a patient's bed. The nurse has partially lowered one crib side so that she can get close enough to the patient to give him a drink.

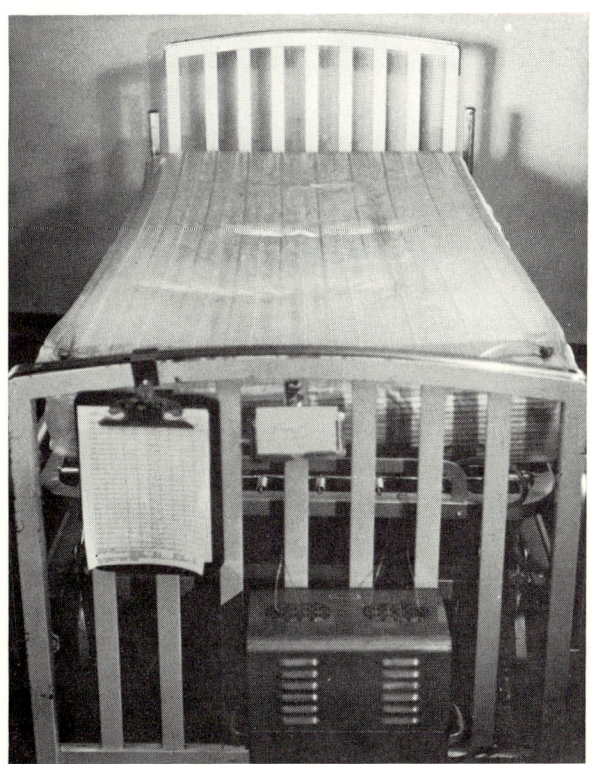

Fig. 7-13. An alternating pressure pad in place over the mattress. Note that the pumps used to inflate and deflate the pad are attached to the foot of the bed.

body presses our foot on that wrinkle? The wrinkle presses against the skin and the blood vessels in our foot, shutting off the circulation of the blood in this area, and we develop a sore spot with a collection of fluid that we call a blister.

The same thing happens to the patient who lies on wrinkled sheets. The patient's blood supply is cut off by the pressure of the weight of his body against a wrinkle in the sheet. A blister forms first. Then a gangrenous spot develops as the pressure continues. This is called a bedsore, or a pressure sore, or a decubitus ulcer.

The most important part of making the patient's bed, then, is to make it smooth—free of wrinkles and uneven surfaces. This means that the bedclothes under the patient must be pulled tight and anchored well under the mattress to keep them tight. If we fail to make the patient's bed smooth and free of wrinkles, we are actually creating a hospital situation that will make the patient get worse, rather than get well.

Second principle of bedmaking

Avoid shaking, waving, and pulling linen about. Such activity permits any bacteria on the linen to be thrown into the air and increases the possibility of your breathing these bacteria into your body. Perhaps the first patients you care for when you start your nursing assistant's job will have little or no disease-producing bacteria on their sheets, but later you will care for many patients who do. Therefore from the start it is essential for your own health to develop safe working habits. This will be discussed more fully in the section on communicable diseases. However, we want to stress here that the floor is not clean, not free from bacteria. Therefore if sheets or pillowcases fall on the floor, discard them in the linen hamper—do not put them on the patient's bed.

Although we would like to give the patient clean bed linen every day, it may be impossible. Therefore be sure that you know which linens are to be changed.

Planning the work

Learn to plan your work to avoid unnecessary running back and forth, and you will find that your feet will not ache so much at night. Each morning find out *what* you are to do, *how* you are to do it, *when* you are to do it, and for *whom* you are to do it. Jotting down your work assignment is the first step in planning your work to save steps. If, for example, you received an assignment to make beds, proceed as follows:

1. Find out what beds you are to make and what bed linens you are to change.
2. Find out what kind of beds you are to make—for example, postoperative beds, beds with crib sides, or beds with cradles.
3. Find out if any special time factor is involved—for example, postoperative bed to be taken to the operating room to receive a patient at 10 A.M., or a bed to be cleaned and made following the discharge of a patient at 11 A.M.

Since this assignment entails only bedmaking, we shall assume that the patients are in a self-care unit or in an extended care facility and out of bed when you start your task.

Now collect all the linen you will need and load it on a wheeled linen cart. Then get a laundry hamper for soiled linen. If the cleanliness of the furnishings of the patient's hospital home (bed, bedside stand, chair) is your responsibility, collect damp cloths, soap, polishing or cleaning materials, and a basin of water and place them on a tray on the linen cart. You are now ready to start. Proceed to your first bed, pushing the linen cart and pulling the laundry hamper.

Take the linen for the first bed off the cart. Two sheets, two pillowcases, a spread, a set of towels, and a washcloth are the routine requirements.

Take the bed linen into the patient's hospital home and place it on his chair. Now remove all of the bed linen that is to be discarded. Remove cases from the pillows and place the pillows on the chair. Fan the spread back and remove the blanket. Fold the blanket in quarters lengthwise, and place it over the back of the chair. Loosen the bedclothes on both sides of the bed and at the top and bottom. Fold them in from the sides, up from the bottom, and down from the top of the bed until they are in a small enough bundle for you to pick up easily and carry to the laundry hamper, which is positioned just at the fringe of your work unit. Damp dust the bed and then remake it. If housekeeping is part of your assignment, damp dust the furniture and wash the bedside stand thoroughly, scouring the top as necessary. Wash your hands thoroughly at the sink in the ward or in the patient's room when you are finished, and then proceed to your next bedmaking job.

The hospital does not have an inexhaustible supply of linen. Before you discard any linen from the patient's unit, take in its replacement. It is much better for the patient to use a pillowcase 2 or even 3 days than to be without one.

BED POSITIONS

Since the patient may be required to stay in his bed 24 hours a day, many different activities of living must be carried on in his bed. *Therefore* the hospital bed is designed so that it can be placed in different positions:

1. The top half of the bed may be elevated to place the patient in a semi-sitting position for eating or for toileting (Fig. 7-14).
2. The bottom half of the bed may be elevated to place the patient in a position in which his head is lower than his feet in order to increase the blood supply to his head (Fig. 7-15).

The bed may be placed in these positions either by electrical or manual operation.

1. In the electrically operated bed, the patient activates the bed himself by pushing a control button.

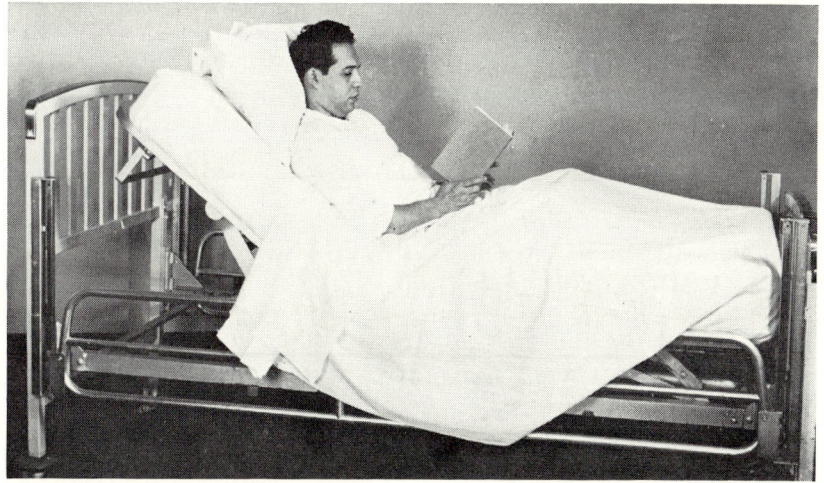

Fig. 7-14. The head of the bed is elevated to place the patient in a sitting position on the bedpan. (Note that the patient is relaxing with a book during defecation.)

38 Nursing assistant meets patient's basic daily needs in health care facility

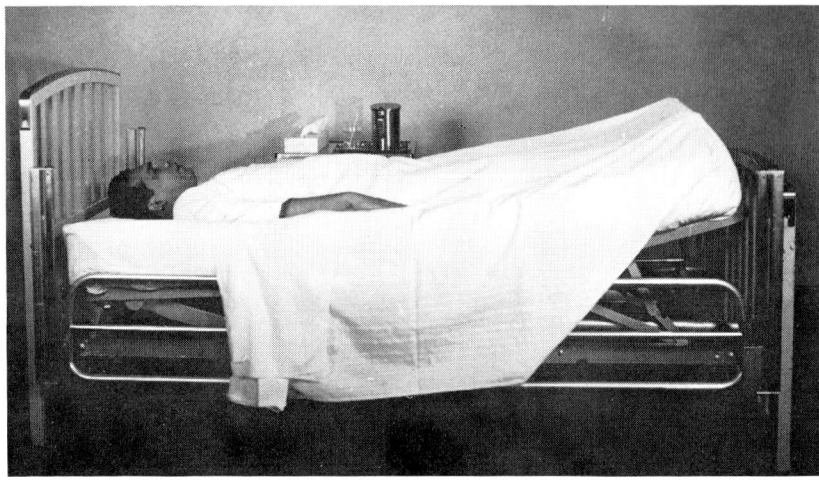

Fig. 7-15. The foot of the bed is elevated to place the patient in shock position. This position causes an increased flow of blood to the patient's head.

2. In the manually operated bed, the nursing assistant manipulates the cranks at the bottom of the bed.

While you are making the unoccupied beds about the ward, manipulate the cranks or the electrical controls and put the beds into several kinds of positions. Later when a bed patient asks you to raise or lower his head, you will know how to do it.

SUMMARY

The patient's bed is equipped with the treatment material he needs to help him get as well as he possibly can. In order to make a patient's bed, it is necessary to know what his needs are. The patient's bed is to him what our shoes are to us. Just as blisters will develop on our feet if the circulation is cut off by the uneven pressure of our weight against a wrinkle in the lining of our shoe, so will bedsores develop on any area of the patient's body in which the blood supply has been cut off because of the uneven pressures of his weight against a wrinkle in the bedclothes. Therefore the first principle of bedmaking is to keep all sheets tight and free of wrinkles.

The second principle of bedmaking is to avoid unnecessary shaking, waving, and pulling of bedclothes. These activities throw bacteria into the air and fill the environment with germs.

The nursing assistant will be given a detailed work assignment each day. He should study this assignment carefully and plan his work effectively to eliminate unnecessary trips around the ward. Two ways in which this can be done are as follows:

1. Study the assignment, collect all the material needed, place it on wheeled carts, and take it around the ward with you.
2. Do all the work you can from one position before moving to another. For example, make up one side of the bed completely and then proceed to the other side. This requires only one trip around the bed to complete it, whereas tucking in each piece of linen as it is put on the bed requires seven trips around the bed.

DISCUSSION QUESTIONS

1 How many kinds of equipment can you find on the hospital beds on your wards? Does the equipment on a bed give you a clue to the patient's condition?

2 Discuss how you would prepare your equipment and supplies if you were assigned to make ten beds on your ward.
3 Feel an alternating pressure pad that is in operation and discuss how it relieves pressure on the patient's back.
4 How does a wrinkled sheet cause a pressure sore?
5 What kind of work assignments do you receive? How could these assignments be made more valuable to you?
6 Why must you wash your hands after you make one bed and before you make another one?
7 Is the bed linen changed every day on every bed on your ward? If not, what is the plan for changing linen?
8 Bed positions can be changed in order to make the forces of gravity help the patient. What other examples of the use of the force of gravity have you seen in the hospital?

VOCABULARY

alternating pressure pad An electrically inflated double-sectioned air mattress. The two sections alternately inflate and deflate for 3 minutes. Although the patient is lying in the same position on this alternating pressure mattress, it alternates the pressure on the pressure-bearing areas of his body every 3 minutes. It is usually used for patients who have difficulty changing position.

bed board A board placed under the mattress to keep the mattress straight and the patient's back straight. It is usually used for all patients with back difficulties, paralyzed patients, and patients who must stay in bed for long periods of time.

bed cradle A wire frame placed over the patient's body or feet to support the weight of the bedclothes. It is usually used for patients with body burns or painful feet and legs.

crib sides Protective rails placed on the sides of the bed to prevent the patient from rolling out of bed. They are usually used for unconscious, restless, confused, or aged patients and for those receiving hypnotics or large doses of sedatives.

decubitus ulcer A gangrenous sore that develops when the pressure of the patient's body against the bed cuts off the circulation of the blood to the skin and it dies.

footboard A board placed at the end of the mattress at the foot of the bed to keep the feet in the standing position. It is usually used for patients on prolonged bed rest or for paralyzed patients.

high-low bed An electrically or manually operated bed that can be raised to the height of the regular hospital bed and lowered to the height of the home bed. The high position permits the staff to carry out patient care easily, while the low position permits the patient's feet to reach the floor when he sits on the side of the bed. It is usually used for patients who need assistance getting in and out of bed and for disabled patients who can get in and out of bed by themselves when and if they can reach the floor with their feet.

hypnotic A sleep-producing drug.

incontinence Loss of bladder and/or bowel control.

lifting sheet A sheet that is folded in half lengthwise and placed under a helpless patient from his shoulders to his hips to enable two assistants to lift him easily.

medical patients Patients who are cared for primarily by the use of drugs.

mitered corner A triangular fold made in bedclothes to hold them in place at the corners.

trapeze Lifting bar suspended over the head of the bed. It is usually used to help patients lift themselves up in bed to use the bedpan or to change their position when they are unable to use their feet for lifting.

SOURCE OF ADDITIONAL INFORMATION

1 Film: Bedmaking (part of bed care series); may be obtained from Encyclopaedia Britannica, 425 N. Michigan Ave., Chicago, Ill. 60611. (*Film is 8 minutes long—8 mm. individual or group teaching visual aid.*)

8/Meeting the patient's need for food

STUDY QUESTIONS

1. What is the digestive system?
2. What is the function of the digestive system?
3. Why is it necessary for us to understand how the digestive system functions?
4. How can disturbances of the digestive system be recognized?
5. How fast can you feed a patient?
6. What is the best position for eating?
7. Why does a patient have difficulty eating if he is short of breath (dyspneic)?
8. Why cannot an unconscious patient be fed orally (by mouth)?
9. Why are patients given different kinds of diets?
10. What is glucose? Why is it given intravenously?
11. Why would a patient with diarrhea be thirsty?
12. Why should a patient's dentures be in place at mealtime?

THE BODY NEEDS FOOD

The body is a complex machine that keeps its organs working day and night, week in and week out, with no holidays, in order to carry on the process of living. Like every machine the body needs fuel, waste removal, and preventive maintenance in order to do this. Unlike other machines, however, it contains separate systems to provide it with these special services. Some of these systems and their specific body services are as follows:

1. *Digestive system.* No matter what we eat, this system will extract the fuel the body needs from it. This fuel will pass into the blood, and the leftover food will be thrown out of the body as feces.

2. *Respiratory system.* Regardless of our activity, this system will push air into the lungs, separate out the oxygen and exchange it with the blood for carbon dioxide, and then exhale or eliminate the remaining air and carbon dioxide.

3. *Circulatory system.* The blood distributes the food and oxygen to all the cells of the body, and in the return trip to the heart the blood revisits each cell and picks up the waste or garbage.

4. *Urinary system.* The kidneys remove the waste from the blood, store it in the bladder, and eliminate it at convenient times.

5. *Intestinal system.* The small and large intestines move the left-over food down to the rectum, store it until a convenient time, and then eliminate it.

UTILIZATION OF FOOD AND OXYGEN IN THE CELL

The cells (the units of body structure) are the machines that generate the forces of life. They use the food and oxygen for the following purposes:
1. To produce energy for the heart to beat, the muscles to work, the brain to think, etc.
2. To produce enough heat to maintain body temperature
3. To produce building materials to replace or repair cells (healing)
4. To produce the substances to build bones, establish electrolyte balance, and maintain health

The food we eat really serves no significant purpose in the body until it has been processed by the digestive system and is delivered to the cells by the bloodstream. In fact, the food we eat, appetizing as it may be, is really a work load on the digestive tract. Why is the diet simplified in illness? Why are oral feedings (mouth) eliminated in patients with acute flare-ups of diseased conditions of the digestive tract such as peptic (stomach) ulcers? How do intravenous feedings give the digestive tract a rest?

DIGESTION

Digestion is the process of preparing the food we eat for distribution, by the bloodstream, to the cells of the body. The body is not able to use eggs, cream, potatoes, or meat floating around in the bloodstream. It needs nutrients in the following forms:
1. Glucose for energy—so all carbohydrates (potatoes, cereals, bread, sugars, etc.) are broken down into glucose
2. Fatty acids and glycerol for heat and energy—so all fats (creams, oils, butter, fatty meat, etc.) are changed to fatty acids and glycerol
3. Amino acids for body building blocks—so all proteins (animal products such as meat, milk, cheese, eggs) are changed to these
4. Calcium for bone building—so the minerals are extracted (from milk, meat, cheese, liver, fish, eggs, whole grains, fruits, vegetables, etc.) and made accessible to the bloodstream
5. Vitamins for health maintenance—so they are separated out of the leafy vegetables and fruits and made accessible to the bloodstream
6. Water to maintain fluid balance—flow ability of body fluids and blood—so it is extracted from the foodstuffs during digestion or obtained from fluids taken orally and made accessible to the bloodstream

DIGESTIVE PROCESS

The digestive system is the part of the body that performs the following functions:
1. Takes in the food
2. Separates out the food that the body can use
3. Changes this food into a form that the cells of the body can use to carry on their living activities
4. Throws this changed foodstuff into the blood (absorbed into the blood in much the same way as a sponge absorbs water)
5. Throws out the unwanted portion of the eaten food as feces

The digestive system, then, consists of a tube that starts at the mouth and ends with the rectum, Any abnormal conditon (disease) in this system will have some effect on the patient's ability to use food or to throw out feces and must be treated by a special diet. Therefore the patient's diet is a very special part of his treatment and is specifically prescribed for him by the doctor.

PARTS OF THE DIGESTIVE SYSTEM AND THEIR FUNCTIONS

Mouth, teeth, and tongue

The *mouth* takes in food, the *teeth* grind it up, and the *tongue* mixes it up and pushes it back toward the throat. The *saliva* wets the food in preparation for swallowing.

Then the food is swallowed. It is pushed back in the throat and it goes past the epiglottis and down into the esophagus on its way to the stomach. Swallowing is not under control of the will. We can swallow only when we have something in our mouth that is ready to be swallowed. Try to swallow five times in succession! Of course, you cannot. This means that when feeding a patient we must feed him slowly and give him ample time to chew his food so that he can swallow it before we attempt to place more food in his mouth. If the patient is paralyzed on one side of his body (hemiplegia), place the food in the nonparalyzed side of his mouth. Just as his paralyzed arm and leg cannot move and have no sensation, so will his face and tongue on the paralyzed side be unable to feel or control any food placed in that side of his mouth.

Throat

The air goes into the nose and food goes into the mouth. However, in the back of the throat, these two passageways become one passageway and remain one for a distance of 5 or 6 inches, after which they again separate into two different passageways or tubes.

We all know that when food accidentally gets into the windpipe (trachea), we cough and choke and tears come to our eyes. However, this is usually avoided, even though we have only one tube for the passage of both food and air in the back of the throat, by the epiglottis (Fig. 8-1), which guards the entrance to the trachea at the point where the one tube again becomes two.

Therefore when we swallow, the epiglottis shuts off the windpipe (trachea), and the food is shunted backward and into the esophagus and then goes on its way to

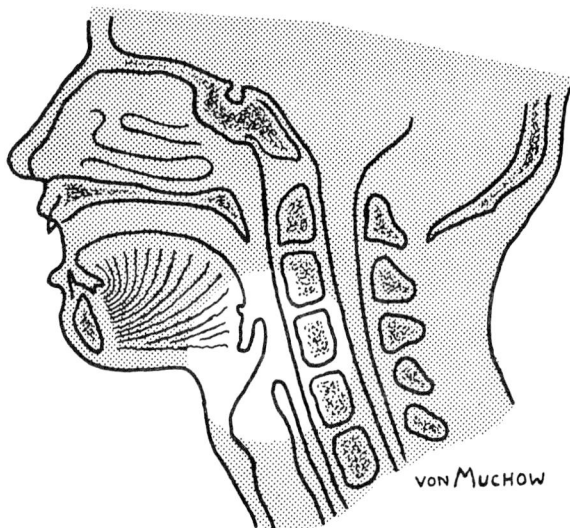

Fig. 8-1. The fingerlike projection (the epiglottis) that closes off the trachea (windpipe) during swallowing.

the stomach. When we breathe, the epiglottis relaxes, the entrance to the trachea is opened, and the air passes into the trachea and on into the lungs. For three reasons this is of significance when feeding the patient:

1. When the patient is unconscious, the epiglottis does not work. Therefore food or fluid placed in the mouth of an unconscious patient will remain there, since he cannot swallow, until it is pulled back into the throat by gravity and pushed into the lungs with the air the patient breathes. Therefore we cannot feed an unconscious patient or any patient who has a paralyzed throat and cannot swallow.

2. The saliva of an unconscious patient who is lying on his back will be pulled to the back of his throat by gravity and pushed into his lungs by breathing. Fluid will collect in his lungs, and pneumonia or drowning will result. Therefore an unconscious patient must not lie in a back-lying position unless he is being constantly attended and his saliva suctioned out by an attendant (during an operation, the anesthetist guards the trachea and suctions out the saliva).

3. A patient cannot breathe and swallow at the same time. Try it. You know how choked you can get when you try to talk with a mouth full of food. The epiglottis is open to let us blow air out over our vocal cords to allow us to talk, and at the same time the food we are attempting to swallow gets into the trachea and we start to choke. Therefore the patient must be fed slowly and given ample time for breathing and swallowing. Incessant chatter to the patient only increases the need for him to talk while he is eating and increases the possibility of his choking. The patient with difficult or rapid breathing will not be able to eat and breathe, so he will give up eating. Therefore see to it that such a patient has a diet requiring little chewing and one that can be swallowed quickly in ample time for the next breath to occur. Remember how you feel when you have a cold. You are so concerned with breathing through your blocked nose that you really are unable to eat.

Esophagus

After the food is swallowed, it passes through a long narrow tube called the esophagus, which is the passageway from the throat to the stomach (Fig. 8-2).

Stomach

The stomach produces the gastric juices and hydrochloric acid that act on the proteins to break them down into simpler substances. The proteins still will not be ready to pass into the blood after this activity in the stomach but will need to be acted upon further in the small intestine. Little or no change (digestion) is made in the fat or carbohydrate foods in the stomach.

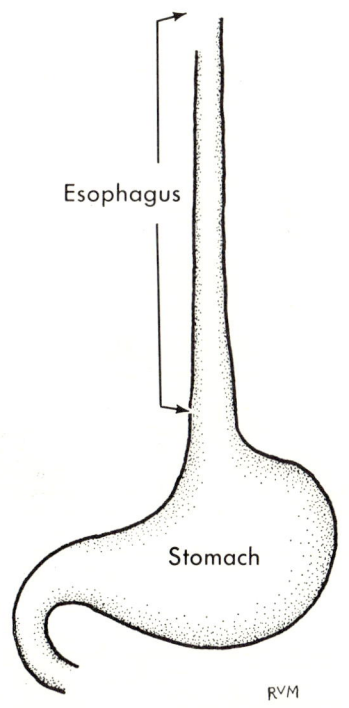

Fig. 8-2. The esophagus and the stomach.

44 Nursing assistant meets patient's basic daily needs in health care facility

The hydrochloric acid also acts as a germicidal agent (germ killer) to cut down on any bacteria taken into the stomach with the food.

Food stays in the stomach for different lengths of time depending on the kind of food it is. Water leaves the stomach almost immediately. Small meals of soft food may remain in the stomach for 1 or 2 hours, whereas the average meal remains there for 3 to 4 hours.

There is a close connection between the brain and the stomach. Therefore emotions play a significant part in stomach activity. Since worry, pain, anger, grief, and fear slow down stomach activity, hunger feelings do not occur, and the patient has no interest in eating. He may even have stomach distress if he is forced to eat. This is due to the decreased secretions of acids and gastric juices.

On the other hand, the tense, jittery, anxious patient may have an increased flow of gastric juices and acids. If there is no food in his stomach, these acids and juices then begin to work on and digest the stomach itself. The patient has pain as an ulcer (hole) develops. As the juices digest more and more of the stomach, the ulcer gets deeper and deeper until it erodes (cuts) into a blood vessel, and then the patient vomits blood. Now he has a bleeding ulcer. One method of helping this patient get relief from his stomach pain is to give him milk and cream (proteins and fats) every hour so that the gastric juices and acids can work on this food in the stomach and leave the stomach lining alone.

A milk and cream diet is prescribed for the patient with an ulcer. Later, when healing begins to occur and the bleeding stops, he will be placed on a smooth food diet

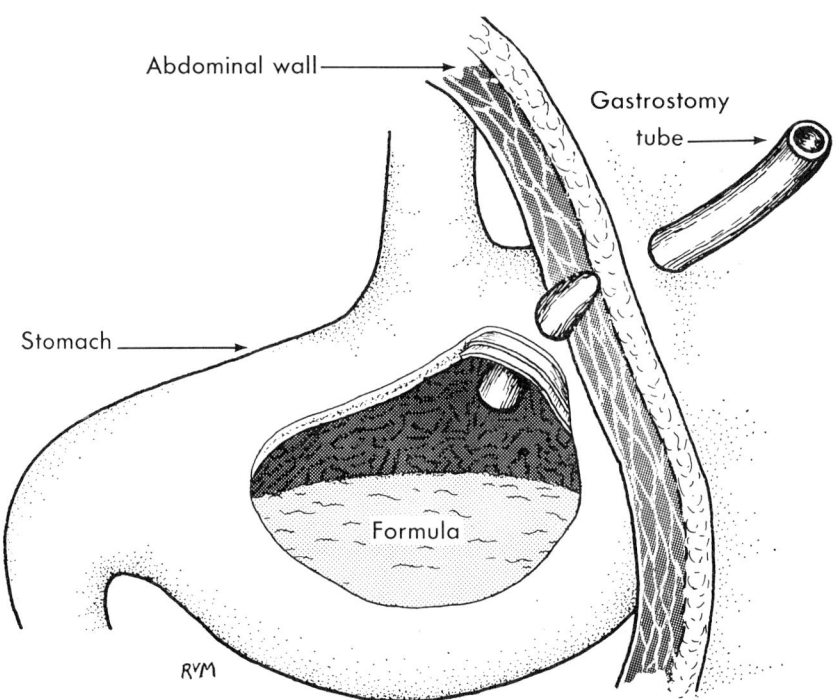

Fig. 8-3. Gastrostomy.

called a bland diet (no rough food to irritate and cause bleeding). A bland diet consists of foods that are not rough and that are not stimulating to the stomach.

The word gastrostomy is made up from the prefix *gastro* (meaning stomach) and the suffix *ostomy* (meaning opening into). Therefore a gastrostomy is an opening into the stomach. It is made by the doctor for feeding the patient.

The gastrostomy opening is made in the top of the stomach, and a short tube is inserted into the opening and is sewed in place (Fig. 8-3). A gastrostomy is usually performed on patients who have the esophagus blocked by tumors, or those who have the larynx removed (laryngectomy) (the larynx is that area in the throat between the back of the mouth and the beginning of the esophagus and trachea that contains the vocal cords), and on patients who are unconscious for long periods of time and so require constant tube feedings.

In order to feed a patient with a gastrostomy, it is necessary to obtain the formula ordered by the doctor from the dietary department. The consistency of this food formula is usually about as thick as watery cereal. When the patient is fed, he is placed in a sitting position in bed or in a chair (Fig. 8-4). A funnel or an Asepto syringe barrel is attached to the gastrostomy tube, and the formula is poured into the tube as prescribed by the nurse or doctor. As the formula enters the stomach, gravity causes it to drop to the lowest position in the stomach (Fig. 8-5). If you feed the patient while he is lying down (Fig. 8-6), the formula splashes all around his stomach, and some comes back out around the tube opening. Since gastric juices and acids would flow out with the formula, the patient would soon develop a reddened, raw, irritated area around the gastrostomy opening.

The gastrostomy formula should be removed from the refrigerator 20 to 30 minutes (to warm it slightly) before it is fed to the patient. The patient should be given his feedings as close to regular mealtimes as possible, with in-between-meal feedings to supplement this diet. For example, the main feedings might be given at 8 A.M., 12 noon, and 5 P.M., with in-between-meal feedings, such as eggnogs and milk shakes, at 10 A.M., 2 P.M., and 9 P.M.

At the beginning and end of each feeding, cool water should be flushed through the tube to prevent its becoming clogged with food. If the patient is able to, he should be taught to give the feedings to himself.

Small intestine

The food passes from the stomach into the small intestine, where digestion is completed (Fig. 8-7). The pancreas pours pancreatic juices into the small intestine. These juices complete the digestion of proteins (break them down into amino acids) and also digest the carbohydrates by breaking them down into simple sugar such as glucose. The liver manufactures bile, which is stored in the gallbladder and emptied into

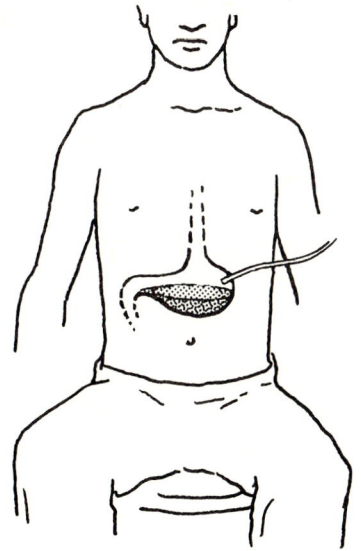

Fig. 8-4. Gastrostomy feeding with the patient in a sitting position.

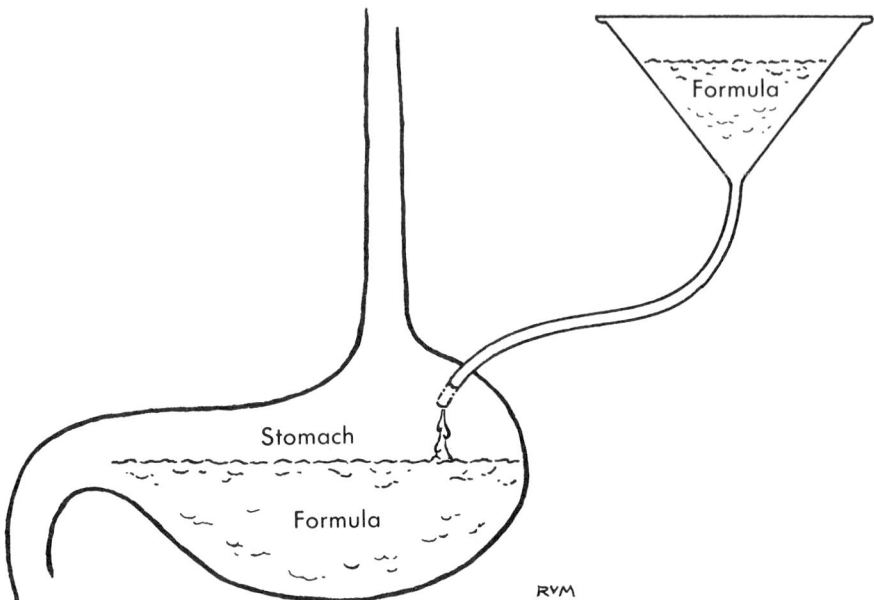

Fig. 8-5. Gastrostomy feeding. Note how the formula drops to the bottom of the stomach and away from the gastrostomy opening.

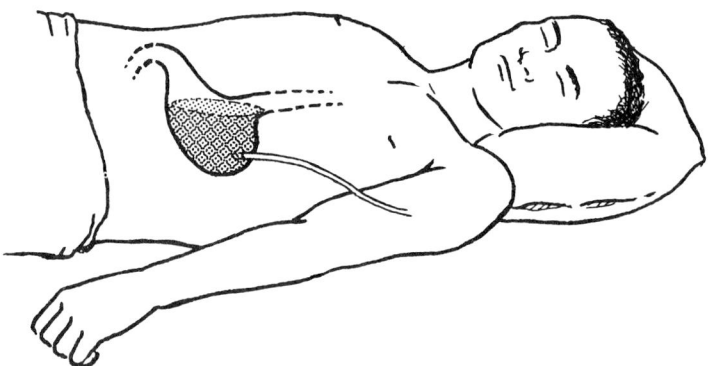

Fig. 8-6. Gastrostomy feeding with the patient lying flat in bed. Note how the formula flows around the tube. It will leak out around the tube opening and cause skin irritation.

the small intestine. The bile and one of the pancreatic juices act together to digest or break down the fats into fatty acids and glycerol. (It is interesting to note here that bile is essential also for the absorption [taking into the blood] of vitamin K; vitamin K is the vitamin that aids in blood clotting.)

In addition to producing several pancreatic juices that break down carbohydrates, fats, and proteins, the pancreas also produces a substance called insulin. Insulin is not poured into the small intestine but is secreted directly into the blood. The insulin is used by the cells of the body to enable them to convert the glucose they get from the blood into the energy to keep them functioning. Insulin functions much

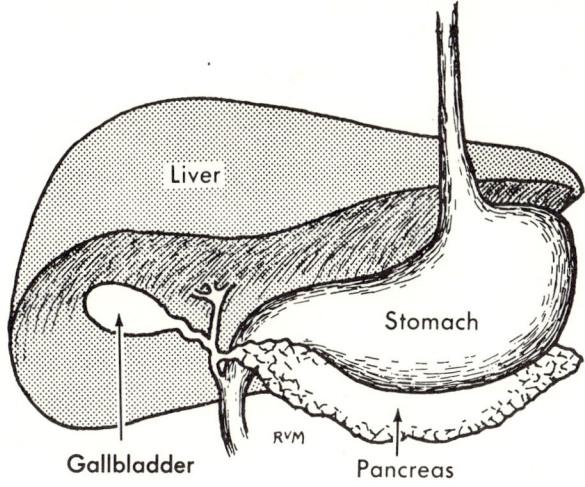

Fig. 8-7. The pancreas, gallbladder, and liver pour digestive juices into the small intestine.

the same way as the spark plug does in producing the spark the car needs to use the gas to run the engine to work the car. The blood could be loaded with sugar, but without the insulin, the body cells would be unable to use this sugar and get the energy to enable our body cells to carry on the activities of living. The patient with a deficiency of insulin is said to have diabetes. The treatment for this condition is twofold:

1. The doctor must determine the amount of energy the patient needs to live, and then he must calculate a diet containing enough carbohydrates (sugar) to produce the energy requirements.
2. The doctor must prescribe the dosage of insulin required by the patient's body to use these carbohydrates and convert them into energy.

Since insulin is normally secreted or poured into the blood directly and does not go into the digestive tract, the nurse must inject the insulin that the doctor orders directly into the patient's body tissues by hypodermic (under the skin) injection. Insulin taken by mouth is rendered inactive by the digestive juices.

The patient with liver disease (inadequate production of bile) has several problems. Since he is not able to digest fats, he will develop actual pain and nausea and vomiting if he eats a diet containing large quantities of fat. Consequently, the patient with liver disease is placed on a low-fat diet. The heat and energy his body needs will be obtained by increasing his carbohydrate intake. Therefore he will be given a low-fat, high-carbohydrate, high-protein diet.

When the flow of bile into the small intestine is blocked, the bile will overflow into the bloodstream (much like a blocked sink will overflow onto the kitchen floor). This backflow of bile into the blood will cause the patient's skin to have a yellowish or bronze appearance (jaundice), and the absence of bile in the small intestine will cause the feces to have a light yellow or sandy-colored appearance.

The jaundiced patient has little or no bile in the small intestine and therefore has difficulty getting vitamin K into his blood. Thus he may bleed easily and even without an apparent cause. Watch jaundiced patients carefully and report any excessive bleeding of the gums when the teeth are brushed or any excessive bleeding of the face if the patient is cut during shaving.

The small intestine is approximately 22 feet long. All 22 feet are contained within the abdomen (area between the umbilicus and the genital region). The small intestine has three parts or sections (Fig. 8-8):

1. The duodenum, which is about 10 to 12 inches long, is the first part.
2. The jejunum, which is about 7 to 8 feet long, is the second part.
3. The ileum, which is about 13 feet long, is the third part.

The small intestine has a sausagelike appearance and contains muscles in its lining. These muscles contract and relax in a rhythmic fashion (peristalsis), pushing the food through the intestines (Fig. 8-9). When the intestines become irritated and contract and relax rather violently, we complain of cramps.

Inside, the small intestine is filled with fingerlike projections called villi. These villi function much like straws in a soda do as they suck the digested food (amino acids, fatty acids and glycerols, glucose, vitamins, and minerals) out of the small intestine through their fingerlike projections and deposit them into the bloodstream. Vitamins are absorbed (pass from the intestine into the bloodstream) primarily in the lower third of the small intestine (ileum). Minerals are absorbed throughout the small and large intestines.

Surgical openings made into any part of the small intestine are named after the section of the intestine involved plus the ending *ostomy*. Thus *duodenostomy* is an opening into the duodenum, *jejunostomy* is an opening into the jejunum, and *ileostomy* is an opening into the ileum.

An ileostomy is a rather common procedure done to remove feces from the body when the large bowel is removed because it is diseased. This will be described in another chapter.

The material in the small bowel is in a

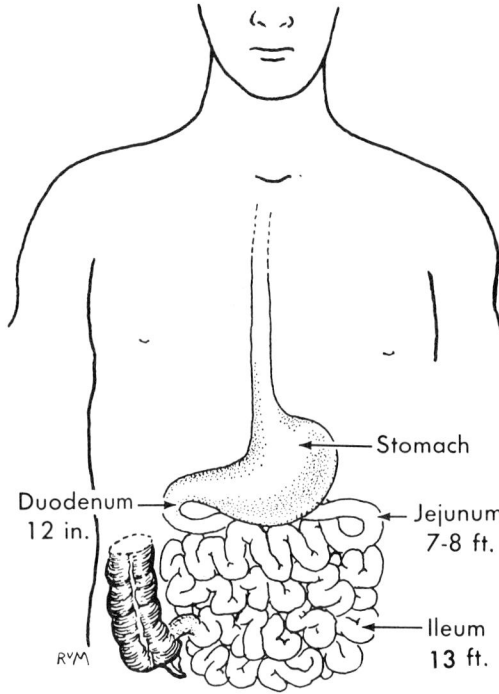

Fig. 8-8. The sections of the small intestine.

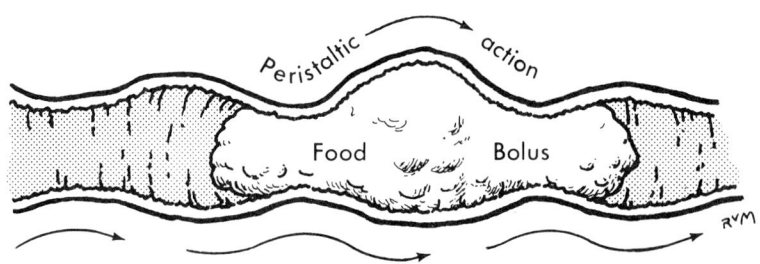

Fig. 8-9. Peristaltic contractions that move the food through the 22 feet of small intestine.

liquid form. Therefore a patient with an opening into the small bowel will have unformed liquid feces draining from this opening.

Large intestine

The small intestine (the portion called the ileum) enters into the large intestine (the portion called the cecum) at the right side of the lower abdomen. The narrow loop of bowel extending from the point at which they join is the appendix. The large intestine is about 5 feet long and consists of the following parts: cecum, the ascending colon, the transverse colon, the descending colon, the sigmoid colon, the rectum, and the anus (Fig. 8-10).

When the food passes into the large intestine from the small intestine, it is in a semiliquid state. However, as it moves through the large intestine, water is absorbed (passes from the large intestine into the blood), and the feces thus becomes less watery, more formed, and quite solid. The large intestine has a muscle in its lining that contracts (narrows and widens) to push the food along. However, this muscle action is less frequent than the muscle contraction (peristalsis) of the small bowel, and it seems to occur in relation to the filling of the large intestine. Therefore the role of the large intestine is to absorb (or take into the blood) water and to push unwanted food (feces) out of the body. The feces collect in the rectum, and eventually it fills and its wall becomes stretched. This stretching creates a feeling of discomfort and pressure that is relieved by defecating (passing feces from the rectum).

When the muscles of the large intestine

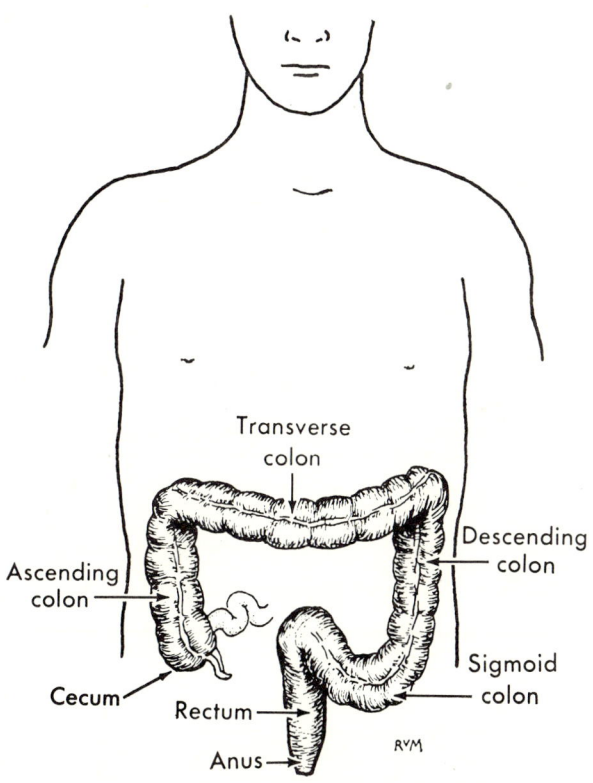

Fig. 8-10. The large intestine and its seven parts.

are sluggish, foodstuffs move along too slowly and too much water is taken out of them, causing the waste material (feces) to become so dry and hard that it is difficult to expel (move the bowels). This condition is called *constipation*.

However, if the muscles of the large intestine (colon) are irritated and contract too often or too vigorously, the foodstuffs move through too fast, little or no water is absorbed, and liquid bowel movements or *diarrhea* occurs.

SIGNIFICANCE OF STRUCTURE AND FUNCTION OF DIGESTIVE SYSTEM IN FEEDING THE PATIENT

Because the digestive system consists of a tube extending from the mouth to the rectum, a sitting position facilitates eating and swallowing food. Therefore we eat sitting on a chair at a table; observe the number of dining rooms in nursing homes. In this way, gravity aids the food to pass down through the digestive system. Inasfar as a patient's condition permits, he, too, should sit on a chair at a table to eat. If this is not possible, he should be placed in a sitting position in bed. If he is not permitted to sit up in bed, his head should be propped up on pillows.

Remember, the patient can swallow only when he has something to swallow and not really at his own will; also, breathing and swallowing cannot be done at the same time. Therefore when feeding a patient, we must give him sufficient time to chew his food properly and prepare it for swallowing. Furthermore, since eating and talking cannot be done at the same time, we should not talk incessantly to the patient while we are feeding him.

Unpleasant emotions such as fear, distaste, worry, and anger block our feeling of hunger, spoil our appetite, and even give us indigestion or discomfort if we eat. Pleasant emotions like joy, happiness, peace, and contentment increase our appetite. Therefore the patient's mealtime should be as pleasant as possible. Frightening news of an impending operation or a painful diagnostic test should be delayed until after mealtime. Unpleasant sights such as bedpans, urinals, and emesis basins should be removed from the patient's bedside before his meal is served. Observe the piped in music in nursing home dining rooms. Why is this done?

The nursing assistant serving meals should be wearing a clean uniform and should be pleasant and friendly. Hurrying and rushing to pass out meals and collect diet trays must be avoided. When the nursing assistant feeds the patient, she should sit (if possible) comfortably at the patient's side and feed him in much the same way as she feeds herself.

Two activities that differentiate an adult from a baby are (1) the ability to feed himself and (2) the ability to care for his own toilet needs. No matter how ill your patient is, he, too, likes to do these activities for himself. When he cannot feed himself or go to the toilet at will, he feels like a baby and is unhappy and depressed. Therefore when you serve the patient his tray, know how much he can do in relation to feeding himself (Fig. 8-11).

If one of the patient's arms is paralyzed, in a cast, or immobilized for an intravenous injection, pour and fix his coffee, cut his meat, butter his bread, and set up the tray so that he can manage to feed himself with his one arm. If the patient is recovering from surgery and is quite weak, assist him by guiding his arm movements or steadying his hand. Give him straws to drink fluids. If the patient is totally helpless, serve his tray last and feed him. Let him help in some way. Perhaps he can manage to hold and eat the bread by himself.

When you serve the tray, tell the patient what is on it, ask him about any special preparation of the food (adding salt or butter, fixing coffee). Place the napkin or bib in place under his chin. Feed him the food in the same order in which you eat

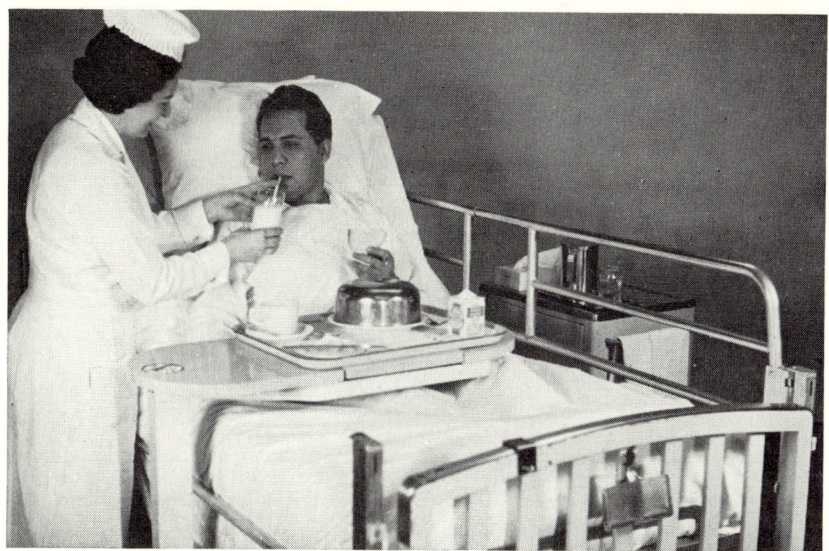

Fig. 8-11. The nurse is feeding an acutely ill patient. Note the patient's sitting position. Note also that the nurse is fostering a feeling of independence in the patient by encouraging him to hold his own bread.

yours. Give him the soup, then the salad, then the main course, and then the dessert. Ask him if he wishes to drink his beverage with his meal or afterward, and serve it in accord with his wishes. Sometimes the liquids, soups, and cereals can be handled by the patient if they are in a cup. At other times the patient can take them best through a straw.

When you know the patient's needs in regard to food, write them on his diet card so that any person serving the tray can assist the patient in the way that he needs to be helped. Examples might be as follows:

1. Cut meat, pour soup in cup, pour coffee, and butter bread.
2. Patient can feed himself the bread, and he likes to do so.
3. Place the food in the right side of the mouth or the patient will choke on it.

Do not increase the patient's feeling of helplessness by serving his tray and leaving him alone to wonder if and when someone will come to help him eat.

Be sure to serve the tray to the patient for whom it was prepared. Remember, the diet is an important part of the patient's treatment. A diet high in fat that is given by mistake to a patient with liver disease will give him a great deal of abdominal discomfort.

Remove the tray promptly when the patient has finished eating. Check to see how much he has eaten. Record your observations on the nurse's notes.

If the patient on a diabetic diet has not eaten all his food, notify the nurse. Remember, this patient is receiving insulin (by injection) in sufficient amounts to cover the glucose in his diet. If he does not eat the food and has already received the insulin, an insulin reaction (dizziness, confusion, sweating, staggering, unconsciousness, coma, death) may occur. This reaction can be avoided by giving the patient a glucose solution (usually orange juice) that is prepared by the dietitian to contain the same number of calories as in the uneaten food. This glucose solution will use up the insulin the patient has taken.

When collecting the diet trays after each

meal, check whether the patient is to have his fluid intake recorded. If so, record it promptly on the intake and output record.

BEFORE-MEAL CARE

It is impossible to eat with a dry, dirty mouth, unclean dentures, and with hands that have just assisted with toileting. Therefore when preparing the patient for his meal, it is necessary to remember his personal needs as well as the factors that help the digestive tract to function well. Find out if he needs a bedpan or urinal. If he does, give it to him and remove it promptly and then wash his hands. Then provide him with equipment for cleaning his mouth and brushing his teeth, especially before breakfast. The ambulatory patient will do this for himself, but the bed patient depends entirely on you to help him with these activities.

AFTER-MEAL CARE

It was pointed out earlier in this chapter that the movement of the feces along the large bowel occurs in relation to its filling. Therefore after meals there may be a movement of feces into the cecum. This stimulates the contracting and relaxing of the bowel muscles and moves enough feces into the rectum to stretch the rectal walls. The stretched rectal walls cause pressure and create the need for the patient to evacuate. Therefore many patients may need a bedpan soon after eating. Knowing this fact assists us in bowel training a patient because we know that he will very likely need to defecate after each meal. Consequently, a bowel-training program would include giving the patient a bedpan after meals.

FOOD TAKES THE BLAME!

One important thing we must remember is that sick patients usually think that the hospital food is terrible. One reason for this is that the patient suffering from pain and worry will have a decreased flow of gastric juices and acids and, consequently, less effective digestion. Another reason, however, is that the sick patient projects his anger about his sickness and helplessness onto the food. He does this because he cannot focus this anger on the doctor, nurse, and nursing assistant, who are trying to help, for he is afraid they may withdraw their help from him if he does so. Therefore he takes out his frustration on the food. It is amazing to observe how the "terrible" food suddenly improves as the patient's condition improves and he approaches being well. One would almost believe the hospital put in an entirely new dietary department. Remember that the patient who hates the food really hates his condition, hates his sickness, hates his helplessness, and that the only way he can really express this acceptably is by complaining about the food.

MEALTIME IN THE NURSING HOME

Like all homes, the nursing home has a dining room where all the patients who are physically able come and eat together. This togetherness in living activities soon makes the nursing home patient a group member —a member of the family and no longer alone and lonely.

FEEDING THE UNCONSCIOUS PATIENT

Although the unconscious patient is lying still, his body requires a great deal of energy to carry on the activities of living and to fight his illness. The energy (fuel) for these activities must be provided by food.

We have seen that it is impossible to feed an unconscious patient by mouth, since his epiglottis is not working, and foodstuffs will get into his trachea and drown or choke him. However, the unconscious patient may be fed by any one of the following methods:
1. Gastrostomy feedings (discussed earlier in this chapter)
2. Levin tube feedings (A Levin tube, or gastric tube, is passed through the

patient's nose and into his stomach; because the tube is quite narrow in diameter, only liquids can be administered through it.)
3. Intravenous feedings

Levin tube feedings

Levin tube feedings are not so safe or comfortable to the patient over a long period of time as is the gastrostomy method of feeding for the following reasons:
1. The tube through the nose hinders the patient's ability to breathe through his nose, so he breathes through his mouth. This means that he will need frequent mouth care because the air dries his mouth.
2. The tube may be pulled up slightly or coughed up slightly by the patient. Then it comes out of the stomach and curls up in the back of the patient's throat. Fluids injected into a tube that has been pulled out of the stomach could be aspirated easily (sucked into the trachea). This means that the position of the tube must be checked before each Levin tube feeding to make sure that it is still in the stomach.
3. The tube will irritate the nose and throat. This irritation increases secretions. These secretions may be aspirated and cause pneumonia.

Levin tube feedings, which are pre-

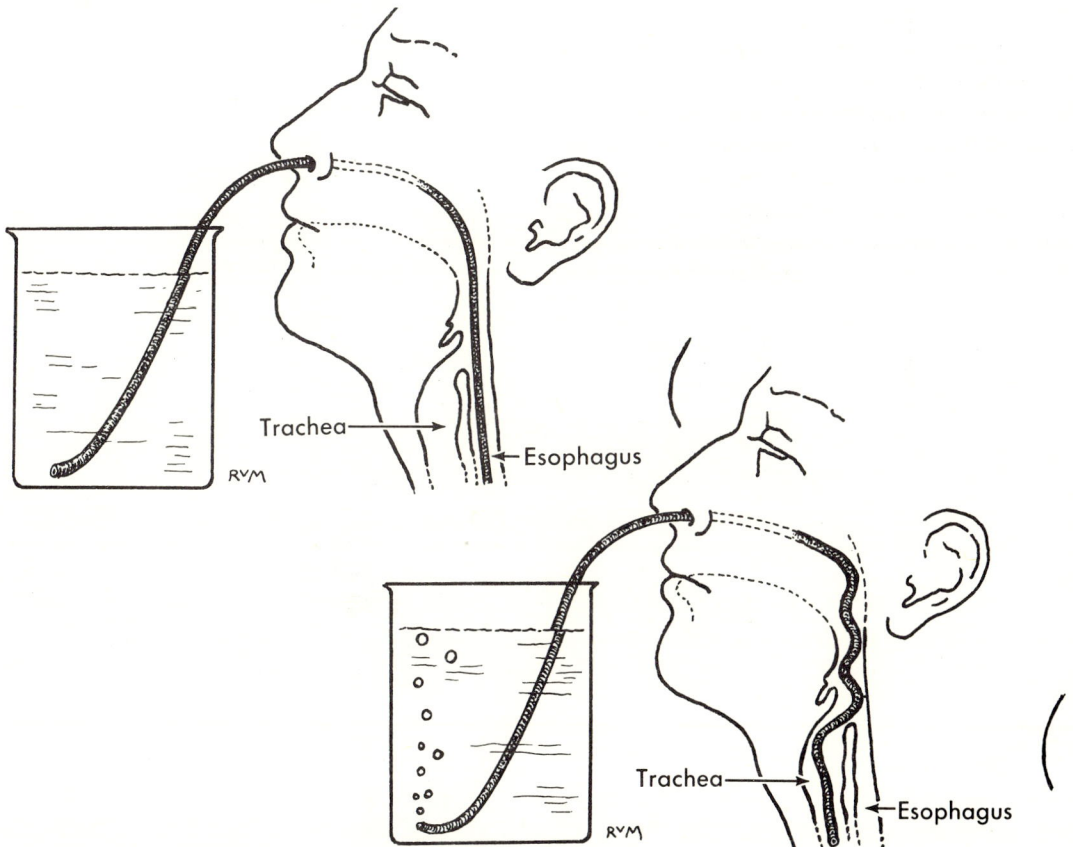

Fig. 8-12. Testing the Levin tube by immersing the end in a glass of water to determine whether the tube is in the stomach or in the trachea.

scribed by the doctor, as are all diets, are ordered from the dietary department. A plan for the patient feedings is developed by the nurse and is written in the Kardex. This plan usually consists of feedings at mealtimes: 8 A.M., 12 noon, and 5 P.M., with in-between-meal feedings at 10 A.M., 2 P.M., and 9 P.M. However, it should consist of six equal feedings of 500 ml. each.

Equipment for a Levin tube feeding usually consists of a pint container (pitcher), an Asepto syringe, and a glass of cool water. The feeding is removed from the refrigerator, poured into the small pitcher, and allowed to stand at room temperature for approximately 20 minutes to warm it. Then it is taken to the patient's bedside on a tray that also contains the Asepto syringe and the glass of cool water. The plug (catheter plug or golf tee) is removed from the end of the Levin tube protruding from the patient's nose, and the tube is immersed in a glass of water (Fig. 8-12). If bubbles are observed in the water, do not give the feeding. Call the nurse to check the tube to determine if it is in the trachea. If bubbles do not appear, the tube is still in the stomach, and the feeding can be given. The barrel of the Asepto syringe is attached to the Levin tube. The tube is pinched off, and cool water is poured into the Asepto barrel from the glass. The pinch (this avoids pushing the air from the Asepto syringe into the stomach) is released, and the water is permitted to flow through the tube into the stomach, thus rinsing the tube of all secretions. Before the Asepto syringe barrel completely empties, the feeding is poured into it from the pitcher or glass. This pouring of the feeding continues until the pitcher or glass is empty (Fig. 8-13). The feeding is then completed by giving the patient the remaining cool water through the tube to flush out all the feeding to avoid clogging of the tube. The tube is then plugged or clamped. The feeding is charted

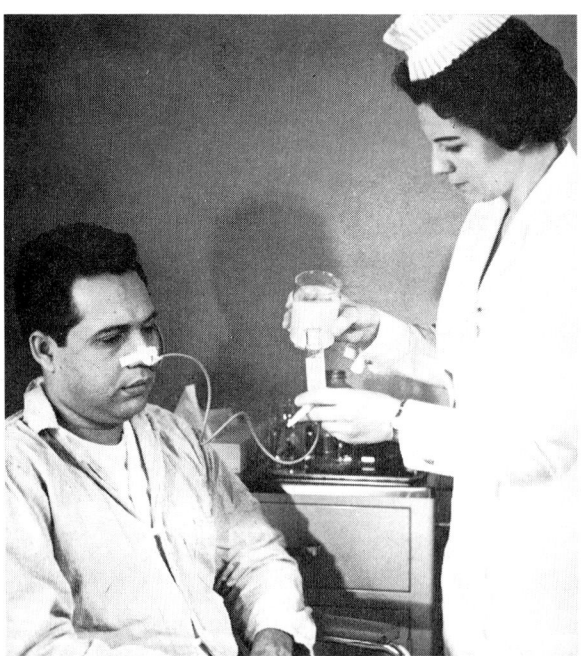

Fig. 8-13. The nurse is giving a Levin tube feeding to a hemiplegic patient who is unable to swallow.

on the intake and output sheet, and the tray is cleaned up and returned to its proper place.

Intravenous feedings

Intravenous feedings contain little food value and are given primarily for their water, mineral, or electrolyte value. An intravenous bottle containing 1,000 ml. of 5% glucose solutions contains only 50 ml. of glucose (less than 2 ounces) and 950 ml. of water. The caloric value of these 50 ml. of glucose is 200 calories. The average caloric need of the patient is 3,000 calories in 24 hours. A calorie is a measure of food value just as an inch is a unit of distance. You can readily see that the food value of intravenous feedings is rather insignificant. The value of intravenous solutions in maintaining electrolyte balance will be discussed later.

Special note

The nursing service in each hospital will identify those procedures that the nursing assistant can do to help take care of the patients. Giving the patient Levin tube or gastrostomy tube feedings may or may not be included in your job description. Check your description carefully and perform accordingly. The inclusion of these procedures in this book does not indicate, in any way, that it is or is not a task that the nursing assistant can do. This decision remains with the nursing service in the hospital in which you are employed.

SUMMARY

Food is the fuel that the body uses to run its complex machine and carry out the activities of living. Food cannot be used by the body cells in the form in which it is taken into the mouth, so the body changes it into the form it needs through the process of digestion.

In relation to food, the digestive system serves much the same purpose in the body as the mother serves in a family. Just as the mother obtains foodstuff from the store and then changes it (through cooking) into the kind of an appetizing meal that the family likes to eat, so does the digestive system take in the foodstuff and then change it (through the process of digestion) into the kind of meal the cells of the body like and use.

Just as the family suffers when the mother is sick or away and does not prepare the food for them, the body too suffers when a part of the digestive system does not prepare the food properly for it. Fatty foods will cause pain and bloating if the gallbladder and liver are not working properly. Weakness, lack of energy, and extreme fatigue may result if the pancreas is not secreting the insulin to enable the body to convert the glucose to energy. Therefore any disease that prevents any part of the digestive tract from functioning properly will manifest itself in bodily discomfort and disease.

The sick patient is not interested in food. This makes our job of seeing that the patient eats a rather difficult one. However, we can help the patient maintain his interest in food by controlling the fear in the hospital environment, by helping the patient maintain his independence by permitting him to do as much as he can to feed himself, and by assisting the patient at mealtimes in the way that he needs to be assisted.

DISCUSSION QUESTIONS

1. Do all patients receive the same kind of a diet?
2. Determine the type of diets your patients receive. Then discuss with the nurse the reason for their diets.
3. Who determines what the patient's diet will be?
4. Is the patient's diet an important part of his treatment? Why?
5. Discuss why it is necessary for you to observe and report the patient's eating habits to the nurse.
6. How do you feed a patient who does not have the strength to feed himself?
7. How is an unconscious patient fed? Why?
8. Which is the more normal type of feeding, Levin tube or intravenous? Why?

9 Why is it necessary for a diabetic patient to follow his diet precisely as prescribed by the doctor?
10 What complication might develop if the diabetic patient vomited his entire meal? What would you do if this complication occurred?

VOCABULARY

absorption Passing into the bloodstream.
aspirated Drawing material such as food, saliva, etc. into the windpipe with the breath.
bland diet A nonirritating, nonstimulating diet given to the ulcer patient.
bowel Another name for intestine.
cell The smallest functioning unit of the body. (The cell is to the body what a brick is to a brick building.)
colon Another name for the large bowel.
digestion Process of changing the food that is eaten into the glucose, amino acids, fatty acid and glycerol, vitamins, and minerals that the cells of the body can use.
energy The ability to do a job (work).
epiglottis A body structure situated in the throat near the opening to the windpipe. When swallowing occurs, it closes off the windpipe and thus prevents saliva, food, etc. from entering the windpipe.
feces Consists of the food eaten that the body cannot use, secretions (juices) from the stomach and intestines, and bacteria from the intestines.
gastrointestinal tract Consists of the stomach, the small bowel, and the large bowel.
gastrostomy A surgical opening into the stomach for feeding the patient.
hemiplegia One side of the body is paralyzed from the face down to, and including, the leg.
ileostomy A surgical opening into the last part of the small bowel to permit feces to leave the body.
organ Many cells bound together such as the heart or lungs to do a body activity.
special diet Those foodstuffs that the patient's body can use. It excludes from the diet those foodstuffs that the body is not able to use due to some disease condition.

SOURCE OF ADDITIONAL INFORMATION

1 Film: Feeding the patient; may be obtained from the U. S. Army Film Service; contact the Commanding General of the U. S. Army Corps Area nearest to you or the Director of the Armed Forces Institute of Pathology, Walter Reed Army Medical Center, 6825 16th St., N.W., Washington, D.C. 20025.

9/Meeting the patient's need for water

STUDY QUESTIONS

1. Why does the body need water?
2. How does the body lose fluids?
3. Does the body always need the same amount of fluids?
4. Would the body need more or less fluid on a very hot day? Why?
5. Why is the fluid intake of some patients limited?
6. Why is a daily weight requested on a patient with edema?
7. Where does urine come from?
8. Where is urine stored?
9. What are the signs of dehydration?
10. What is the average patient's fluid need in 24 hours?
11. What is an intake and output record?
12. When are notations made on an intake and output record?
13. Why does the nursing home patient limit his own intake?

THE BODY NEEDS WATER

The body needs about 3,000 ml. (3 quarts) of water each 24 hours to carry on its activities. When this need is not met in a conscious patient, extreme thirst occurs, and the patient is quite uncomfortable. All of us have seen movies showing people lost in the desert without water and how they searched with frenzy for the water to wet their dry, parched, swollen lips. Some of us have had operations and can remember the extremely dry mouth and the intense thirst of the postoperative period.

Thirst is the way the body lets us know of its need for water. Every important function in the body is carried on in a liquid environment. The food is digested into a liquid form before it can pass through the small intestines into the blood. Food must also be in a liquid form in the blood so that it can be carried around to the cells of the body. The blood circulating around the body carrying food and collecting waste is also in a liquid state. The waste material from the cells that the blood collects must also be liquid. Emotion (crying, for example) is also expressed with drops of water called tears, and body cooling is achieved through perspiring and the evaporation of this perspiration from the body. Even the air we breathe is moistened to avoid drying out and irritating our breathing tubes. As you can easily see, the body cannot live long without liquids. In fact, without them the body cannot carry out the activities of living longer than 3 days.

HOW MUCH FLUID DOES THE BODY NEED?

The body must be maintained in a state of fluid balance. Therefore the amount of fluid the body needs depends on the amount the body is losing. Under normal conditions (that is, in a patient with a normal temperature on a cool day, who has no excessive fluid loss such as drainage from the body or diarrhea), the usual fluid loss is about 2,500 ml. This fluid loss is from the following sources:

Skin	400 ml.
Breath	400 ml.
Urine	1,400 ml.
Perspiration	100 ml.
Feces	200 ml.
Total	2,500 ml.

However, fluid loss is increased in many ways. On a hot day the amount of perspiration will be increased and fluid loss may be increased as much as 1,500 ml. This increased perspiration and increased fluid loss may also occur if the patient's temperature is greatly elevated (103° to 104° F.) Fluid loss is also increased if the patient hemorrhages, has diarrhea, or has drainage from any part of the body. Loss of fluid from a draining bedsore may be great enough to cause a severe disturbance of body functioning. *Therefore* it is impossible for us to determine what the patient's fluid needs are unless we know the needs of the patient's body.

The doctor knows the needs of the patient's body best. He knows the fluid needs in relation to the patient's temperature, the weather, and the body fluid loss; therefore he prescribes the amount of fluid the patient should have. But the prescription for fluids is not enough. The doctor wants to know how much the patient is actually receiving and how much he is losing each day, so we record these amounts on an intake and output record. This means that all the fluids taken into the patient's body, as well as all those lost from the patient's body, will be measured and the amounts recorded every 24 hours. Each day the doctor will study this record to determine whether or not the patient is kept in fluid balance. If imbalance occurs (fluid losses are greater than fluid intake) or if the fluid intake is inadequate for living, the doctor may give intravenous fluids or he may instruct us to encourage the patient to drink more. However, if intake or output recordings are done incorrectly, the patient may be treated incorrectly by the doctor.

LIMITING FLUID INTAKE

In some patients, the doctor may want to limit the patient's fluid intake. This is true in those patients whose cells retain the water and do not give it back to the blood so it can be excreted (removed from the body) by the kidneys. This may occur in a patient with heart failure whose heart is not pumping the blood around the body adequately. The blood slows down, or stagnates, in the blood vessels until the blood vessels are so full of liquids that they can take no more from the cells. In much the same way that a plugged pipe will cause your sink to overflow on the kitchen floor, the liquids (serum) in these overfull blood vessels will overflow into the tissues of the body. Because the feet are below the level of the heart, gravity helps the blood get to them easily, but gravity also makes it difficult to get the blood back from them to the heart. Therefore an early sign of heart failure is fluid escaping from the blood vessels into the tissues of the feet, and the patient develops edema (swelling because of waterlogged cells) in the feet and ankles. As the heart failure increases, this edema may increase and involve the entire lower half of the body (legs, thighs, scrotum, and abdomen).

In a patient who has this swelling

(edema) because of watery fluid escaping from the blood vessels into the tissues, the doctor may limit the fluid intake. He may also give the patient a heart strengthener (like digitalis) and a diuretic (like Hydrodiuril) to stimulate the kidneys to take more fluid out of the blood. As the heart becomes stronger and pumps the blood around more effectively, the diuretic will stimulate the kidneys to take the excess fluid out of the blood. In this way the patient's output (urine) will be greatly increased, and the edema will be lessened and will gradually disappear entirely.

Intake and output will be recorded daily, and the doctor will determine the effectiveness of the diuretic by studying how it increases the patient's urinary output and decreases the edema. If our intake and output recordings are inadequate, the doctor will get false information from us and may continue ineffective or even undesirable treatment.

Sometimes the doctor also orders daily weight measurements of patients receiving diuretics so that he can determine the daily loss of retained fluid (fluid in the tissues causing edema). The doctor may want the intake-output and weight measures because of the dangerous drugs he has prescribed and therefore the need for accuracy, or he may be requesting the weights because he cannot rely on the accuracy of our intake-output recordings.

A pint of fluid weighs approximately 1 pound. Therefore a patient who has a loss of 1,000 ml. of fluid (in excess of his intake) should lose 2 pounds. Accurate determinations of the patient's weight can be obtained only if he is weighed at the same time each day and under the same conditions (before breakfast, before daily bowel movement, before getting out of bed, etc.).

URINARY OUTPUT

The body cells take food out of the blood, use it for energy or to rebuild themselves, and throw out the waste material into the blood. The food in the cells leaves a waste product just as any fuel leaves a waste such as ashes when it is burned:

$$\text{Wood} + \text{Fire} = \text{Heat} + \text{Ashes}$$
$$\text{Food in cell} + \text{Oxygen} =$$
$$\text{Heat} + \text{Energy} + \text{Waste} + \text{Water}$$

The waste material (urea and water) thrown into the blood by the cells is carried to the kidneys where it is removed from the blood at the rate of about 60 ml. (2 ounces) per hour, and then it is stored in the bladder as urine. When 250 ml. (about ½ pint) of urine accumulates, the patient develops a feeling of fullness in the bladder, which, he has learned, means that he needs to void (pass urine to the outside). The average urinary output is approximately 1,500 ml. of urine in 24 hours.

When the kidneys fail to work properly and water and urea are not taken out of the blood, the patient has an overloading of water and urea in the blood. The overloaded blood will not be able to take up any more water from the cells, so the cells become waterlogged, with the result that the patient becomes swollen (edematous). Excess urea in the blood is called uremia (*-emia* means in the blood), and this causes the death of the patient, just as overloading a stove with ashes puts out the fire or as overloading an engine with carbon gums up the engine.

The urinary output of the patient is a very important measure of how effectively the kidneys are eliminating waste from the body. Remember how your own physical examination included a urine examination. Observe that each new patient admitted to the hospital has a routine examination of his urine.

RECORDING INTAKE AND OUTPUT

Inform the patient that measurements of his intake and output have been requested by the doctor and that all liquids taken or voided are to be measured and recorded. Instruct him also as to whether he is to drink large amounts of fluid or whether he is to limit his fluid intake. If he is to drink large amounts of fluids, encourage him to take a glass of liquid each hour. If the patient is on limited fluids, instruct him to drink only those fluids given to him by members of the hospital staff. If the patient is ambulatory, show him how to measure and record the fluids he drinks and voids. If he is confined to bed or to a wheelchair or is otherwise unable to keep his own record, place an "intake and output" sign on his bed and then attach a clipboard holding an intake and output record to the foot of his bed.

Each time you collect diet trays from the patients, look for the sign at the foot of the bed. If there is one, determine how much liquid the patient has had and record it on the intake record. Also do this each time you give the patient a glass of water or a glass of liquid nourishment such as fruit juice or eggnog. Each time a urinal is taken from a patient, look on the bed for an intake and output sign. If there is such a sign, measure the urine voided and return to the bedside promptly to chart the amount on the output record. Recording intake when you feed the patient* or give him liquids (Fig. 9-1) and recording output each time you empty a urinal make your intake and output records accurate.

Remember also to measure and chart output resulting from diarrhea, vomiting, blood loss, and drainage from all tubes in the patient. Chart also excessive perspiration that necessitates changes of bed linen.

Once every 24 hours, the intake and output records are collected and totaled, and the amounts are recorded on the patients' charts. A fresh intake and output record is then attached to the clipboard at the foot of each patient's bed. This might be done at midnight. However, it is usually done at 5 A.M. or 6 A.M. so that the intake and output record accurately depicts the patient's condition at the time the doctor makes his rounds and observes it. Then he takes the medical action that he decides is indicated. A more accurate account of the

---

*Foods contain a high percentage of fluid also. However, fluid from food sources is not recorded on the intake record.

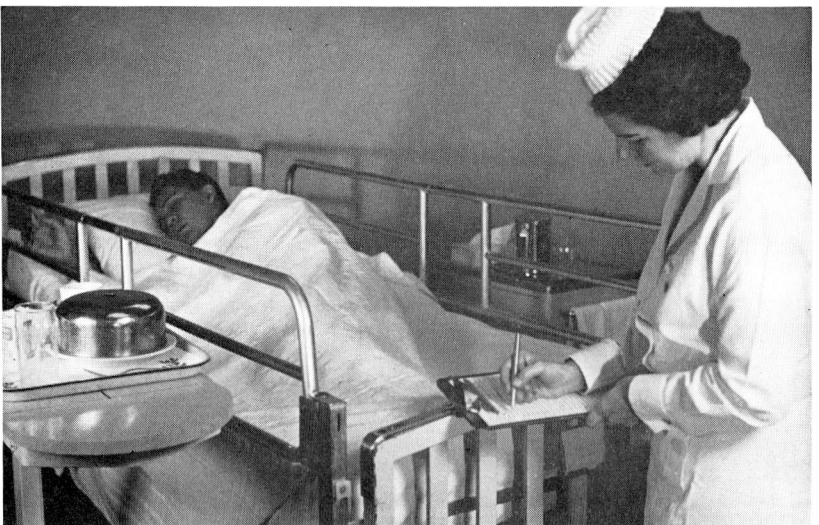

Fig. 9-1. The intake is recorded immediately after the patient is fed and before his tray is removed. Note how comfortably the patient has been positioned after his meal.

Patient's name									
	Intake					Output			
	Oral		Parenteral					Emesis	
Time	Type of fluids	Amount	Type	Started	Absorbed	Urine	Tube	Diarrhea	Other
6 A.M.	24-hour total								

Our utensils contain the following:

    Water glass 240 ml.   Cup   150 ml.   Pitchers 1000 ml.
    Juice glass   120 ml.   Bowls 200 ml.

Fig. 9-2. Intake and output record.

patient's intake can be maintained when the amount of fluid in each fluid-containing receptacle used on the patient's tray is printed on the bottom of the intake and output record (Fig. 9-2).

EXTRA FLUIDS

The name of the patient who is to be encouraged to drink large amounts of liquids should be added to the nourishment lists and he should receive appetizing drinks as in-between-meal feedings (Fig. 9-3). He should be visited hourly and encouraged to drink a glass of fluid.

DRINKING WATER

Fresh drinking water should be distributed to each patient in a clean pitcher each morning. A clean glass should also be provided. Each afternoon and evening the old drinking water should be replaced by fresh water. Avoid collecting and taking all the patients' water pitchers to a central place in the utility room for refilling unless each pitcher is labeled with the patient's name. Why? This practice of mass collection of unlabeled pitchers would result in one patient receiving another's pitcher, and this could result in a spread of infection throughout the hospital.

Keep drinking water covered so that germs cannot get into it. Do not give the patient on limited fluids a large supply of drinking water; give him only what he is permitted to have on his tray at mealtimes.

WHO IS THE PATIENT WHOSE INTAKE AND OUTPUT MUST BE RECORDED?

The doctor orders measurements of intake and output for all patients about whom there is a question of whether or not they are being maintained in a state of fluid balance. These patients might include all those who are unable to take fluids freely by mouth or those who are losing large amounts of fluid. Therefore intake and output measurements would very likely be ordered for the following patients:

1. Patients receiving nothing by mouth
2. Patients in the immediate postoperative period
3. Patients who are seriously ill
4. Patients with extremely high temperatures

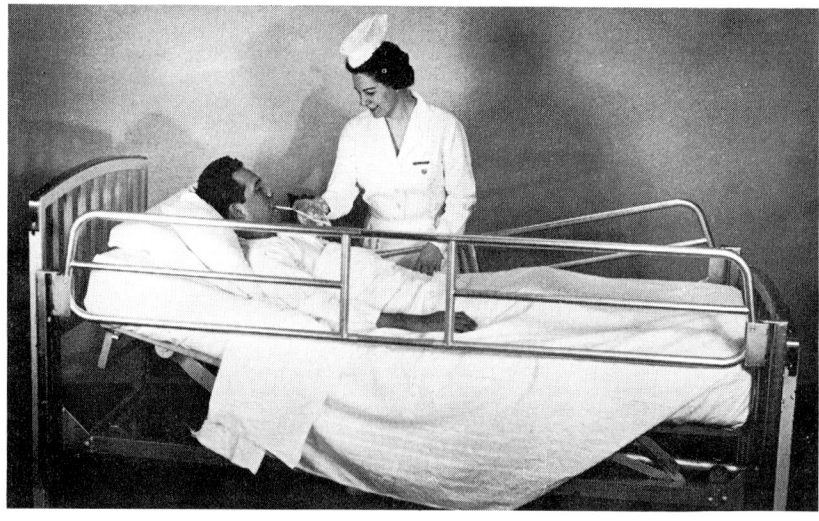

Fig. 9-3. The patient is given an in-between-meal drink to increase his fluid intake.

5. Patients with drainage from the body (such as those with drainage tubes connected to bottles)
6. Patients with persistent vomiting or diarrhea
7. Patients who are bleeding
8. Patients losing fluid from denuded areas on the body such as draining bedsores or burns
9. Patients who appear to be in fluid imbalance
10. Patients who depend on others for drinking and/or bathroom assisting

SIGNS OF EXTREME FLUID LOSS

Patients who are in a state of fluid imbalance (that is, who are losing more fluid than they are taking in) are said to be dehydrated. Signs of dehydration (excessive loss of water from the body tissues) include the following:

1. Dry mouth
2. Reddened, dry tongue, which is sometimes covered with dark brown, thick, dried secretions called sordes
3. Dry and cracked lips
4. Dark yellow-brown and concentrated urine
5. Loose and dry skin that retains a pinch mark for a few minutes because skin elasticity is lost
6. Confusion, disorientation, unconsciousness, and death in extreme dehydration

SUMMARY

Fluid balance is essential in the body if activities of living are to be carried out effectively. The amount of fluid the patient needs is determined by studying the amount he is losing. Since the doctor knows how the patient's body is functioning and what it needs, he prescribes the amount of fluid the patient should receive. The doctor will order a daily measurement and recording of intake and output for those patients he wants to observe to determine their fluid needs.

The patient whose intake and output are being recorded should be informed of this and told what it means and how it is to be done. A sign should be placed on his bed. In this way all personnel caring for him will be aware (either by the patient or the sign) of the need to record the intake and output.

If the intake and output are not recorded accurately, serious errors in the patient's treatment may occur. In order to avoid this, the doctor may order daily determinations of the patient's weight to validate the intake and output reports. Daily weights must be checked at the same time each day and under the same conditions if they are to be accurate. Patients are usually weighed each morning about 7 A.M., before breakfast and before their daily bowel movement, but after voiding.

DISCUSSION QUESTIONS

1 Observe the patients assigned to you carefully for signs of edema in the feet and legs. Discuss these patients with the nurse in relation to the effect, if any, this edema has on their fluid intake.
2 How many of your patients must have their intake and output recorded? Discuss this with the patient's doctor in relation to the value of the accuracy of these recordings.
3 When do you record intake on the record? Is this the best time to record it?
4 Do any of the patients chart their own intake and output measurements and recordings? Who taught them how to do it? If you did, how did you teach them?
5 How do you encourage the patient to take as much fluid as he possibly can?
6 When is fresh water distributed on your hospital unit? How do you avoid getting the patients' water pitchers mixed up when you are refilling them?
7 Does the dietary department wash the patients' pitchers and glasses? If not, who does? Why?
8 How are your patients given fluids if they are unable to swallow?
9 Check the mouth of each of your patients. How many signs of dehydration did you find?
10 What facilities should you provide for the patient who is receiving diuretics? Why?

VOCABULARY

dehydration Insufficient water content in the cells. Fluid imbalance exists when fluid loss is greater than fluid intake. Clues to this condition might be dry, loose skin, dry mouth, reddened tongue, and dark yellowish-brown urine.

digitalis A drug given primarily to slow and strengthen the heartbeat. Because it strengthens the heart and therefore causes the circulation of the blood around the body to be improved, it will also increase the urinary output.

diuretic A drug to stimulate the kidneys to take more water out of the blood. This excess water is excreted as urine; therefore a diuretic would increase the urinary output.

edema Swelling due to waterlogged body cells.

fluid balance The condition in which the patient's body is adequately hydrated (has an adequate amount of fluid). Fluid intake and fluid output are balanced.

heart failure A condition in which the heart fails to do its job of pumping the blood around the body. Stagnation of blood occurs in the body's lowest part (the feet). As the stagnation continues, the blood vessels become so congested that fluid leaks out of them into the body tissues and edema occurs. Diuretics and digitalis are the drugs frequently used for treatment.

Hydrodiuril A diuretic.

intake Fluid taken into the body. The amount must be recorded on the intake record after the patient has drunk the fluid, received it through a tube, or received it by an intravenous infusion. All fluids taken into the body are measured and recorded. The average need is approximately 3,000 ml.

milliliter (ml.), cubic centimeter (c.c.) A unit of liquid measure. Approximately 15 drops = 1 ml. There are approximately 30 ml. in 1 ounce.

output All fluids lost from the body through urine, perspiration, diarrhea, drainage, vomiting, etc. The average patient with a normal temperature loses about 2,500 ml. of fluid on a cool day.

serum Watery portion of the blood containing foodstuffs, water, and the waste materials from the cells.

uremia Failure of the kidneys to remove the waste of food used in the cells from the blood. Urea (one of the waste materials) is retained in the bloodstream.

void Excrete urine from the bladder to the outside of the body.

SOURCE OF ADDITIONAL INFORMATION

1 Pamphlet: The artificial kidney, Public Health Service Publication No. 1409; for sale by the Superintendent of Documents, United States Government Printing Office, Washington, D. C. 20402; price, 15 cents. (*Cartoons illustrate how the kidney and the artificial kidney work.*)

10/Meeting the patient's need for cleanliness and movement—complete, partial, and out-of-bed baths

STUDY QUESTIONS

1. Why is the patient bathed daily?
2. What are the normal arm and leg movements?
3. What happens to an arm or leg that the patient does not move because of pain or paralysis?
4. What are the four areas of the body that require special attention during the bath?
5. How do you massage the patient's back?
6. How do you change the bed linen if the patient is unable to get out of bed?
7. How often should mouth care be given?
8. What kind of patient observations do you make while giving the bath?
9. How many different kinds of baths could a patient receive?
10. How does the nurse determine how the patient is to be bathed?
11. Can a patient determine the kind of bath he would like to receive? If not, why not?
12. How does a complete bed bath differ from a partial bed bath?
13. How do you assist a patient into the bathtub?
14. What is a bath stretcher? For what kind of patient is it used?
15. What is the best time to give the patient his bath?

WHY BATHE THE PATIENT

The patient likes to have a bath. It makes him feel better. Even more significant, however, is the fact that the bath may help him get well. It is difficult for us to think of the bath in a therapeutic way (as part of the patient's treatment), since we usually think of the bath as a means of removing dirt and body odors—and the patient certainly does not get dirty. Although the latter is true, the patient needs the bath even more than we do.

Let us think for a moment what happens during a bath. The skin is lathered with soap and water, rinsed, and dried. This process removes dirt and also removes body odors by removing the bacteria (which cause the odors) from the skin. During this process of washing (rubbing the skin with an antiseptic solution called soap), the circulation is stimulated and the blood supply is increased. Furthermore, in order to reach and wash all parts of the body, the patient's body and limbs are moved. In the process, pressure is relieved, blood flow is reestablished, and the patient's limbs go through all the movements necessary to help him live comfortably.

If you have ever gone on a long trip by automobile or train, you know how stiff, how swollen, and how numb your feet become from inactivity. The patient will have these problems too if he lies still for long periods. Notice the pain a patient has in his arm and the difficulty he has in moving it after it has been immobilized (splinted) on an arm board for 12 to 24 hours while he was receiving an intravenous infusion. If the patient lies still (inactive) for periods longer than 24 to 48 hours, he will develop even more difficulty. Since the muscles that bend the body are stronger than those that straighten it, the patient who does not use his body constantly will develop bent limbs (flexed limbs) and will lose the ability to straighten them. This condition is called a contracture. The bent, flexed or contracted arm is a fixed arm and is of little or no use to the patient in carrying on his daily living activities.

The purposes of giving the patient a bath therefore are as follows:
1. To reduce bacteria on the body
2. To stimulate circulation of the blood and thus prevent pressure sores
3. To maintain normal body movement and thus prevent contractures and deformities

NORMAL BODY MOVEMENT

Before we discuss bathing the patient, it is essential to know what normal limb movement is. You can learn this by observing the range of movement in your own body.

Stand up. Prepare to explore all the possible movements of your shoulder. Since the shoulder is a *ball-and-socket* joint, it is possible to move your arms about to make a full circle. Try it. Now try the following:
1. Hold one of your arms up straight over your head.
2. Bring it down to your side.
3. Bring it across your chest, being sure to move the shoulder.
4. Extend it away from your chest as far as possible, as if you were trying to touch your back (keep elbow straight).

Since the hip is also a *ball-and-socket* joint, the legs can also be moved about in a full circle. Try to do the following movements:
1. Lie flat on your back.
2. Bring one of your legs up perpendicular to the body, and then lay it down flat on the floor.
3. Bend one of your knees and swing it across the other knee, which is flat on the floor.
4. Then swing the bent knee as far as possible to the other side.

Now let us look at the knee and elbow. These are both *hinge* joints and therefore have only two motions: bending and straightening. The fingers and toes are also hinge joints. Try the following:
1. Touch one of your shoulders with the fingertips of one hand and then straighten your arm.
2. Bend and straighten one of your knees.
3. Bend and straighten a finger and a toe.

The wrist and ankle are *sliding* joints. They do not have the circular movement of the ball-and-socket joint, but they have more movement than the hinge joint. Try the following:
1. Bend your wrist back and forth and then rotate it from side to side.
2. Bend your ankle back and forth and then rotate it from side to side.

All these limb movements are necessary for comfortable living. Try to do the following movements:
1. Bend the elbow of your right arm, bring your arm across your chest, bend your wrist down, and bend your fingers into your palms. Now try to make the movements necessary to feed yourself, to comb your hair, and to cut your meat.

This is the deformed position a paralyzed arm will stiffen into if it is permitted to lie still.
2. Bend your knee and bend your foot, bringing your heel as close to the calf

of your leg as possible. Now try to walk.

This is the position of the contracted knee and dropped foot that are common complications of the paralyzed leg.

The patient's condition does not remain the same. If we do not work hard to maintain the normal hand and leg movements (the normal range of motion of the arm and leg), the patient's condition will worsen. He may develop deformities and contractures such as a fixed shoulder or hip, a bent knee or elbow, a dropped wrist or foot, and bent toes and fingers.

THE COMPLETE BED BATH

Let us think about how we take a bath. Can we take a bath with our clothes on? Of course not, so we must remember to take off the patient's clothing before we bathe him. Do we want privacy when we are taking a bath? Well, so does the patient. Keep him covered when he is being bathed in bed. Do not take all the covers off and leave him exposed before the other patients and before any doctor or nurse who may walk into the area to give medicine or a treatment. Do we leave the bathroom door wide open while we are bathing, or do we close or lock it for privacy? Do this for the patient, too. If he is in a private room, close the door. If he is in one of the ward areas or in a semiprivate room, screen his bed carefully.

Upon receiving an assignment to bathe a patient, collect all the equipment and linen needed and take it to his bedside. The bathing equipment includes a basin of warm water, soap, back rub lotion or alcohol, and toothbrushing equipment (cup and emesis basin). Since the hospital gives each new patient a set of disposable toilet articles and bathing equipment, these items will be at the patient's bedside in his stand. The linen and clothing needed include bedclothes (sheets, spread, and pillowcases), towels, a bath blanket to cover him during the bath, and gown or pajamas. Take these to the patient's bedside on a cart, and do not forget to take along the laundry hamper.

As soon as we reach the patient's bedside with the linen, we must tell him what we are going to do and ask him if he would like a bedpan or urinal before we start. All of us need to go to the toilet soon after awakening, so this offer of a bedpan or urinal is usually accepted, and it permits the patient to be comfortable (free from the urgency to void or to move his bowels) during the bath. It also permits us to proceed without interruption.

Close any open windows and then get the patient ready for his bed bath. This bed bath is to be given as the nurse prescribes it and not as the patient wants it done. Strip the bed of all unnecessary linen, including the top sheet, spread, and blanket, and cover the patient with the bath blanket.

Fold the sheet, spread, and blanket in half lengthwise, then in half again, thus folding them in quarters widthwise, lift them off the bed by grasping them in the middle and folding them in half lengthwise, and place them over a chair if they are to be used in remaking the bed. If the linen is not to be reused, remove it from the bed as in making an unoccupied bed.

Now think about the parts of the body that need special attention. Certain parts of our body will have unpleasant odors if not kept clean.

Mouth care

The mouth is the dirtiest part of the body from the point of view of bacteria present there. You all know how dangerous a human bite is. This is only because of the bacteria present in the mouth and the great danger of infection. Therefore one of the most important areas to clean is the patient's mouth. Cleaning the mouth removes food particles and lessens the number of bacteria there. Failure to clean the mouth permits bacteria to grow, and a severe mouth infection may develop. If the patient breathes through his mouth, as many patients do, the bacteria will be pulled down into the lungs with the air, and pneumonia may occur. The mouth is a freeway for germs to enter the body.

Remove the patient's gown or pajamas. Roll up the head of the bed (if the patient's condition permits) and get the patient's toothbrush and toothpaste. Then assist the patient to brush his teeth (Fig. 10-1). Give him a cup filled with warm water to rinse his mouth and an emesis basin in which to expectorate (spit). If the head of the bed cannot be raised, turn the patient's head to the side and follow the procedure just described. A side-lying position allows the mouth-rinsing water to run out the side of his mouth into the emesis basin.

If the patient is unable to brush his teeth, brush them for him. Give him the mouth-rinsing solution through a drinking tube if he is unable to take it from the cup. If the patient is unaware of his environment (unconscious), brush his teeth for him, and then rinse his mouth for him as follows: dip a tongue blade, around which a compress has been securely wrapped, into water or mouthwash, and swab the mouth out well (Fig. 10-2). Repeat the swabbing as often as necessary. Be sure the patient's head is turned to the side, since gravity will then permit excess water to flow out of the mouth. Remember, an unconscious patient cannot swallow.

If the patient has false teeth (dentures), ask him to remove them. Then take them to the sink and brush them thoroughly

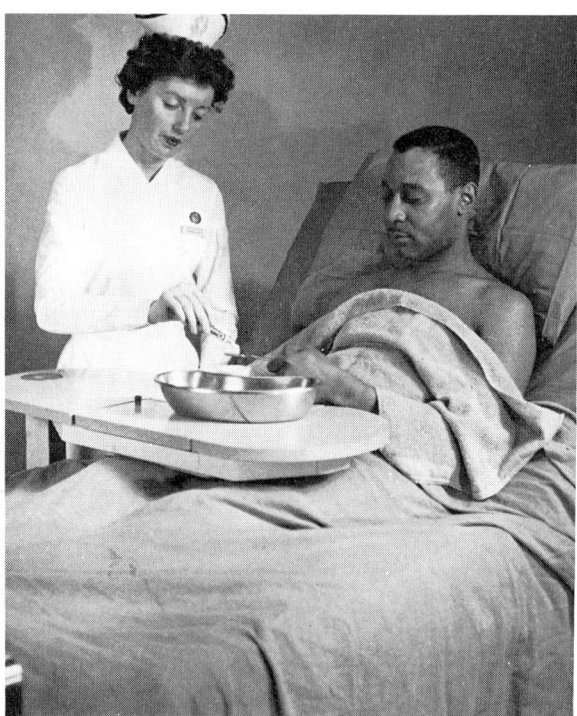

Fig. 10-1. The nurse demonstrating how to assist the bed patient get ready to brush his teeth.

under running water and over a basin of water. Why? Permit the patient to reinsert his dentures only after he has thoroughly rinsed out his mouth.

Frequency of mouth care. Before breakfast, the night nursing assistant helps the patient to clean his mouth. It is impossible to have a good appetite and eat with a dry, foul-smelling and foul-tasting mouth. As stated previously, mouth care, including brushing the teeth, is a very important part of the bath, but this is not enough. Mouth care must be given at least three times a day if the patient is not able to eat, if he is breathing through his mouth, or if he is unconscious. Poor mouth care or lack of mouth care can easily be recognized by the following: a dry tongue coated with a thick, brown, sticky covering (sordes), swollen glands below the ears, or a beefy red, dry tongue.

Body care

Wash the patient in the same manner as you do yourself. Wash the area around his eyes first. (Do not use soap on the washcloth when washing this area. Why?) Then proceed to wash his face, ears, and neck. Wash each part with soapy water, rinse well, and dry thoroughly. Remember, the bath procedure massages the patient's body, keeping the muscles in good condition and keeping the blood circulating, as well as cleans the patient. Therefore use large circular motions, going up and down the entire area to be bathed.

In addition to the mouth, the other areas of the body that give rise to foul odors from

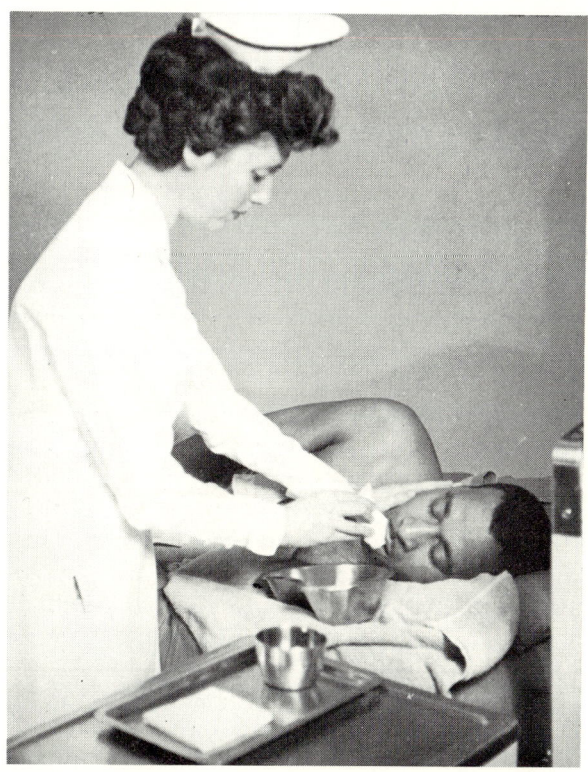

Fig. 10-2. The nurse demonstrating how to clean out the mouth of the unconscious patient who is in a side-lying position. Gravity helps fluid drain out of the patient's mouth in this position.

the growth of bacteria are those areas in which two skin surfaces contact each other, where darkness and moisture exist, allowing germs to grow. Not only will odors occur, but soreness, redness, irritation, and raw, oozing surfaces may result. The body areas in which skin surfaces are in contact are as follows:

1. Under the arm (armpits; axillary region)
2. Between the legs in the groin (genital region)

Washing the arms and axillary area. Wash the patient's arms thoroughly with warm soapy water, using long, massagelike motions up and down the arms from the wrist to the shoulder.

Give special attention to the axilla (armpit). Do not try to squeeze the washcloth into the small space between the body and the arm. Lift the patient's arm and place it on the bed beside his head. This makes the underside of the arm and the axilla easy to reach and wash, and it also helps the patient maintain his normal arm movements.

Rinse the arm well and dry it thoroughly. Grasp it at the wrist and take the patient's shoulder, elbow, wrist, and fingers through the range of motion exercises that were described earlier in this chapter. Then wash the patient's other arm. Take it through the range of motion also. Watch the patient carefully. Never force the arm to move. Stop the range of motion exercises as soon as the patient experiences pain or you feel any resistance.

Next, place the bath basin on the bed. Place the patient's hands in the basin, and wash them thoroughly. Then remove them from the basin and dry them. The patient will appreciate this, since he uses his hands to eat and to wipe his body after elimination without any good opportunities to wash them thoroughly. Clean and trim the patient's nails as required.

Wash the patient's chest and abdomen, including the umbilicus. Then wash his legs thoroughly just as you did his arms, paying special attention to the groin. Place the feet in the basin of water one at a time and wash them as you did the hands.

Now move the hips, knees, ankles, and toes through the range of motion exercises described earlier in this chapter. Watch the patient carefully. Stop if you feel any resistance or if the patient experiences pain.

Washing the genitalia. The penis of the male and the vulva of the female have openings in them that provide germs with a freeway into the body. Therefore the genitalia is the third area of the body requiring special attention during the bath.

If the patient is able to wash his own genitalia, move the bath basin, washcloth, and towels into an accessible position near the bed and leave the patient alone to afford him privacy. If the patient is unable to wash his own genitalia, wash the area thoroughly for him when he is of the same sex as you are. If the patient is of the opposite sex, request assistance from another nursing assistant who is of the same sex as the patient to accomplish this job. This makes it less embarrassing for the patient. (Male nursing assistants do not give such personal care as the bath to female patients.)

Completing the bed bath. By now the bath water is cold. Discard it in the sink and refill the basin. Proceed to the opposite side of the bed and prepare to turn the patient. Bring the arm on the side to which the patient is to be turned across his chest, then cross his legs in the direction in which he is being turned (Fig. 10-3). Grasp the patient firmly at the shoulder and hip and turn him toward you while you stand as close to the bed as possible (Fig. 10-4). This prevents any possibility of his falling out of bed. Guide the patient's uppermost hand to the bed frame and permit him to grasp it firmly to support himself.

When you are sure that the patient is comfortable and safely positioned, walk around to the opposite side of the bed and wash his back, including the area around the anus, using large up-and-down circular motions. Rinse the area well, and dry and massage the back with alcohol or, better still, some skin-protecting lotion. Sprinkle the lotion generously on your hands and massage the patient's back well to reestablish the blood flow that pressure has interrupted.

Start at the buttocks with your hands together in the middle of the back. Then move your hands up the middle of the back, swing them across the shoulders, with each hand going in an opposite direction, and bring them down the sides to meet again in the middle of the back at the buttocks. Repeat these massage motions until the redness and the pressure imprints of the sheets on the patient's back have disappeared. Sprinkle more massage lotion in the palm of your hand and massage the area

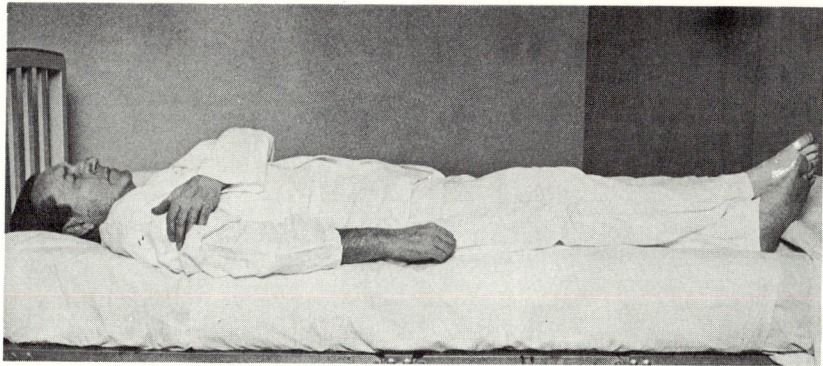

Fig. 10-3. The patient is positioned for a left-side turn: (1) the legs are crossed in the direction of the turn and (2) the arm on the side of the turn is brought across the patient's chest.

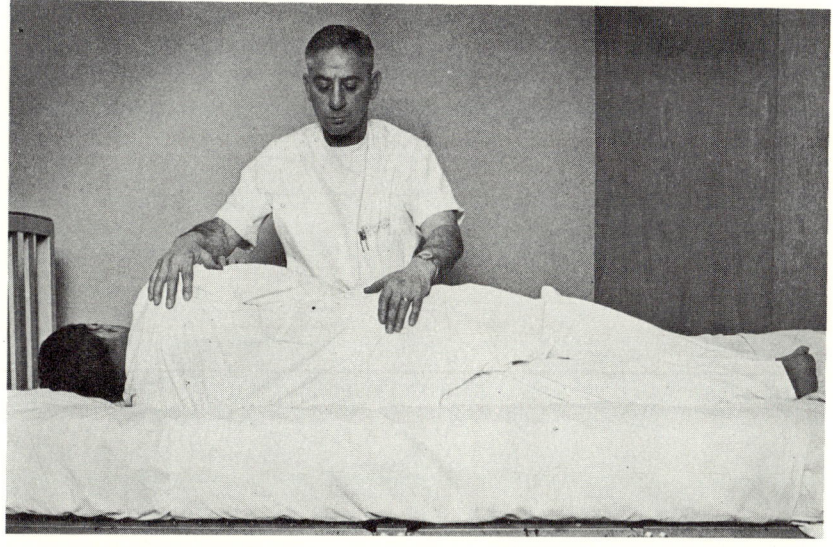

Fig. 10-4. The nursing assistant rolls the patient to his left side.

at the top of the patient's buttocks (Fig. 10-5). Then massage both buttock areas and both hips. These areas of the patient's body are subjected to the most pressure and are very likely to develop bed sores. Therefore they comprise the fourth area requiring special attention during the bath.

Keep the patient lying on his side. Loosen the sheets at the side of the bed and fold those to be removed in as close to the patient as possible in as small a lump as possible. Put the clean sheets on the same way you do on the unoccupied bed, tuck them in on your side of the bed, and fold the other half for the opposite side in as close to the patient as possible.

When you have completed making the first side of the bed, grasp the patient by the shoulder and hip and return him (over the lump of linen) to a back-lying position. Position him to turn by bringing the arm that will be under him after the turn across his chest and the leg that will be on top after the turn across and over the other one. Grasp the patient by the shoulder and hip and turn him toward you. Brace him securely as before (Fig. 10-4). Walk to the opposite side of the bed, remove the used linen, and discard it in the hamper. Pull the clean linen through (under the patient), pulling it tight and free of wrinkles, and tuck it under the mattress the same way as when making an unoccupied bed.

Return the patient to a back-lying position. Put on his gown or pajamas. The hospital gown (much like a coat put on backward) is usually put on patients who are seriously ill. Put your hand up in the sleeve (from the bottom of the sleeve). Then grasp the patient's hand at the palm and fingers and draw it into the sleeve as your hand comes out backward. Repeat this procedure with the patient's other hand. Tie the gown at the neck, and roll up the gown sleeves as desired by the patient.

Put the top sheet on the bed over the patient and remove the bath blanket. Tuck in the sheet as described previously, and put on the bed blanket and bedspread as you do in making the unoccupied bed. Put on clean pillowcases and position the pillows at the head of the bed. Lift the pa-

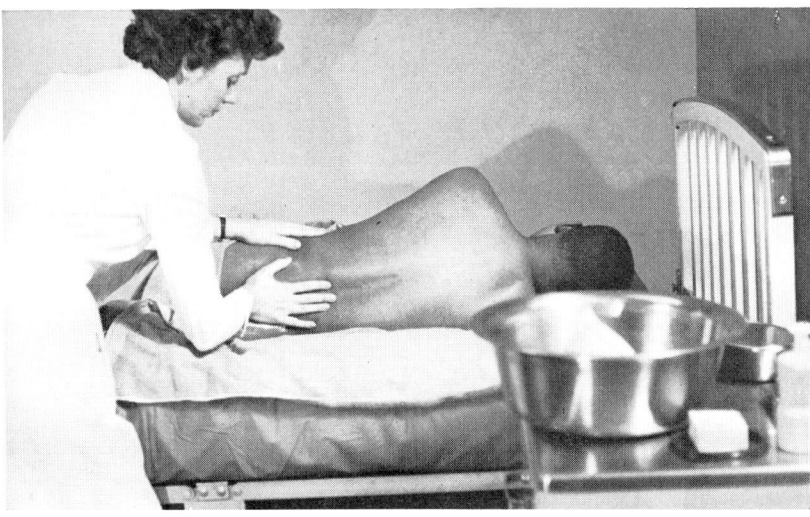

Fig. 10-5. The nurse demonstrating how to massage the patient's back with the heel of her hand in the area just above the buttocks. This is one of the areas in which bedsores are most likely to develop.

tient's shoulders and head with your left arm and hand while you position the pillows with your right hand.

If the patient wishes to be placed in a more comfortable position with the head of the bed elevated, crank up the head of the bed or push the electric button to raise it, depending on how the bed is operated.

When the patient is comfortable, collect all the equipment you used and wash it thoroughly. Return the washed personal care equipment to the patient's bedside stand. Disposable personal care equipment (basins, water pitcher, soap dish) is discarded only on discharge of the patient and then usually by giving it to the patient to take home with him.

Obtain a damp cloth and damp dust the bed, bedside stand, and chair. Position the call bell cord or intercommunication microphone within easy reach of the patient. Adjust the windows and window shades for the patient's comfort. Bring the patient fresh drinking water unless it has already been distributed by the ward maid. Wash your hands thoroughly in the patient's room or unit or in the first handwashing facility available.

After you leave the patient's unit, make notations on the following observations on your assignment sheet (the personal one with you) for reporting to the nurse or for charting at a later time:

1. What the patient said to you about his uncomfortable body or worried mind
2. What you saw (redness, swelling, etc.)
3. What you heard (noisy breathing, coughing, etc.)

Avoid writing your personal opinions. The doctor is the only one permitted to write such opinions on the chart.

Then proceed to bathe your next patient, repeating the procedure just described.

• • •

As soon as you have bathed your last patient, return ward equipment and laundry cart to their proper places. After the equipment is cleaned and returned to its proper place, record your observations on the patient's chart or in the book provided for communications to the nurse. Proceed to your next assignment.

When you have more than one patient

Collect enough linen on your work cart for your entire assignment, one setup for each patient assigned. Take work cart and laundry hamper with you as you give patient care, positioning them just outside your work area.

When the patient can help

Remember, our job is to help the patient get well. Know how much the patient is able to do for himself and encourage him to do those self-care activities.

When the patient cannot help

Even though the patient may look well, he may not be able to do any self-care activities. This is particularly true of a patient with a coronary thrombosis. This patient may want to bathe himself. He may feel like a big baby with you bathing him, and he may insist on doing it himself. The nurse will tell you what care each patient is to be given, how it is to be done, and whether or not the patient can get out of bed. The patient does not know what his medical and nursing care should be. He does not know what his sick body is able to do. He only knows what he does not want, and he really does not want any part of the hospital or his illness. Therefore nursing care is prescribed by the nurse, not the patient.

Patient exercises

Although we have discussed at great length the need for arm and leg exercises for the patient, I want to stress here that these should be given only on the nurse's direction. It is true that they are essential to maintain the arm and leg movements the patient has. However, a patient may have such severe heart disease that his heart is barely able to pump enough blood around for his body needs when he is at complete rest. In such a patient, the exercises would keep the arms and legs in good condition, but they *could* kill the patient by overtaxing his heart.

THE PARTIAL BED BATH

Sometimes the nurse may prescribe a partial bed bath for the patient instead of the complete bed bath. The reasons for giving the patient a partial bed bath rather than a complete one may include the following:

1. There may be insufficient personnel on the ward to give each bed patient a complete bed bath each day. Therefore the patient may receive a complete bed bath one day, a partial bed bath the second, a complete bed bath the third, and so on.
2. The patient's skin may be quite dry, and daily baths would further rob the skin of the remaining body oils and increase its dryness. This is especially true in older patients.
3. The patient's energy may have to be conserved. The patient may have such severe heart or lung disease that he is unable to tolerate any extra activity. Bathing and moving him may cause an extra strain on his heart or lungs, which would increase his breathing difficulty and pain and discomfort. Therefore minimal bathing with maximum conservation of patient energy is the rule.
4. The patient may have improved to the point that he is able to do some of his self-care activities.

The partial bed bath is given in much the same way as the complete bed bath, and the same equipment is used. However, there are these two basic differences:

1. In the complete bed bath the entire body of the patient is washed, whereas in the partial bed bath only those parts are washed that will cause illness, odor, or discomfort if they are neglected.
2. In the complete bed bath all of the patient's bedclothes and the bed linen are changed, whereas in the partial bath only soiled linen is changed.

Giving the patient a partial bed bath

The bathing equipment (wash basin, emesis basin, mouthwash, massage lotion, or alcohol and soap) is found in the patient's stand. Check to see what bed linen needs changing and then get the required bed linen and bring it to the bedside.

Prepare the patient for the bath. Since the bed linen is not to be changed, it may be sufficient to fanfold the top linen to the foot of the bed while you cover the patient with a bath blanket at the same time. The patient's pajamas (or gown) are then removed, and the bath is begun. Bathe only those parts of the patient's body that will have an unfavorable effect on his illness or increase his discomfort if they are not bathed. These parts are as follows:

1. Mouth
2. Eyes and face
3. Hands
4. Underarms and genitalia
5. Back

After the bath is completed, massage the patient's back. Then remake the bed by pulling tight all the linen in the foundation of the bed (bed covers under the patient). Change all soiled linen. Then put on the patient's gown or pajamas, and pull the top covers into place as the bath blanket is removed. Straighten the top covers, remake the corners as necessary, and clean the patient's unit (damp dust) as described previously.

OUT-OF-BED BATH
Bathing the patient in the bathroom

As soon as the patient has sufficient physical strength to be out of bed and to bathe in the usual way in the bathroom, the doctor will prescribe on his order sheet that the patient is to do so. Since the doctor is the only one who knows the condition of the patient's body (its strength and weakness), he is the only one who can say that the patient is strong enough to resume this out-of-bed bathing safely.

If the patient has regained sufficient strength to be out of bed and resume the care of his own body, he may go to the bathroom and bathe at the sink. However, you should provide him with linen and towels as needed, and you should prepare the bathroom for him by closing the windows and turning up the heat. If the doctor thinks that the patient is able to resume bathing in the bathtub or shower, he will write this on the order sheet. In such an instance, you should instruct the patient how the bathroom fixtures work so that he will not burn himself. Stress also the safety factors about getting in and out of the bathtub and shower carefully, so that he will not slip and fall. Stress also that he is to use water that is not so hot that it could cause weakness or burn him. Show the patient the call bell in the bathroom whereby he can summon aid if he needs it.

Usually, however, the patient who can have a bath in the tub or shower cannot take it without assistance. The patient who is in the hospital with an acute illness for a short time and then recovers will probably receive bed baths and then graduate to self-bathing at the bathroom sink. The patient who is chronically ill and, because of this, in the hospital for a long period of time will probably be the one who will be bathed by you in the tub or shower.

Tub bath. The nurse will probably assign you to give a tub bath to the extended care facility patient or to the patient who has been in the hospital for a long period of time and who is recovering from a stroke (hemiplegia). This patient will be paralyzed on one side and will be unable to give himself a tub bath.

The nurse may also assign you to give a tub bath to a patient with multiple sclerosis, or some other chronic disease, who is becoming progressively more helpless. This patient may be perspiring a great deal, may be incontinent, and may have some skin irritations. The patients you bathe in the tub may have any one of a number of different diseases or disorders. However, none of them will be able to get into the tub or shower by himself, and each will need the soaking in the water to clean the skin and prevent further skin irritations. The preparation of the bathroom for tub bathing the patient would include:

1. Closing the bathroom windows
2. Turning up the heat in the bathroom
3. Hanging an "in use" sign on the ward bathroom to prevent personnel from opening doors and invading the privacy of the patient and permitting drafts to blow in on him
4. Collecting a clean set of clothing and towels for the patient
5. Placing a laundry hamper in a convenient spot to receive soiled clothing and towels

After these preparations are completed, take a wheelchair to the bedside and assist the patient out of the bed into the wheelchair. Then collect his personal toilet articles, such as soap, toothbrush and toothpaste, razor, etc., and take these with the patient into the bathroom. Permit the patient to brush his teeth at the bathroom sink while you are running the water for his bath. Half fill the bathtub with warm water, approximately 100° to 105° F. (The water should feel warm and comfortable when both hands are completely immersed in it.) If necessary, test the temperature of the water with a bath thermometer to avoid getting water hot enough to burn the patient.

When the tub is ready and the patient has finished brushing his teeth, take him to the tub area. Close the bathroom door or screen the tub area. Help the patient to undress. Push the wheelchair as close to the side or back of the tub as possible and brake the chair. Lift the patient's legs over the side of the tub and into the water. Assist the patient into the tub by lifting and supporting his body at the level of his arms. Guide the patient's hands to grasp the sides of the tub (one hand on each side) so that he can support himself during the move from the wheelchair into the tub.

Encourage the patient to wash himself. Assist him by washing those parts of his body he is unable to reach. Do not waste time. The water will cool quickly, and it is unsafe to add water by turning on the water faucets while the patient is in the tub, since the hot water may burn him.

Some patients may complain that the water is too cool. This is especially true of the older patient with circulatory disturbances (poor blood flow), who has some loss of feeling or sensation. In fact, these patients have such loss of feeling that they will burn themselve with hot water without even knowing they are burned until they see the blister. Therefore you cannot take the patient's word for the correctness of the water temperature. You must be sure that it is the safe temperature yourself.

At home we run the water and jump into the tub. If the water is too hot, we jump right out again fast. However, the patient cannot jump into and out of the tub. If he could, he would not need you to help him with the bath. Therefore if you assist the patient into a tub of water that is too hot, he will be burned before you can get him out.

After the patient's body is completely washed, let the water run out of the tub, and dry the upper part of the body. Position the patient's hands on either side of the tub. Then grasp the patient below the arms and assist him while he helps himself to sit on the back or side of the tub. Dry the rest of his body thoroughly. Support him (at the back) while he repositions his hands on the arm supports of the wheelchair. Be sure the wheelchair is braked. Assist the patient to slide backward off the tub into the wheelchair. Lift his legs out of the tub.

Finish drying the patient and help him dress. Discard soiled clothing and towels in the laundry hamper. Scour and rinse the tub. Mop up any water on the floor. Collect the patient's personal articles and return them with the patient to his room.

In order to give the patient a bath in the tub safely (safe for the patient and safe for you), he must be able to lower himself into the tub and raise himself out of the tub with your assistance. If he cannot do this but must be lifted in and out of the tub, a lifting device such as the mechanical lift must be used to avoid the back injury you will get from the awkward lifting required and the strain that this places on your back.

A combination of a mechanical lift—a transport chair and a relaxing massaging bath—is found in the Century Tub. Here, the only lifting or patient transfer required is from bed to transport chair. The Century Tub lift then attaches to the chair and hoists it into and out of the tub. Washing the patient is also simplified and more therapeutic. The friction is accomplished by whirlpool water currents rather than by hand motions. Nursing home patients enjoy the ease of transfer and the massaging water currents.

Shower bath. Perhaps the patient who is unable to assist himself in and out of the tub because of paralyzed or weak muscles might be bathed more effectively in the shower (if the Century Tub is not available).

The bathroom is prepared for showering a patient in the same way as for tub bathing, except that the shower is turned on at the desired temperature (warm to the arms and 100° to 105° F.) and left running before you go for the patient. The patient is assisted out of the bed into the shower chair (rustproof chair) and taken, with his personal toilet articles, to the shower room.

The patient brushes his teeth and then undresses (with your assistance). Just before he is pushed into the shower in the shower chair, test the running water again. If the temperature remains correct (as tested by a thermometer or your hands), push the patient under the shower and bathe him. If the patient is unable to bathe himself, you should change your uniform to the clothing supplied by the hospital (bathing suit), which will enable you to assist the patient in the shower. When the shower is completed, dry the patient, dress him, and return him to his room, along with his personal toilet articles.

Bath stretcher. Some patients are unable to maintain themselves in a sitting position because of paralyzed back and abdominal muscles. They are unable to sit in the bathtub or the shower, and yet they need the soaking in water because of the irritation to the skin caused by incontinence, perspiration, and pressure. These patients may be bathed in running water in a lying-down position on a bath stretcher (Fig. 10-6) (rather like taking a shower while lying down).

Prepare the bathroom as for a tub bath. Close the windows and turn up the heat. Then take the bath stretcher to the bedside, and transfer the patient from the bed to the stretcher. Cover him with a bath blanket and take him to the bathroom. Regulate the bath spray to warm. Remove the bath blanket, and bathe the patient in much the same manner as in the shower, except that he is now lying down rather than sitting or standing and the spray is a movable one in your hand rather than the fixed shower head. When the bath is completed, turn off the water, dry the patient, cover him with a bath blanket, and return him to his bed. The patient is moved from the stretcher to a bath blanket on the bed. This bath blanket absorbs any moisture under the patient and completes drying him. It also avoids getting the freshly made bed wet.

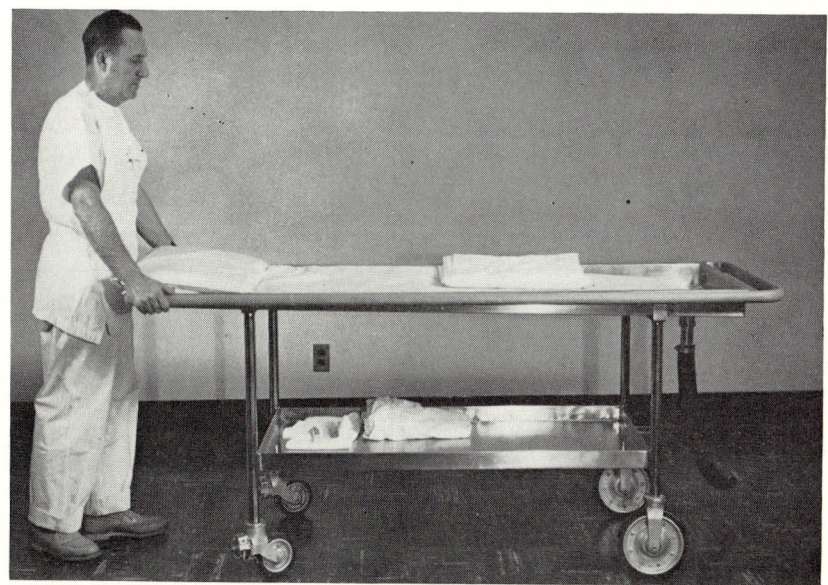

Fig. 10-6. The nursing assistant is going for the patient with the bath stretcher. Note the linen on the bottom of the stretcher.

Time of out-of-bed bath

The best time to bathe the patient depends on the patient's needs. If the patient gets a tub bath, he needs a warm, draft-free, private bathroom. This might be easier to obtain in the afternoon than in the morning. If the patient is in a busy rehabilitation program starting with occupational therapy at 8 A.M. and ending with physical therapy at 3 P.M., he might be freer to take and enjoy a bath in the evening after supper. If the patient has been lying in bed for the past 24 hours, he probably needs a bath and a back massage early in the morning.

Some nursing assistants feel that all baths are to be given before 10 A.M., but you can easily see that a routine of this sort ignores the patient and his needs. Therefore if you work in a ward in which the patients spend most of their 24 hours in bed, you may give the baths in the morning. If, on the other hand, you work in the rehabilitation ward, you may give mostly tub baths and showers in the evening after supper. If you work in a psychiatric ward where the patients are relearning how to live effectively, you may model the patient's day after one of your own (since we are models for the patients), and you may give the patient his tub bath or shower just before bedtime. The patient and his need determine the plan of care.

OBSERVATION OF THE PATIENT'S BODY DURING THE BATH

Whether the patient is bathed in bed, in the shower, or in the tub, you must observe changes in his body (swellings, rashes, bruises, irritations, etc.) as well as changes in his mind (discouragement, depression, disgust, hope, elation, etc.) and report these observations to the nurse or team leader. Remember, when the nurse assigns you to use your hands and your friendliness to care for the patient's body and his mind, she also expects you to use your eyes and ears to gather clues for her concerning the patient's progress.

SUMMARY

There is no set way of giving a bath to all patients, since each patient's needs determine the method of the bath. When the patient does not have the body strength to tolerate a complete bed bath, he may receive only a partial one (for example, the patient with a severe heart attack). However, the role of the hospital is to help the patient resume normal living insofar as he is able. Therefore when the doctor feels that the patient is able to resume the usual methods of bathing, the patient will be permitted to bathe himself in the bathroom.

Some patients who are in the hospital for long periods may have a tendency to develop skin irritation from pressure, perspiration, and incontinence; these patients may be bathed in the tub, in the shower, or on the bath stretcher, depending on their degree of dependence.

DISCUSSION QUESTIONS

1. In your patient care today, how were all the baths you gave similar? How were they different?
2. Did you observe any patients with deformities (contractures) of the arm and leg from too little movement? If so, what do you plan to do about it?
3. Which patients on your unit are receiving nothing by mouth? Check their mouths.
4. To which patients on your unit can you give arm and leg exercises during the bath? Are there any patients on your unit who must avoid these exercises?
5. Why do mouth and body odors occur? How can they be avoided?
6. What observations did you make about your patient today? Of what value were these observations to the nurse? To the doctor?
7. Which patients on your unit can do some of their own personal care activities during the bath? Do they want to do it? If not, why not?
8. *Discuss the comment:* I give all my patients the same care.
9. Should all patients get a complete bed bath every day?
10. Should all patients get a very vigorous back rub?

11 Which patients on your unit should not get a vigorous back rub? Which patients on your ward should get a vigorous back rub?
12 Why is it up to the doctor to decide whether the patient should stay in bed or get out of bed?
13 Who determines whether or not the patient should be bathed in bed or in the bathtub? Why?
14 Demonstrate how to put a patient in the bathtub from a wheelchair.
15 Who determines the temperature of the shower —you or the patient?
16 When are the baths given on your unit? Is this the best time for the staff or the patients? Explain.

SOURCES OF ADDITIONAL INFORMATION

1 Pamphlet: Strike back at stroke; may be obtained from local heart association. *(Gives a visualization of the bed exercises described for the patient during his bath.)*
2 Phibbs, Brendan: The human heart, ed. 2, St. Louis, 1971, The C. V. Mosby Co. *(The layman's guide to heart disease.)*
3 Films: Bed care series: (a) Bedbath, (b) Mouthcare (self-care and helpless patient), and (c) Incontinent patient; may be obtained from Encyclopaedia Britannica, 425 N. Michigan Ave., Chicago, Ill. 60611. *(Films are 8 minutes long— 8 mm. individual or group teaching visual aids.)*

11/Caring for the patient's toilet needs

STUDY QUESTIONS

1. How does the patient know he needs to defecate?
2. What is involved in holding the feces in the rectum until toilet facilities are obtained?
3. What is involved in a child's toilet training?
4. Is peristalsis (contractions of the muscles in the intestines) under the control of the will (voluntary)? Is this desirable or undesirable?
5. What is the involuntary nervous system and what are its functions?
6. What is the voluntary nervous system and what are its functions?
7. What is the most desirable position for defecating?
8. How can you help the patient meet his toilet needs?
9. How can you put a helpless patient on the bedpan?
10. Why is the seriously ill cardiac patient sometimes permitted to get out of bed to use a commode?
11. Can an incontinent patient be helped to regain his continence? How?
12. Which is more difficult to control—the bowels or the bladder? Why?
13. How does the patient know that he needs to void?
14. Which patients may have increased voiding needs?
15. How can a bladder-training program be conducted?
16. How does the incontinent patient feel? Why?

The patient has two toilet needs: the need to excrete feces from the rectum and the need to excrete urine from the bladder.

THE PATIENT'S NEED TO DEFECATE

After water and foodstuffs are absorbed from the digested food, the remaining waste material, called feces, is pushed along the intestines by peristaltic waves until it reaches the end portion of the large intestine (the rectum), where it is stored. When the rectum is full, the stretched rectal wall activates a nerve in the autonomic nervous system, which takes the message to the brain that the rectum needs to be emptied. Immediately another nerve brings back the message to empty the bowel, and this nerve helps to do this by relaxing the anal sphincter muscle at the end of the rectum and by stimulating the muscles of the intestines to propel the feces to the outside.

This happens automatically in much the same way that swallowing occurs. The nerves in the mouth send the message to the brain that the food is properly chewed and ready to be swallowed, and so swallowing occurs. In fact the entire functioning of the body, including getting the heart to beat, moving the lungs to bring in air, moving the feces along through the bowel, and stimulating the kidney to take waste material out of the blood, occurs automatically without our conscious efforts or control.

Bowel training

The automatic process of emptying the rectum, or defecation, occurs in infancy and early childhood, but it must be modified and brought under some control of the will as we grow up. The process of interrupting the automatic emptying of the rectum and having it empty at the time and place we want it to is called bowel training.

As the child becomes aware of his surroundings and his body needs, he is taught that the fullness in the rectum and its discomfort are not to be relieved immediately but are to be inhibited until the right facilities for moving the bowels are available.

Therefore the higher centers of the brain are brought into this process as the child learns to send a message from his brain to his anal muscle to hold tightly closed until he gets to the toilet. This is difficult to do because the anal muscle is trying to relax and the intestinal muscles are working hard to propel the feces from the body. But the pleasure and satisfaction the child derives from pleasing his parent and from staying clean overcome the discomfort of rectal pressures and the child acquires bowel control. The trained bowel sends the same urgent messages that it is full and needs to be emptied, but the brain sends down a stronger message to the anal muscle to remain tightly closed until toilet facilities are obtained with a minimum of delay.

The educated or trained bowel

When the proper facilities are obtained, the brain ceases to send down its strong message to hold the feces by tightening the anal muscle. Then the messages from the autonomic nervous system function to relax the anal muscle and to stimulate the peristaltic movements in the large bowel, and defecation occurs.

Nervous control of body functions

As mentioned previously, we have two nervous systems: one that functions automatically without control of the will (involuntary) and one that functions under the control of the will (voluntary).

Involuntary nervous system control. The involuntary or autonomic nervous system controls and regulates the activities occurring within our body, such as heartbeat, breathing, peristalsis, formation of urine, sweating, and temperature regulation. This automatic control of these vital processes of living leaves us free to work and play without the need to consciously keep our body working at keeping us alive.

It is a nerve from this system that takes a message to the brain that the rectum is full. It is also a nerve from this system that brings back the message to empty it. This occurs without any conscious control in infancy. Of course, as we grow from infancy to childhood, we are taught to control the bowels by interrupting automatic defecation and bringing it under some limited control of the will.

Voluntary nervous system control. The voluntary nervous system controls and regulates those activities in the body over which we have conscious control. Running, jumping, thinking, learning, feeling, talking, and moving, as well as retaining urine or feces until we find a toilet, are all activities regulated by the voluntary nervous system.

Toilet training helps us feel the bowel and bladder pressures, helps us learn what these pressures mean, and then helps us inhibit or block bowel and bladder emptying until the proper facilities are obtained with a minimum of delay.

Facilities for defecation

Since the sitting position permits gravity to assist the feces to move through the intestine and out of the body, it is the most desirable position for defecation. The individual should be as comfortable and as relaxed as possible. If he is uncomfortable or emotionally distressed (embarrassed, etc.), the autonomic nerves work to protect the body from the threat of discomfort or fear and cease to work on stimulating the peristalsis necessary for bowel movement. Then constipation and discomfort will occur.

The patient, until the time of his hospitalization, has been accustomed to caring for his own bowel needs. Now he must ask you for help. This is distressing. He feels embarrassed and ashamed about asking you for a bedpan or a bedside commode, and he feels worse about having you take the used bedpan away and clean it. He wishes that he could go to the bathroom himself, and he will every chance he gets. It makes no difference how much the doctor and nurse stress the need for him to stay in bed; he still sneaks off to the bathroom. Using the bedpan makes him feel like a child.

Think of yourself in the patient's situation and do for him what you would like done for yourself. Upon admission, instruct the patient how his toilet needs are to be met. If he is ambulatory, show him where the bathroom is located. If he is a bed patient, explain to him the use of the bedpan and urinal; also explain how he can summon you to get them for him. If the patient is a bed patient who is permitted to use the bedside commode, tell him about this. Then on the Kardex write out the plan for meeting the patient's toilet needs. It is very distressing to the patient to try to explain that he does not get the bedpan but that he can use the bedside commode, and it is downright discouraging if he has to do this explaining every time he needs to defecate.

Now remember all that we learned about the process of defecation. In the discussion on digestion in an earlier chapter we learned that eating frequently causes the contents of the bowel to move along faster and that the need to have a bowel movement occurs frequently after eating. We have just learned in this chapter that emptying the bowel occurs automatically and that a conscious effort to hold in the feces must be made in order to interrupt this process. This means that you will need to offer the patient a bedpan after meals. It also means that when a patient asks for a bedpan or for assistance in getting on a bedside commode, you must meet his request with a minimum of delay.

Remember, too, how you sit on the toilet seat in the privacy of the bathroom with perhaps a magazine or a book to help you relax. Provide these things for the patient too. If he receives a bedpan in bed, raise his bed to a comfortable sitting position, screen him well to give him all the privacy available, and do not rush him. Be sure he has an ample amount of toilet paper and that he is well propped up in bed so that there is no danger of his falling. If the bed has crib sides, pull them up into position to support the patient. When the patient signals you that he is finished, cover and remove the bedpan promptly. Return to the patient with a basin of water and permit him to wash his hands while you put the screens back in their proper place and the bed back in its original position (Fig. 7-14).

Assisting the patient with the bedpan

Some patients may be too weak to bend their knees and lift up their buttocks so that you can slip the bedpan in place under them (Fig. 11-1). In these instances, you can place the patient on the bedpan in the following way:

1. Roll the patient toward you and then move to the opposite side of the bed.
2. Place the bedpan in the correct position, tightly pressed against the patient's buttocks, and hold it there as you roll the patient back toward you and onto the bedpan (Fig. 11-2). (Be sure that a crib side is in place on the bed before you roll any patient away from you because he may roll out of bed.)

Adjust the bed so that the patient is raised to a sitting position. Screen him, place the call bell nearby, and leave him in privacy. Be sure that he has an adequate supply of toilet paper before you leave.

In removing the bedpan, steady it by holding it with one hand while with the other hand you roll the patient away from you (or toward you if there is no crib side) and off the bedpan. (The bedpan will tip and spill if it is not held steady.) Wipe the patient's buttocks area clean with

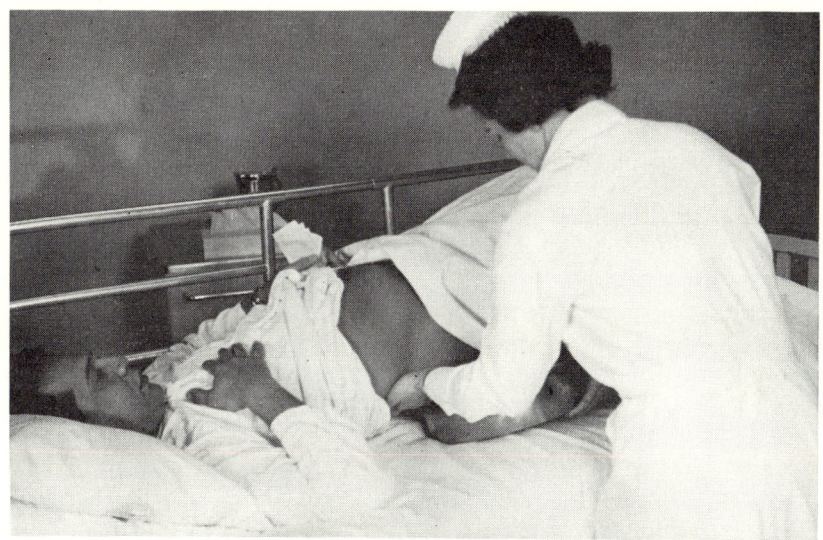

Fig. 11-1. The patient bends his knees and presses his feet firmly against the bed to lift up his buttocks in preparation for receiving a bedpan. The nurse helps to lift up the patient's back with one hand while she slips the bedpan into position under him with the other hand.

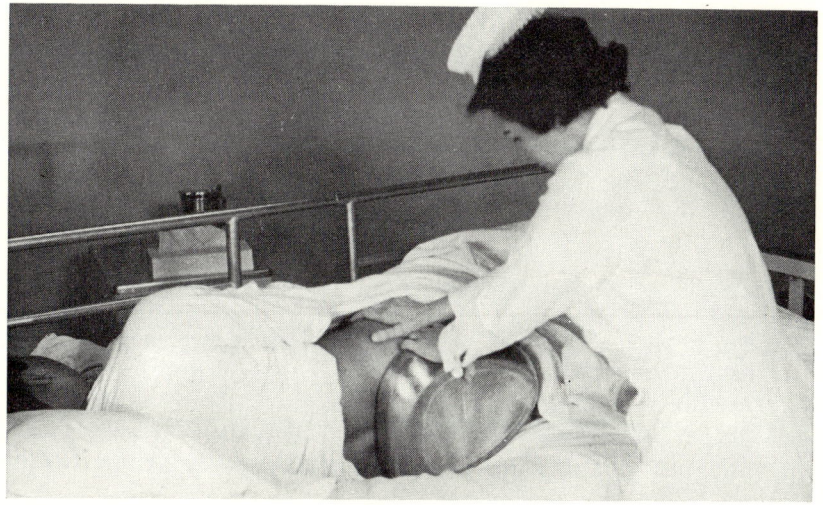

Fig. 11-2. The nurse assists the helpless patient to roll back onto the bedpan.

toilet paper, put the paper in the bedpan, remove the bedpan to a safe position near the bottom of the bed, and return the patient to the back-lying position. The patient may be quite embarrassed about his need for you to give him such personal care, so avoid any remarks about odor and any facial expressions that register disgust. Cover and remove the bedpan from the patient's unit, and then promptly empty and clean it in the utility room. Note any unusual odor, color, or consistency of the fecal material when you empty the bedpan. (This will be discussed more fully in the chapter on giving the patient an enema.)

Bedside commode

Many bed patients may be permitted to use a bedside commode once a day in order to decrease the physical effort involved in having a bowel movement. On the bedside commode, gravity helps the feces to move out of the body. In the lying position, strong muscular forces must be exerted to expel the feces. Therefore the doctor may permit a seriously ill cardiac patient the use of the bedside commode once daily because the patient is too ill to use the bedpan in bed.

The patient with lack of muscle control

The patient who has paralyzed arm and leg muscles or the patient with extreme muscle weakness from disease or from old age also has muscle weakness inside his body and in his intestines. Therefore we can expect the patient who is too weak to walk without assistance to be too weak to control his bowel movements without assistance. We can expect the patient who is unable to move his paralyzed arm and leg to also have trouble moving his bowels. We can also expect the patient who has difficulty knowing where he is or what is happening to him also to have difficulty in knowing what the pressure in his rectum means and how he must inhibit emptying of the bowel until he obtains the proper facilities.

In all these instances our job is simply that of retraining the patient's bowel.

Bowel retraining. Retraining the bowel may be done in the following way:

1. Place the patient on the toilet, bedside commode, or bedpan (which ever is permissible) after each meal and especially after breakfast.
2. Tell the patient that you are placing him on the toilet, commode, or bedpan and ask him to consciously try to have a bowel movement.
3. Do this each day at the same time.
4. Report the results to the nurse.
5. If the patient does not have a bowel movement, the nurse may stimulate the intestines to work by giving the patient a suppository each morning or by giving him prune juice the night before. Usually a suppository stimulates the intestines, and, aided by gravity, will help the patient have a bowel movement within 30 minutes.
6. When the patient has established a regular habit of having a bowel movement each morning after breakfast, the suppository may be eliminated and the habit will continue.
7. This bowel control may be accomplished even in patients who are unconscious. With these patients the method might be one of irrigating the rectum daily or every other day as ordered by the doctor. You will soon find that the patient will have bowel movements only at the time of irrigation.

THE PATIENT'S NEED TO VOID

On the average, approximately 1,200 ml. of blood pass through the kidneys each minute. The kidneys remove the waste material from the blood. This liquid waste, which amounts to approximately 1 ml. per minute, consists of waste material dumped into the blood by the cells (urea, uric acid, and creatinine) and any other substance in the blood that the body does not need. This means that excess amounts of water and electrolytes are removed from the blood by the kidneys in order to keep the body in a state of balance. Electrolytes will be discussed later. It is sufficient to say here that electrolytes are chemicals in the body that carry the positive and negative electrical charges essential to keep the heart beating, the brain working, and the nerves carrying their messages.

Each minute, the kidneys sends 1 ml. of liquid waste down the ureter to the bladder, where it is stored (Fig. 11-3). After 2 hours there are about 120 ml. or 4 ounces of urine in the bladder, and the bladder wall begins to stretch.

Emptying the bladder is controlled in much the same way as emptying the rectum. The stretched bladder wall sends a message to the brain by means of the involuntary nervous system that the bladder is stretched, and the brain sends back the message to empty it by way of the same system. Another nerve from this system also assists in emptying the bladder by relaxing the urinary sphincter muscle and by stimulating the bladder muscle to force the urine out. Like emptying the rectum, this occurs without awareness in the infant and small child. However, when bladder training is given, the child learns to understand what the fullness in the bladder means, and he learns how to send down a message from the brain to the bladder sphincter muscle to hold tightly closed until toilet facilities are obtained. Of course, toilet facilities are then obtained with maximum haste.

Facilities for voiding

As mentioned in the discussion on facilities for defecation, the patient needs privacy and a comfortable position. For the female patient, this would be a sitting position on the bedpan, on the bedside commode, or on the toilet seat in the bathroom. Female urinals that can be used by the patient in a lying position seem to be most inadequate, since leakage usually occurs around them. The leakage can be minimized if the head of the bed is elevated slightly. However, it is wise to place an absorbent pad or small rubber sheet covered by a towel under the female patient when she is using a urinal. A bedpan is much better, because it utilizes the sitting position that is the usual voiding position for the female.

For the male patient, the urinal can be used in the back-lying position, the side-lying position, and in the sitting or standing position.

However, it should be remembered that here, too, gravity helps the urine flow from the bladder to the outside, and for those patients who have difficulty voiding, success may be obtained if the standing position is used for the male or the sitting erect position is used for the female.

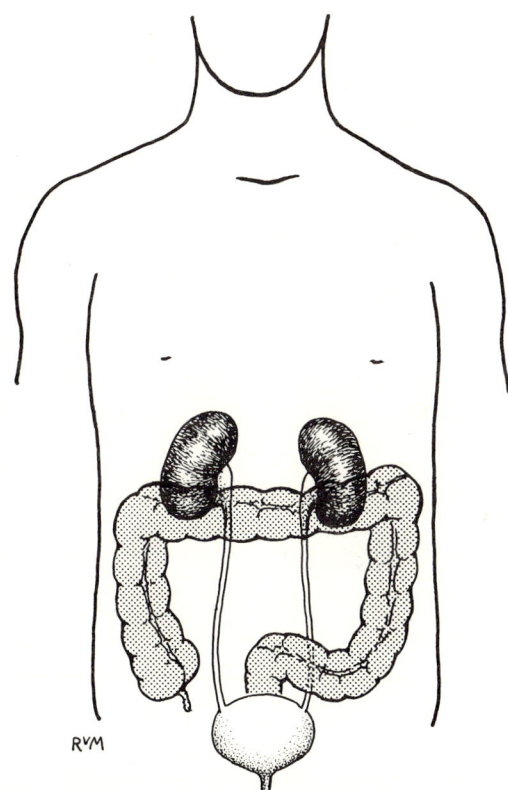

Fig. 11-3. Kidneys, ureters, and bladder. Note that the bladder is located just in front of the rectum.

Since the involuntary nervous system also works to relax the urinary sphincter muscle and to contract the bladder muscle to squeeze out the urine, the patient must be free of any tense, frightening, or embarrassing situations during voiding. If the patient is hurried, upset or embarrassed, the involuntary nervous system sets up its mechanism to protect the patient and forgets the voiding. Remember that since voiding is automatic, it takes willpower to inhibit it and that this inhibiting is possible only for a short time. Therefore plan to meet the patient's needs for voiding even before he asks. This can be done by developing a schedule for offering the patient voiding facilities. Such a schedule might consist of offering the patient a urinal or bedpan at the following times:

1. Upon his awakening (Remember that urine has been collecting in the bladder all night at the rate of 2 ounces per hour.)
2. Before meals
3. After meals
4. At his bedtime

A schedule of this sort permits the patient the security of knowing that his needs to void will be met and that he can drink water freely and take all the fluids on his meal tray without any fear of needing a urinal or bedpan and failing to get it. It also enables you to care for all the patients assigned to you without being constantly interrupted.

The patient with increased urinary output

Some patients may have doctor's orders for increased fluid intake (forced liquids). These patients should also have increased facilities for voiding. A plan to adequately meet this patient's needs would be to offer him a urinal each time you offer him fluids. Since an intake-output record is also ordered for such a patient, the time and the amount he voids will be recorded. After 2 days, a definite plan of *his* voiding needs can be obtained by studying his output record. These voiding times can then be written on the patient's nursing care plan on the Kardex. Then the urinal need be offered only at these times.

The patient who has received a diuretic (a drug to stimulate the kidneys to remove excess water from the blood) will also have increased voiding needs. If such a patient is ambulatory, move him as close to the bathroom as possible. If he is a bed patient, plan to offer him a urinal or bedpan every 2 hours. Since an intake and output record is also kept on this patient, the record of his output will give you an indication of his voiding needs for the next time he receives a diuretic. The patient may receive diuretics by mouth each day or by injection two or three times a week. Listen carefully in the team conference for a report on your patients and the medications they are receiving. Ask the nurse if any of your patients are receiving diuretics. Plan with the nurse to meet their voiding needs effectively.

The patient on continuous intravenous injections of fluid may also have increased needs for voiding. However, he may be so seriously ill that he will not be aware of bladder pressure, and he may void automatically in the bed unless you plan to offer him the urinal or bedpan at 2-hour intervals.

After the patient voids, always remove the urinal or bedpan promptly, take it to the utility room, empty it, and flush and sterilize it in the flusher provided. For the following reasons, do not permit a used urinal or bedpan to sit on the patient's bedside stand:

1. A strong unpleasant odor permeates the room and ruins the patient's appetite, which may be already poor.
2. Waste material in the urine settles and clings to the sides of the urinal or bedpan and is very difficult to remove.
3. Waste material is to be disposed of and should not be sitting in the patient's unit to be a source of em-

barrassment for patients and visitors.
4. A full urinal or bedpan will be spilled in the bed the next time the patient attempts to use it.

However, it should be removed primarily for the same reason that you and I would not eat our dinner in the bathroom. Remember, the patient's tray is placed on his bedside stand.

Cleaning urinals

Even when urinals are removed promptly and cleaned thoroughly, they have a tendency to develop a strong, unpleasant ammonia-like odor. This odor is easier to prevent than to correct. Prevention may be accomplished by establishing a regular time each week for thorough cleaning of all urinals. The hospital pharmacist will give you a preparation, together with directions for its use, which will dissolve urinary salts that collect in urinals. Soaking urinals in this preparation for the designated time, followed by a thorough washing in soapy water and adequate rinsing, will certainly keep the ward free of urine odors. One solution for soaking urinals that removes salts and odor is a 25% vinegar solution.

Bladder training

The bladder is not so easy to control as is the bowel. This is rather obvious when we consider that voiding occurs eight or nine times every 24 hours, whereas defecation may occur only once and, indeed, this is about the ratio of difficulty. The bladder is about nine times as difficult to control as is the bowel. If you have had any experience in helping a child learn bladder and bowel control, you already know this.

One method of achieving bladder control is to study the patient. Place an intake and output record on his bed and record all intake of fluids and all voiding. Every hour on the hour give the patient a glass of fluid and offer him a urinal or bedpan. Chart the results. Repeat this for 2 or 3 days. Study the patient's voiding pattern.

Now write down your ideas about the times that you expect the patient to void. Develop a plan to offer him the urinal or bedpan approximately a half hour before the time you expect him to void. Calmly and carefully instruct the patient as to what you want him to do each time you give him a urinal or bedpan and assist him as necessary. Screen the patient and place him in a comfortable position. Minimize his failures and praise his successes. Do not give up.

Following are two exercises that will help the patient strengthen his bladder control muscles:
1. Stopping the urinary stream during the act of voiding and holding it for a few seconds
2. Squeezing the buttocks muscles together as tightly as possible

This program of bladder training should be started only with and under the direction of the doctor and nurse. However, identify those patients who are having trouble controlling their bladder. Study the situation to be sure that the incontinence is due to the fact that the patient is unable to control the bladder and not to the fact that no one answers the patient's call for a urinal or bedpan. Then discuss these patients with the head nurse or team leader.

Urinary difficulties

The patient who has difficulty with his walking muscles or his eating muscles may certainly also have difficulty with his bladder control muscles. The patient who is confused, disoriented, and unaware of who or where he is will certainly have difficulty understanding and controlling the pressures of urine in his bladder.

THE PATIENT HAS A PROBLEM CONTROLLING HIS BOWELS

The patient's problem in moving his bowels and ridding his body of intestinal waste material may be related to one or more of the following factors:

1. If the patient is unable to get a nursing assistant when he feels the urge to defecate, he may tighten up his anal muscle and inhibit defecation. Even though the rectum is full of feces, the urge to defecate soon leaves the patient. The feces stored in the rectum lose all their water (it is absorbed into the bloodstream) and become a dried, hard mass. Soon, it is too large a mass to pass through the small anal opening. Eventually the patient's bowel becomes full of feces. However, the large, hard, fecal mass in the rectum is too large to pass through the anal opening, and the patient has marked discomfort and a feeling of pressure in the rectum. The bowel may attempt to empty itself through the mouth by reversing peristalsis and causing severe vomiting (usually fecal).

2. The patient may have such weakened bowel muscles and paralyzed abdominal muscles that he is unable to bear down effectively to help force the feces out of the body.

3. The patient may have a tumor in the intestines or rectum that is blocking the movement of feces to the outside.

4. The patient may have weakened bowel muscles that move the feces through so slowly that too much water is taken out and the waste material becomes caked, hard, and dry and plugs up his bowel.

5. The patient may have a disease affecting the nerves that carry the message to the brain that the rectum is full of feces. The brain never gets the message and therefore never sends down a message to the anal muscle to relax and to the intestine muscles to squeeze down and push the feces out of the rectum.

6. The patient may have a brain disease that has destroyed the functioning of his brain so that it cannot interpret or understand the message that his rectum is full.

7. The patient may have brain or nerve disease that prevents him from sending down the message to hold the bowel movement until the proper facilities are reached, and so his bowel habits revert to those of a child in that he moves his bowels anytime he develops rectal pressures.

Therefore the patient may have a problem controlling his bowels because of brain disease (does not get the message that his rectum is full and so fails to send down a holding one), because of nerve disease (messages are blocked), or because of muscle disease (does not have the muscular power to squeeze down and push the feces out of the body). All these diseases affect the patient's ability to move his bowels normally.

THE PATIENT HAS A PROBLEM CONTROLLING HIS BLADDER

The same conditions affecting the bowel would also affect the bladder. For example, the patient with a severe spinal cord injury (injury to the nerves of the back) would probably be unable to move his legs. He would also have difficulty receiving the message that his bladder was full and sending one to the muscles to squeeze down and empty. So urine would collect in the bladder until the overstretched bladder could hold no more, and then it would start to dribble out at about the rate of 30 to 60 ml. per hour. The patient would be wet constantly. You should suspect a full bladder with a dribbing overflow in your patient if he is wet each time you visit him or if he voids small amounts (30 ml.) frequently (every 30 to 60 minutes). Report your observations to the nurse immediately so that proper treatment (emptying the bladder by catheterization) can be started and serious complications (bladder and kidney infections) avoided. Then, too, the patient will be dry and comfortable.

The patient with a stroke, with hemorrhage into and destruction of the brain would have hemiplegia, but he would also have urinary incontinence because he would have destruction of that area in the brain that sends down the "hold" message to the bladder. Every 2 hours, when the bladder collected enough urine to stretch it and so send a message to the brain, he would be incontinent.

The best answer to incontinence, then, is not placing a bedpan or urinal at the bedside but retraining the bladder in the diseased body to function again.

SUMMARY

Waste material (feces) is stored in the rectum until it is full. The stretched rectal wall activates the involuntary nervous system in the same way the distended bladder does. Lack of bowel and bladder control is to be expected in those patients who have general muscular difficulties or difficulties in understanding their environment.

Urine is stored in the bladder at the rate of 1 ml. per minute until the bladder wall is quite stretched. This stretching stimulates the nerve in the involuntary nervous system that takes the message to the brain that the bladder is full. Immediately a second nerve, also from the involuntary nervous system, sends a message to the bladder to empty. This nerve assists the bladder in empting by relaxing the urinary sphincter and by stimulating the bladder muscle to squeeze down. Bladder control is a matter of training the person to recognize bladder pressures and to send down a message from the brain to the urinary sphincter to hold tightly closed until adequate facilities for voiding are obtained with a minimum of delay. This message must be sent down to the bladder by the voluntary nervous system.

Bladder and bowel retraining is possible in most patients. Bowel control is accomplished quite readily; bladder control is much more difficult to achieve.

The full rectum and bladder usually empty automatically unless conscious effort is directed toward inhibiting the response until toilet facilities are made available with a minimum of delay. Therefore the hospital patient must have his toilet needs met or he will have much pain and discomfort and will be incontinent.

Incontinence may be due to the inability to control the bladder or bowel or to the inability to get the urinal or bedpan on time.

DISCUSSION QUESTIONS

1. Do you have any incontinent patients on your unit? Study these patients and try to find out why they are incontinent.
2. Why would a patient with a severe head injury or a stroke have the problem of incontinence?
3. Select an incontinent patient on your unit. Make a plan, in conference with your team leader, for helping the patient develop continence.
4. Why would a plan to leave the urinal or bedpan on the bedside stand of a patient with urinary incontinence be entirely ineffective?
5. Why does the patient with a severe injury to his back and back nerves have difficulty controlling his bladder and bowel?
6. What is the best possible bed position for the patient who is having a bowel movement?
7. What amount of urine should a patient excrete each 24 hours?
8. How do you clean the urinals and the bedpans on your unit? Are they free of odors? Contact the hospital pharmacist and ask him about a method of cleaning that will free them from odors.
9. Why is it harder for the patient to regain control of his bladder than it is to regain control of his bowels.
10. Which patients on your unit are on limited fluids? Why? Discuss these with the head nurse in team conference.
11. Which patients on your unit are receiving diuretics? What plan will you make to help these patients meet their increased voiding needs?
12. How does the bed-lying position cause constipation?
13. Which patients on your unit receive a bedside commode for defecating? Why?

VOCABULARY

ambulatory Walking.
anal sphincter muscle Circular muscle in the anus. This muscle opens and closes the anus.
anus Opening from the large intestine to the outside of the body.
autonomic nervous system The nervous sytem that controls those body functions not under control of the will, such as peristalsis or heartbeat.

bedside commode Toilet chair.
bladder Body organ that stores urine.
bowel training Bringing the automatic emptying of the rectum under the control of the will so that it empties when the patient wants it to empty.
buttocks Area of the body on each side of the anus.
constipation Inability to expel the feces from the rectum because the feces have become a hard, dry mass.
defecation Act of excreting feces from the rectum.
forced fluids High fluid intake (amounts in excess of 3,000 ml.).
incontinence Loss of voluntary control over the bladder and bowels or both.
involuntary nervous system Same as the autonomic nervous system.
kidney Body organ that removes waste materials from the blood.
paralysis Inability to move part of the body at will.
peristalsis Rhythmic contracting (squeezing down and relaxing) of the intestinal muscles to move contents along the intestines.
rectum End portion of the large intestine where feces are stored; it is about five or six inches long.
retention with overflow An overfull-overstretched bladder from which urine dribbles almost constantly at the rate of about 30 to 60 ml. per hour.
stool Feces.
suppository Form of medication that melts at body temperature and which is inserted about 2 inches into the rectum.
ureter Tube connecting the kidney to the bladder.
urinal Receptacle into which the patient voids.
voiding Excreting urine from the body.
voluntary nervous system The nervous system that controls those body functions under control of the will, such as talking, walking or holding urine.

SOURCE OF ADDITIONAL INFORMATION

1 Bowel training manual and professional nurse lectures available from Geigy Pharmaceuticals. Ardsley, N. Y. *(No charge.)*

12/Caring for the patient's need to move

STUDY QUESTIONS

1. Why is it so difficult to sit still in a confined place?
2. How will a bed-lying position actually make the patient's condition worse?
3. How does the bed act like a body splint?
4. Why do lung complications occur frequently in the bed patient?
5. What is a decubitus ulcer?
6. What are contractures and how do they occur?
7. Why are kidney stones a complication in bed-ridden patients?
8. Why does the doctor keep the patient in bed if it is so dangerous?
9. What is the average patient's minimum need for physical movement?
10. How can you change the position of a helpless bed patient?
11. How can the entire unit staff be kept aware of what the patient's next position change should be?

THE BODY'S NEED TO MOVE

All of us have experienced the bodily discomfort that occurs from immobility. Perhaps you can remember your last long train or auto trip and the actual pain associated with sitting still in a confined place over a long period of time. First your buttocks ached as the weight of your body pressed against the car or train seat and interrupted or interfered with the blood circulation to the muscles there. As the pressure continued without any relief, the ache turned to numbness. Your knees also ached and became stiff. Your feet suffered too. As the veins, which depend on the movement of the leg muscles to bring the blood back to the kidneys and heart, became overextended with waste-laden blood, your feet became swollen and numb. Your shoes fitted too tightly, and perhaps you removed them. However, the pressure of the seat against the back of your knees further impaired the return of blood from your legs by acting very much as a tourniquet on the veins there. Soon the overfilled veins in your feet spilled the waste-laden serum (watery portion of the blood) back into the cells of the feet. Swelling increased in the feet and actual pain occurred.

When your destination was reached and you attempted to put on your shoes, it was impossible. Standing and walking, too, were difficult on your stiff, swollen, painful feet; all this may have occurred on an 8-hour or 10-hour trip. It usually requires even less time for immobility to cause discomfort. Think of how difficult it is to sit through a 2-hour class without an opportunity to get up and stretch (relieve the pressure) after an hour or so.

Now, let us think of the effect that lying still has on the patient who is confined to bed for 24 hours every day for a period of a week or a month. We know how difficult it is for him to move the painful, stiff arm that has been immobilized on an arm board for 24 hours while he received an intravenous infusion, but there are many complications of the lack of physical movement that we cannot see. If we think of the patient's bed as a body splint, much the same as the board that splints the arm for an intravenous infusion, we can begin to understand how the bed position limits body movement and causes difficulty.

THE BED ACTS AS A BODY SPLINT

The weight of the patient's body against the bed holds the patient on this splint (bed) and limits his movements. The chest muscles are not able to expand and stretch the chest, so the patient's lung movements and breathing abilities are lessened. Leg movements are not required to support the patient. As the leg veins become distended with blood, there is an overflow of serum back into the cells of the motionless legs, causing edema. The bony skeleton is no longer needed to support the patient; the bed splint does this, so minerals like calcium (which keeps the bones firm) are removed from the bones and are thrown into the blood for excretion from the body. The bones lose their strength, becoming soft and less rigid. The kidneys suffer, too. Clumps of calcium plug up the kidney tubules, and kidney stones occur.

Movement of the blood through the body is interrupted in those areas in which the blood vessels are closed off (as if a tourniquet were applied) by the pressure of the body's weight against the bed. Without blood, these body areas die. The dead areas are called bedsores or decubitus ulcers. In the back-lying position, body weight is greatest at the back of the head, the buttocks, and the heels; therefore these are the areas where decubitus ulcers most frequently occur. In the side-lying position, body weight is greatest at the ear, shoulder, hip, knee and ankle, so these are the areas most frequently affected by decubitus ulcers. In the face-lying position, the areas most frequently affected are the forehead, nose, chin, chest, knees, and toes (Fig. 12-1).

The bed does not act as a splint that keeps the body in a functional position (a position that permits standing and walking), but it does *splint* the body in that it limits mobility. Because of this limitation the strongest muscles of the body (the

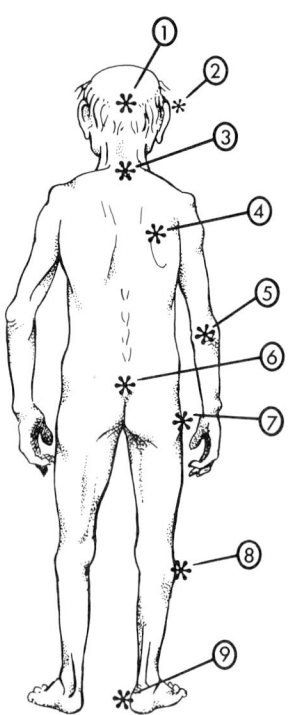

Fig. 12-1. Body areas most frequently affected with decubitus ulcers.

benders) begin to shorten and tighten while the weakest ones (the straighteners) let go and permit deformities to occur. The feet drop, the knees and hips bend (flex), the fingers bend so that the hand becomes a fist, the wrist bends, the elbows bend, and the shoulder bends. Even the back muscles bend, and the patient develops a curved back. When such changes occur, we say that the patient has contracture deformities.

In the discussion of bathing the patient in bed (Chapter 10), the body movements that you must do for the patient when you bathe him were described. Now you can understand how important it is to do the range-of-motion movements. Perhaps they are the most important part of the bath.

COMPLICATIONS OF LYING IN BED

The doctor will order bed rest when he believes that the patient's body is not able to carry out the essential activities of living adequately and that the patient's living must be made as simple and easy as possible. Therefore bed rest means a lessened load on the heart, a lessened load on the lungs, a lessened load on the muscles and bones, and a lessened load on the voluntary nervous system. It also means that there is a greater load on the digestive system, a greater load on the intestinal system, and a much greater possibility of complications occurring from bed rest.

Decreased activity may result in the following complications:

1. Lessened activity of the lungs means not only less breathing, but also less ability to get up the 3 pints of secretions (mucus) normally produced in the lungs and known to us as sputum. Therefore these secretions collect in the lungs, resulting in pneumonia, and plug up breathing tubes or the air sacs, resulting in atelectasis.

2. Lessened assistance from gravity in the elimination of waste from the intestines, together with the emotional distress or embarrassment as well as the discomfort of the bedpan, causes constipation.

3. Decreased muscle movement in the legs causes the blood to stagnate, the veins to overload, and serum to spill back into the cells of the feet, resulting in swelling and edema. Another danger is that a clot may form in the stagnated blood. This blood clot (thrombus) may remain in the leg and interfere with that circulation only, or it may move when the patient increases his activity by getting out of bed.

The clot moves through the veins back into the heart. Since the veins going to the heart are usually larger than the one in which the clot forms, little difficulty occurs. However, after the clot gets into the heart, it is pumped out into the arteries. Now it becomes a floating plug going into smaller and smaller blood vessels. Usually this floating plug (embolus) gets stuck in the lungs (pulmonary embolus) or in the brain (cerebral embolus). In the brain the embolus blocks the arterial blood supply to a section of the brain and the patient may have a stroke. In the lungs it also blocks the blood supply to a section of the lungs, and the patient has a sudden episode of shock, shortness of breath, blueness (cyanosis), and death.

4. With lessened use of the bones for body support, calcium is removed from the bones, and bone softening (osteoporosis) occurs.

5. Large amounts of calcium are removed from the bones and are dumped into the blood, and the kidney tries to excrete them. However, the kidneys frequently get plugged up with these calcium deposits, which are called kidney stones.

6. Because of decreased muscular activity, the muscles weaken and shorten. This results in bending deformities.

7. Lessened amounts of body weight are borne by the feet and greater amounts are borne by the body surfaces. Pressure on body surfaces that is not relieved at

2-hour intervals will permit decubitus ulcers to develop.

8. Lessened weight-bearing movement of muscles is required, and weakness results.

9. Less assistance is obtained from gravity to move food from the mouth to the stomach. Therefore eating is more difficult, and interest in food declines.

10. With a reduction in the patient's ability to care for his own needs, greater concern over his own body functions occurs, and the patient limits his interest in life and living to his worries about the bedpan, the urinal, eating, drinking, and having the nursing assistant present to help him in ever-increasing ways.

MEETING THE PATIENT'S NEED TO MOVE

Teaching the patient why he needs to move about in bed, exercising his feet, changing his position, straightening his arms, and encouraging him to breathe deeply should be sufficient to meet this patient need, but there are three reasons why it is not:

1. The patient may have such an immediate problem of pain, of difficulty in breathing, or of fear of dying that he has little time to remember the threatened complications of lying in bed. He is concerned with relief of his present condition and has no time to worry about what might happen.

2. The moving about in bed may, and frequently does, cause the patient some discomfort or pain. Therefore the patient is more interested in avoiding the pain that moving brings than he is about preventing the "maybe" complications.

3. The patient may be unable to move. Therefore you must know what body activity movements he needs, and you must make an actual plan for carrying them out. This plan may be written on the patient's nursing carecard, or it may be written on a plain card attached to a clipboard on the bed. We have found that by attaching a nursing care plan to the clipboard at the foot of the seriously ill patient's bed, the entire ward staff is kept more aware of the patient's nursing needs. (See Fig. 12-1.)

The patient's need for movement depends, to a great extent, on his disease. In a patient who has such severe heart disease that maintaining enough force in the heart to adequately pump the blood around the body is a big problem, movement will be limited. In the patient who has just been operated on for removal of the stomach (a gastrectomy), the breathing exercises and leg movements might be required every hour. In the patient who has paralysis of one side of his body (hemiplegia), bed position changes would be required every 2 hours, and arm and leg exercises would be done three times a day. Therefore the plan for meeting the patient's need for physical movement should be developed carefully in collaboration with the team leader, head nurse, or ward doctor. However, some general rules are the following:

1. The patient's position should be changed every 2 hours. Experiments have shown that pressure on a body surface for periods longer than 2 hours is sufficient to start the formation of a decubitus ulcer.

2. Disuse (lack of movement of a body part) causes loss of the ability to move. Therefore arms and legs must be moved if muscle strength and ability to move are to be maintained by these parts, and the patient's arms and legs should be put through their normal range of motion at least once a day during the bath.

3. Softening of bones occurs when weight bearing is not required by the skeleton. Therefore a footboard must be placed at the foot of the bed to maintain the feet in the standing position and to enable the patient to exert pressure against it (simulate weight bearing).

4. The bed splints the chest and limits lung expansion and activity. Therefore

NURSING CARE PLAN

OBSERVATIONS				NURSING CARE		
VITAL SIGNS	SIGNS/ SYMPTOMS OF PATIENT	ADVERSE EFFECT OF DRUG	TUBES	PHYSICAL CARE	POSITION	SAFETY MEASURES

NOTIFY CHARGE NURSE AT ONCE:
1. If changes in vital signs occur:
   a. T
   b. P
   c. R
   d. B/P
2. If symptoms develop
	TEST OR TREATMENTS SCHEDULED:

breathing exercises should be done by the patient at least three times a day. Changing the patient's position every 2 hours helps to prevent lung complications.

5. Bending contractures or deformities occur in the limbs when disuse occurs, especially in the limbs of paralyzed patients. Therefore limbs must be put through a normal range of motion in all patients at least once a day and at least three times a day in the paralyzed patient.

Considering the patient's need to move and the complications that result when this need is not met, a plan for a bed patient might include the following procedures:
  1. Turn the patient to the left every 2 hours. This would mean the following positions for the patient:
  a. 8 A.M.—turned from the back-lying to the left side-lying position
  b. 10 A.M.—turned from the left side-lying position to the face-lying position
  c. 12 noon—turned from the face-lying to the right side-lying position
  d. 2 P.M.—turned from the right side-lying to the back-lying position
  e. 4 P.M.—turned from the back-lying to the left side-lying position
  f. 6 P.M.—repeat (b)
  g. 8 P.M.—repeat (c)
  h. 10 P.M.—repeat (d)

2. Take arms and legs through normal range of motion each morning during the bath and each evening during evening care.
3. Place a footboard on the bed and encourage the patient to exert the force of his body weight against it each morning during the bath and each evening during evening care.
4. Encourage the patient to take ten deep breaths every 2 hours at the time of position changes.

If the patient is able to move about in bed easily, your job may be only to remind him to move and to breathe deeply and to exercise his limbs. However, if the patient is unable to move, you will need to turn his body and move his limbs.

Occasionally, you may encounter patients who cannot be moved into a certain position. For example, the patient who had a large tumor removed from the left side of the brain may not be permitted to turn on his left side, or the patient who had the left lung removed may not be permitted to lie on his right side. To avoid moving a patient into positions that are not permitted because of the condition of his body, label his bed with the sign, "do not turn on left side" or "do not turn on right side."

Unless you have been specifically instructed otherwise (as you would be in the case of a patient with a bone graft in his back), the patient should be turned from the back-lying to the side-lying position in the following manner:

1. Cross the patient's feet in the direction of the turn.
2. Bring the arm on the side to which the patient is turning across his chest.
3. Stand on the side of the bed to which the patient is turning, grasp the patient at the hip and shoulder, and roll him toward you (Figs. 10-3 and 10-4).

Now the job is only half done. If the patient was able to maintain himself in this position, you would not have needed to assist him in turning. Therefore it is necessary to support the patient in this position. The correct side-lying position is one that would permit the patient to stand erect in

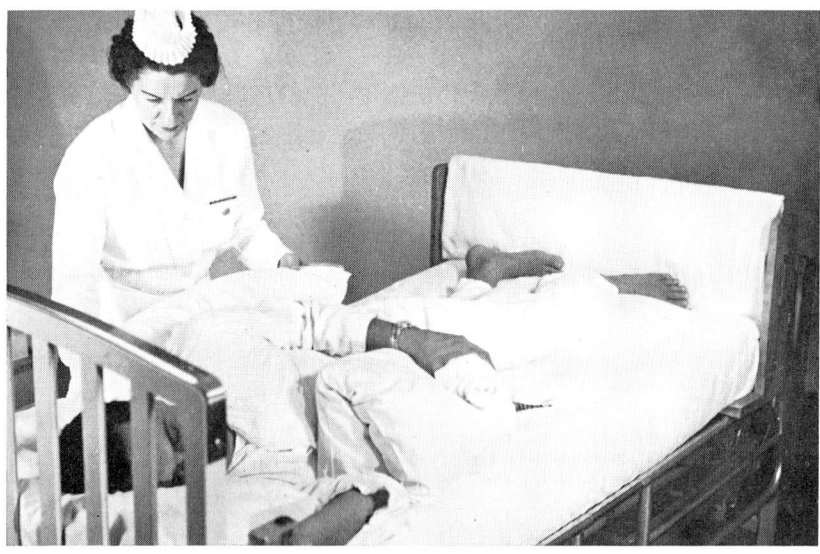

Fig. 12-2. The nurse positions and supports the patient in a side-lying position. Note the rolled-up towel in the patient's left hand to prevent bending contractures of the fingers.

the position of taking a step if you lifted him out of bed and onto his feet. In order to attain this position and to maintain the patient in it, you will need to support him with three pillows as follows (Fig. 12-2):

1. Place the first pillow under the uppermost leg.
2. Place the second pillow as close to the patient's abdomen as possible. Be sure that it is supporting his body and that it will prevent him from toppling over on his face. Support his arm and hand on the pillow.
3. Place the third pillow as close to the patient's back as possible. Be sure it is supporting his back and that it will prevent him from falling backward.

The pillows should be covered with rubber or plastic pillowcases, since the patient who cannot control his body muscles will probably be unable to control his bowel or bladder.

Of course, it is essential that a footboard be placed on the bed to support the patient's feet in the standing position. Crib sides should be in place on the bed of any patient who is unable to move. These sides will keep the patient from rolling out of bed. Crib sides should also be in place on the beds of those patients who need assistance in turning. They provide him with a firm support to grasp and pull on.

To turn the patient from a side-lying position to a face-lying position or from a face-lying position to a side-lying position, it is necessary to move the patient as close as possible to that edge of the bed opposite to the one to which he is being turned. If you fail to do this, you will find that the turn has moved the patient so dangerously close to the edge of the bed that the possibility of his falling out is too great for him to remain in the position.

The easiest and safest way to move the patient on the bed is to lift and slide him on a lifting sheet. Put this lifting sheet on the bed by placing a half sheet or a regular-sized sheet folded in half lengthwise under the patient (in much the same way as you put a regular sheet on the bed) from his neck to his thighs. Now the patient can be moved from a side-lying position to a face-lying position easily in the following way:

1. Get another nursing assistant to help you.
2. Place the patient in a back-lying position.
3. Both nursing assistants (one on each side of the bed) grasp the ends of the lifting sheet and slide the patient in the sheet as close as possible to the edge of the bed opposite to the one to which he is going to turn.
4. Place a pillow on the bed at the level of the patient's chest.
5. Place a second pillow on the bed just above the level of the patient's ankles.
6. Turn the patient on his side by grasping him by the shoulder and hip as discussed previously.

   The patient can be turned with the use of the lifting sheet by rolling one side of the sheet as close to the patient's body as possible and then grasping the top and bottom edges of the sheet and lifting the patient on the sheet from the back-lying position to a side-lying position. One nursing assistant turns the patient. However, since the assistant is turning the patient away from himself and toward the opposite edge of the bed, the second nursing assistant must be prepared to receive and support the turning patient.
7. Continue turning the patient over from a side-lying to a face-lying position.
8. Lift the patient on the lifting sheet and slide him over to the center of the bed.
9. Adjust the pillows under the patient's chest and legs.
10. Turn the patient's head to the side

and support it with a small pillow or a folded sheet.
11. Free the patient's arms from the weight of his body, and bring them up along his body to rest at both sides of his head (Fig. 12-3).
12. Place crib sides on the bed.

Although the face-lying position is an extremely valuable one for preventing bending deformities of the legs and for promoting the drainage of secretions from the lungs, it is the one in which it is most difficult to eat and defecate. Plan your patient's turning schedule in such a way that the patient is not in the face-lying position at mealtimes. Also, before turning the patient into this position, offer him a bedpan and/or urinal and a drink of water so that he can remain comfortably in this position for 2 hours.

Turning a helpless patient to a face-lying position with the use of a lifting sheet requires two nursing assistants. A device that permits one nursing assistant to turn the helpless patient is the Foster frame. This device consists of two separate frames with canvas-type mattress supports and a stand. The patient lies on one frame. When his position is to be changed, the second frame is placed in position over the patient and attached to the frame stand. The patient is sandwiched between these two frames and is turned by loosening the lock on the stand and reversing the position of the sandwiched patient. However, only two positions are available for a patient in a Foster frame: the back-lying and face-lying positions (Figs. 12-4 to 12-9).

As in any sandwich, the top and the bottom, or the two frames, are well supported but the sides are not. Therefore the patient's arms and legs may slip out between the frames and be injured if they are not prevented from doing so. One easy method of preventing the arms and legs from slipping out is to fold two sheets in quarters (widthwise) and then wrap one sheet around the frame at the level of the patient's knees and the other around the frame at the level of his elbows and pin the sheets in this position.

Develop a time plan for changing the

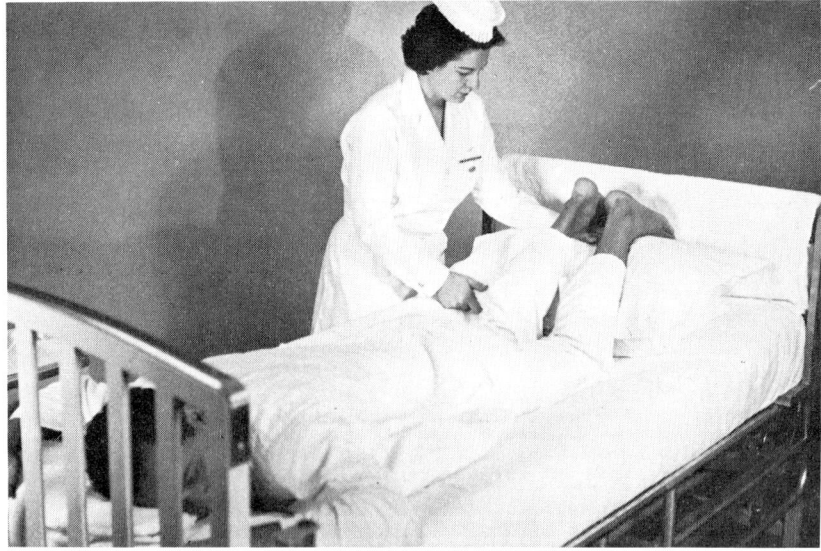

Fig. 12-3. The nurse has placed the patient in a face-lying position. Every 2 hours the patient should be turned to a different position.

Caring for the patient's need to move 99

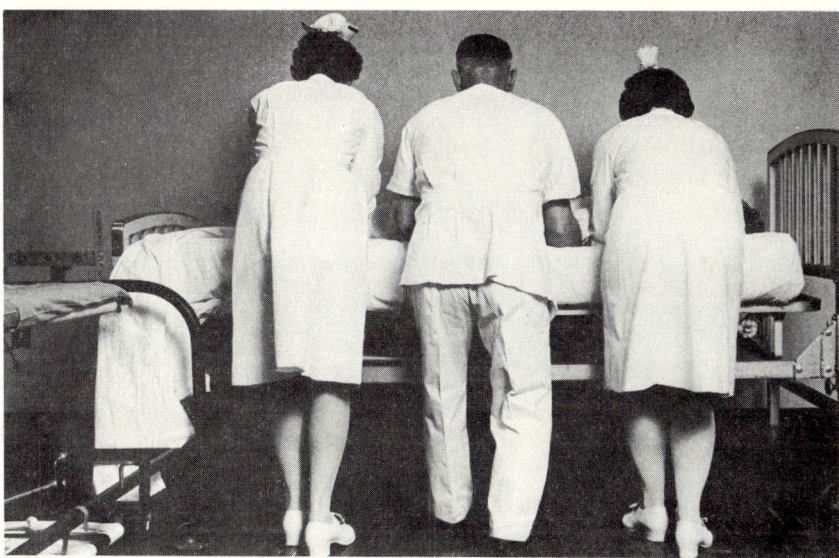

Fig. 12-4. Nursing personnel preparing to lift the patient to the Foster frame by a three-man carry. Note that the Foster frame is placed at a right angle to the bed.

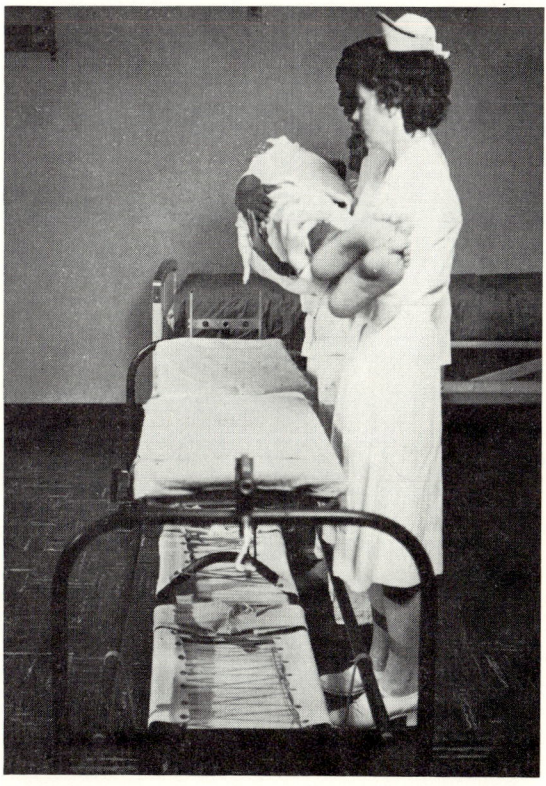

Fig. 12-5. The patient is being lowered onto the Foster frame.

100 Nursing assistant meets patient's basic daily needs in health care facility

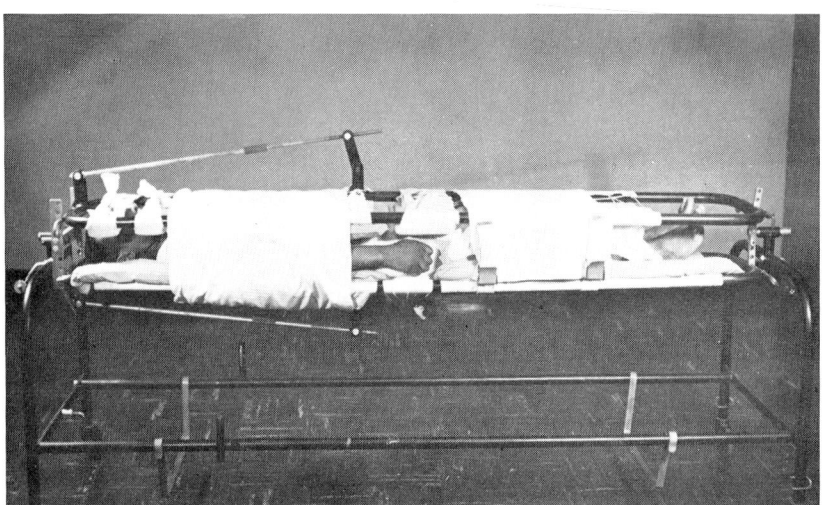

Fig. 12-6. The patient is sandwiched between two frames and is prepared to be turned. Note the protective support at elbow level and at knee level.

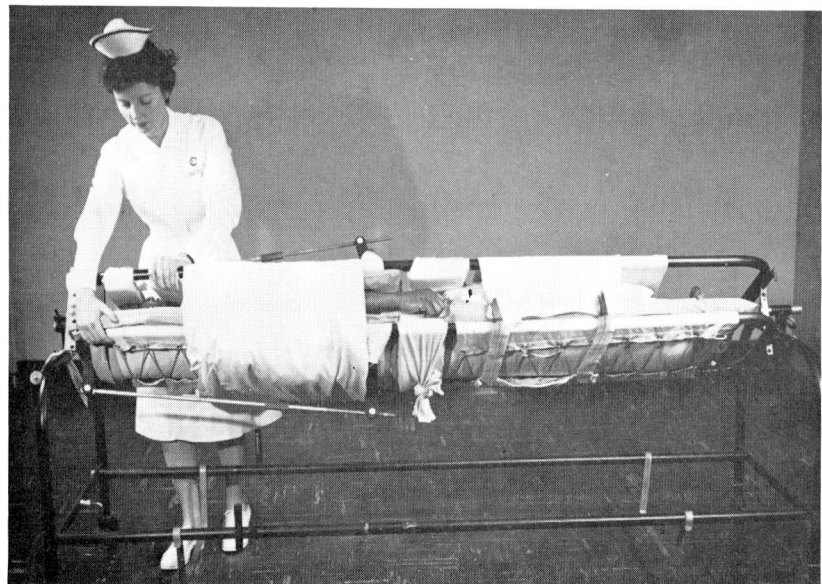

Fig. 12-7. One nurse turns the completely helpless patient on the Foster frame. Note that the nurse stands at the head of the frame.

Caring for the patient's need to move 101

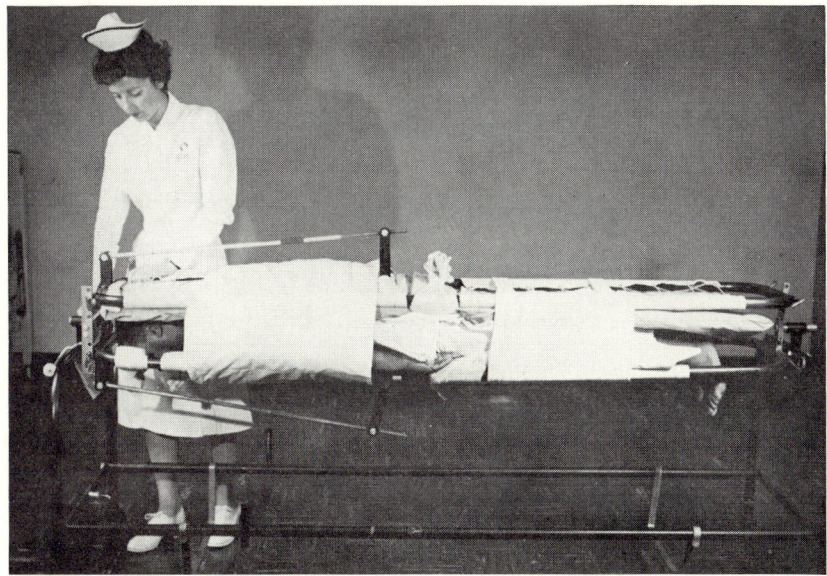

Fig. 12-8. The patient has been turned to a face-lying position, and the nurse is locking the frame in this position.

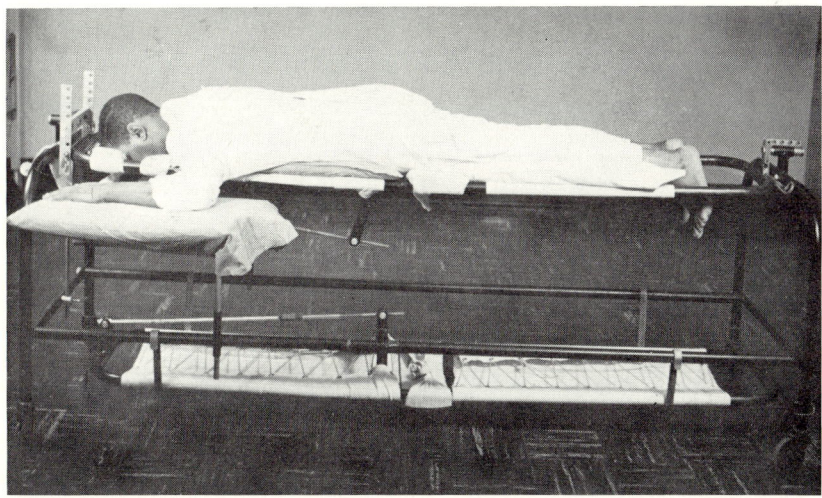

Fig. 12-9. The top frame and supports are removed, and the patient is made comfortable in a face-lying position.

patient's position. Write it on the Kardex and attach it to a clipboard on the frame. Keep in mind the patient's mealtimes and remember that the patient is unable to eat in the face-lying position. If the mealtimes on the unit are 8 A.M., 12:30 P.M., and 5 P.M., the plan for turning the patient might be as follows:

    7:30 A.M.—back-lying position
    9:30 A.M.—face-lying position
   11:30 A.M.—back-lying position
    1:30 P.M.—face-lying position
    3:30 P.M.—back-lying position
    5:30 P.M.—face-lying position
    7:30 P.M.—back-lying position

Nursing care for the patient on the Foster frame should be planned around his position changes and should not interfere with them. The daily bath should be started about 30 minutes before the position change. The body surface uppermost is washed first, then the patient's position is changed and the other body surface is washed to complete the bath. Treatments such as enemas must be planned for and given when the patient is in a back-lying position. A bowel-training program is important for this patient, too; otherwise, bedpan needs will interrupt the patient's positioning. The bowel movements of an incontinent patient on the frame would create quite a serious problem, since they would run down under the patient when he was in the face-lying position.

CIRC-O-LECTRIC BED

Another two-frame turning device that operates much like the Foster frame in that it turns the patient from a back-lying to a front-lying position and back again is the Circ-O-lectric bed. However, this bed differs from the frame in that it turns the patient over from head to foot rather than from side to side. Then, too, it is wider, more comfortable, and electrically operated (Figs. 12-10 to 12-14).

Two advantages of this bed over the frame are its extreme mobility, which permits transporting helpness patients to diagnostic or therapeutic activities via the bed,

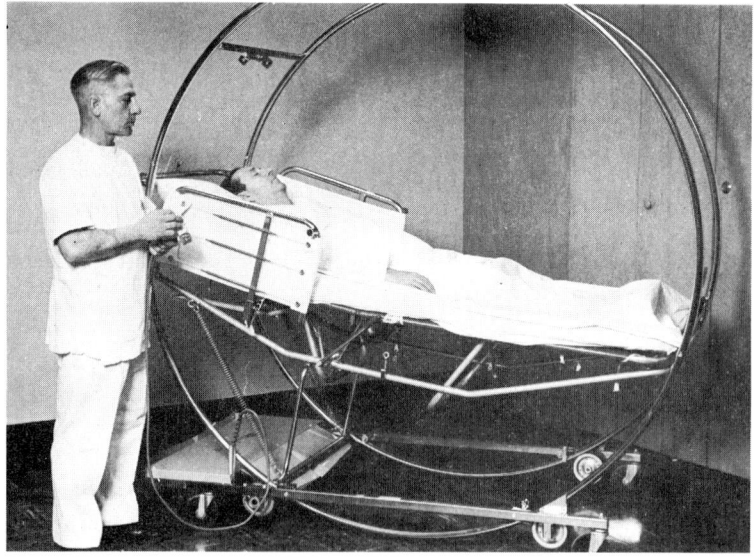

Fig. 12-10. The nursing assistant is tilting the patient into a position with the head higher than the feet by rotating the frame 10°. Note how carefully he observes the patient while he operates the controls on this electrically operated frame.

Caring for the patient's need to move 103

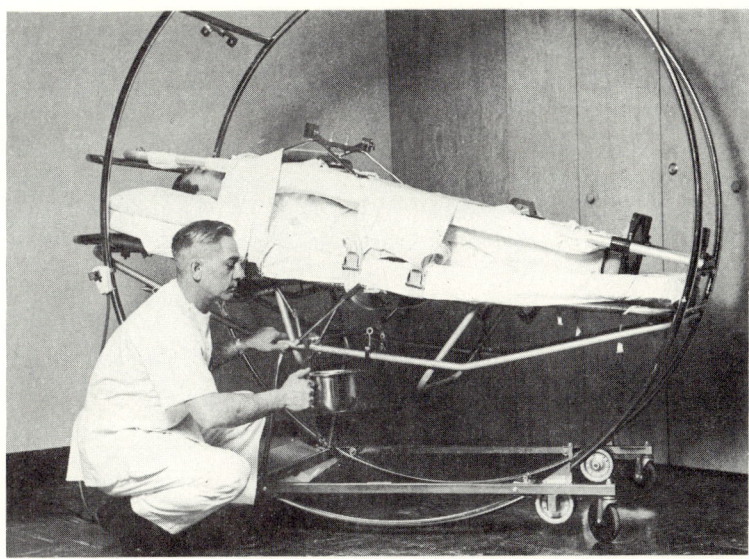

Fig. 12-11. The patient is prepared for the turn: (1) the top frame is bolted (end bolts) into position over the patient; (2) the feet are supported on a board; (3) the arms and legs are maintained in position by protective supports; and (4) the nursing assistant is removing the frame pot.

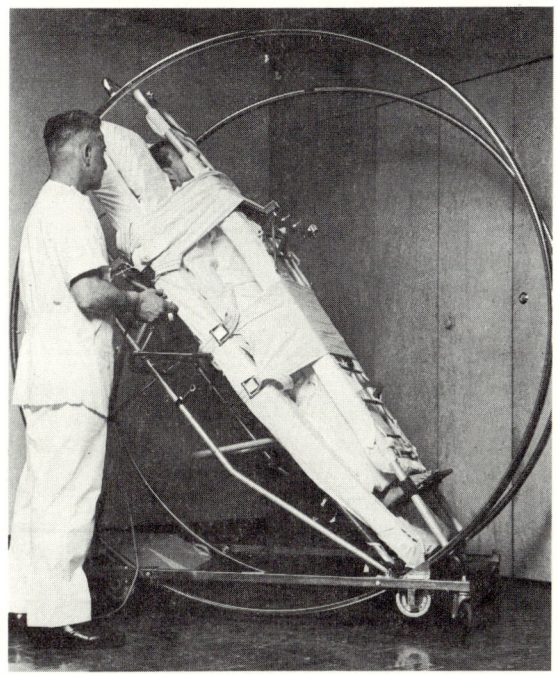

Fig. 12-12. The nursing assistant is rotating the patient from a back-lying to a front-lying position. Note how the footboard supports and anchors the patient during the turn.

104 Nursing assistant meets patient's basic daily needs in health care facility

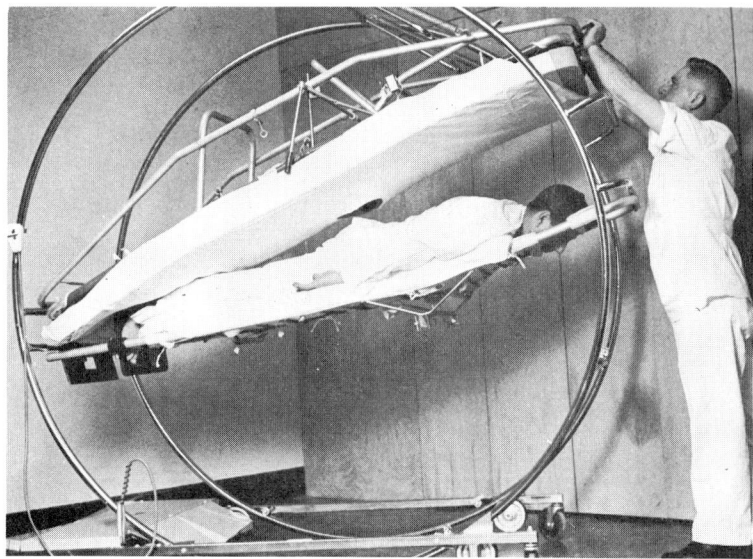

Fig. 12-13. The patient is now in a front-lying position, and the nursing assistant is tilting the back-supporting frame up into its attachment on the circle. Note that the back-supporting frame (unlike that in the Foster frame) does not need to be removed completely during the front-lying phase of patient care.

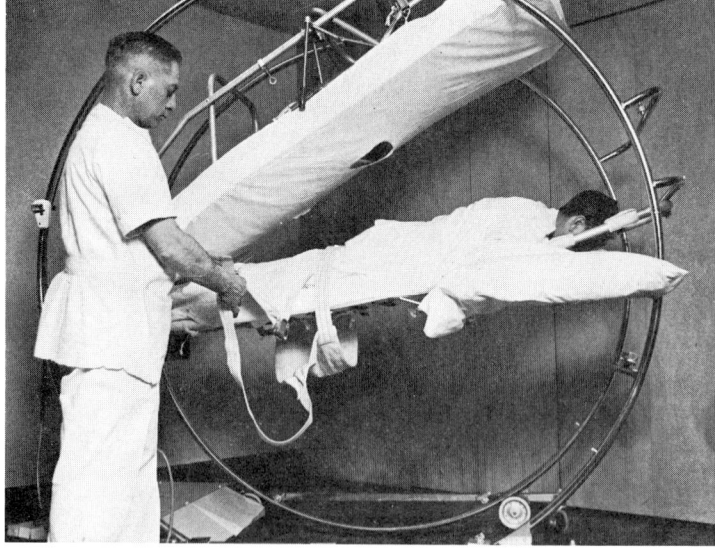

Fig. 12-14. The nursing assistant is making the patient's front-lying position safe and comfortable. He has placed the arms on pillow-covered supports and is now putting on a protective leg restraint.

and its head over foot turning mechanism, which permits tilt board type standing and weight-bearing exercises during each position change.

Nursing care of the patient, however, is planned in the same way as it is for the patient on the frame.

ALTERNATING PRESSURE MATTRESS

The alternating pressure mattress is actually two air mattresses in one. A pump attached to the mattress inflates one section of the mattress with air, and the patient's body weight is supported by only one area for 3 minutes. Then this section is deflated and the second section is inflated. Now the patient, without moving or changing his position, has his body weight supported by a different area of his body on the second section of the mattress for the next 3 minutes. Therefore the patient on the alternating air pressure mattress supports his body weight on two areas of his body—one area for 3 minutes, and then another area for the next 3 minutes, then the first area again for 3 minutes, etc.

In this way, the patient's need for 2-hour position changes is altered to 4-hour position changes by the alternating pressure mattress.

ENCOURAGE THE PATIENT TO MOVE

In the previous paragraphs we have discussed how a helpless patient is positioned. However, the nursing assistant's responsibility does not end as soon as the patient is able to move his own body; he must encourage the patient to move.

Everyone feels silly doing exercises that consist of apparently purposeless movements, such as kicking around the legs or waving the arms. The patient will think these exercises are purposeless, too. Instead of asking him to perform such exercises, encourage him to do as many of his self-care activities as possible. Encourage him to comb his hair and wash his face. Ask him to push himself up in bed by grasping the back of the bed with his hands and pulling himself up as he bends his knees and uses his feet and legs to push up. Let him hold his own glass of water when he drinks. Permit him to do as much as he can to feed himself. Remember that you are not going home with the patient, even if you are his muscles and arms and legs while he is sick, and that you must help the patient strengthen his own muscles so that he can regain the ability to care for his own needs.

SPECIAL NOTE

The nursing service in your hospital will identify those patient care skills that you are to do to help them take care of the patients. You will find these patient care skills in your job description. Perform accordingly. The inclusion here of the procedures in moving and positioning the helpless patient on a Foster frame and in a Circ-O-lectric bed does not imply that these procedures should or should not be a nursing assistant activity.

SUMMARY

The bed splints the body, limiting physical movement to such an extent that complications will occur to make the patient's condition worse unless we develop and execute a plan of nursing care to prevent them.

The doctor orders the patient to stay in bed, knowing that complications may occur, only because the patient's body is having difficulty carrying out the minimum activities of living. But the doctor knows also that the nursing personnel will work hard to avoid these complications.

Complications that result when the patient must lie in bed for prolonged periods include the following:

1. Decubitus ulcers
2. Stagnation of blood in the feet and legs
3. Softening of bone
4. Kidney stones
5. Bending contractures of the limbs

6. Formation of blood clots in the legs
7. Muscle weakness
8. Sputum plugs in the lungs with development of lung infections
9. Emotional regression of the patient until he is concerned only with his physical needs for food, water, bowel movements, and constant attention.

The nursing assistant should find out from the nurse what kind of physical movements the patient's body needs and can tolerate. Then a nursing care plan must be developed to carry out these patient movements.

As the patient recovers from his illness, he must be encouraged to do these physical movements for himself not by doing purposeless exercises but by doing self-care activities.

DISCUSSION QUESTIONS

1 Are all your patients who are confined to bed permitted the same amount of physical movement?
2 What determines whether or not the patient's physical activity is to be limited or encouraged?
3 Try to find a patient on your unit who has a beginning bedsore (decubitus ulcer). Plan a schedule for changing his position every 2 hours and observe the effect on the bedsore.
4 Check the nursing care plans for the acutely ill patients. Do they contain a plan for changing the patient's position? If not, discuss these patients with the team leader or doctor and determine what the patient's needs are.
5 Imagine sitting completely still in one chair for 2 hours. What effects do you think would result from this pressure of your body against the chair?
6 Study your patients. How many have difficulty moving? Do all these have aids on their bed to help them move? If not, why not?
7 In what areas of the body are decubitus ulcers most likely to develop?
8 Discuss how a back massage as well as a position change is a method of preventing decubitus ulcers.
9 Select the most helpless bed patient on your unit and plan a schedule for his physical activities.
10 What observations of your patients should you make each day in order to discover complications that might be developing?

VOCABULARY

atelectasis Collapse of a part of the lung. This usually occurs because a plug of mucus has blocked the air tube to that part of the lung.
contracture A condition in which a limb is fixed in a bent position.
decubitus ulcers Bedsores.
embolus A blood clot that is moving around the body in the blood.
flex Bend.
gastrectomy Removal of the stomach.
hemiplegia Paralysis of one entire side of the body.
intravenous infusion Injection of a sterile solution into the vein.
kidney stones Mineral deposits in the kidneys. These mineral deposits plug up the kidneys and interfere with the removal of waste materials from the blood.
mucus Clear, jellylike material secreted by the linings of body cavities (for example, the air tubes secrete approximately 3 pints normally in a 24-hour period).
osteoporosis A condition in which spaces (holes) occur in the bones.
pneumonia Inflammation of the lungs. Since pneumonia may be of so many types, the doctor usually uses a descriptive word with the term pneumonia. Examples are the following:
  acute pneumonia Inflammation of the lungs caused by bacteria (germs).
  aspiration pneumonia Inflammation of the lungs usually caused by food, fluid, saliva, or vomit that is inhaled into the lungs.
  hypostatic pneumonia Inflammation of the lungs caused by lying in bed for long periods.
  lobar pneumonia Inflammation of a lobe (section) of the lungs caused by bacteria. The inflamed lobe (section) of the lungs becomes solid with germs—pus and fluid—and air cannot get in. The patient develops a high temperature, chest pain, and shortness of breath.
serum Watery portion of the blood.
splint A device to immobilize a part of the body.
sputum Material spit out the mouth, usually consisting of mucus.
thrombus A blood clot in a vein.

SOURCES OF ADDITIONAL INFORMATION

1 Film: *Positioning the patient* (part of bed care series); obtained from Encyclopedia Britannica, 425 N. Michigan Ave., Chicago, Ill. 60611. 8 mm. 8-minute visual aid.
2 Film: *Use of turning frames*; may be obtained from Audio-Visual Support Center of the Army area in which you reside. *(Demonstrates Stryker, Foster, and Circ-O-lectric frames and their use in patient care.)*

13/Caring for the patient's need to get out of bed

STUDY QUESTIONS

1. What does bed rest mean? How does bed rest differ from absolute bed rest?
2. Why would a patient on absolute bed rest be permitted the use of a bedside commode?
3. What does B.R.P. mean?
4. How can you get a patient with hemiplegia out of bed?
5. How can you get a patient with paraplegia out of bed?
6. What does dangle mean? Why is it done?
7. What is the two-man carry?
8. How can a helpless patient be maintained in a sitting position in a wheelchair?
9. Can decubitus ulcers occur from sitting in a wheelchair?
10. What is a mechanical lift? How is it used?
11. What is a Davis roller? Why is it used?
12. How long should a patient sit in a wheelchair?

THE PATIENT WHO MAY GET OUT OF BED

In the previous chapter we learned that continuous bed rest is dangerous for the patient and that he needs to get out of bed as soon as possible. The doctor keeps the patient in bed only because the patient's body is not able to carry out the activities of living effectively and living must be made as simple and easy as possible. However, as soon as the patient's body regains the ability to carry out the minimum activities of living, the doctor will write an order to get the patient out of bed. The patient who is allowed out of bed, therefore, may not be cured. In fact, he may still be seriously ill, but he may be allowed out of bed because a complication of lying in bed is occurring or because a complication may be such a dangerous threat to life if it occurs that the doctor cannot take the risk of keeping the patient in bed. Because of this, you must know what your patient's condition is, how he is to get out of bed, and how long he is to remain out of bed. You cannot assume that a doctor's order to get the patient out of bed means that the patient is getting well, that he needs no further help from you, and that he is now perfectly able to take over his own care. If you do assume this, many serious accidents may occur.

DOCTOR'S ORDERS

The patient is to receive the care that the doctor prescribes exactly as he prescribes it. Therefore it is essential for you to understand what the following orders mean.

1. *Bed rest* means that the patient is to remain in bed throughout the 24 hour period and that all the patient's living activities are to be carried on in bed. This means the patient eats in bed, uses the bedpan to void and defecate, etc.

2. *Absolute bed rest* means that the patient remains in bed throughout the 24 hours of each day just as the patient on bed rest. However, it means too that the patient's body is so affected by disease that it is having difficulty carrying out the minimum activities of living. Therefore this patient's energy must be conserved. You will have to do everything for this patient—feed him, give him a drink, bathe him, turn him, etc. His diet will consist of foods that require little or no chewing and that are easily digested. His bath should involve a minimum of activity, and range-of-motion exercises as well as the vigorous back massage will be omitted. An example of a patient on this regimen might be a patient with a heart attack who has marked difficulty in breathing (dyspnea) and marked cyanosis (blueness of lips, fingernails, earlobes, and nose tip) and whose dyspnea increases with the slightest exertion.

3. *Bathroom privileges* means that the patient may get out of bed to urinate and defecate but that he must remain in bed at all other times throughout the 24 hours of each day. Bathroom privileges (B.R.P.) may be permitted by the doctor when the patient who is quite ill is having serious problems in using the bedpan.

4. *Out of bed to use bedside commode* means that the patient may get out of bed to defecate in the commode at his bedside (not in the bathroom). The patient who is allowed to do this is usually one who is seriously ill with a severe heart condition and is permitted out of bed to defecate in order to utilize gravity and thus minimize the stressing and straining (with the increased load that it places on the heart) required to have a bowel movement in bed. Usually the patient needs assistance to get out of bed. One doctor may order the patient to be lifted out of bed, whereas another may permit the patient to step out of bed and to pivot into position on the commode.

5. *Dangle* means that the patient is to be assisted to a sitting position on the side of the bed. Usually this dangling of the feet over the side of the bed is maintained for 15 minutes. Dangling assists the patient's body to regain its ability to carry on the activities of living in the sitting position and soon in the standing position. Usually it is ordered for those patients who are being prepared to get out of bed after they have been on a long period (2 weeks or more) of bed rest. The dangling position gives the heart and blood vessels time to adjust their functioning so that an adequate supply of blood will be maintained in the brain when the patient gets out of bed. Usually the patient gets a little light-headed, sweaty, and dizzy and may even faint when he dangles his feet for the first time. This is due to the fact that the heart and blood vessels are having difficulty pumping the blood uphill to the head after the long period during which the head was on a level with the heart. It is essential that you stay with the patient who is dangling, that you stand in front of him, and that you return him to his bed-lying position after 15 minutes unless he becomes so dizzy, pale, or sweaty that it is necessary to place him in the lying position before that time. The doctor usually orders all patients who have undergone serious operations to dangle before they are permitted to get out of bed.

Dangling is an effective method of preparing the patient to get out of bed, since it gives the body time to adjust to the increased activities. Getting the patient out of bed suddenly, without adequate time for the heart and blood vessels to adjust, may cause the patient to become weak and sweaty. He may even faint.

6. *Out of bed in chair for 30 minutes* means that the patient's body can tolerate only this short period of time out of bed. Therefore you should assist the patient to get out of bed and make him comfortable in a chair. Stay with him or, if this is not possible, check him frequently. Keep the call bell within his reach. Return promptly at the end of 30 minutes to assist him back into bed. Usually he is quite exhausted by this time. If he becomes lightheaded, dizzy, sweaty, or faint, call for help and return him to bed even if 30 minutes are not up. Place the patient in bed with his head on the same level as his heart. Elevate his feet, and summon the doctor or nurse immediately.

7. *Out of bed walking* means that the patient is to spend his time out of bed walking (not sitting) about the ward to stimulate the circulation in his legs. This may be ordered to prevent blood stagnation in the feet and the formation of a blood clot there. When the patient is tired of walking, he should return to bed.

8. *Ambulatory or out of bed ad lib* means that the patient is permitted to be out of bed whenever he wishes. He may be able to care for his own needs in the bathroom and may even go off the ward to the hospital coffee shop, the dining room, or the library.

9. *Out of bed on stretcher* means that the patient may be out of bed but must maintain the lying-down position, so he is placed on a stretcher. This order is usually written for patients in body casts or for patients with paraplegia who have developed a decubitus ulcer on the buttocks and must avoid the pressure of sitting. Although this long-term hospital patient does not get out of the lying-down position, moving him to a stretcher does permit him to go to the dayroom and visit with other patients. It relieves boredom.

10. *Out of bed—no weight bearing on right (left) leg* means that the patient is to get out of bed by supporting all his body weight on the left leg (or the right, as the case might be) while the other leg (free of the need to help support the body) hangs freely and rests lightly on the floor. This order is written for those patients whose broken leg bones have not healed sufficiently to support body weight. This is quite easy to teach the younger patient. However, in the older patient you may find that the broken leg was the patient's strongest body support (perhaps the reason why he broke it) and that the unaffected leg is weakened by arthritis. This patient—terrified of falling again and unable to support his weight on the leg weakened by arthritis—will require a great deal of assistance, emotional assurance, and encouragement before he will be able to get out of bed easily.

ASSISTING THE PATIENT OUT OF BED INTO A CHAIR

Determine what the patient is able to do to support his own weight and how much assistance he will require from you. If the patient is weak but able to support himself on his own feet, you can get him out of bed by the following procedure:

1. If the patient is in a high-low bed, lower the bed to its lowest position. If he is in a regular bed, get him a footstool.
2. Crank up the head of the bed until the patient is sitting upright in bed.
3. Place the patient's chair at the foot of the bed, facing toward the head of the bed. Lock the wheels if a wheelchair is used.
4. Get the patient's robe and slippers and place them on the chair.
5. Place one arm under the patient's

ankles and the other under his shoulders.

6. Pivot your body one-half turn until you are facing the foot of the bed. At the same time that you pivot, bring the patient's legs over the edge of the bed and lift his shoulders up so that he is in a sitting position on the side of the bed. Permit the patient to sit on the edge of the bed a few minutes so that his body can adjust to this changed position. Then assist him in putting on his bathrobe and slippers.
7. Ask the patient to place his hands on your shoulders as you slip your arms under his and around his chest, locking them there by grasping one of your hands firmly in the other. If the patient is in a low bed, you may have to lower your body by bending your knees, but you must keep your back straight.
8. Raise your body by straightening your knees and at the same time lift the patient out of the bed to a standing position on the floor. Maintain your hold on the patient.
9. Turn your body around one-half turn by taking several small steps of a shuffling type, keeping both your feet on the floor, and at the same time bring the patient with you. Now you are facing the wheelchair, and the patient's back is toward it.
10. Permit the patient to take his hands from your shoulders and to reach back and grasp the arms of the wheelchair. Maintain your hold on the patient.
11. Lower the patient into the wheelchair by bending your knees while you keep your back straight.
12. Place the patient's feet on the foot supports of the wheelchair.
13. Make the patient comfortable by placing a pillow at his back, etc.
14. Give the patient his glasses, newspaper, etc., and take him to the ward dayroom.

The patient can be assisted back into the bed by reversing the process just described.

If the patient is paralyzed on one side of his body (hemiplegic), he can still be assisted out of bed in this way. However, you will need to keep his paralyzed leg from buckling and causing him to fall by splinting it with your leg. You can do this by assuming the following position:

1. Place your foot along the outer side of the patient's paralyzed foot.
2. Keep your knee pressed firmly over the paralyzed knee. As you assist the patient out of bed to a standing position, stabilize his paralyzed leg by pressing your foot against his foot and your knee over his knee. As you turn sideways to face the chair at the foot of the bed, use a shuffling gait. Keep your foot and knee in position to splint the patient's paralyzed leg. Turn his splinted leg by pushing your foot against his as you pivot. Lower him into the chair as described previously.
3. Support the patient's paralyzed arm on a pillow or, better still, on an arm support attached to the wheelchair (Fig. 13-1).

When you help a hemiplegic patient out of bed, always place the wheelchair in the position that will enable him to use his functioning arm to help himself. This means that the chair should be placed at the foot of the right side of the bed or at the head of the left side (Fig. 13-1) if the patient has right-sided hemiplegia and at the foot of the left side or at the head of the right side of the bed if the patient has left-sided hemiplegia. Then the patient's functioning arm will be available to grasp the arm of the chair and enable him to help himself.

The patient who is unable to support himself on his legs, such as a paraplegic patient who is paralyzed from the waist down, will need to be lifted out of bed.

Caring for the patient's need to get out of bed 111

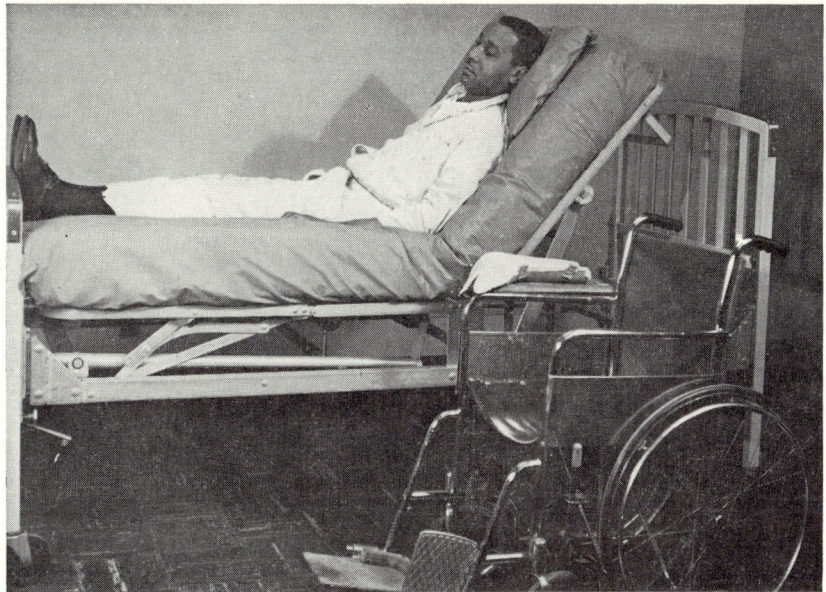

Fig. 13-1. The wheelchair is placed at the head of the left side of the bed in readiness to receive a patient with right-sided hemiplegia. Note the right arm and right foot supports attached to the chair. This patient will be able to use his left hand to grasp the chair to support himself during the transfer from the bed to the chair.

Since you cannot safely lift more than 35 pounds by yourself, you will need the help of another nursing assistant or the help of a mechanical lift.

If you are getting the patient out of bed with the help of another nursing assistant you can do it by using the two-man lift. This is done as follows:

1. Assist the patient into a sitting position on the side of the bed, as described previously.
2. Position the wheelchair at the foot of the bed with enough space between the bed and the chair for one of the lifters to step around the chair.
3. Lock the wheels on the wheelchair.
4. Stand on one side of the patient, with the other nursing assistant on the other side, so that you are facing each other.
5. Lower your body (by bending at the knees) as the other nursing assistant lowers his, and each place one arm under the patient's knees. Lock your arms in this position by grasping each other's arm firmly about the wrist.
6. Each place the other arm around the patient's back and lock these arms in position as described in step 5.
7. Ask the patient to put his arms over your shoulders.
8. Stand as close to the patient's body as possible.
9. Together lift the patient off the bed as you each raise your body to the erect position by straightening the knees (Fig. 13-2).
10. Turn halfway around, one assistant walking to the right and the other to the left, until the patient is suspended over the chair.
11. Lower the patient into the wheel-

112 Nursing assistant meets patient's basic daily needs in health care facility

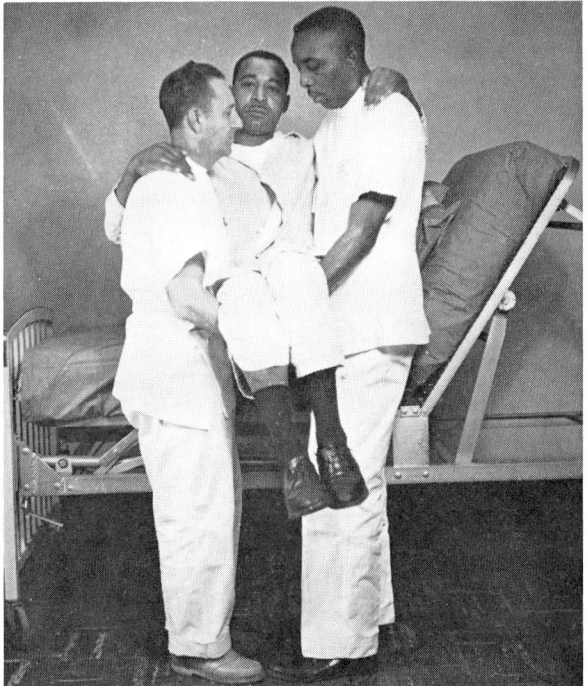

Fig. 13-2. Patient is lifted off the bed as the two nursing assistants straighten their knees and rise to an erect position.

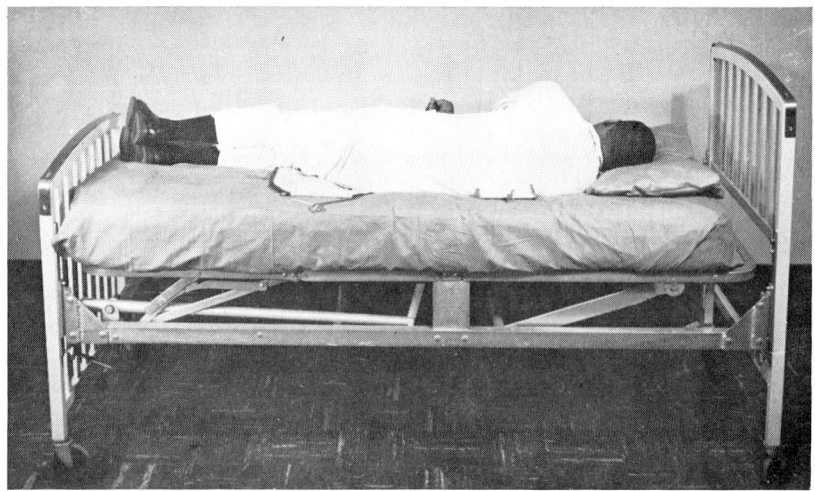

Fig. 13-3. The seat and back supports in position under the patient.

chair by both bending down from the knees. (Be sure that each of you keeps your back straight.)
12. Position the patient in the chair as previously described.

Although the procedure just described requires two people, one nursing assistant can get the heaviest patient out of bed with the use of a mechanical lift. The mechanical lift looks something like a swing in a frame. The patient is rolled onto his side, the seat of the swing is placed under the patient at the level of his thighs (from the back of the knee two thirds of the way up the thigh), and the back of the swing is placed under the patient at the level of his shoulders (Fig. 13-3). The patient is rolled over onto his other side, and the seat and back supports are pulled through under the patient in much the same way as a sheet is put under a patient. Now the patient's bed is cranked up a few times, and the seat and back supports are attached to the frame of the mechanical lift. Then the head of the bed is raised completely, thus sitting the patient upright. Check the release valve on the mechanical lift to be sure it is closed. Manipulate the pump handle to raise the patient in the seat clear of the bed. Raising the bed to a sitting position bends the patient in the bed, thereby making it unnecessary to lift up the patient's head and shoulders as the mechanical lift frame raises the patient clear of the bed.

When the patient clears the bed, lift his feet over the side of the bed and back the mechanical lift away from the bed. Then manipulate the lever on the left to spread its supports so that you can bring a wheelchair between them and into position under the patient. Ease the release valve open gently (about one sixth of a turn), and guide the descent of the patient in the swing so that he is lowered into the wheelchair (Fig. 13-4). Unlock the seat and back supports from the lift frame and leave them in position under the patient.

When the patient is to be returned to bed, rehook the seat and back supports to the frame and reverse the procedure just described.

One caution in the use of the mechanical lift is to be sure that the release valve is opened cautiously. This is a hydraulic jack, and the rate of descent is determined by the weight of the patient. Therefore the heavier the patient, the greater the need for care in manipulating the release valve.

The lift can also be used to lower the patient into the bathtub or to lift him out of it. Seat supports with large openings in the center can be purchased with the mechanical lift. These can be used for those patients who are to be lifted on and off the toilet. It is necessary for you to place the back and seat supports under the patient

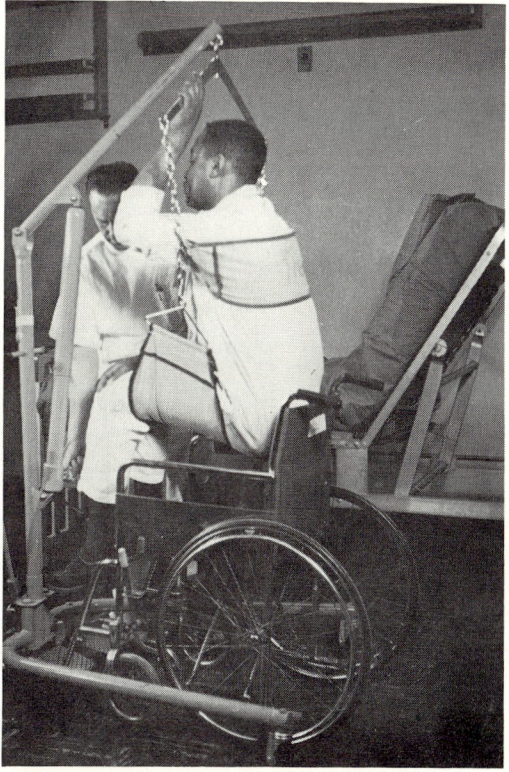

Fig. 13-4. Patient in a mechanical lift is being lowered into a wheelchair.

while he is in bed and to leave them under him while he sits in the chair. Therefore each patient who is assisted in and out of bed with the lift needs his own set of supports.

A full-length (head-neck-back) support is used, instead of the two pieces in Fig. 13-4, if the patient is unable to maintain himself in a sitting position.

The bilateral amputee (patient with both legs amputated) is able to get himself in and out of bed by using a bed trapeze. The patient must be taught how to bring his wheelchair close to the bed and how to lock it in position. Then he can get himself out of bed by lifting himself up and around until he is sitting backward on the edge of the bed and in front of the wheelchair. Then he reaches back, grasps both arms of the chair, and with his hands lifts himself back into the wheelchair.

The paraplegic patient also can be taught to do this after his arms have been sufficiently strengthened through exercises to lift his body.

Some paraplegic patients can be taught to get out of bed by bringing the wheelchair alongside the bed and removing one arm support from the chair. Then they place a sliding board in position from the bed to the chair. The patient then lifts himself onto the sliding board with the help of the trapeze and slides from the bed (over the wheel of the chair covered by the board) into a sitting position on the chair.

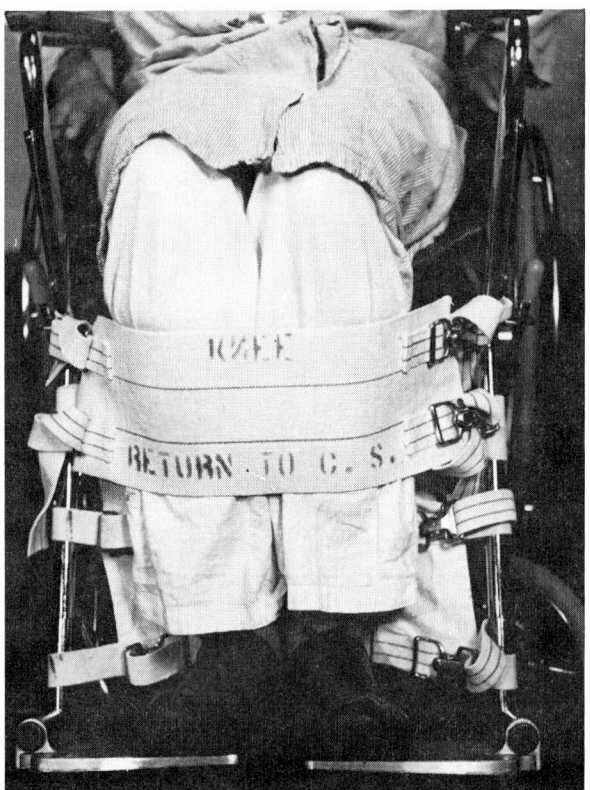

Fig. 13-5. Shin supports to maintain the patient's feet in position on the wheelchair. These supports will keep the patient from sliding down and out of the chair.

Check to be sure that the wheels are locked before you attempt to get a patient out of bed into a wheelchair. Locking the wheels is also an essential part of teaching patients to help themselves in and out of wheelchairs.

A patient who needs a great deal of help in getting in and out of bed will also need some help to maintain him in a comfortable sitting position in the wheelchair. Since the feet are the supports for the body, maintaining the patient in a sitting position in a chair can be accomplished easily by keeping his feet in the correct position to support him. This can be done with shin supports (Fig. 13-5) and foot supports. The patient cannot be prevented from sliding down and out of the wheelchair by any type of chest support. Such supports only keep the patient's arms up while his legs and buttocks and body slide out of the chair.

Try this simple experiment yourself. Sit in a chair. Ask a friend to stand behind you and support you in the sitting position by placing his arms under yours and around your chest. Permit your legs to slide. Soon your buttocks begin to slide off the chair. How effective are your friend and his bear hug in holding you up?

Large arteries and veins pass through the axilla as they take blood to the arms and carry it back to the heart (Fig. 13-6). The support that is wrapped around the patient's chest and under his arms actually becomes a tourniquet, shutting off the blood supply to the arms, as the patient slides down in his chair. The support then is not only useless, but also dangerous.

We have found that a helpless patient in the wheelchair can be maintained in a sitting position effectively with foot supports. However, he may topple forward out of the wheelchair unless he has a vest-type support to keep him back in the chair. The vest-type support is illustrated in Figs. 13-7 and 13-8.

ASSISTING THE PATIENT OUT OF BED ONTO A STRETCHER

The patient who is able to move himself with assistance can be helped onto the stretcher by the following method:

1. Bring the stretcher alongside the bed.
2. Lock the stretcher wheels, reach over

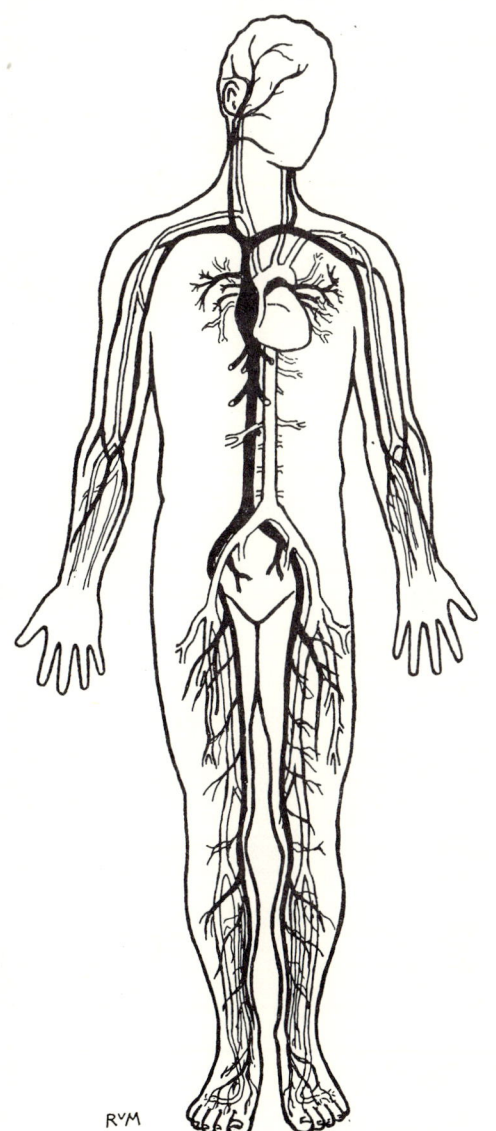

Fig. 13-6. Large arteries (outlined) and veins (filled in) of the body. Note how the arteries and veins pass through the axilla.

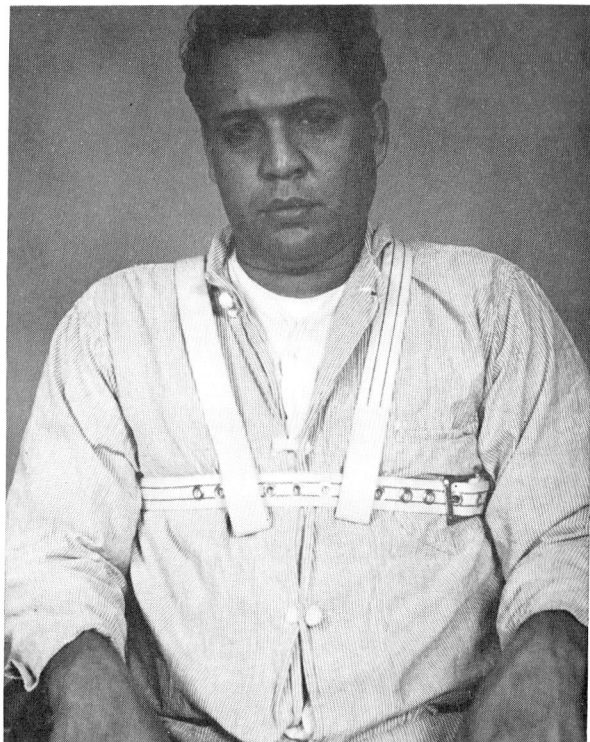

Fig. 13-7. Front view of a vest-type chest support for wheelchair patients.

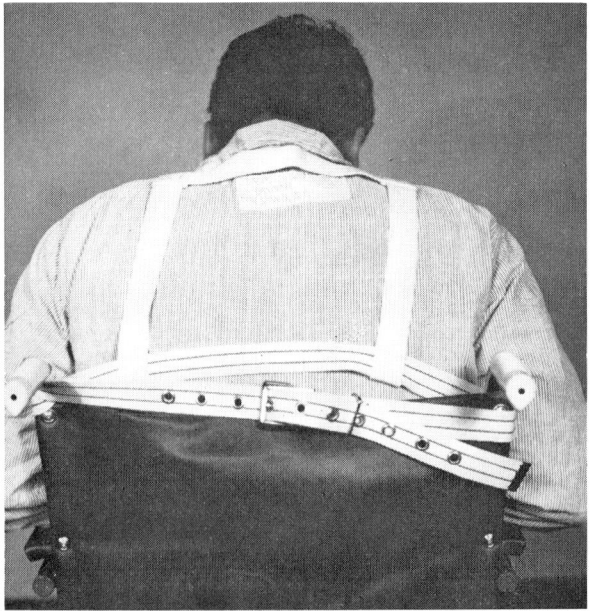

Fig. 13-8. Back view of a vest-type chest support for wheelchair patients.

the stretcher, and grasp the patient's hand farthest from the stretcher.
3. Permit the patient to support himself as he moves over by using the arm closest to the stretcher to support his body. You stand on the side of the stretcher opposite to the bed.

The completely helpless patient may be rolled (like a log) from the bed to the stretcher. This can be done rather simply when the patient is already lying on a lifting sheet:

1. Put another folded lifting sheet on the stretcher (remember, the patient will have to be moved off this, too).
2. Then bring the stretcher alongside the patient's bed.
3. Lock the stretcher wheels.
4. Check to be sure that the bed wheels are locked.
5. Go to the opposite side of the bed, fan down the top covers, and place a sheet over the patient.
6. Loosen the lifting sheet on that side of the bed and throw it over the patient.
7. Return to the side of the bed where the stretcher is in place.
8. Reach over the stretcher, grasp the lifting sheet, and pull it toward you, rolling the patient onto the stretcher.

The seriously ill patient with a breathing difficulty, the patient who has recently been operated on, or the one receiving an intravenous infusion cannot be moved to the stretcher in the manner just described. This patient should be moved to the stretcher by using the Davis roller. This is accomplished as follows:

1. Fan the top covers down to the foot of the bed and cover the patient with a sheet. Then get another nursing assistant to help you.
2. Have your helper turn the patient.
3. Loosen the lifting sheet on your side of the bed, throw it up over the patient, and place the Davis roller as close to the patient under the lifting sheet as possible (Fig. 13-9). Be sure that the roller will be under his head and feet when he moves.
4. Now return the patient to a back-

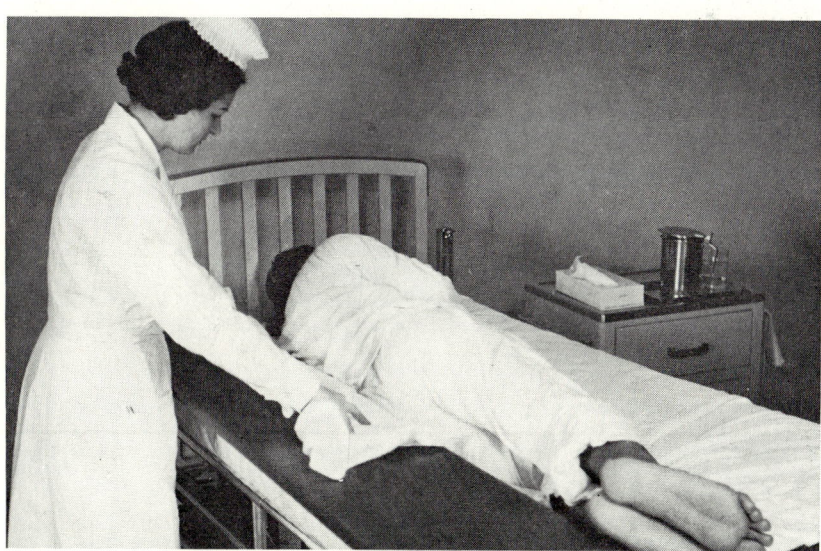

Fig. 13-9. The nurse places the Davis roller on the bed as close to the patient as possible. Note that the lifting sheet is placed over the roller loosely.

lying position, half on and half off the roller covered by the lifting sheet.
5. Position the stretcher at your side of the bed as your helper loosens the lifting sheet on his side of the bed.
6. Lock the wheels on the stretcher and on the bed.
7. Reach across the stretcher and grasp the lifting sheet, which is under the patient but on top of the roller (Fig. 13-10).
8. Pull the lifting sheet toward you with a quick, steady pull as your helper tilts the patient onto the roller by lifting up on the lifting sheet. The patient rides over on the roller as you pull on the lifting sheet, and your helper elevates his end and holds it steady. If your helper did not do this, the patient would slip off the sheet rather than go over with it. It is impossible to use the Davis roller to move the patient from the bed to the stretcher without the lifting sheet.

If you had difficulty moving the patient onto the stretcher, you will have the same difficulty moving him off of it in the x-ray department, in the operating room, or in any therapy department to which you are taking him. Therefore it might save you a great deal of heavy lifting if you made a shelf for the Davis roller on the stretcher so that you could take it with you and use it at off-ward areas to move the patient.

STAYING OUT OF BED

Remember your last long train or auto trip and how uncomfortable you were sitting in a confined place. Sitting in a wheelchair is no different. After 2 hours the patient will have aches in the buttocks that will turn into numbness in a short time. As this occurs, circulation is being impaired, and decubitus ulcers (pressure sores) may result. These can be avoided in the following ways:

1. Change the patient's position in the

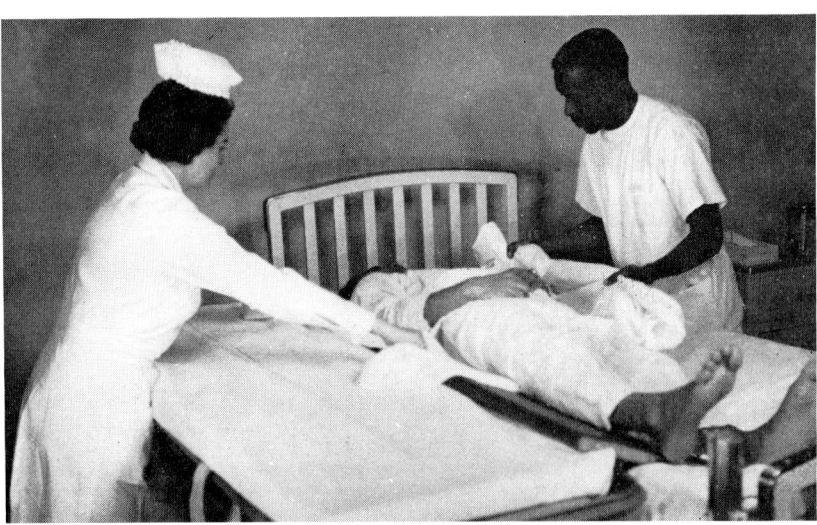

Fig. 13-10. The nurse and nursing assistant are transferring the patient from the bed to the stretcher on the Davis roller. The nursing assistant is tilting the patient onto the roller, and the nurse is ready to pull him over onto the stretcher with a steady pull on the lifting sheet.

wheelchair every 2 hours. This can be done by teaching the amputee or paraplegic patient to raise his buttocks up off the chair at frequent intervals, by raising the hemiplegic patient to a standing position for short intervals every 2 hours, or by returning the patient to bed for rest periods throughout the day.
2. Use a chair alternating pressure pad under the helpless patient, and then change his position every 4 hours by one of the methods described previously.

Sitting a helpless patient in a wheelchair in the same position without any relief of pressure on his buttocks and without any movement of his legs will certainly result in venous congestion and swelling in the legs, as well as the development of decubitus ulcers on the buttocks.

THREE-MAN CARRY

Lifting the patient by means of a three-man carry (Fig. 12-4) is done when the helpless patient is to be moved quickly from the bed to a treatment device such as the Foster frame or the Drinker respirator or when the patient has a broken bone in his back and must be moved as a log (with no bending of his body) so that the broken bone will not move and cut his spinal cord or his spinal nerves.

This lift is done in the following way:
1. Place the device to which the patient is being moved at right angles to the foot of the bed, with the head of the device tightly against the foot of the bed. This device might be a Foster frame, a respirator, a stretcher, or a rocking bed.
2. Get two other nursing assistants to help you.
3. Stand at the side of the bed with the other two nursing assistants—on the same side where the device is placed against the foot of the bed. One nursing assistant should stand at the level of the patient's ankles, the other at hip level, and the third at shoulder level.
4. Together, bend from the knees and place your arms flat on the bed.
5. Slide your arms under the patient in the following way:
    a. The first nursing assistant slides his arms under the patient's legs beneath the ankles.
    b. The second one slides one arm under the buttocks at the level of the patient's hands and the other arm under the back at the level of the patient's elbows. Be sure this nursing assistant slides his arms under the patient far enough so that his hands can come through under the opposite side and support the patient's hands and elbows.
    c. The third nursing assistant slides one arm under the patient's shoulders and the other under the patient's head. The arm under the head bends at the elbow to form a support for the patient's head and the hand grasps the patient's shoulder.
6. At a given signal, together slide the patient (like a log) as close as possible to the edge of the bed on the side where you are standing.
7. At a given signal, holding the patient securely in your arms, each raise your body by straightening the knees while the back is held straight and lift the patient up and off the bed.
8. Tilt the patient toward you, permitting him to roll slightly toward your chest. (In this way the patient is supported partly by the lifters' arms and partly by their bodies.)
9. At a given signal, synchronize your movements and move backward and around one-half turn until you are at right angles to the bed and facing

120 Nursing assistant meets patient's basic daily needs in health care facility

the device on which the patient is to be placed.
10. At a given signal, walk slowly, in unison, toward the device on which the patient is to be placed.
11. When the device is reached (you can feel it with your shins), lower the patient slowly (like a log) as you each lower your body by bending at the knees (Fig. 12-5).
12. When the patient is placed on the device, keeping your arms in position, check to be sure that the patient is in the correct position—that his head is where it should be, etc.
13. Keeping your arms flat against the device, each slowly step back, and at the same time withdraw your arms.

ONE-MAN CARRY FOR EMERGENCIES

Emergency does not mean an impatient x-ray department waiting to make an x-ray examination or an impatient surgeon waiting to operate, but it does mean a life-threatening situation such as a hospital fire.

In the case of a hospital fire, you may be required to remove patients from a burning, smoke-filled ward to safety very quickly. You probably will have no one to help you get the patient out of bed, since everyone will be busily evacuating patients. You can get patients out of bed the following way:
1. Place a blanket (from the patient's bed) lengthwise on the floor alongside the bed.
2. Kneel on one knee at the patient's bedside and slide both arms under the patient, one at the level of his shoulders and the other at the level of his thighs.
3. Slide the patient along the bed toward you until he is lying on the edge of the bed.
4. Pull the patient's buttocks out of bed to your elevated knee.
5. Pull the patient's shoulders out of bed as you lower his buttocks to the floor by lowering your bent knee.
6. Lower the patient's head and shoulders to the floor.
7. Remove your arms from under the patient's body, stand up, and go to the head of the blanket.
8. Grasp the head of the blanket firmly in both hands and drag the patient who is lying on the blanket out of the ward to the safety area (Fig. 13-11).
9. Proceed to evacuate the next patient with this blanket drag.

It is imperative that you know what to do in case of fire—how to send in the alarm, how to evacuate the patients, how to direct fire-fighting personnel to fire-fighting equipment, and how to shut off

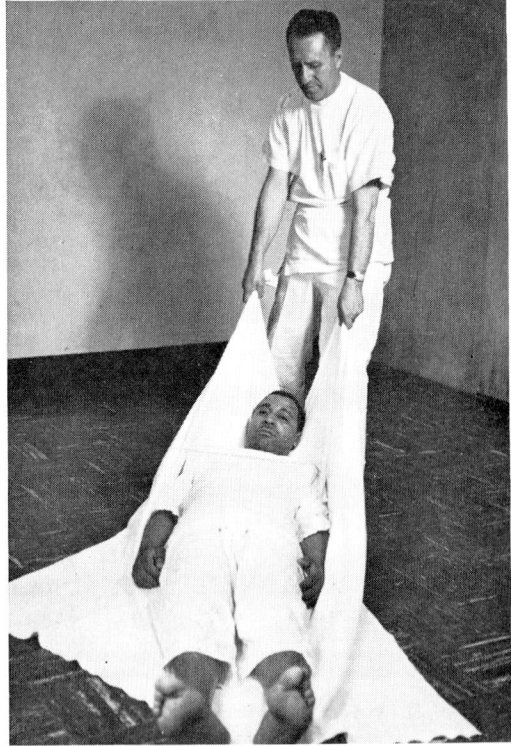

Fig. 13-11. The nursing assistant demonstrating the blanket drag, which is used for emergency evacuation of patients from a ward.

ward or floor oxygen supply valves. If you do not know what the hospital expects of you in case of fire, find out today. Check with the head nurse immediately.

DISCUSSION QUESTIONS

1 Is there a mechanical lift available in the hospital for lifting helpless patients out of bed? Do you use it? Explain your answer.
2 What patient do you have difficulty assisting out of bed? Make this problem the subject of your next nursing rounds or team conference.
3 How long do you expect the helpless patient to stay out of bed in the wheelchair?
4 How do you relieve the pressure on the buttocks of those helpless patients who stay out of bed most of the day?
5 Discuss with the team leader the possibility of building a trapeze in the dayroom so that wheelchair patients might be taught to use this to lift themselves up frequently and relieve the pressure on their buttocks.
6 What patients on your unit are on absolute bed rest? Why? Discuss your method of giving them nursing care and how you conserve their energy.
7 Why should the patient who feels dizzy, lightheaded, or faint be put back into bed with his head flat (not supported by a pillow) and his feet elevated?
8 How can you splint the leg of a hemiplegic patient when you are getting him out of bed? Demonstrate.
9 How could foot supports be made for your unit wheelchair?
10 How are the trays served to wheelchair patients on your unit? What type of over-the-wheelchair device could you provide to make it easier for the patient to eat?
11 Why is it dangerous to attempt to keep a patient in a sitting position by placing a sheet around his chest and under his arms and tying it to the wheelchair?
12 Read the morning paper to all your wheelchair patients as they sit quietly in the dayroom. Do this every morning for a week. Discuss your observations during this project.

VOCABULARY

amputee A patient who has had a limb or limbs removed surgically.
bilateral Occurring on both sides.
cyanosis Bluish color to lips, nail beds, tip of the nose, and earlobes. This is a sign that the blood is not getting enough oxygen to the cells of the body.
Davis roller Device for moving a patient from the bed to a stretcher, to another bed, or to an examining table.
dyspnea Difficulty in breathing.
mechanical lift Device for lifting a helpless patient out of bed to a chair, a bathtub, etc.
paraplegia Paralysis from the waist down. The paraplegic patient is unable to control the movements of his legs, his bladder, and his bowels.

SOURCES OF ADDITIONAL INFORMATION

1 Film: Emergency removal of patients; may be obtained from Abbott Laboratories Medical Film Service, North Chicago, Ill., 60064.
2 Film: Lifting and moving the patient (part of bed care Series) may be obtained from Encyclopaedia Britannica, 425 N. Michigan Ave., Chicago, Ill. 60611. 8 mm. 8-minute film. *(New and interesting Australian lifting technique demonstrated.)*
3 Film: Strokes; may be obtained from your local heart association.
4 Film: Stroke—early restorative measures in your hospital; may be obtained from Public Health Service Audiovisual Facility, Chamblee, Ga. 30005, Attn: Film Distribution.

14/Meeting the patient's need for sleep

STUDY QUESTIONS

1. How much sleep does a person need?
2. Do all patients need the same amount of sleep?
3. Of what value is sleep to the body?
4. How can you help the patient to sleep?
5. What causes the patient to awaken?
6. Can worry keep the patient awake?
7. What effect do prolonged periods of wakefulness have on the body?
8. What are the strongest arousal messages?
9. Why does the patient with breathing difficulties have trouble sleeping?
10. How does a sleeping pill help the patient sleep?
11. Why is the use of hypnotics avoided in a patient with breathing difficulty and sleeplessness?
12. Why should the patient who has received a hypnotic have crib sides in place on his bed?

THE BODY'S NEED FOR SLEEP

The body has two nervous systems—involuntary and voluntary. The involuntary nervous system regulates and controls those body functions not under the control of the will, such as heartbeat, breathing, blood pressure, digestion, and body temperature. The voluntary nervous system controls those body functions under the control of the will, such as walking, talking, moving, and seeing. These two systems are constantly monitoring the condition of the body, and they send messages to the midbrain immediately if a part of the body needs something. An example of this would be the way in which the involuntary nervous system to the rectum is stimulated and sends a message to the brain when the need to empty the rectum by defecation occurs. The voluntary nervous system determines the need to obtain facilities and stimulates the body to move—to sit up, get out of bed, and run to the bathroom. While this is occurring, the brain sends down via the voluntary nervous system a message for the anal sphincter to clamp down tightly and hold the feces until facilities are available. Another example of the workings of these systems might be the way in which the higher centers of the brain (those concerned with thinking, worrying, getting ideas, remembering, etc.) get the idea that a left-sided chest pain is a heart attack, and send this message to the midbrain. Immediately the midbrain sends a message to the nerves of the chest to watch this area carefully, and it alerts itself to focus its attention on that part of the body. Soon the individual becomes highly aware of his heartbeat, his breathing, and his pain, and he even begins to fear death, which he thinks is rapidly approaching.

The midbrain is constantly being informed of body needs and feelings by the higher brain centers and by the nerves of the body. As long as messages flow freely, the midbrain is extremely active and the person is awake. However, when all the body needs have been met and the messages have ceased to flow, the midbrain ceases to be excited and the person falls asleep. Wakefulness, then, is the result of stimulation of the midbrain by those nerves that carry the messages of body needs, whereas sleep results when body needs are met and the brain stimulation subsides.

However, sleep will be interrupted and wakefulness will recur when the brain becomes stimulated again by nerve messages of body needs. The strongest arousal messages are those of pain and of body needs such as the need to breathe, the need to void, and the need to defecate. Wakefulness does not occur automatically. The body has to be awakened by exciting the midbrain with messages of body need. The body needs sleep to restore the balance in the nervous system. It needs sleep to permit the nervous system to rest, free from the need to carry messages, so that it can regain its acute awareness of body need and its ability to control and regulate body functioning. Prolonged periods of wakefulness disturb the functioning of the nervous system and may result in symptoms such as sluggishness of thought, irritability, confusion, slow and exaggerated reactions, and psychosis.

During sleep the voluntary nervous system stops sending messages to the midbrain, and those muscles of the body under the control of the will (for example, the arms, legs, and back) are completely relaxed. However, the involuntary nervous system remains alert to control and regulate those activities of living not under the control of the will. The involuntary nervous system has two parts: the sympathetic part and the parasympathetic part.

The sympathetic part of the involuntary nervous system controls involuntary activity when the body is under stress. When the body is under the control of this part, the heart beats faster, the blood pressure rises, the gastrointestinal activity slows, the mouth dries, the pupils dilate, and the blood flow to the arm and leg muscles increases. The body is now ready to meet the emergency situation causing the stress.

The parasympathetic part controls involuntary activity when the body is relaxed, comfortable, and free of stress. The parasympathetic part controls the body under the usual conditions of life. The blood pressure falls, pulse rate decreases, breathing slows, and gastrointestinal activity increases.

During sleep the parasympathetic section of the involuntary nervous system functions to control the activities of living.

WAKEFULNESS

Sleep will be interrupted and wakefulness will occur as soon as the midbrain receives the message of a body need, such as one of the following:

1. To be relieved of pain
2. To breathe more effectively
3. To void
4. To defecate
5. To be relieved of fear
6. To be turned in order to relieve a tired back

When wakefullness occurs, it is maintained for a period of time, perhaps 15 to 30 minutes, even after the need is met. It takes this much time for brain activity to decrease so that sleep can recur.

THE BODY FOCUSES ITS ATTENTION ON THE SICK PART

When a nerve carries a message to the midbrain that a part of the body is in difficulty, the midbrain immediately focuses all its attention on that part, much as a mother focuses all her attention on a sick child. This mechanism of the midbrain, which permits it to select that part of the body in trouble for all its attention, tends to have the individual forget everything but his trouble. For example, the patient with a particle of dust in his eye thinks of nothing but his eye. The patient who cannot pass urine thinks of nothing but his inability to void. This usually creates behavior in the patient that is greatly exaggerated and out of proportion to the actual pain and distress caused by the affected body part.

One way to determine the actual level of the patient's discomfort and pain is to distract his attention from the sick body part by asking him to tell you about his difficulty. As you listen to his explanation, your concern and attention usually lessen his fear and worry, and he will be able to give a more accurate and less exaggerated description of his problem.

HOW MUCH SLEEP DOES THE PATIENT NEED?

If you asked your classmates how much sleep they needed, they would each give a different answer. Each person is different and has different needs. This fact is frequently forgotten when we are caring for patients. We forget that the patient is a person, just like you and me, who has some disease and who is now in the hospital because of it. However, his stay in the hospital will be only a temporary one. Soon he will move from his patient status in the hospital to resume his person status in the community. Therefore you should make his life in the hospital as similar to his life in the community as possible. On admission, ask the patient what his usual hour of sleep is and what his usual hour of awakening is. Tell him that you hope he can continue this sleep pattern in the hospital. This sleep pattern should also be written on the Kardex for the information of the entire unit staff.

The patient usually has difficulty adjusting to his illness, to the strange environment of the hospital, and to the enforced inactivity of lying in bed all day. Because of this, he may have difficulty going to sleep for the first night or two that he is in the hospital. If this difficulty does occur, the doctor and the nurse should be made aware of it so that they can give the patient a sleeping pill to help him sleep. When the patient is permitted to maintain his usual sleeping pattern at night and is provided with interesting activities (such as reading, television, or radio) during his waking hours, this sleeplessness quickly disappears and he soon sleeps well without the sleeping pill.

If you expect all the patients to change their sleeping patterns and go to sleep the minute that the lights go out, you will be greatly disappointed to find most of the patients awake, tossing restlessly about the bed, when you make rounds. Your critical remark of "Why aren't you asleep?" will only tell the patient that he should be asleep and may create a false need for a sleeping pill.

The acutely ill patient whose body is exhausted by fighting disease or the postoperative patient who is receiving hypodermic injections of narcotics to dull the brain's ability to receive the pain messages will sleep most of the 24 hours in each day. The patient who is convalescing will resume his usual pattern, which may consist of 7 or 8 hours of sleep in every 24 hours. The older patient, whose body tires more easily and who has less physical energy as well as fewer interests to occupy his attention, will sleep about 12 to 16 hours a day. The patient who has little stimulation of his midbrain from his higher brain centers, who has little interest in living, who has nothing to do all day long, and who is bored will sleep all day long. (What do you do when you are bored?) Therefore the patient who stays in bed all day when he should be up or the one who lies in a chair in the dayroom sleeping really needs some "life" put in his living.

PREPARING THE PATIENT FOR SLEEP

Preparing the patient for sleep consists of taking care of all his needs so that his body will not keep his brain awake with messages about its problems. Preparing the patient for bed is done in exactly the same way we prepare ourselves for bed and would include the following:

1. Make the patient's body comfortable.
   a. Just as you wash your body and brush your teeth, the patient should have his face and hands and back washed and his teeth cleaned.
   b. Just as you lie down in bed to take the weight off your feet, the patient's position should be changed and his back massaged well with alcohol or back-rub lotion to relieve the pressure on his back.
   c. Just as you go to the toilet to empty your bladder and bowels, the patient should receive a bedpan and/or a urinal to empty his bladder and bowels.
   d. Just as you take a drink of water before going to bed, the patient should receive an adequate supply of fresh water.
2. Make the patient's mind comfortable.
   a. Just as you check the stove and lock the door to be sure you are safe, the patient should be checked to be sure that his call bell or communication system is within easy reach so that he can call you if he needs something.
   b. Tell the patient that you will come around every 30 minutes to see him. This lets him relax because he is sure of your attention and care. Instruct the patient that there is no smoking in bed, especially at night.
3. Make the patient's unit comfortable.
   a. Just as you open your windows, put warm covers on your bed, and darken the room, give the patient extra blankets, turn out his overhead lights, and turn on the night lights in his area.
4. Be sure the nurse knows all about the patient's condition.
   a. Report to the nurse all the observations that you made about the patient while you were preparing him for sleep. This might include any complaints of pain, any trouble with breathing, any worries he expressed about himself, etc.
   b. As you make rounds every 30 minutes, go into the patient's area and observe him carefully. Is he sleeping? Is he breathing easily and noiselessly? Does his condition appear unchanged? Is he complaining of pain? Report these observations to your nurse at once.

Most of the chapters in the next section of this book will be concerned with such diagnostic and therapeutic techniques as checking temperature, pulse, and respiration, taking blood pressure, and giving treatments. Here it is sufficient to say that diagnostic or therapeutic measures ordered for the patient should be done before you prepare him for bed so that you will not need to awaken him for them. Remember that wakefulness will be maintained for a long period of time before the brain activity quiets down and permits sleep to recur.

When you make rounds and find a patient still awake, sit down in a chair near his bed and try to determine what body need is keeping him awake. Ask the patient how he is, and listen while he talks to you.

If you have adequately prepared the patient for sleep, the body need that is now keeping him awake will probably be fear—fear of what his hospitalization will mean to him in bills and expenses, fear of coming tests, fear of cancer, fear of an operation, or fear of dying. Stay with the patient and comfort him with your listening presence.

After you discover what his problems are, discuss them with the nurse. The nurse is frequently able to minimize the patient's apprehension and fear by explaining the tests or the operation. Sometimes the nurse may find it necessary to give the patient a sleeping pill, and at other times she may find it necessary to have the doctor see the patient. A sleeping pill helps the patient go to sleep because it decreases or lessens the ability of the midbrain to receive nerve messages from the body.

OBSERVATIONS OF THE SLEEPING PATIENT

Make rounds every 30 minutes, check the patients carefully, and answer patients' signals promptly. A patient who seems quite comfortable when you prepare him for bed may have a serious worsening of his condition 30 minutes later. Therefore know what the nurse expects you to observe in each patient and make these observations faithfully every 30 minutes during your rounds.

The patient may be awakened by some new pain or ache or some strange, frightening sound that makes him extremely apprehensive. Every second that he waits for you to answer the signal increases his fear and apprehension a hundred times. Therefore answer signals promptly at night. This will prevent the patient from becoming distraught and will increase the possibility of his returning to sleep easily. Remember, the patient does not awaken for no reason; he has been awakened by some body need.

The patient who has marked breathing difficulties will be afraid to sleep. Perhaps he will doze off for short periods, only to be awakened by his need for oxygen. Therefore he will be extremely apprehensive, because of his shortness of breath, each time he awakens. Visit such a patient frequently. Answer his call signal immediately. Once he is sure that you are watching him closely, he will be less frightened and more able to sleep for short intervals throughout the night.

This patient will probably not receive a sleeping pill (hypnotic) from the nurse because the sleeping pill will decrease the ability of the midbrain to receive the message from the body that it needs more oxygen. If the brain is so dulled that it does not receive the message, it will not set in motion the patient's increased breathing to bring in more oxygen. Therefore the patient will be unable to meet the oxygen need of the body and may even die.

SLEEPING PILLS

Hypnotics, or drugs given to induce sleep, do so by dulling the midbrain's ability to receive nerve messages from the body about its needs. The patient who has received this hypnotic or sleeping pill may be jolted only half awake by the body messages of pain or the need to void. He may not know where he is, or how he got there, or what is happening. All that he does know is that he has a pain or a need to void.

In his half-awakened state the patient may think that he is at home, and so he may attempt to get out of bed to meet his need. If so and if the bed is high, he may fall. Safe nursing practice therefore is to place crib sides on the beds of all patients who receive hypnotics and to make rounds to their rooms frequently. This is especially indicated in all patients over 50 years of age, since hypnotics tend to make the older patient confused at night.

Sleeping pills do nothing to relieve pain. In fact, they tend to excite and confuse the patient with pain, since the midbrain gets the message but is sluggish in interpreting it and in putting into action those activities necessary for the body to get the help it needs.

Each evening, ask the nurse for a list of those patients who need the protection of crib sides on their beds because they have received hypnotics. Visit these patients promptly and pull the crib sides into position.

SUMMARY

Sleep occurs when the midbrain becomes quiet because the body is comfortable and the nerves are no longer carrying messages of body needs. Wakefulness occurs when a part of the body sends the message of its need to the midbrain. Wakefulness occurs as the brain sets the body into action in an attempt to satisfy the need of that body part in difficulty. In this way, the patient always awakens with a problem. The strongest arousal messages are sent by the following body needs:

1. Relief of pain
2. To breathe
3. To void
4. To defecate

Preparation of the patient for sleeping involves satisfying all the patient's needs. Then his comfortable body sends no messages, and the midbrain decreases its activities and sleep occurs.

DISCUSSION QUESTIONS

1 Do you receive a list of the bed patients on your unit each afternoon as you get the evening report?
2 How do you set up your "patient preparation for sleeping" cart?
3 Does the nurse give you a list each evening of those patients who have received hypnotics?
4 What is the policy in your hospital about putting crib sides on the beds of patients who have received hypnotics?
5 What patients on your ward awaken frequently throughout the night? Discuss these patients with the nurse and try to determine what body needs are awakening them.
6 Why do patients need a urinal or bedpan on awakening?
7 What time are the lights turned out in your unit? What happens to the patient who does not feel like sleeping?
8 How do you know that a patient is having difficulty sleeping?
9 Check those patients on your ward with breathing difficulty. Do they awaken frequently? Develop a plan for giving them the assurance that you are watching them closely so that they can sleep.

VOCABULARY

body reaction to stress Changes in the body brought about by the sympathetic nervous system in answer to a threat. These include (1) dilation of the pupils, (2) quickened heartbeat, (3) increased pulse, (4) elevated blood pressure, (5) increased blood flow to the arms and legs, (6) decreased production of saliva in the mouth, (7) decreased intestinal activity, (8) excitement of the brain, and (9) released energy. Pain, worry, fear, and anger are all stressful situations that make the body function in this manner. The patient's body has prepared him to fight or flee. This explains the basis for the unusual behavior of the patient with these emotions.

hypnotic Drug that produces sleep by dulling the brain so that it does not receive messages from the body.

parasympathetic nervous system That part of the involuntary nervous system that under usual conditions controls and regulates body processes not under control of the will.

stress A situation that threatens the security of the individual. The body reacts to this stress (threat) by speeding up the body processes to enable it to fight or flee.

sympathetic nervous system That part of the involuntary nervous system that in times of stress takes over, controls, and regulates body processes not under control of the will.

SOURCES OF ADDITIONAL INFORMATION

1 Film: Nursing care: evening and morning care; may be obtained from Director, Medical Film Library, United States Naval Medical School, National Naval Medical Center, Bethesda, Md. 20014.
2 Film: Pain and its alleviation; may be obtained from University of California Film Service; rental charge, $18.50 for three days. *(Shows how nerves carry messages to the brain and how the body responds to the pain message. Depicts reactions of several patients to pain. Nurse is shown in each case listening to the patient, determining the cause of pain, and using appropriate nursing techniques to relieve it.)*

THE NURSING ASSISTANT MEETS THE PATIENT'S PARTICULAR NEEDS IN THE HOSPITAL AND EXTENDED CARE FACILITY

SECTION III

Chapter 15 Receiving the patient on the ward
15 Receiving the patient on the ward
16 Caring for the patient's emotional environment
17 Maintaining a safe physical environment for the patient
18 Identifying, recording, and reporting the patient's needs
19 The vital signs
20 Taking the patient's temperature
21 Taking the patient's pulse
22 Counting the patient's respirations
23 Taking the patient's blood pressure
24 Observing the patient's level of consciousness
25 Charting temperature, pulse, and respiration
26 Collecting specimens from the patient
27 Giving the patient an enema
28 Caring for the patient with a colostomy
29 Caring for the patient with an ileostomy, a "wet" ileostomy, or ureterostomies
30 Applying heat to the patient's body in the presence of infection
31 Reducing the patient's temperature
32 Internal and external urinary drainage

15/Receiving the patient on the ward

STUDY QUESTIONS

1. What clues do you get about the patient:
   a. From the way he is admitted to the ward?
   b. From his vital signs?
   c. From his physical signs?
   d. From his symptoms?
2. What is a sign of illness?
3. What is the difference between a sign and a symptom?
4. What questions can you ask the patient to elicit his symptoms?
5. How can you discover the signs of illness without creating apprehension on the part of the patient?
6. What observations would you make about the patient's mouth?
7. Should you chart whether or not the patient has false teeth? Why?
8. What observations should you make about the patient before you put him in bed?
9. What clues can you get during the admission of the patient that will help you to know how to care for him?
10. What is included in the admission note on the chart?
11. How do you help the doctor examine the patient?

THE PATIENT COMES TO THE WARD

After checking to be sure that a bed is available, the admitting department informs the head nurse that a patient is being admitted. Usually enough information is given about the patient to enable the personnel to set up the kind of unit the patient needs. The head nurse or team leader will then assign one of the nursing assistants to stand by to receive the patient and to take him to his already prepared hospital unit. The patient who is received in this manner feels that the nursing staff members are really concerned about him and that they want to help him, and much of his fear and apprehension about coming to the hospital begins to subside.

However, if the head nurse is not aware of the fact that a patient is coming and the unit is not ready for him, the patient will be forced to remain in the hall while members of the staff rush about getting facilities ready. As he sits, stands, or lies in the hall and watches the ward staff gather linen, clean the unit, and make the bed while he remains there alone in his pain, he feels lonely, unwanted, and in the way. A feeling of helplessness and hopelessness overcomes him as he realizes that the ward staff does not care about him. As a result he may become quiet and depressed, or he may decide to fight for the care he needs by becoming an aggressive, demanding patient. Therefore you must recognize how important this person, your patient, is. You must receive him on the ward in a quiet and efficient but friendly manner. You must be pleased to see him and as concerned about his comfort as you are about the comfort of guests you receive in your own home.

THE TRIP TO THE WARD

The patient arrives on the ward with an escort from the admitting service. The way he comes will depend on his condition. If he is seriously ill, he may be brought on a stretcher. If he has difficulty walking or standing but is not seriously ill, he may be brought in a wheelchair. However, if he is able to walk without any serious pain or danger to himself, he may walk up to the ward. Therefore you receive a clue to the seriousness of the patient's illness or physical discomfort by the manner in which he is brought to the ward.

ADMITTING THE PATIENT TO THE WARD

If the nurse assigned you to admit the patient on the ward, greet him, introduce yourself, and take him to his already prepared unit. Take his chart from the escort assistant and give it to the head nurse or ward clerk.

Observe the patient carefully to determine whether or not the bed is adequately prepared to meet his needs before you put him in it. Make the following observations and take the appropriate nursing actions:
1. Does the patient move about easily? Will he need help to move? If he will need help, put a lifting sheet on the bed.
2. Does the patient understand what is said to him? Does he give appropriate answers? If he does not, put crib sides on the bed.
3. Does the patient have a broken bone or a backache? If he does, check with the nurse to find out if a bed board is to be placed under the mattress.
4. Is the patient paralyzed? Is he unconscious? If he is, put a rubber sheet covered by a drawsheet on the bed, since he will probably be incontinent.
5. Does the patient have difficulty breathing? Is he short of breath? Crank up the head of the bed if he has difficulty breathing.

After he has been observed, screen him to ensure him privacy. Assist him in undressing and help him into bed. Handle his clothing carefully. Remember, he will be wearing it to return home. List each item on the proper hospital form, and then hang the clothing in his closet if he is in a private room or send it to the hospital clothing room if he is in a ward. Get it ready for his family if they are going to take it home. Also check and list the patient's valuables on the proper hospital form. Inform the patient of the hospital facilities for safeguarding his money and valuables. Ask him if he would like to use these facilities.

When the patient is comfortably in bed, proceed with the next part of the admission procedure, which is gathering as many clues about his illness as you can. Take his vital signs—temperature, pulse, respiration, and blood pressure. Jot them down on a piece of paper. If the patient is confused, unconscious, or dyspneic (short of breath), be sure to take his temperature rectally.

Observe his body for signs of illness. These signs would include any of the following:
1. *Head:* bumps; cuts; scratches; lice (suspect lice if scratches present)
2. *Face:* flushed; pale; cyanotic; cut; bruised; scarred; grimaces of pain; tics (twitchlike movements)
3. *Eyes:* jaundiced (white part is yellow); ecchymotic (hemorrhage under the skin, commonly called black eye); difficulty in seeing
4. *Lips:* cyanotic (blue); dry, cracked;

presence of cold sores (herpes simplex)
5. *Ears:* draining; difficulty in hearing
6. *Tongue:* dry; red; swollen; evidence of being bitten; presence of sordes (dark brown dried material)
7. *Skin:* hot; cold; dry; moist; jaundiced; scarred; cuts; presence of ecchymosed areas
8. *Teeth:* absence; dentures; number of plates or bridges
9. *Arms:* evidence of paralysis (inability to move) or paresis (weakness; compare one arm with the other for strength); fingernail beds cyanotic; joints swollen (shoulder, elbow, wrist, finger)
10. *Chest:* coughing, expectorating blood or mucus (describe as green, yellow, or white, thick or watery)
11. *Abdomen:* distended (enlarged with skin taut; sometimes distention so great that umbilicus may be pushed out)
12. *Genitals:* edematous, swollen penis or scrotum; groin raw and excoriated
13. *Legs:* evidence of paralysis or paresis (weakness); edematous ankles; brownish discoloration above ankles; leg ulcers; black discoloration of toes (gangrene); open areas (sores) on heels or soles of feet; swollen joints (hip, knee, ankles, toes)
14. *Back:* reddened areas on sacrum; decubitus ulcers

These observations can be made easily, without creating any apprehension on the part of the patient, while you are undressing him.

Then ask the patient to tell you about this illness that brought him to the hospital. These discomforts or interruptions in normal body functions that the patient tells you about are called symptoms. Sometimes the patient is so frightened or upset about his hospitalization or is in so much pain that he does not know what to say. You can help him get his thoughts in order by asking him some questions about how his body functions. Listen carefully as he relates his symptoms and ask him to describe them fully. These questions and their possible answers might include the following:

1. Do you have any difficulty moving? (Patient will then relate symptoms of paralyzed or weak limbs, pain on movement, or difficulty standing, walking, or sitting.)
2. Do you have any difficulty eating? (Patient will then relate symptoms of inability to tolerate certain foods and of distress after eating such as belching, gas, nausea, and vomiting; be sure to ask him to describe any vomitus. He may also complain of loss or increase in appetite and of excessive weight gain or loss.)
3. Do you have any difficulty with bowel movements or urination? (The patient will then relate symptoms of constipation, diarrhea, bloody stools, or pain on defecation. He may also relate symptoms of difficulty starting his urinary stream, dribbling after urination, increased urination together with the need to get out of bed at night to void, or of pain on voiding.)
4. Do you have any difficulty breathing? (The patient may then relate symptoms of dyspnea on exertion or dyspnea when he lies flat. He may also relate symptoms of pain on breathing. Ask him to describe the position that makes his breathing easiest. He may also relate symptoms of coughing and of expectorating.)
5. Do you have any discharges from your body? (The patient may relate symptoms of bleeding from the rectum or the genitals or of expectorating or vomiting blood. He may also describe discharges of pus from the rectum or genitals.)
6. Do you have pain? If so, describe it. Do you know of anything that makes it better? Anything that makes it

worse? (The patient may then describe, if he has not done so previously, sharp, dull, throbbing, pressing, or squeezing pains in an area of his body.)
7. Are you receiving treatment for any medical condition? (The patient may quickly answer "no" because all chronic illness may be forgotten in the pain of his present problem. Pursue this point by asking specific questions such as follows: Do you have diabetes? Do you have any allergies to drugs such as penicillin?)
8. Do you have difficulty sleeping? (The patient may tell you that he slept well until he developed this present condition but that he is unable to sleep now. Ask him to tell you about his usual sleeping pattern.)

You may not need to ask all these questions of the patient who comes to the hospital with a rather obvious local disease (affecting one part). A patient who comes to the hospital because he has fallen and broken his arm is an example. However, if you do ask these questions, you may find that the patient has had bleeding from the rectum for the past 8 months but that he did not seek medical care because he was too embarrassed. You may also find other symptoms that will lead the doctor to discover diabetes, ulcers, or a venereal disease such as gonorrhea. Since the doctor is busy, often the patient hides many symptoms that he feels are unimportant, but he will tell them to you if you take the time to listen and if you show him that you are interested.

The conversation just described between you and the patient (about his symptoms) may reveal a history of a previous hospitalization. However, if it does not, ask the patient if he has ever been in the hospital before. If he has, ask what hospital he was in and what they did for him there.

Do not stand over the patient with a pencil and paper and ask these questions as though you were a newspaper reporter having an interview. Sit facing the patient. Try to show him by your manner that nothing else matters at that moment but him. Ask your questions in a way that shows your concern for the patient and your interest in helping him get well. Jot down briefly those facts that you want to chart later.

Explain to the patient how the hospital functions to give him care. Tell him when meals are served and where he will eat. Show him the bathroom facilities if he is permitted out of bed. Explain how he can notify you of his needs if he is a bed patient. Demonstrate how the call bell or communication system operates. Explain the rules about smoking in the hospital. Give him the names of the head nurse and his doctor. Tell him when the doctor will come to see him. Introduce him to the other patients in the area. This introduction consists of names only and does not include a history of illnesses. Remember, everything that the patient tells you is confidential material shared only with other members of the ward staff.

Check with the nurse to find out if the patient is permitted to have water. If he is, get him a pitcher of ice water and a glass. Make him as comfortable as possible. Be sure his call system is within easy reach, and then return to the nurse's station and give the nurse a report of your findings about the patient. Then chart your observations on the nurse's record on the patient's chart (see sample admission form on p. 140). These observations would include all those clues you discovered about the patient and his illness, such as the following:
1. Vital signs
2. Signs you observed
3. Symptoms described to you by the patient

Then chart all the information the patient gave you that will affect his care in the hospital. This would include the following:

1. Previous hospitalizations
2. Allergies (such as penicillin)
3. Diseases other than the one for which he is now in the hospital (such as diabetes)
4. Prostheses (such as false teeth)

Make no statement about the patient's degree of illness. Chart only what you saw or heard and what the patient has told you.

Communicate to other members of the ward staff those clues that will help them care for the patient by writing them on his nursing care plan in the Kardex (see sample Kardex notations on p. 139). These clues would include the following:
1. Foods the patient cannot eat
2. Difficulties the patient has in seeing or hearing
3. Factors that increase the patient's pain, his breathing difficulty, or his physical discomfort
4. Allergies other than food allergies that the patient possesses
5. Fears
6. Nature of the patient's physical problem

Some specific examples of the kind of clues that will help the nursing staff care for the patient are the following:
1. Patient is hard of hearing—Talk loudly and stand in front of him as you speak to him.
2. Patient cannot talk but does understand—Explain what you want him to do and he will cooperate fully.
3. Patient is confused; he does not seem to understand what is said to him and he thinks he is at home—Keep the crib sides in place.
4. Patient is paralyzed on his right side —Keep the bedside table on his left side, serve food from the left side, and feed him from the left side.
5. Patient talks constantly about the lump in his throat and feels sure that it is cancer.
6. Patient usually slept from 11:30 P.M. to 6:30 A.M. before his illness.

These clues will be expanded into an individualized nursing care plan for the patient by the entire nursing team during the evaluation rounds. (See Chapter 3.)

HELPING THE PATIENT ADJUST TO HOSPITAL LIVING

Continue with your other work after you have admitted the patient and charted all your findings, but do not forget him. He has been thrust into this new frightening world of the hospital where he has to depend on others for his every need. He lies in bed wondering and fearing what will happen to him next. Hospital sounds are magnified and may frighten him with their strangeness. He sees patients wheeled off the ward on stretchers and wonders where they are going and if he will have to go too. He watches these stretcher-borne patients return and he strains to see if the trip caused them more pain or discomfort.

He watches the ward staff go about their work and he searches their manner and their actions for signs that they care about the patients. "If the staff members care about the other patients," he reasons, "they will also care about me." However, he knows no one but you, so he will evaluate the entire hospital staff on the basis of how you take care of him. If you stop by his bed or visit his room frequently to see how he is and to determine if he needs anything, his apprehensions about the hospital and the staff will be relieved by your caring. However, if you come only when he calls, he may become more and more frightened and worried about what will happen to him if he needs you and cannot reach the signal cord or talk into the communication system.

The patient's mind is extremely active, and since it is not activated by meeting the needs of living, it becomes concerned with the problems of illness. One of two behavior patterns may develop: (1) the patient may focus all of his attention on his illness, which may cause him to exaggerate his symptoms to such an extent that he needs constant attention from you, or (2) the patient may deny the fact that he is ill and may refuse to accept the doctor's treatment or to follow his advice. On one hand, the patient's worry and fear may cause him to become a demanding patient who always needs something. On the other hand, his worry and fear may threaten him so that he does the exact opposite of what the doctor tells him. He does this in an attempt to prove that the doctor is wrong and that this illness is not serious. Then the members of the nursing staff label the patient as uncooperative. However, your frequent visits and your constant attention will show the patient that he is in capable hands, and his overconcern about himself will be transformed into anticipation of your next visit.

THE PLAN FOR THE PATIENT'S CARE

The doctor will come to see the patient as soon as his work load permits. He will read your notes on the chart and then go to see the patient. First, he will take a detailed history of that aspect of the patient's life that may have an effect on his health. Then he will examine the patient thoroughly. The physician will need a female nursing assistant to help with the examination and to chaperon the female patient. A physician will also need a male nursing assistant's help when a male patient is being examined.

The physician usually needs the following equipment:
1. Stethoscope (usually the doctor has his own)
2. Blood pressure apparatus
3. Tongue blades
4. Flashlight
5. Ophthalmoscope
6. Reflex hammer
7. Draping sheet
8. Pair of rubber gloves or finger cots and lubricant

When the doctor asks you to assist him or when the head nurse assigns you to assist him, collect all the equipment just listed. Test the flashlight and the ophthalmoscope. Take the equipment to the patient's bedside. Fold the patient's bedcovers to the foot of the bed and cover him with a sheet.

Assist the doctor as follows:
1. Lower the window shades and turn out the lights as the doctor examines the reaction of the patient's eyes to light.
2. Discard the used tongue blade after the doctor examines the patient's throat.
3. Expose the patient's front chest; then, if the patient is a woman, hold up the left breast while the doctor listens to the heart.
4. Assist the patient to sit up in bed and then expose the back of the chest. Direct the patient to follow the instructions the doctor gives such as "breathe through your mouth" or "hold your breath."
5. Help the patient lie down and then cover the front chest and expose the abdomen. Instruct the patient to bend the knees slightly to relax the abdominal muscles.
6. Then cover the abdomen and expose the legs. This can be done easily by bunching the sides of the sheets together and placing them between the patient's legs (Fig. 15-1).
7. Position the patient for a pelvic (internal) and rectal examination.
    a. For the pelvic examination, have the patient assume a back-lying position and bend up both knees. Pull the sheet over the patient in such a way that it is diamond shaped. Cover both legs with the sides (corners) of the sheet and expose the genitalia by lifting up the bottom corner.
    b. For the rectal examination this same position may be used. However, if only a rectal examination

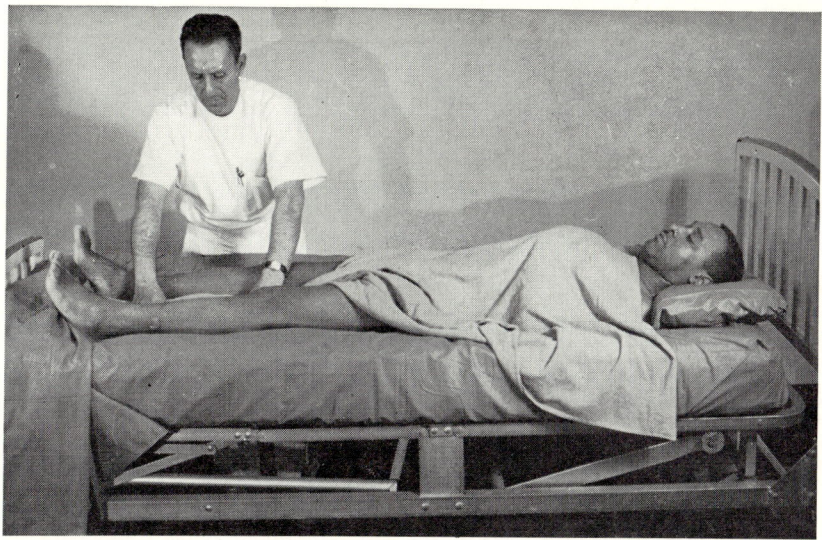

Fig. 15-1. The nursing assistant exposing the patient's legs while assisting the physician with the examination of the patient.

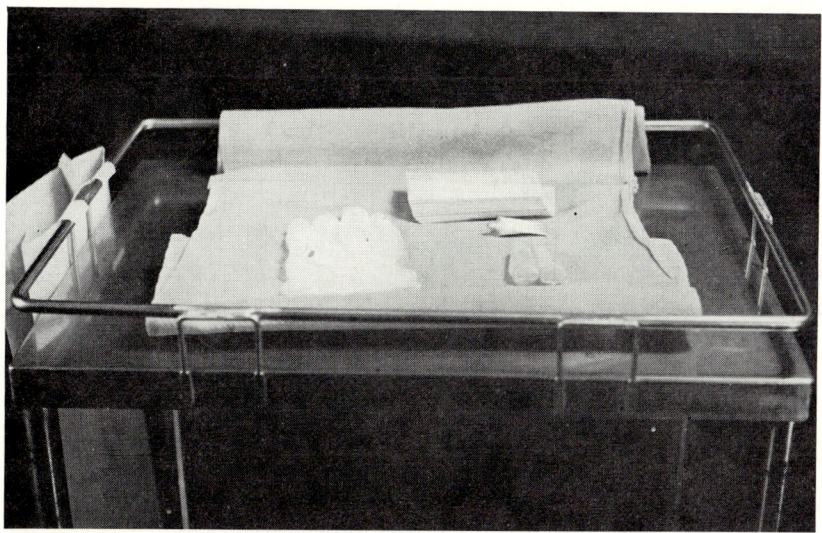

Fig. 15-2. Rectal examination tray containing gloves and/or finger cots, lubricant, and toilet paper.

is done, the patient may be turned to a side-lying position.
8. Assist the doctor in putting on his rubber gloves (or finger cot) and squirt some lubricant on the doctor's rubber glove–covered hand. (See Fig. 15-2.)

This usually completes the examination, and the doctor will return to the office to write up the chart. You remain with the patient. Remove the draping sheet, pull up the top bedclothes, and help the patient into a comfortable position. Collect all the examining equipment and take it back to the doctor's office or to the treatment room.

The doctor may ask you to weigh the patient. Take the standing scale (if the patient is permitted to get out of bed and stand on it) or the bed scale (if the patient is unable to get out of bed) to the patient's room and weigh him. Look at the measurements on the scale carefully. Measurements on the standing scale usually are in pounds and ounces, whereas those on the bed scale usually are in kilograms (2.2 pounds equal 1 kilogram) and tenths of a kilogram. Report the weight in the measure on the scale. Do not attempt to convert pounds to kilograms or kilograms to pounds.

The patient is placed on the overbed scale by turning the patient to the side and by positioning the scale over the bed on the opposite side. The patient is rolled back onto the stretcherlike carrier of the scale that is over the bed (Fig. 15-3). Then the carrier is raised until it is free of the bed, and the scale is manipulated to determine the weight. Report the weight to the doctor and chart it.

The patient's weight may be important to the doctor in calculating medication doses or in evaluating the patient's progress. If the patient is edematous and the doctor has prescribed diuretics, he will gauge their effectiveness by the patient's weight loss. If the patient is hemorrhaging, the doctor may gauge the degree of bleeding by the weight loss. For the weight to be significant, it must be determined each day at the same time and under the same conditions. Daily weights are usually taken each morning after the patient voids and before he has breakfast and a bowel movement. The patient must wear the same amount and type of clothing at each weighing.

After the patient has been examined and weighed, the doctor will prescribe the diagnostic measures to be taken, the laboratory tests to be made, the medications to be given, the treatments to be carried out, and the vital signs to be observed. The head

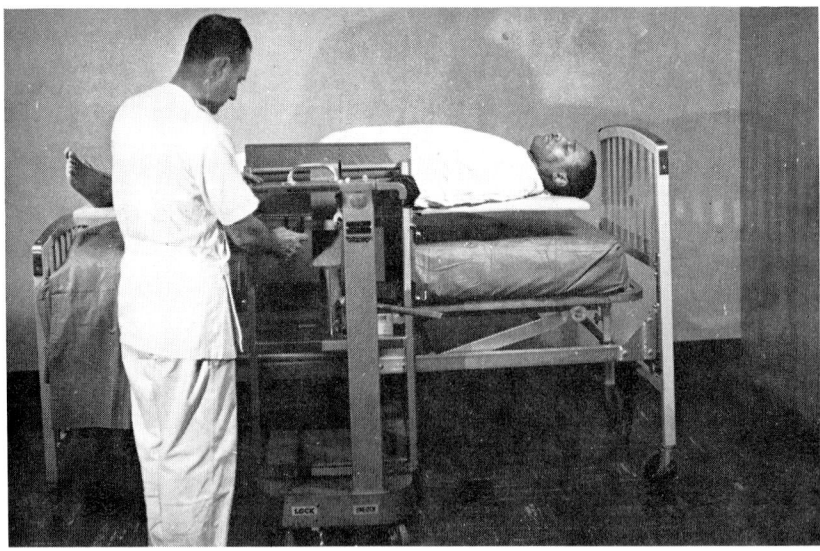

Fig. 15-3. The nursing assistant weighing the bed patient on the overbed scale. Note the scale lock.

nurse or team leader will meet the team and together they will develop a plan of nursing care for the patient. You will be assigned to do those nursing care activities in this plan that you are able to do. Part of the responsibility of the care of the patient is in your hands, and the doctor and nurse expect you to do it in the very best way that you know how and to keep them informed of any changes in the patient's signs or symptoms. You can do all these things easily if you care for this patient in the same way that you would want him to care for you if your positions were reversed.

OBSERVATIONS OF THE PATIENT

Many diagnostic studies and laboratory tests will have to be done before the doctor makes a diagnosis. Therefore, during your care of the patient, you will have to look at the patient's body for new signs of illness and listen to his symptoms for improvement or worsening of his condition. Chart these signs and symptoms that you observe daily as soon as you make them.

SPECIAL NOTE

The nursing service in your hospital will identify those patient care activities that you are to do when admitting a patient. They may or may not include taking blood pressures, charting, and assisting the physician. The inclusion of these procedures in this book does not imply that these tasks should be delegated to nursing assistants. Perform according to your own job description when admitting a patient to the hospital in which you are employed.

SUMMARY

The patient is a person who comes to the hospital for medical and nursing care because he is unable to go on living comfortably with his painful body. The signs and symptoms that he presents will give you many clues about his difficulty and many clues about how you can help him during his stay in the hospital.

The doctor will examine the patient thoroughly soon after his admission, but he will be unable to establish a diagnosis

SAMPLE KARDEX NOTATIONS OF ADMISSION OBSERVATIONS*

	NURSING CARE PLAN	
DATE	PATIENT'S NEED	NURSING ACTION
10/28/72	Patient has difficulty hearing.	Speak loudly and stand in front of the patient when you talk to him.
10/28/72	Patient is very restless; moves around the bed constantly.	Keep crib sides in position on bed. Visit patient frequently and sit with him as much as possible.
10/28/72	Patient complains of severe pain when right leg is moved.	Handle right leg carefully.
10/28/72	Patient states that he is allergic to penicillin.	Chart marked with notice that patient is allergic to penicillin.

*These admission observations will be expanded into a therapeutic nursing care plan for the patient during the team meeting.

SAMPLE ADMISSION FORM

	HOUR		
DATE	A.M.	P.M.	OBSERVATIONS
			NURSING NOTES
			Admitted to unit _____ Via _____
			Admission diagnosis _____
			X-ray taken on admission _____
			Sex _____ Age _____ Race _____
			TPR _____ B/P _____
			HT _____ WT _____
			Patient's complaints _____
			Clinical observations _____
			Known allergies _____
			Prosthetic appliances _____
			Money _____ Valuables _____
			Smoking regulations _____
			Doctor _____ Notifed of admission and condition of patient by _____
			at _____ A.M. / P.M.
			Signature of admitting nurse _____

Patient's identification   Unit No.

until many studies and tests are done. Therefore he will depend on you to observe the patient's signs and symptoms.

The patient is a frightened person entering a strange new world of examinations, tests, treatments, and medicines. He does not know what the doctor will find out about his body and he does not know whether the illness is curable or not. He is frightened and he needs you.

Receive the patient on your ward as you would a guest in your own home, and care for him as you care for yourself. Remember that you are his muscles, legs, and arms.

DISCUSSION QUESTIONS

1 How is the patient's clothing safeguarded on your unit?
2 How do you care for the patient's clothing if he is admitted at night?
3 Which patients are sicker—those admitted during the day or those admitted at night? What significance would this have for you if you were on night duty?
4 Do patients ever lose their false teeth on your unit? Why?
5 Think about the last patient you admitted. How could you have done it better?
6 Check the Kardex on the last patient admitted to your unit. What clues does it give you about caring for him?
7 Read the admission note on that patient whose Kardex you checked in question 6. What further information could have been written on the Kardex?
8 Ask the nurse to let you admit the next patient to your unit. Ask the nurse to help you with the admission note and Kardex notes.
9 What is the difference between a sign and a symptom? Give examples of each.
10 Help the doctor do a physical examination. Notice how carefully he checks the patient's body. Do you observe the patient carefully when you give him a bath?
11 How many times do you visit your patients when you have nothing to do for them?
12 How helpful are your admission observations to the team planning the therapeutic nursing care for that patient?

VOCABULARY

aggressive Striking out constantly; usually refers to an angry, fighting patient.
ambulatory Walking.
confused Not responding appropriately to what is said or asked.
cyanotic Having a bluish tinge to lips, fingernail beds, earlobes, or tip of nose; signifies oxygen want.
demanding Continually asking for things.
distention Filling of the abdominal contents with gas or fluid so that the abdomen becomes greatly enlarged and the skin over it becomes taut and shiny.
ecchymosed Showing bluish discoloration due to blood under this skin. (A black eye is really an ecchymosed eye.)
excoriated Skin rubbed off, watery fluid oozing out through broken skin.
expectorating Spitting.
gangrene Death of tissue.
incontinent Unable to control voiding and/or defecating.
jaundiced Characterized by yellowish color; whites of eyes and skin may be yellow.
Kardex Patient care plan card.
signs Clues to the patient's illness that you can see or hear.
symptoms Things that the patient tells you about his illness.
umbilicus Navel.

16/Caring for the patient's emotional environment

STUDY QUESTIONS

1. What are the emotional needs of the patient?
2. Why is the patient fearful of each new test or treatment?
3. How can you dispel this fear?
4. What can you tell the patient about his forthcoming test?
5. What are the emotional needs of the convalescing patient?
6. How does the convalescing patient express his emotional needs?
7. Is the hospital boring to patients? Does it have to be?
8. How can you make your unit more interesting and more livable for the out-of-bed patient?

THE PATIENT COMES TO THE HOSPITAL

The patient comes to the hospital because his body or mind is causing him so much discomfort that his living has become painful and he needs the relief that medical and nursing care can give. He is concerned about himself and may be fearful of dying, of having cancer, or of being helpless. He is confused by the mysteries of his pain. With each diagnostic test he worries about what the doctor might find and about the pain associated with the test.

During the acute phase of illness, when he is being examined and tested constantly, the patient needs explanations of what is being done for him, why it is being done, how it will be done, and the results that can be expected. The patient is vitally concerned about himself. Therefore he must have this kind of information because all that he does not know frightens him.

When you are caring for the patient, you will need to listen to his conversation carefully and ask yourself why he is telling you about himself. Is the patient who tells you that he is having a heart study (EKG) telling you this because he thinks you do not know, or is he telling you because he does not know anything about it and wants you to explain what is going to happen? Is the patient who tells you that he is having his stomach removed (gastrectomy) giving you information, or is he asking for it?

The patient is well aware of the fact that you know what tests or treatments are scheduled for him. Therefore the patient's telling is really his asking. Once you understand this, you will be able to remove much of the patient's fear during his hospital stay by explaining away the mystery and the worry that causes it by fully preparing him for each hospital experience with an adequate explanation.

Each morning as soon as you receive your patient care assignment from the head nurse, which will indicate any special tests or studies scheduled for your patients, ask her what kind of explanation you should give to the patients about them. Also, since explanations to patients will be much easier to give when you know what happens during the different diagnostic tests and studies, observe as many different kinds of studies as possible. However, it is extremely important for you to check with the doctor or the nurse regarding just what kind of explanation the patients are to have. The doctor or nurse will help you to understand that the patients must have enough information about the study to remove their fears but that they should not be told all the painful details.

For example, a patient who is having a spinal tap should be told that he will have to roll over on his side and curl up in a ball while the doctor takes a specimen of spinal fluid from his back. The specimen of spinal fluid will be taken, you can explain, in much the same way as a blood specimen is taken from the arm. The patient does not need to know the size of the needle or how deeply it is inserted. He will receive a local anesthetic that will deaden his pain. All that the patient really needs to know is what he has to do during the test, when the doctor is doing it, and what discomfort he can expect from it. The patient who receives a good explanation is not frightened, his muscles are relaxed, and the study can be accomplished easily. Therefore you help the patient and you also help the doctor when you prepare the patient well.

THE CONVALESCING PATIENT

After the diagnosis has been made and the treatment is started, the improving, or convalescing patient may be transferred from the acute care hospital to a nursing home or an extended care unit. The mystery and fear and pain of the acute hospital is over, but the long waiting for recovery is very boring. The patient may be out of bed, but he has no place to go and nothing to do. He becomes restless, irritable, and full of complaints of his boredom. During this phase of his hospitalization, the patient, who was a busy person before his illness, again needs something to keep him busy.

The following are some ways that you might make the patient's environment more interesting:

1. Contact the librarian and have him visit the patient, or, better yet, take the patient to the library.
2. Arrange for the patient to eat in the patients' dining room (Fig. 16-1). If there is no dining room for patients, arrange to set up a ward dining room in the patients' lounge. After mealtimes, the tables could be used for recreational activities. Take a look at the patients' lounge. Does it have anything in it besides chairs?
3. Obtain recreational equipment for the patients' lounge. This might consist of a television set, a card game, and even a record player. Take a survey of the out-of-bed patients and find out what kind of activities would interest them. This information will give you a good idea of what kind of equipment to get.
4. Take the out-of-bed patients to the hospital barber shop or beauty parlor.
5. Request assistance from the volun-

teer service and set up special programs for the long-term helpless or blind patients. Perhaps a volunteer could come to the patients' lounge each day to read and discuss the daily paper. Perhaps a volunteer could conduct an afternoon or evening program, such as card game sessions or motion picture programs.

6. Schedule patient teaching programs

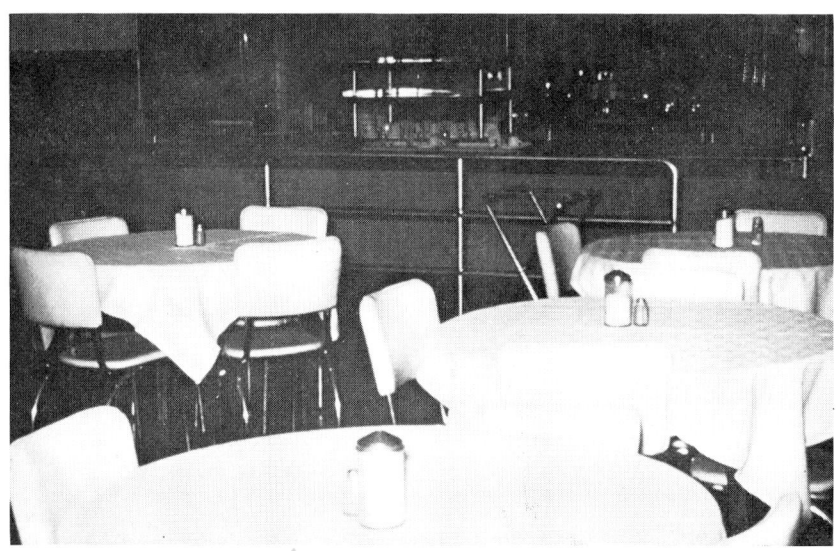

Fig. 16-1. Patients' dining room. Note the serving counter where the patient is able to select his own food.

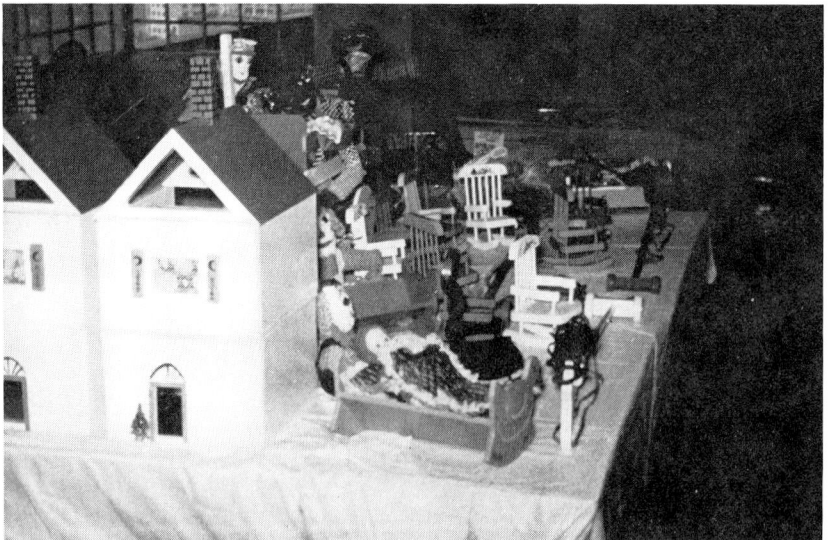

Fig. 16-2. Toys built by long-term patients for a nearby crippled children's hospital. This project was done under the direction of the occupational therapy department.

in the patients' lounge. This type of program would need to be conducted by the nurse. However, as a result of your observations of patients' problems and the questions they ask you, you might make the doctor or the nurse aware of this need. Such scheduled programs might offer the patients opportunities to learn more about their illness, their diet, and their care after discharge so that they can maintain their health.

7. Secure the consultation and the participation of the occupational therapy department. Perhaps they will be able to provide a therapist at a regularly scheduled time each day to conduct a program in arts and crafts in the patients' lounge (Fig. 16-2).
8. Provide opportunities for patients to make trips to the hospital cafeteria or gift shop.
9. Visit the patients' lounge often and engage the patients there in the kind of friendly conversation you have with friends.
10. Set up and stock a rack in the patients' lounge with health education materials. Pamphlets on smoking, sensible eating, mental health, exercise, and foot care may be obtained from local insurance companies or health agencies. Pamphlets specifically related to the rehabilitation and health maintenance of the patients on your ward should also be stocked here. These might include publications such as the following:
    a. Rehabilitation of the patient who has had a stroke
    b. Living with heart disease
    c. Control of diabetes
    d. Living with arthritis
    e. Colostomy care
    f. Care of the stump
11. Set up a bulletin board on the unit and post announcements of significant health teaching programs in the patients' lounge.
12. Invite recovered (discharged) patients to return to the hospital to participate in ward motivation and rehabilitation programs for hospitalized

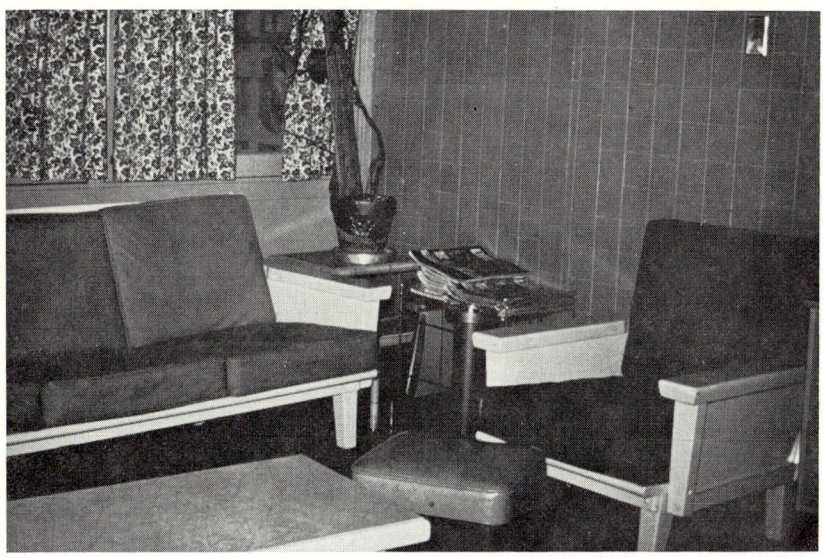

Fig. 16-3. A corner of the patients' lounge.

patients. Associations such as Alcoholics Anonymous, Larynget's Society, the Colostomy Society, and the Ileostomy Society will be glad to send members to the patients to help them relearn how to live with their changed bodies. The addresses of the local organizations can be found in the telephone directory or by contacting the national associations. If you need assistance in locating them, consult your local visiting nurse society.

13. Conduct refreshment breaks in the lounge at regularly scheduled times (Fig. 16-3). Morning coffee breaks, afternoon fruit juice refreshers, and evening warm milk soothers will certainly interrupt the long waits between meals. They will motivate conversation, too. These breaks will make the day much more interesting, and soon the patients will become bound together in friendship.

All of these ways of making the environment more interesting will not apply to every extended care unit, but some of them will. Members of the staff on each unit should study the needs of the particular patients and then plan to develop the recreational activities to meet these needs. If you work with surgical patients, you may find that refreshment breaks, health education pamphlets, and patient association meetings will make up an adequate program. However, if you work with neurological or geriatric patients, you may find that all of the forementioned techniques will need to be utilized in order to put some life back into the helpless patient's living.

SUMMARY

During the acute phase of illness, when the diagnosis is being established and treatment has not yet begun, the patient is filled with fear and apprehension. He needs an emotional environment in which the mysteries of his strange new world and its effects on him are explained away. In the convalescent stage, when treatment is controlling the illness and recovery is occurring, the patient is bored with his dull and uninteresting life in the extended care or convalescing unit. He now needs an emotional environment that will remotivate his interest in living. The patients' lounge will need to be changed from a sitting room to a living room, where interesting activities of living occur.

DISCUSSION QUESTIONS

1. Visit the patients' lounge on your ward. Observe the patients there. Are they doing something or are they just sitting?
2. Where do your out-of-bed patients go and what do they do all day?
3. Conduct a survey of your patients to determine:
   a. Whether they are interested are bored.
   b. What kind of activities they would like to do on the unit.
4. Conduct a survey of the unit staff members to find out how they feel about making the unit an interesting place for the out-of-bed patients.
5. How can the Kardex be used to help you understand how to explain the scheduled studies or treatments to the patients?
6. How can the Kardex be used to help you understand what the patient has been taught or if the patient has been taught?
7. Listen to your patients carefully today. Jot down those statements that you think are request for explanations.
8. Accompany a patient who is going to have a diagnostic test made and observe the procedure. Write out the explanation you would give to a patient who was scheduled to have the same kind of test tomorrow.
9. How do you know when a patient is bored?
10. Why do some patients become even more demanding as their condition improves?

SOURCE OF ADDITIONAL INFORMATION

1. Film: The eye of the beholder; may be obtained from Audio-Visual Support Center, Armed Forces Institute of Pathology, Washington, D. C. 20305. (Dramatizes the fact that man sees what he wants to see and that no two people ever see anything in the same way.)

17 / Maintaining a safe physical environment for the patient

STUDY QUESTIONS

1. What is the cause of most accidents sustained by patients in the health care facility?
2. How can the nursing personnel know all of their patients when there is a rapid turnover?
3. Why do patients wear wristbands labeled with their name?
4. Why should the nursing assistant make rounds to all of the patients when he comes on duty?
5. What are the typical characteristics of the patient who falls out of bed?
6. What hours are the most dangerous in the health care facility from the standpoint of patient falls?
7. How can the bed patient be protected from falling out of bed?
8. What patients should have crib sides on their bed?
9. How are restraints applied?
10. How are wheelchair supports applied?
11. Why is it dangerous to tie a patient in a wheelchair with a sheet?
12. Why do patients fall off of stretchers or treatment tables?
13. How can the patient be safeguarded while he is on a stretcher?

The patient who is in a health care facility can be injured in two ways: (1) by receiving the medications or the treatments prescribed for another patient or (2) by falling out of bed, out of a chair, or off of a treatment table.

Injuries that occur from receiving medication or treatment intended for another patient or from falling out of bed, out of a chair, or off of a stretcher may result in an increased stay for the patient, permanent disability, or even death. These injuries can be avoided easily if you give the patient the kind of nursing care that you would like to receive if you were the patient and he were the nursing assistant.

THE RIGHT PATIENT MUST GET THE PRESCRIBED TREATMENT

Today there is a rapid turnover in the patients in health care facilities. Modern operative procedures and new drugs have decreased the length of illnesses and have speeded up the recovery rate. Therefore a large number of patients are discharged and a large number admitted each day. This means that you will have to make rounds to each patient when you come on duty. During these rounds you should spend enough time with each newly admitted patient to get to know him. Then check the roster of patients on the unit and be sure that the names of discharged patients are removed and the names of new ones inserted. Check the temperature, pulse, and respiration chart as well as the diet roster and bring these up to date by removing the names of the discharged patients and by adding those of the new ones.

Personnel from the various services will depend on the nursing personnel to direct them to right patients (Fig. 17-1). The laboratory technician will draw blood from the patient you identify. The dietary aide will take the dinner tray to the patient you say is in room X or in bed 10. The operating room runner will take the patient you designate to the operating room for a surgical procedure. Therefore you must know your patients by name, and you must be sure that the name tag on a bed is the correct one for the patient who is in that bed.

The rapid turnover of patients and the constant changes in the nursing staff (due to turnover, days off, sickness, etc.) have made health care facilities places filled with strangers. The nursing assistant who

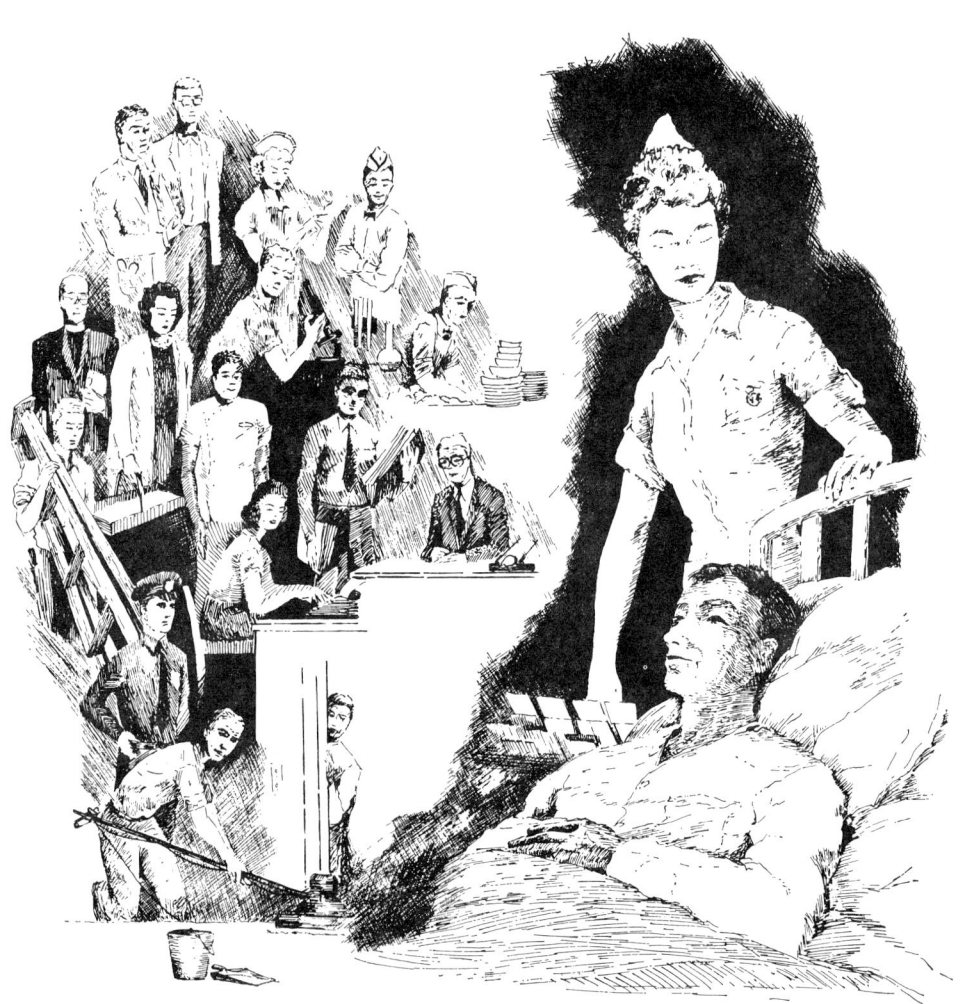

Fig. 17-1. Members of the entire hospital team depend on the nurse and the nursing assistant to identify the patient for them.

is returning from a few days off does not know the patients, and the patients do not know him. Instead of making rounds to get to know the patients and to check the accuracy of the name tags and ward rosters, all too many nursing assistants have resorted to calling the patients by numbers. This has resulted in so many cases of mistaken identity in which patients were given the wrong medicine, the wrong diet, or the wrong operation that most hospitals and extended care facilities have adopted a plan whereby each patient is labeled upon admission with a wrist band containing his name.

This labeling of patients with a wrist band is done to avoid errors resulting from mistaken patient identification. Therefore each time you care for a patient, you must check his wrist band to be sure that you are giving the care you were directed to give to the patient you were assigned to give it to. However, this labeling may give the patient the impression that he is unknown and friendless in the health care facility. The procedure was not intended to have this effect, and you must not let the patient get the wrong impression. You can use the wrist band for positive patient identification when giving treatments or taking patients to diagnostic services, but you must get to know your new patients each day during rounds at the beginning of the tour of duty. Know each patient's name and always use the name when addressing the patient. Remember that your friendliness and your caring about the patient will reduce his fear, worry, and pain. However, using the wrist band for positive patient identification will assure the patient that he will always get exactly what is prescribed for him.

Talk with some of the members of your family or with your friends who have been patients recently. Ask them if they received a diet or a medication intended for another. Ask them also how many times they were incorrectly identified and whether or not this was frightening.

The court records are filled with too many cases of injuries to patients that occurred because the wrong patient was operated upon. This hospital error is really the error of the nursing staff members who sent the wrong patient to the operating room and not the error of the surgeon who performed the operation. Patients all seem to look alike in operating room garb. The patient who is anesthetized and asleep on the operating room table cannot tell his own name, nor can he watch the operation to be sure that he is having the one he was supposed to have. He depends on you, and you must be dependable enough to always send the right patient to the operating room. Regardless of the emergency, there is always enough time to check the wrist band or to check the patient's name verbally and to be sure that the right patient is getting the drug or treatment or is going to the operating room.

THE PATIENT WHO FALLS

Falling is an all too common patient accident, and it can be prevented easily when you understand why it occurs. A study of hospital accidents reveals that the patient who falls out of bed usually (1) is over 50 years of age, (2) is under the effects of a sedative or hypnotic (sleeping pill), and (3) is trying to get out of bed to go to the bathroom. This study further reveals that most falls occur between the hours of 5 A.M. and 8 A.M.

These facts indicate that the patient who falls out of bed usually is the older patient whose brain is dulled by a drug. However, his need to void or defecate awakens him and he attempts to get out of bed. He does not fully realize, because of the dulled brain activity, that he is in the hospital and in a high bed, so he attempts to step out of bed and, of course, falls. Frequently he bangs his head on the bedside stand and cuts his scalp or twists his leg and breaks a bone. The patient who is partially paralyzed by disease or by a spinal anesthetic may also fall out of bed by just turning over. As he turns his body over from a back-lying to a side-lying position, his heavy paralyzed limbs flop over, pull him forward, and throw him out of bed.

The ambulatory patient who slips to the floor or who faints and falls is usually the patient who is out of bed for the first time. He is usually very glad to be out of bed so that he can go to the bathroom. He sits on the bed and dangles his legs for only a minute and then rushes off to the toilet. Usually he arrives at the bathroom all right but he uses up his remaining energy defecating and thus becomes quite weak. Then he topples off the toilet onto the bathroom floor, either banging his head or breaking his leg as he falls.

The ambulatory patient who is receiving large doses of tranquilizers falls for still another reason. The tranquilizers calm and quiet his fears or his worries, but they also lower his blood pressure. The patient may complain of feeling lightheaded but may not think this is important. He walks around the unit or goes to the bathroom. As he stands, his blood pressure drops so low that blood cannot be sent up to the brain. Since the brain stops working when it is deprived of blood, the patient faints and falls. When you find him you will notice that he is cold and sweaty and that his pulse is rapid and weak.

The patient who falls out of a chair is usually one who is too weak to maintain himself in a sitting position or one who has paralyzed limbs that prevent him from doing so. This patient sits in the chair and slides down until he slips right out of it and onto the floor. Occasionally, the weak, elderly patient who is confused also falls out of a chair. He cannot understand why he is in the hospital, and he constantly tries to get away and go home. However, he is too weak to walk and falls as soon as he gets out of the chair. Sometimes such a patient may even try to go home in the wheelchair and may attempt to wheel the chair away from the ward and even down the steps.

SAFEGUARDING THE BED PATIENT

The bed patient can be protected from falling out of bed by the following nursing measures:

1. Place side rails on the beds of all those patients who are over 50 years of age and on the beds of those patients who are under the effects of a spinal anesthetic.
2. Pull the side rails up into the protective position when the nurse gives the patient a sedative or a hypnotic, and when you are preparing the patient for sleep, before you put out the lights.
3. Make rounds every 30 minutes after the lights are out. Visit each patient during these rounds. If a patient is awake, offer him a urinal or bedpan and a drink of water. Then try to find out what has awakened him. Report this wakefulness to the nurse.
4. Expect patients who are on forced fluids, those who are receiving intravenous infusions, or those who have received a diuretic to need to void frequently. Check these patients on each round and offer them a urinal or bedpan if they are awake.
5. Expect patients to wake up early in the morning because of the need to void. Listen carefully for signs of patient activity and visit the patient as soon as you hear any. Do not wait for the patient to call you; many times he does not even remember that he is in a hospital or extended care facility.
6. Answer the patient's bell immediately. Remember that the need to void has probably awakened him. When you are busy collecting specimens or taking temperatures in the early morning and you do not answer the patient's call promptly, he may be forced to get out of bed to go to the bathroom.
7. Make early morning rounds and offer urinals or bedpans to the patients

who are awake. Do not try to take temperatures or give morning care before you give the patient an opportunity to void. He will not be able to hold his urine until you finish taking the temperatures and have the time to get him a urinal or bedpan.

8. Be available to the patients all night. Do not prop urinals or bedpans on bedside chairs. The patient may easily fall out of bed in the middle of the night when he is reaching for this bedpan or urinal.
9. Be sure that the call bell is available to the patient. When you prepare the patient for bed, place it where he can reach it and reposition it in an easily available position each time you give the patient any care.

Sometimes the patient may become so restless and confused at night that additional measures are needed to keep him safely in bed. When you observe this confusion and restlessness in the patient, stay with him and use the patient's call bell to signal for the nurse. The nurse will notify the doctor, who may order some drug to help the patient sleep or some protective measure to keep the patient in bed. The protective device may be a safety belt, a safety net, or arm and leg restraints. It is much better to have someone stay with the patient and keep him in bed than to resort to using a protective device. However, when the staffing does not permit this, a protective device may be ordered by the doctor to help keep the patient in bed.

Safety belt

A safety belt is placed around the patient's waist and the ends of the belt are tied to the side of the bed. Crib sides must also be placed on the bed when a safety belt is used. If they are not, the patient's head and shoulders or his legs may come out over the sides of the bed. Then as the patient attempts to get out of bed, he may upset the bed on top himself. The safety belt is valuable because it keeps the patient in bed without limiting his ability to sit up or to turn from side to side. Therefore it does not permit him to develop the complications that can result from lying still.

Chest harness

A chest harness, which is similar to a vest, can also be used to keep the patient in bed. The patient slips his arms into the harness, and the ends are crossed over the chest and tied to the bedsprings at each side of the bed. Crib sides must also be used on the bed when the patient wears the harness, or the lower half of his body will slip out and over the side of the bed. A disadvantage of the chest harness as a protective device is that it does limit chest movement, and because of this it may interfere with the patient's breathing. This is particularly true in the older patient in the extended care facility who may already have some breathing difficulties because of heart disease.

Safety net

A safety net can be put on the bed and tied into position over the crib sides if the patient is constantly attempting to get out of bed over the crib sides. It gives the bed the appearance of a tent. Its advantage is that it permits the patient to move about the bed freely but prevents him from climbing out over the crib sides. A disadvantage is that it frequently gives the patient a feeling of being closed in, so that he tries harder to get out of bed. Another disadvantage is that the net is strong enough to be used effectively only for the weak, confused patients and not strong enough for the restless, disturbed ones.

Arm and leg restraints

The patient's arms and legs can be held on the bed by linen, muslin, or leather protective devices. These restraining devices are usually made in such a way that the attachments that fit around the wrists and around the ankles do not tighten when the patient pulls on them. This is an important feature of these restraining devices that protect the patient by keeping him in bed while preventing any complications due to interference with the circulation in the hands and feet. With arm and leg restraints, too, the patient should have crib sides on the bed because his restlessness and his thrashing about may cause him to throw his body over the side of the bed. If the patient does this, the restraining devices may cause him to dislocate the shoulder and hip on the side opposite to the one hanging out of the bed, or they may cause the patient to be injured by holding him just off the edge of the bed in such a way as to cause the bed to tilt over sideways and fall on top of him. The leather arm and leg restraining devices should be put on the patient in the following way:

1. Collect the equipment, which consists of two wristlets, two anklets, and three straps.
2. Take the equipment to the patient's bedside.
3. Explain to the patient that you are protecting him from falling out of bed.
4. Place a wristlet on the patient's wrist. Have this wristlet loose enough to permit you to slip two fingers between the restraint and the patient's wrist. Buckle it in this position. Place the leather strap through the wristlet buckle and attach it to the bedsprings at the side of the bed. Check to be sure that the wristlet is loose enough to permit you to slip two fingers between the wrist and the restraint. If it is not, loosen it immediately.
5. Repeat step 4 and put the second wristlet on the patient.
6. Loosen the bedclothes at the foot of the bed and fold them back to expose the patient's ankles.
7. Place an anklet on each leg. Place these on so loosely that you can slip two fingers between the ankle and the leather anklet. Buckle the anklets in this position. Place the leather strap through the buckle in both anklets and attach it to the bottom of the bed. Check to be sure that the anklets are loose enough to permit you to slip two fingers between them and the ankle.
8. Remake the bottom of the bed by tucking in the bedclothes loosely.
9. Place crib sides on the bed.
10. Check the patient every 15 minutes to be sure that he is comfortable and safe.
11. Give the patient the following care every 2 hours:
    a. Offer the patient a bedpan or urinal.
    b. Give him fluids to drink.
    c. Check his wristlets and anklets to be sure they are not too tight.
    d. Remove one wristlet, massage the patient's wrist with alcohol or massage lotion, and reapply the wristlet. Repeat this step on the second wrist. Then remove the anklets, massage the patient's ankles, and reapply the anklets. Rub the patient's back well.
    e. Change his position. (The patient may be placed in a side-lying position with both arms restrained to one side of the bed if crib sides are in place.)
12. Remember the patient is helpless, so provide for the patient's needs as follows (Fig. 17-2):
    a. Remove the restraints and permit him to feed himself, or, if this is not possible (the nurse directs you as to what nursing actions to take), feed the patient.
    b. Remove the restraints and permit the patient to wash himself or do this for him.
    c. Remove the restraints and per-

Maintaining a safe physical environment for the patient 153

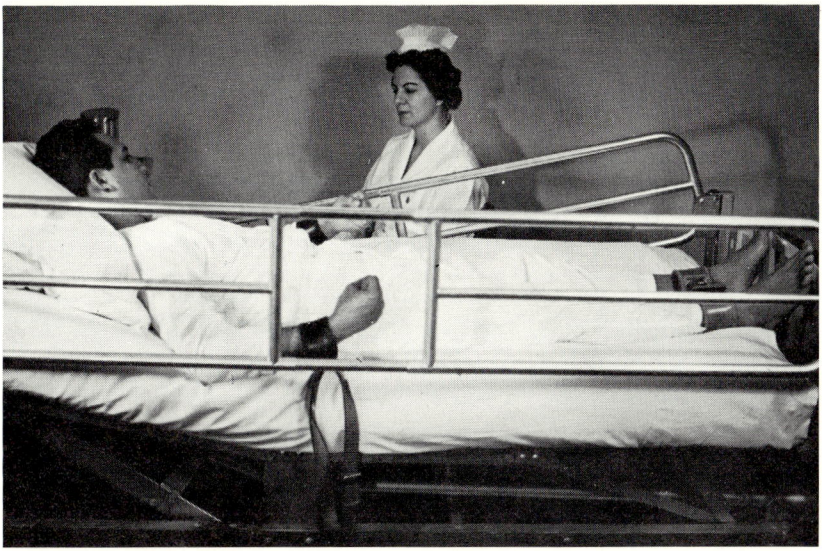

Fig. 17-2. The restless, disturbed patient in leather protective devices. A nurse or nursing assistant should spend as much time as possible with such a patient in order to remove his fear and help him develop trust in the hospital staff. Note in this illustration that the nurse has lowered the crib side on the left side of the bed so that she can be close to the patient.

mit the patient to wipe himself after his toileting or do this for him.

d. Follow the nurse's directions carefully. Apply or remove the restraints only as she directs you to. Remember, however, that the patient who is in restraints is just as helpless in meeting his own needs as the paralyzed patient. Therefore you will have to be his arms and legs and muscles and provide all his care.

13. Spend as much time as you can with the patient. Soothe and comfort him with your caring and your presence. Soon the patient will begin to understand (even in his confusion) that you are trying to help him, and his fear and restlessness may begin to subside.

14. Remember that restraining devices are used to protect the patient. However, they may become devices of torture if you do not continue to care for the patient that you have made helpless by their application.

15. Keep the restraint key available to all ward personnel so that the device may be removed promptly if a ward emergency, such as fire, occurs.

Protective devices also restrain, and so they deprive the patient of his freedom. Because of this, they can be applied only on a medical order. The nurse will receive this order and direct you to apply the specific protective device that the patient needs.

SAFEGUARDING THE PATIENT DURING A TREATMENT

The seriously ill patient may become confused or disoriented and may try to discontinue the treatment that the doctor has prescribed for him. He may become irritated by the tube in his nose or in his bladder, and he may grab at it and try to pull it out. He may thrash about in bed and wave his arms so wildly that the needle and tubing through which a blood transfusion or an intravenous infusion is being given is jerked out of his vein and is forced to run into the tissues in his arms. He may pull off the dressings protecting an operative site, and he may even injure his body by banging it against the crib sides on the bed.

The patient must receive the treatment that the doctor prescribed for him. He must be prevented from discontinuing or interrupting this treatment by his restless grabbing or thrashing about. This can be accomplished by immobilizing the patient's hands in one of the following ways:

1. Place boxing gloves on the patient's hands so the fingers are no longer able to grab and hold on to tubes, to intravenous tubing, or to dressings.
2. Place stiff muslin restraint mitts (Posey type) on the patient's hands and fasten them firmly about his wrists.
3. Place the patient's arms (palms down) on arm boards, and bandage the hands and fingers to the boards with elastic bandages.
4. Place the patient's hands in pillows and pin or tape the pillows closed over his hands (splint the hands).
5. Place a folded towel in the patient's palm. Bandage the hand, over the towel, into a fistlike position with an elastic bandage. Repeat on the other hand.

These devices should be removed at least once daily, and the hand should be exercised. As soon as the treatment is over, these protective devices should be removed.

The patient's arm can be immobilized to prevent him from pulling a tube out of his nose by one of these measures:

1. Splint the arm, from the elbow down to and including the hand, in a pillow. This prevents the arm from bending at the elbow.
2. Splint the arm in an inflatable plastic splint that encircles the arm, and cover the fingers with a restraint mitt.

These devices immobilize the arms only and permit the patient to move about in bed, thus preventing those complications that occur from lying still in bed.

Complications occurring from the use of restraining devices

All restraining devices that immobilize the patient's arms and legs seem to terrify the patient and increase his restlessness by forcing him to try in every way he knows to get them off. Therefore these devices should be used only after all other nursing measures to quiet and protect the patient have failed and only after the use of the restraining devices has been thoroughly explained to the patient. Although the patient is confused or disoriented, he may be able to understand that in applying restraints you are really helping him. Of course, this understanding must be reinforced by your nursing care of visiting him often, providing for his toileting needs every 2 hours, changing his position frequently, and massaging his sore wrists and ankles. This understanding will be lost quickly, however, if you tie him in bed, make him helpless, and then forget about him.

The complications that the restrained patient may develop and measures to prevent them from developing are listed in Table 17-1.

Remember, only the doctor can decide that the patient is hurting himself and that he must be protected from this self-inflicted harm by the use of restraints.

SAFEGUARDING THE HELPLESS PATIENT IN A CHAIR

The helpless patient who is out of bed in a chair can be protected from falling out of the chair by the following nursing measures:

1. Position the patient in the kind of a chair that he needs. Use a chair with

Table 17-1. Possible complications from restraining patients and preventive measures

Complication	Preventive measure
Swelling in the hands and feet. May occur if the circulation in the hands and feet is shut off by the restraints. Even though the wristlets and anklets are put on loosely, the patient may strain against them so continuously that the circulation will be interrupted.	Remove the anklets and wristlets every 2 hours and massage the body parts well in order to restore the circulation.
Linen burns on the elbow, back, hips, and heels. May occur because of the constant wriggling motions of the patient as he attempts to get the restraints off.	Make frequent visits to the patient to care for his needs for fluid and for his needs to void and defecate.
Constantly mounting fear and eventually panic develops, causing the patient to strain at the straps to break them. If this fails, he may attempt to get his razor and razor blades out of his bedside stand in order to cut the straps. If he fails in this, he may scream and thrash about wildly until he becomes exhausted and dehydrated. However, if he succeeds in removing the straps either by breaking or cutting them, he may jump out of the window in his panic and in his need to escape.	Explain to the patient why the restraints are necessary and visit him constantly during his period of restraint, to care for his needs. However, if the restrained patient continues to thrash about the bed and becomes wilder and wilder, the nurse and doctor must be notified promptly. Watch the patient's pulse closely, and keep the nurse informed of its rate. Keep the bedside stand out of the restrained patient's reach.
Death sometimes occurs during ward emergencies, such as fires, because the ward personnel cannot find the restraint key in time to free the patient.	Have a key to restraint devices on the ring with the keys for narcotic supplies.

a high back if the patient has weak back and neck muscles. Use a chair with foot supports if the patient has paralyzed legs. Determine the patient's needs and discuss them with the nurse. The nurse will probably get the hospital repair or brace shop to adjust the chair to meet the patient's needs.

2. Determine what, if anything, causes the patient to slip out of this position in the chair. The following are some of the usual causes:
   a. The feet slip off the foot supports on the chair, permitting the patient to slide down and out of the chair.
   b. The weak or paralyzed side of the body causes the patient to tilt over toward the weak side until he tips the chair over.
   c. The patient becomes tired and sore from sitting, so he gets out of the chair and attempts to walk around. Since he is unable to walk, he falls.
   d. The patient gets tired of sitting and tries to get out of the chair so that he can go back to bed.
   e. The patient is so confused that he is constantly wandering off as he tries to find his way home.
3. Apply the correct supportive measure to keep the patient in the chair.
   a. If the patient is sliding out of the chair, the proper support is one that stabilizes his feet on the foot supports of the chair. This can be

done by placing a toe and heel support on the chair's footrest and a leather strap (the patient's belt padded by a sheet will suffice) over the patient's legs and around the chair (Fig. 13-5). This will keep the patient's legs under him on the foot supports of the chair and will prevent him from sliding down and out of the chair. If the patient is weak, he may tip or lean over frontward so far that he upsets the chair. This can be avoided by placing a vestlike support over his chest and by anchoring this support to the back of the chair (Figs. 13-7 and 13-8).
b. If the patient is tilting over sideways toward his paralyzed side, an arm support (splint) should be attached to the wheelchair and the paralyzed arm should be stabilized on this arm support. A pillow or a rolled blanket can also be placed along the patient's weak side to support it in the chair.
c. If the patient attempts to get out of the chair because he gets sore from sitting, place an alternating pressure pad under him in the chair. Plan his time out of bed in such a way that he is out to eat and defecate, but permit him to return to bed in the morning and afternoon for a rest.
d. If the patient attempts to get back into bed frequently, follow the directions in step 3 (c), but also try to find some interesting activity in which he can participate when he is out of bed.
e. If the patient is confused, either support him in the chair with feet and leg supports and with a vest-type support or keep him in bed until you have the time to take him for a walk to the cafeteria, to the library, or to the area outside the health care facility. Then take him back to the ward and put him to bed. This walk will give him some interesting activity, and it will tire him enough so that he will be glad to rest when he returns to the ward.

Complications from the use of devices that support the patient in a chair

The complications discussed here do not really result from the device itself but rather from the use of an improper device or from the incorrect use of the devices described previously.

The improper device that is used most frequently is a sheet placed under the patient's arms and chest and then tied to the chair at the back. The patient's legs slip off the foot supports on the chair and his body slides down. Then the sheet rides up the patient's chest until it is pressing tightly on the underarm area, or axilla. Since all the blood vessels and nerves enter the arm at the axilla, the circulation to the arm is cut off by the pressure of this sheet and the nerves are injured. Soon the patient develops swelling and numbness in his arms. The irony of all this is that the sheet does not hold the patient up anyway, and he slides out of the chair until he is caught in a position halfway in and halfway out of the chair with his arms hung on the sheet. Needless to say, this sheet also constricts the patient's chest movement and leads to the development of chest infections.

Another complication occurs when the vestlike support and the arm and leg straps are so effective in maintaining the patient in a good sitting position that the ward nursing personnel allow the patient to sit in the chair all day. Then the patient develops the same kind of decubitus ulcers on his buttocks that would occur if he lay in bed all day in the same position. His feet also swell because the lack of movement in them prevents the blood from getting back to the heart through the veins. These complications can be prevented by giving the patient morning and afternoon rests in bed.

SAFEGUARDING THE AMBULATORY PATIENT

The ambulatory patient can be protected from falling by the following nursing measures:

1. Explain to the patient who is getting out of bed for the first time just what he is able to do and why his activities must be limited. Place his call bell near him, and ask him to call you if he wants to go to the bathroom or if he wants to walk around the ward. Visit him frequently to observe his progress. Return promptly and put him in bed when his out-of-bed time is up. Tell him when he is permitted to get out of bed again and when you will return to help him out. Offer to take him to the bathroom when he gets out of bed and stay with him until he is finished. Then help him back to bed.

2. Know those patients on your ward who are receiving large doses of tranquilizers. Assist them in getting out of bed. Check on their condition frequently. Return them to bed immediately, and check their blood pressure if they complain of feeling lightheaded or dizzy. Keep the nurse informed of the patients' complaints. Send these patients to off-ward treatments or tests in a wheelchair.

Complications of ambulating the sick patient

Although the bed-lying position is filled with dangerous complications, ambulating the sick patient has the danger of falls.

Falls may occur when the patient gets out of bed after a long period of lying flat because his heart fails to adjust the force of its beat and the size of its blood vessels in order to get the blood to the brain. Then the patient gets light-headed and dizzy, and he faints from an inadequate blood circulation to the brain. Then, too, the fears of illness and the uncertainty of the diagnosis may so disturb a patient that the physician may need to prescribe large doses of tranquilizers to soothe and quiet his involuntary nervous system. These drugs have the intended soothing effect, but they also widen the blood vessels and reduce the blood pressure so that an inadequate blood supply to the brain may occur when the patient stands. If this happens, the patient will faint and fall.

The falls that complicate ambulation can be prevented if we remember that the patient is allowed out of bed as soon as possible because of the dangers of the bed-lying position. We must accept the fact that the out-of-bed hospital patient is sick and needs as much of our nursing care and our skilled observations as the bed patient.

THE PATIENT WHO FALLS IN OFF-THE-WARD AREAS

The patient who is taken off the ward to a treatment or diagnostic area usually is prepared for this trip with a sedative or a hypnotic or both. Therefore he is usually drowsy and a little confused from the medicine. Actually, that is why it is given—to depress or slow down his thinking, worrying, and feelings of pain. However, this means that the patient may forget what you told him about lying still on the x-ray table, or lying flat on his back on the stretcher, or lying quietly on the operating table. He may turn over quickly or jump up suddenly at the slightest noise. Of course, such movement will throw him off the narrow stretcher or treatment table and he will be injured. Therefore all stretchers and treatment tables should be equipped with safety straps, and these safety straps should be fastened over the patient's body as soon as he is put on the table or stretcher.

It is impossible to anticipate what a patient under the influence of a drug might do, but it is easy to protect him if you always apply the safety straps promptly. Do not let the patient convince you that he will not need these protective straps. He does not know what drug he has received, nor does he know how this drug will affect him. You must be sure that he is safe. Always utilize all of the safety devices available when you care for patients.

SUMMARY

The hospital and extended care facility patient is injured by falling or by receiving treatments or drugs intended for someone else. These injuries can be prevented by protecting the patient from errors of mistaken identity by labeling him with a wrist band, and by protecting him from falling by supporting him in the position that he is to maintain.

The patient may be maintained in bed by eliminating the need for him to get out of bed or by applying those protective devices necessary to keep him there. The patient may be maintained in a wheelchair by using those foot and leg supports that keep his feet under him on the chair and thus prevent him from sliding.

The ambulatory patient is actually a sick person who needs careful nursing observation and care. When members of the ward staff fail to recognize this fact, the patient may be forced to carry out activities far beyond his physical abilities, and he may faint and fall and injure himself.

The patient who goes to off-the-ward diagnostic and therapeutic services usually is prepared for the tests or treatments by a sedative or a hypnotic drug. These drugs depress brain activities, and they may cause the patient to become confused and even disoriented. This may result in his forgetting your explanations and directions and may cause him to become rather restless. This restlessness may result in falls from treatment tables and stretchers unless the patient is well protected by safety straps.

DISCUSSION QUESTIONS

1 How many of your patients fell last week?
2 Where did the patients fall?
3 Were the patients injured in these falls?
4 Discuss at your team meetings the ways in which these patient falls might have been avoided.
5 What is your health care facility policy about crib sides on the patients' beds?
6 What is your health care facility policy about putting crib sides on the beds of the patients who receive a sedative or a hypnotic?
7 How do you support the helpless patient in a wheelchair?
8 Why should an effective wheelchair support be applied to the patient's feet instead of to his chest?
9 How many of your patients are receiving tranquilizers? What observations do you make on these patients before you get them out of bed?
10 What signal or patient call device do you have in the patients' bathrooms? How could a patient call you if he became weak in the bathroom?
11 Why should a patient have wrist and ankle restraints removed every 2 hours? Why should his wrists and ankles be massaged every 2 hours when the restraints are removed and before they are reapplied?
12 Where do you keep the key to the locked restraints on your ward? Do all ward personnel have easy access to it? Why is this necessary?
13 Who determines that restraints are to be applied? Why?

VOCABULARY

ambulatory Walking.
confused Inability of the patient to correctly interpret what is going on in his surroundings. The response of the confused patient to his surroundings will be incorrect. He may try to get out of bed and go home, he may feel that he is kept in the hospital against his own wishes, etc.
hypnotic A drug that causes sleep.
panic An emotional state of overpowering fear that occurs when an individual feels trapped and cannot escape from a danger that is real (a fire) or from a danger that he imagines (an attempt by the hospital personnel to kill him).
restraints Devices that limit the patient's ability to move in order to protect him from injury.
spinal anesthetic A drug injected into the spinal fluid to deaden the patient's ability to feel pain. This drug also causes a paralysis for the duration of its action.
tranquilizers Drugs given to soothe, calm, and quiet the frightened or the distressed patient. These drugs also lower blood pressure.
wheelchair supports Devices that maintain the patient in the correct sitting position.

18/Identifying, recording, and reporting the patient's needs

STUDY QUESTIONS

1. How do you answer the doctor who asks how the patient is today?
2. How do you know whether the patient's condition is changing?
3. What does "observe the patient closely" mean?
4. When are the observations of the patient made?
5. What observations would you make to determine whether or not the patient is receiving enough fluid?
6. Where are the observations about the patient recorded?
7. How are these observations recorded?
8. What observations are you permitted to record on the chart?
9. How can you tell that the patient feels miserable?
10. Each morning, during the assignment conference, the nurse focuses your attention on those special observations that need to be made on the patients. Why does she do this?

HOW IS THE PATIENT TODAY?

What this question really means is how are the patient's diseased body and troubled mind functioning today. The answer is given by describing failures of the body and mind to function in the way that is required for comfortable living. Actually, the answer is given by stating how the body fails to meet the needs that have been discussed in previous chapters.

OBSERVATION OF THE PATIENT

The doctor and nurse will want to know about any clues showing that the patient's body and mind are not meeting the needs of living. Each time a patient is given care, these clues must be looked for and, if found, must be reported to the doctor and/or nurse so that the proper medical and nursing care can be started immediately.

These clues about the patient's condition cannot be our thoughts about him. They must be actual observations of ineffective body functioning or actual statements (quotes) from the patient, describing how his body functioned ineffectively. The doctor is the only person who has sufficient medical knowledge to have valuable thoughts about the patient. The physician's personal opinion about the patient's illness is really the diagnosis.

THE CLUES WE REPORT

The body is not effectively meeting the patient's need for food if one or more of the following situations exist:

1. The patient is unconscious. The patient is unable to be awakened and he cannot swallow, so food cannot be given by mouth.
2. The patient is unable to swallow. Each drink of water or each bite of food that he puts into his mouth slips into his windpipe (trachea) and causes severe coughing and choking.
3. The patient vomits the food he eats.
4. The patient has severe discomfort and pain after eating.
5. The patient has diarrhea.
6. The patient is vomiting blood or passing blood by rectum.
7. The patient is unable to move his bowels.
8. The patient's bowel movements cause severe pain.
9. The patient does not eat his food.
10. The patient's bowel movements are black, green, or yellow.

The patient's body is not adequately meeting his need for water if one of the following observations is made:

1. The patient vomits all the water he takes by mouth.
2. The patient drinks less than 2 to 3 quarts of water daily.
3. The patient's mouth, tongue, and lips are dry, coated, and swollen.
4. The patient's skin is dry and its elasticity (ability to spring back into place after being pinched) is lost.
5. The patient's urine is dark yellowish brown.
6. The patient's urinary output is less than 1,500 ml.

We receive a clue that the patient's body is not effectively removing waste if one of the following observations is made:

1. The patient voids less than 1,500 ml. of urine.
2. The patient fails to void.
3. The patient's urine is dark yellowish brown.
4. The patient has pain on voiding.
5. The patient's body becomes edematous (feet, legs, and abdomen become swollen).
6. The patient voids where he is and not in the proper facilities (is incontinent).
7. The patient fails to defecate.
8. The patient's bowel movement is so hard and dry that he is unable to expel it from the rectum.
9. The patient has pain on defecation.
10. The patient defecates where he is and not in the proper facilities (is incontinent).

Clues telling us that the patient's body is not meeting his need for physical movement include the following:

1. The patient is unconscious (not able to be awakened).
2. The patient is developing pressure sores (decubitus ulcers) on his body at the base of the spine (sacral area), at prominences over the backbones, or at the bony prominences of the shoulders, elbows, hips, knees, and ankles.
3. The patient is unable to move all parts of his body (is paralyzed). Paralysis may be hemiplegia (paralysis of one side of the body from the face down to and including the leg), paraplegia (paralysis of the body from the umbilicus [navel] down), or monoplegia (paralysis limited to one part such as the arm or the leg).
4. The patient is unable to change his position in bed.
5. The patient's lungs are splinted by the bed, and thus the movement of the lungs is so limited that they retain sputum. The breathing tubes are plugged. Air cannot get in through the sputum-plugged tubes, and the patient develops some type of breathing difficulty such as dyspnea, short-

ness of breath, cyanosis (blueness of fingernail beds, lips, earlobes, or tip of the nose due to lack of oxygen in the blood), or noisy, gurgling breathing due to air being sucked into the sputum-filled lungs.
6. The patient develops bent limbs that cannot be straightened easily (contracture deformities).
7. The patient's ankles and wrists drop.
8. The patient's feet and legs swell as serum seeps out of the waterlogged veins.
9. The patient develops pain in the calves of his legs (blood clots due to blood stagnation [thrombophlebitis]).

The patient's body may not be functioning adequately to meet his need for cleanliness if one of these signs is observed:
1. The patient develops a foul-smelling mouth with a brown-coated tongue.
2. The patient has thick white secretions collecting in the inner corners of the eyes.
3. The patient has a foul-smelling, red, raw, irritated area under the arm or in the genital area.
4. The patient has a foul-smelling drainage from the umbilicus.
5. The patient is dirty.
6. The patient develops body lice, head lice, or maggots.

Clues that the patient's body is not effectively meeting his need for freedom from discomfort may be obtained from any of the following signs:
1. The patient has pain.
2. The patient is coughing.
3. The patient has difficulty in breathing.
4. The patient is frightened.
5. The patient seems worried.
6. The patient becomes quiet and wants to be alone.
7. The patient wishes that he were dead.
8. The patient begs for relief.
9. The patient is constantly calling for the nurse, doctor, or nursing assistant.
10. The patient refuses food, medicine, treatments, etc.

The patient's body is not fulfilling his need to feel dignity and self-worth if ineffective functioning of the body results in one of the following conditions:
1. The patient has to be fed.
2. The patient is incontinent.
3. The patient needs to have the intimate, personal aspects of his care done by you.
4. The patient is helpless.
5. The patient's body is changed in such a way as to change his living. For example, he is blind, he has an amputated leg, he has a colostomy, he has a foul-smelling drainage area, or he has a facial deformity (lost his nose because of cancer).
6. The patient is mentally ill.
7. The patient has a venereal disease.
8. The patient is an alcoholic.
9. The patient believes that the members of the ward staff do not like him.

The patient's body is not functioning well enough to meet his need for sleep if the patient is unable to carry out his usual sleeping pattern. Clues to this would include the following:
1. The patient cannot sleep at night.
2. The patient asks for a sleeping pill at night.
3. The patient knows that he will not be able to sleep and asks you to be sure to remind the nurse to bring in his sleeping pill.
4. The patient gets a sleeping pill each night, followed by a repeat dose soon after midnight.
5. The patient awakens frequently throughout the night.
6. The patient stays awake all night, calling you frequently, and then he sleeps all day.
7. The patient has so much pain that he is unable to sleep.

8. The patient is having so much difficulty breathing that he is afraid to sleep.
9. The patient is so worried that he cannot fall asleep.

As you make your rounds during the late evening and night, visit the patients and make the following observations:

1. Note whether or not the patient is sleeping.
2. If the patient is not sleeping, what is keeping him awake? If you can remove the obstacle to his sleeping by taking care of the body need that is keeping him awake, do so. Give him the urinal or bedpan so he can void, or change his position to rest his tired back. If he is afraid to sleep, stay with him for awhile and then come back to see him frequently. If you cannot remove the obstacle, report to the nurse the fact that the patient is unable to sleep and give her all the clues you can about the body needs that are keeping him awake.

Sleeplessness causes the patient to lie alone in a darkened area with nothing to occupy his attention but the one personal problem that is keeping him awake. He focuses on this problem and magnifies and distorts it until it becomes overwhelming. The patient's pain becomes unbearable, the impending surgery becomes (in his mind) a life-threatening operation, and the troubled breathing seems to him to make life unlivable and suicide a must for relief. Therefore the sleeplessness of the patient that continues after you have tried all the ways mentioned in the previous chapter to help him sleep should be reported to the nurse promptly.

In the morning when the night nurse reports how your patients spent the night, listen carefully for accounts of how they slept, whether or not they needed sleeping pills to help them sleep, and whether or not they stayed awake most of the night. A report of sleeplessness might be your first clue that the patient is troubled. Observe him carefully for more clues. Discuss these with the doctor and nurse.

You can either see or hear most of the clues to illness. However, those clues related to the patient's feeling that he is not a worthwhile person cannot be seen or heard. That is, you cannot see them or hear them unless you first suspect that they might be present; then you diligently search for them.

However, these clues become easily recognizable when we mentally put ourselves in the patient's place and try to figure out how we would act. The patient acts very much like we would act if the situation were reversed. Think of how you would act if you were caught redhanded in an embarrassing position. More than likely, you would become quiet, avoid your wife or husband, have a desire to be alone to hide, avoid answering questions, or wish to escape. Perhaps you would talk incessantly or blame the situation on someone else.

When he finds himself in an embarrassing situation, the patient also acts in one of two ways: he may become quiet and stay in his room alone, avoiding all companionship because of his imagined worthlessness, or he may become extremely talkative, blaming the world and berating it for what it did to him. Remember that it is impossible to behave miserably and feel good, just as it is impossible to feel good and behave miserably. The patient's actions speak loudly to tell us how he feels. Observe these actions and describe them to the doctor and nurse, who will then assist you in understanding how to help the patient.

REPORTING THE CLUES

The doctor and nurse need to know a great deal about the clue. They need to know to whom it happened, what happened, when it happened, where it happened, and how it happened. It is not sufficient to say that Mr. Jones vomited. This really tells very little. It is essential that your report include information like that given in the following example:

Who: Mr. Jones.
What: Vomited 4 ounces of bloody liquid
When: Immediately after lunch
Where: On the floor
How: Suddenly—came out like an explosion

Having received such a report, the doctor has all the information we could possibly give him, and he proceeds to gather the medical information that will give him the answer to the remaining question—why?

Each morning as you get your patient care assignment, the head nurse or team leader will tell you about the special clues to look for in your patients. These clues will, no doubt, include some of those listed earlier in this chapter. However, the nurse may call your attention to a specific clue so that you will look for it especially diligently because it has vital meaning to the doctor. Perhaps this is the clue that determines the need to operate, the need to prepare more blood for transfusions, the need to tube feed the patient, or the need to give him an enema.

How to report the clues

On each patient's chart there is a nurse's record on which are recorded the clues you observed about the patient's condition and the treatment that you gave him. Since nursing assistants are part of the nursing team, they record the patient observations they make and the patient care they give on the nurse's record. Remember that the chart is a legal document. This means that entries must be written in ink, that recordings must be accurate, and that spelling must be correct. It means, too, that crossing out or erasing is forbidden.

Look at the nurse's records on your patient's charts. Observe how the nurse gives a word picture of the patient's day. She describes what his physical condition was like, the clues of illness observed, the nursing care he received, the off-the-ward trips he made, and doctors' visits to the patient.

Avoid making comments on the nurse's record that mean nothing, such as "no complaints," "usual day," or "in good spirits." Remember, describe what you see, how the patient acts, or what he says. If you have nothing to say about the patient, record nothing.

SPECIAL NOTE

The nursing service in your hospital will identify, in your job description, whether you should chart your observations on the chart or in a special ward report book. Perform according to your job description. The inclusion of charting in this book was intended to reinforce the need for you to observe your patient and was not intended to determine where these observations should be written.

SUMMARY

The signs that the body is not meeting its needs for living effectively are really the clues or symptoms of illness. We must observe the patient carefully for any of these clues of illness in each contact that we have with him.

These clues must be reported to the doctor and nurse, and they must be recorded on the nurse's record on the patient's chart. Since this record is a legal document, all observations and nursing care must be recorded on it accurately in ink. The observations of the patient recorded here are the actual descriptions of the clues of illness that you observed, the patient behavior you saw, or the patient complaints you heard. Only the doctor has the medical information that enables him to record his personal opinion, which is really the diagnosis, on the chart. We record the observation that the patient's nose is draining a watery substance; the doctor records the opinion that the patient has sinusitis. We may have thought the patient had a cold, but then we really do not have sufficient medical knowledge for recording our thoughts.

DISCUSSION QUESTIONS

1 Observe the nurse's records on the patients you cared for yesterday. Would these records give you a picture of the patient's day?
2 Observe your sickest patient carefully. What clues of illness do you observe?
3 Observe the intake and output record on your sickest patient. What clues to his illness does this record give you?
4 What special observations did the nurse assign you to make today? Why did she want these observations made?
5 Select that patient in your care with whom you would least like to spend 30 minutes. What are his problems?
6 Put yourself in the position of the patient you selected in question 5. Would you act differently?
7 Ask the nurse to help you chart that patient care you gave and the observations you made today.
8 Why is the patient in a dangerous situation if the nursing assistant just gives bedpans, passes out ice water, etc., and never observes the patient?
9 Observe as many clues of illness as you can. Write them down. Ask the team leader or doctor to tell you what they mean to the patient and why they appear. If you observe and learn the meaning of one clue to illness each day, you will soon be a valuable, observant nursing assistant.

VOCABULARY

contracture deformities Bending of the limbs that cannot be corrected.
cyanosis Blue tinge to fingernail beds, lips, earlobes, etc.
defecation Bowel movement.
dyspnea Difficult breathing.
hemiplegia Paralysis of one half of the body, including the face, arm, and leg.
incontinence Loss of control over bladder and/or bowels.
monoplegia Paralysis of one limb (arm or leg).
paralysis Loss of ability to move.
paraplegia Paralysis of the lower half of the body from the umbilicus down.
thrombophlebitis Inflammation and blood clot formation in the veins (*thrombo*, clot; *phlebitis*, inflammation of the vein).
trachea Windpipe.
umbilicus Navel.
unconscious Not aware of or responding to surroundings.

SOURCE OF ADDITIONAL INFORMATION

1 Film: Nursing: the cardiac patient; may be obtained from Director, Film Library, United States Naval Medical School, National Naval Medical Center, Bethesda, Md. 20014. (*Illustrates the hospital corpsman's part in the care of a patient suffering from a myocardial infarction. Covers taking vital signs, giving oxygen, bathing, and feeding. Particular attention is given to observation and charting.*)

19/The vital signs

STUDY QUESTIONS

1. What are the vital signs?
2. Which vital signs are routinely taken together?
3. How often are the vital signs taken?
4. Who determines how often the vital signs should be taken?
5. Why are the vital signs "vital"?

The vital signs are those measures of body functioning that indicate how effectively the body is carrying out the essential activities of living. These measures include the following:

1. Temperature
2. Pulse
3. Respiration
4. Blood pressure
5. Level of consciousness

Any serious attack on the body by germs or any failure of an organ to function adequately will be evident through changes in the vital signs.

The vital signs of temperature, pulse, and respiration are taken together because they give significant clues to the condition of the patient's body. The temperature tells whether or not germs have invaded the body, the pulse tells the condition of the heart, and the respiration tells the condition of the lungs. Taken together, these signs show how the body is working to maintain life by maintaining body temperature, pumping around the blood, and bringing in the oxygen essential for life.

The vital signs you take help the patient only if you report abnormal findings to the doctor or the nurse. Therefore, the following observations should be reported:

1. Temperature above 98.6° or below 97.6° F.
2. Pulse rate above 120 or below 60

3. Respiration above 28 or below 12
4. Irregular pulse rates
5. Noisy breathing
6. Cyanosis

The vital signs give the doctor a great deal of information about the patient's body and how it is functioning to maintain life. Because of this, he will ask you to take the patient's vital signs at regular intervals throughout every 24-hour period. The frequency of these intervals will depend upon how much difficulty the patient's body is having in maintaining life or upon how much information the doctor wants about the patient. If the patient has a temperature so high that it threatens his life, the doctor will order medications and treatments to reduce it. However, he will also ask you to take the patient's temperature every 15 minutes, so that he will know that the medications and treatments are effective.

When a patient is admitted and the doctor wants to collect all the information possible so that a diagnosis can be made quickly, he will request that the patient's vital signs be taken every 4 hours.

The vital signs give an accurate picture of how the patient's body is functioning even while he is unconscious. This is true because the activities of life that they measure are under the control of the involuntary nervous system. Therefore the seriously ill unconscious patient or the anesthetized patient who has recently been operated on is observed for changes in his condition primarily through the taking of his vital signs.

DISCUSSION QUESTIONS

1 How often are vital signs taken on your patients?
2 Are the vital signs taken with the same frequency on all patients?
3 How does the taking of vital signs help the patient?
4 How is the unconscious patient's condition observed?
5 What vital sign determinations would you report to the nurse?

SOURCE OF ADDITIONAL INFORMATION

1 Film: Vital signs. Part I: Cardinal symptoms; may be obtained from Director, Film Library, United States Naval Medical School, National Naval Medical Center, Bethesda, Md. 20014. (*Explains how vital signs present a picture of the patient's condition.*)

20/Taking the patient's temperature

STUDY QUESTIONS

1. What does the patient's temperature measure?
2. How is the patient's temperature taken?
3. How is the body heat normally regulated to maintain a body temperature of 98.6° F.?
4. Why does our face flush during exercise?
5. Of what value is perspiration?
6. What is a fever?
7. What does a fever indicate?
8. How many ways can the patient's temperature be taken?
9. How do you know which one of these ways is best for your patient?
10. Which method of taking the temperature is the most accurate? Which is the least accurate?
11. What do the little lines on a thermometer mean?
12. How is a rectal thermometer inserted?
13. What is the normal range of a patient's temperature?
14. What temperatures are considered abnormal and must be reported to the nurse?

DEFINITION OF BODY TEMPERATURE

Temperature is defined as a degree of heat. A high temperature indicates the presence of a great deal of heat, whereas a low temperature indicates the presence of little heat. A thermometer is an instrument for measuring temperature or heat. Normal body temperature is considered to be 98.6° F. However, the activities of the body vary throughout the 24-hour period, and the body temperature varies, too. During the day when the body is seeing, thinking, working, digesting food, and moving about, the temperature is normally about 98.6° F. At night, when the activities of the body are at their lowest ebb and the body is at rest, the temperature, too, is at its lowest point (normally), which is about 97.6° F. In this way, the temperature changes normally throughout the 24-hour period, varying about one degree from a low of 97.6° F. at night to a high of 98.6° F. during the day.

Body heat

Body heat is obtained from the metabolism (utilization) of food by the cells of the body. As the cells in the muscles utilize the food, heat and energy are produced and waste material is left. This is much the same as the process we use to heat our home. Fuel (oil, wood, gas) and fire in the furnace produce heat and waste material such as carbon (ashes). Food (changed by digestion) and oxygen in the cell produce heat and energy and waste material.

In your home, the heat does not collect in the basement around the furnace. Instead, it is used to heat air or water. This hot air or water is then circulated throughout the house in a system of pipes. In the body, heat warms the blood, which is then circulated around the body in the blood vessels in order to maintain body heat or a body temperature of 98.6° F.

NORMAL BODY TEMPERATURE

Since 98.6° F. is the temperature that permits the body to carry out its activities of living most effectively, this is the body temperature that the heat-regulating center in the brain tries to maintain. It does this by throwing off heat when too much is produced or by conserving heat when too little is being produced.

An example of this regulation might be the way in which the body functions during exercise. During strenuous exercise such as playing football or handball, the cells in the muscles use more food to get energy. Therefore the energy for the exercise is produced, but heat is also produced and the body gets warm. The heat-regulating system in the brain will get rid of this excess body heat in two ways—widening of blood vessels and perspiration.

It will widen the blood vessels close to the body surface so that more blood is brought close to the outside of the body and is cooled. (Notice how flushed the face becomes when the body is warm.)

It will also get rid of the excess heat through perspiration. Water is secreted by the sweat glands and expelled onto the surface of the body. This perspiration evaporates by taking enough heat from the body to convert the water (perspiration) into a water vapor that then disappears into the air. (This is similar to the process by which boiling water takes enough heat from the stove to change into water vapor or steam, which then passes into the air.) On a humid day when the air already contains a great deal of water vapor, it will be unable to take up any more. Then perspiration cannot evaporate from the body, and so the body will become extremely hot, sweaty, and uncomfortable. Fans cool the body by circulating air around so that the air filled with perspiration is moved away from the body and dry air is moved in to absorb more moisture.

When too little heat is being produced, the body conserves it. The heat-regulating center narrows the blood vessels close to the surface of the body, thus bringing less blood to the surface for cooling.

The heat-regulating center is located in the brain and is kept aware of the body temperature by the nerves of the involuntary nervous system that are located throughout the body.

FEVER

Fever is defined as any temperature above the normal 98.6° F. Fever occurs when so much heat is produced that the body is unable to get rid of the excess or when the heat-regulating center in the brain stops functioning effectively.

Although the patient may be lying quietly in bed, his body may be engaged in a tremendous fight—a fight for his life. Germs, or disease-producing bacteria, may have invaded his body, and all his body defenses may be fighting to overcome these germs and permit the patient to recover. Fever indicates to the doctor that germs have invaded the patient's body and that a battle is raging. The fever does not tell the doctor where the germs are. This he determines by studying the patient. Is the patient coughing? Where does the patient have pain? Is the patient's operative site draining?

Since fever usually indicates that the patient's body has been invaded by germs, the doctor will direct the nurse to give these patients antibiotics. Antibiotics are medications that inhibit the growth of germs in the patient's body and permit the body defenses to overcome them. It is interesting to note that *anti* (against) *biotics* (life) are really bacteria raised in the laboratory and prepared in a form that can be given to the patient as a medication. These antibiotics work against the germs in the body by preventing them from getting the foodstuffs they need to grow, in much the same way that a cat works against rats and curtails their activities or a dog works against cats.

Since antibiotics are also bacteria, the patient may have some reactions to them. When you give the patient his morning bath or evening care, observe him carefully for any evidence of rashes, joint pains, nausea and vomiting, or diarrhea. Report these signs of a reaction to the nurse as soon as you observe them.

WHAT TEMPERATURE TO REPORT

Taking the patient's temperature, in itself, does not help the patient. The patient's temperature merely tells you something about the patient's body. What helps the patient is what is done for him because of the information obtained by taking his temperature. Therefore it is not enough to just take the temperature. You must look at this information you get about the patient and decide whether or not it indicates that his condition is changing—worsening or improving. Then you must decide how to notify the nurse about these changes.

If a patient's temperature is not markedly changed from the previous one, it may be sufficient for you to mark it down in the record. Then you can continue taking the temperature of the remaining patients. When you are finished taking temperatures, take this record to the nurse's station and give it to the nurse. However, if a patient's temperature is markedly changed from his previous one, do not wait until all the temperatures are taken, but notify the nurse immediately of this change.

Since the normal temperature range is 97.6° to 98.6° F., abnormal temperature readings are those below 97.6° F. and those above 98.6° F. The nurse can wait until you take the temperatures of all the patients on the ward to learn about the readings below 100° F. However, any temperature over 100° F. should be reported immediately.

THE VERY HIGH OR THE VERY LOW TEMPERATURE

Although it is normal to make a mistake in giving a patient nursing care, mistakes must be avoided. You can avoid them only by constantly checking your own work. Therefore any temperature that is extremely high or extremely low should be verified by taking it over, preferably in another way. After you verify the correctness of the temperature reading, record it so that the doctor and nurse will know you checked it. Otherwise, they will ask you to verify the temperature before they institute medical and nursing measures to treat the patient. A verified temperature can be recorded by marking a V opposite the temperature on the record.

Checking your own work is a good habit to develop. Perhaps it will save you the embarrassment of calling the doctor at 3 A.M. for a patient with a temperature of 103° F. that turns out to be 99.2° F. when the doctor rechecks it.

METHODS OF TAKING TEMPERATURES
Oral method

An oral thermometer is placed in the patient's mouth under his tongue and kept there for 3 minutes. The patient is asked to keep his mouth closed and to breathe through his nose.

Rectal method

The rectal thermometer is placed in the patient's rectum and kept there for 3 minutes. The nursing assistant keeps his fingers on the end of the thermometer protruding from the rectum while it is in place.

Axillary method

An oral or rectal thermometer is placed in the patient's dried axilla, and his arm is brought down to his side and over it. The arm is held close to his body (to keep the thermometer in place) for 10 minutes.

• • •

The most accurate means of taking temperatures is the rectal method and the least accurate is the axillary method. It is interesting to note that axillary temperatures require the longest time to take (10 minutes) and are far from accurate.

Normal rectal temperature is 99.6° F. (one degree above the normal oral temperature of 98.6° F.), and the normal axillary temperature is 97.6° F. (one degree below the normal oral temperature). Since the normal rectal temperature is one degree above the oral and the normal axillary temperature is one degree below the oral, it is necessary to mark R after rectal temperatures and Ax after axillary temperatures on the temperature record. If there is no R or Ax after the temperature, it is assumed that it was taken orally.

WHICH METHOD TO USE IN TAKING THE PATIENT'S TEMPERATURE

The oral method is used in taking the temperatures of the following patients:
1. Patients who can understand the directions to keep the mouth closed over the thermometer and to breathe through the nose and who can be trusted to do this without biting the thermometer
2. Patients who can follow the preceding directions and who can breathe adequately with the mouth closed

This means that the patient who has his temperature taken orally is conscious, alert, able to follow directions, and able to breathe adequately through his nose when his mouth is closed.

Temperatures are taken rectally in the following patients:
1. Patients who cannot understand and follow directions
2. Patients who are receiving oxygen
3. Patients who are obviously short of breath
4. Patients who are unconscious or confused
5. Patients who are too young to understand and follow directions, such as infants and small children.

Temperatures are taken by the axillary method in those patients who cannot have their temperature taken orally or rectally. This means that axillary temperatures are taken only when the temperature cannot be taken in some other way. An example of this situation might be the case of a patient who has had his rectum removed and who is still unconscious from the anesthesia. However, as soon as this patient regains consciousness, the method of taking the temperature will be changed from axillary to oral.

READING A THERMOMETER

Look at the thermometer closely and you will find that the two ends are different. One end is silver colored and tapers in from the body of the thermometer, whereas the other end appears white and is of the same width as the body of the thermometer.

Rotate the thermometer in your fingers by holding it at the untapered end. Notice that on one side of the thermometer there is a broad white strip going from one end to the other. This is the back of the thermometer. Now turn this side away from you and look at the front of the thermometer. Notice the lines at the top of the thermometer barrel and the numbers at the bottom (Fig. 20-1).

Before you can read the thermometer, it will be necessary for you to know that the

Taking the patient's temperature 171

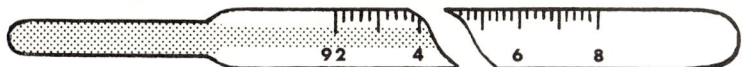

Fig. 20-1. The left part of the thermometer illustrated here shows the correct side for reading it, and the right part shows the back of the thermometer. When you look at the back of the thermometer, you will be unable to see the mercury (silver streak) and thus will be unable to get the temperature reading. Note the tapered silver-colored end of the thermometer. This is the end that is inserted into the patient's mouth or rectum.

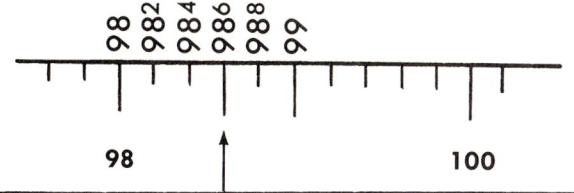

Fig. 20-2. The parts of the degree from 98 to 99. Note the long line and arrow at 98.6° F. (normal temperature).

Table 20-1. Comparison of parts of a dollar and parts of a degree

Dollar	Degree	Parts of the degree from 98 to 99
.20	.2	98.2
.40	.4	98.4
.60	.6	98.6
.80	.8	98.8
1.00	1.0	99.0

lines really indicate a part of a degree. Each degree of the thermometer is divided into five parts, and each part is actually one fifth of a degree (Fig. 20-2). In order to make the measurement of temperature easier to write and to understand, we adopt much the same system in reading the thermometer as we do in talking about money. Instead of saying or writing one fifth of a dollar, we would say or write $.20; instead of saying or writing two fifths, we would say or write $.40. We do this in reading the thermometer, too. Instead of one fifth of a degree, we say and write .2.

The range between 98° and 99° is one degree on the thermometer. This degree, like all degrees, is divided into five parts, and each part is marked by a small line. Actually the degree is divided just like the dollar, except that we drop the zeros (Table 20-1).

Now hold the thermometer at the untapered end (the tapered end is silver colored because it contains mercury) and rotate it slowly between your thumb and index finger. Hold the thermometer at eye level. Observe the area between the lines and the numbers 98 and 100 until you can see a silvery streak of mercury in this space between the lines and the numbers. Notice where the mercury ends. Rotate the thermometer to see what number is closest to

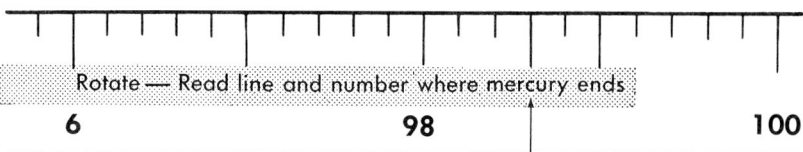

Fig. 20-3. Thermometer reading 99.2° F.

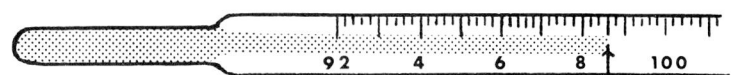

Fig. 20-4. Thermometer reading 98.6° F. Note the long line and arrow at 98.6° F. to signify that this is normal temperature.

the end of the mercury. Then rotate the thermometer slightly to see how many lines the mercury extends past 99 (Fig. 20-3). Check your reading by rotating the thermometer quickly to see the position of the mercury in relation to the numbers and the lines.

Notice the arrow and the long line at 98.6 on the thermometer (Fig. 20-4). This reading has the long line (the only place on the thermometer where a part of a degree is marked by a long line) and the arrow because it is normal temperature.

Now try to read a few thermometers. Remember that each small line indicates (stands for) two tenths of a degree, not one degree. You cannot get a reading with an odd part of a degree such as 103.3° because there is no .3 or .1 or .5 or .7 on the thermometer. Remember that each degree is marked at intervals of .2, .4, .6, and .8. If you see the mercury between two small lines, read it at whatever line it is closest to (Table 20-1).

Be careful when you are reading the thermometer to state the whole number and the parts of the degree correctly. There is a great deal of difference between a temperature of 102° and one of 100.2° F. or 104° and one of 100.4° F.

TAKING THE PATIENT'S TEMPERATURE

Collect the equipment for taking the patient's temperature, which would include the following:
1. Oral thermometer tray with wipes
2. Rectal thermometer tray with lubricant and wipes
3. Temperature record
4. Pencil

Be sure that you have a clean thermometer for each patient whose temperature you are going to take. However, if each patient has his own thermometer in a receptacle in his room, your equipment would consist only of the following:
1. Temperature record
2. Pencil
3. Container of wipes
4. Container of lubricant

Place all the equipment on a movable table and go to the patient's area. Take the oral temperatures of four patients at a time. Check to be sure that the thermometers register below 94° F. Then have each patient open his mouth so that you can insert the thermometer under the tongue. Be sure that the patient is not smoking. After placing four thermometers, return to the first patient and count his pulse and respirations. Remove the thermometer (when 3 minutes have elapsed) and read it. Question the patient about how many times his bowels moved in the preceding 24 hours. Chart the temperature, pulse, respiration, and bowel movements on the temperature record. (Bowel movements are usually charted only with the morning temperature.) Wipe the thermometer and place it in the container for soiled thermometers on the tray, or return it to the receptacle in the patient's area. Go to the next patient and repeat this procedure. When all four of these thermometers have been collected, take the temperature of four more patients.

When the temperature roster indicates that a patient's temperature is to be taken rectally, take this temperature by itself. Check the thermometer to be sure it registers below 94°. Squirt some lubricant on a thermometer wipe and lubricate the thermometer by rotating it in the wipe. Then roll the patient onto his side and insert the thermometer into his rectum, directing it toward the patient's mouth. Keep the fingers of your one hand on the thermometer while you take the patient's pulse with the other. Now count the patient's respirations. After 3 minutes remove the thermometer, clean it with a wipe, and read it. Question the patient about his bowel movements. Return the patient to his correct position, and place the thermometer in the proper receptacle on the tray or in the patient's room. Wash your hands thoroughly. Record the temperature, pulse, respiration, and bowel movements on the temperature record.

Do not shake the thermometer after you remove it from the patient's mouth or rectum until you have read it. This thermometer is different from the weather thermometer in that it registers the patient's temperature and then it sticks at this point until it is shaken down. If this did not occur, we would be unable to get an accurate reading of the patient's temperature. However, after you read the thermometer, hold it firmly at the untapered end (end that does not contain the mercury), between the thumb and index finger, and flick the wrist with quick, short, jerking movements. This will shake the mercury down to 94° F. If the patient has his own thermometer in a receptacle of antiseptic solution in his room, it is essential to shake down the thermometer before replacing it in the receptacle. If the thermometers are cleaned in a central service unit, they may be shaken down by a centrifuge, making it unnecessary for you to do so. However, if you clean the thermometers on your own ward by soaking them in an antiseptic solution, it may speed up the process if you shake each one down after you use it.

Remember the following when taking temperatures:

1. Oral thermometers can be distributed to four patients, but rectal thermometers can be distributed to only one patient at a time when you are taking patients' temperatures.

2. The oral thermometer is placed under the patient's tongue. The rectal thermometer is inserted approximately 2 inches into the rectum. When inserting rectal thermometers, remember that the rectum is part of the digestive system, which starts at the mouth. Then insert the thermometer into the rectum by directing it toward the patient's mouth.

3. Place the silvery end (the tapered end of the thermometer containing the mercury) into the patient's mouth or rectum as indicated.

4. Handle the clear end (the untapered end without the mercury) when inserting or removing a thermomoter.

5. Wash your hands thoroughly after taking a temperature rectally and before proceeding to take another temperature. Inserting, holding, and removing the rectal thermometer will bring your hands in close contact with the patient's rectum and with fecal material. Therefore handwashing is essential after each rectal temperature to

avoid carrying organisms and fecal material from one patient to another.

It is extremely desirable to plan your temperature-taking assignment in such a way so that you take all the oral and axillary temperatures first and the rectal temperatures last.

6. Check the thermometer to be sure that the mercury registers below 94° F. before you insert it. Shake down the thermometer and retake the temperature if you get an extremely high or low reading. Better still, get another thermometer and take the temperature by another method. For example, if you get a high or low reading when you take the temperature orally, get a rectal thermometer and take the temperature rectally.

7. Taking the patient's temperature in itself does not help him. What you do about the temperature, however, should help him.

DOCTOR'S ORDERS FOR TAKING THE PATIENT'S TEMPERATURE

The doctor may write an order on the chart stating how many times he wants the patient's temperature taken in every 24-hour period. He may designate this frequency by the following abbreviations:

    o.d.   Once a day
    b.i.d. Twice a day
    t.i.d. Three times a day
    q.i.d. Four times a day
    q.4h. Every 4 hours (day and night)

The hospital has a routine time for taking temperatures. This time was selected because it is the best possible time to meet the patients' nursing care needs. The time for taking temperatures may be just before the doctor makes his morning, afternoon, and evening rounds.

SUMMARY

The patient's temperature may be a symptom. It is a measure of his body heat. His body heat (and therefore his temperature) increases when germs invade his body (infection occurs) or when the heat-regulating system fails to function adequately.

The patient's temperature can be taken by the oral, rectal, or axillary method, depending upon the patient's condition. However, the axillary method requires the longest time and is the least accurate of the three methods.

Taking the temperature does not help the patient; what is done with the information may help the patient to recover. Temperatures above 98.6° F. and those below 97.6° F. are considered abnormal and should be called to the nurse's attention.

DISCUSSION QUESTIONS

1 At what time are temperatures taken routinely on your unit?
2 Does your unit have any special policy about how many times a day certain patients (for example, patients just admitted or postoperative patients with elevated temperatures) should have their temperatures taken?
3 Who cleans (disinfects) the used thermometers for your unit?
4 What abnormal temperatures should you report to the nurse promptly?
5 Do your patients have individual thermometers in containers on their bed or in their room? If so, how are these thermometers and receptacles cleaned?
6 What patients assigned to you have their temperatures taken rectally? Why?
7 Why is it necessary to remain with the patient and to hold onto the end of the thermometer when the temperature is being taken rectally?
8 How can you determine if the patient had a bowel movement when he is unable to understand your directions about holding the thermometer in his mouth?
9 Why should you wash your hands after you take a temperature rectally?
10 Observe the patients on your unit who develop an elevated temperature. Discuss these patients with the nurse and attempt to find out what caused the elevation.
11 Why is it a good policy to take the patient's temperature as soon as he complains about pain? (Assume that he is not having his temperature taken routinely.)

VOCABULARY

antibiotics Bacteria that are raised in the laboratory and used as medications to help the body kill germs.

axilla Underarm (armpit).

decimal point (.) Indicates a part or fraction of a whole number. For example, $.50 means $\frac{50}{100}$ or one half of a dollar; .2 means $\frac{2}{10}$ or one fifth of one degree.

Fahrenheit (F.) System of measuring heat.

fever Temperature elevation above 98.6° F.

metabolism Working of the cells of the body to carry on the activities of living.

oral Concerning the mouth.

perspiration Fluid secreted to the surface of the skin by the sweat glands in an effort to cool the body.

pulse Heartbeat measured at the artery.

rectal Concerning the rectum.

respiration Breathing rate.

temperature Degrees of heat.

thermometer Instrument to measure temperature.

vital signs Signs of life. These are the temperature, pulse, respiration, blood pressure, and level of consciousness.

SOURCE OF ADDITIONAL INFORMATION

1 Film: Vital signs; part 2: Taking temperature, pulse and respiration; may be obtained from Director, Film Library, United States Naval Medical School, National Naval Medical Center, Bethesda, Md. 20014. *(Shows Navy corpsmen taking temperatures [oral, rectal, axillary], pulses, and respirations in a variety of patients.)*

21/Taking the patient's pulse

STUDY QUESTIONS

1. What is the pulse?
2. How is the pulse related to the heartbeat?
3. Where is the pulse taken?
4. How is the pulse taken?
5. When can a pulse be taken for 15 seconds?
6. When are 15-second pulse observations so inaccurate that the pulse must be counted for a full minute?
7. What is the normal pulse rate?
8. What pulse rates are abnormal and must be reported to the nurse?
9. What factors cause changes in the heartbeat?
10. What would a very rapid pulse indicate?

THE PATIENT'S PULSE

The pulse is defined as the beat you feel at the artery as the heart pumps the blood around the body. As the heart pumps out a ventricle full of blood, the artery widens. When the ventricle is filling and there is no output of blood, the artery narrows (Fig. 21-1). When you put your fingers on an artery that lies over a bone, you can feel this widening of the artery as the heart pumps out a ventricle full of blood and the narrowing of the artery as the ventricle of the heart is filling. This widening and narrowing of the artery is called the pulse. The pulse, then, is actually a measure of the heartbeat.

WHERE THE PULSE IS TAKEN

The pulse can be counted by placing the fingers on any artery that lies close to the surface of the body and over a bone. The most common places to count the pulse are the following:

1. *At the radial artery,* at the thumb side of the wrist about 1 inch above the base of the thumb
2. *At the dorsalis pedis artery* on the instep of the foot (Fig. 21-2)
3. *At the carotid artery* on either side of neck just in front of and below the earlobes
4. *At the temporal artery* in the temple areas about 1 inch above the outer end of the eyebrow

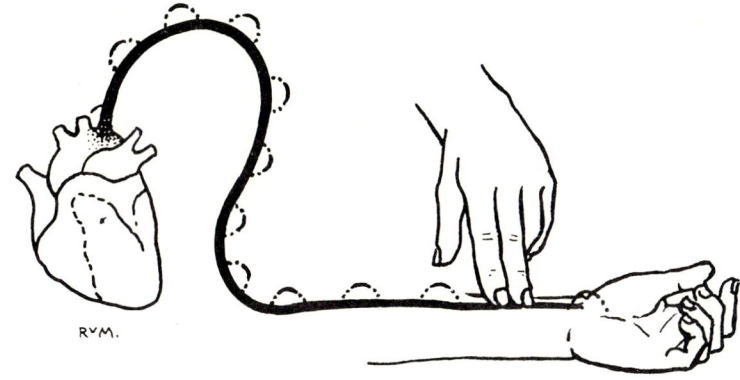

Fig. 21-1. The artery widens with the increased flow of blood in it with each heartbeat and narrows as the flow decreases between the beats. This widening and narrowing of the artery is called the pulse.

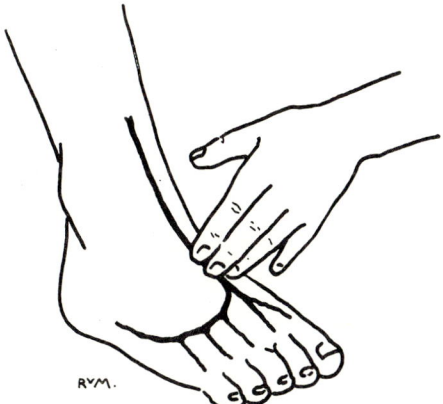

Fig. 21-2. Taking the dorsalis pedis pulse.

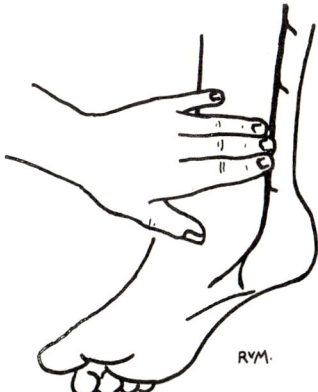

Fig. 21-3. Taking the posterior tibial pulse.

5. *At the posterior tibial artery* on the inner side of the foot about 1 inch below the ankle (Fig. 21-3)

WHEN THE PULSE IS TAKEN

The pulse is usually taken along with the temperature. However, if the patient appears to be extremely apprehensive or if he complains of chest pains, the pulse should be taken at that time.

The pulse is usually taken along with the blood pressure also. If the blood pressure (the force exerted by the heart to pump the blood around the body) is changing because of blood loss or heart failure, the pulse, too, will change. The heart tries to maintain life as long as it can. If the patient has heart failure or a hemorrhage, the heart will attempt to make up for the weakened pump or the blood loss by beating faster and faster. Although the heart beats faster, each heartbeat will be weaker and less effective than the normal one. Therefore there is a relationship between the blood pressure and the pulse rate; both are usually taken when the patient is being observed closely.

Since the number of heartbeats is increased with exercise, nervousness, tension, and discomfort, the patient should be sitting quietly in a chair or lying comfortably in bed when the pulse is taken. He must be at rest if an accurate measure of heart activity is to be obtained through a measurement of the pulse.

HOW THE PULSE IS TAKEN

The patient is placed in a comfortable position sitting at the bedside or lying in bed. He is not permitted to smoke. Then three fingers are placed lightly over the artery at the patient's wrist and the pulse beats are counted for 1 minute. This number of beats per minute may be counted in two ways: (1) the pulse may be counted for 15 seconds and the number of beats multiplied by four or (2) the pulse may be counted for a full minute.

In the 15-second pulse observation, the pulse is counted for 15 seconds and the number of pulse beats obtained is multiplied by four to obtain the number of pulse beats for 1 minute.

For example: 18 (number of pulse beats in 15 seconds) × 4 (number of 15-second periods in 1 minute) = 72 pulse beats in 60 seconds.

Then the pulse is counted for 15 more seconds and the result is multiplied by four again. This rechecking of the pulse is a method of checking your accuracy. If the pulse beat you obtained in the first calculation is the same as the one you obtained in the second, you are probably correct and you can record that pulse rate.

If, however, the pulse rate you obtained the first time differs greatly from the one you obtained the second time, something is wrong. You may have counted the pulse incorrectly, you may have multiplied incorrectly, or the pulse may have an irregular rhythm. If an error does exist in your counting or calculation, it can be corrected by using the second method for counting the pulse rate.

Count the pulse for an entire 60-second period and record this pulse rate on a piece of note paper. Recount the pulse for another 60-second period and compare the results. If you are taking the pulse correctly, they should be the same.

Occasionally you will have difficulty feeling the pulse. This usually is due to the fact that you are pressing on the artery with too much force. In fact, your fingers may be acting like a tourniquet that is closing off the artery. Relax, loosen your fingers, avoid using too much pressure, and try again.

OBSERVATIONS OF PULSE RHYTHM AND VOLUME

After the pulse rate is counted for a period of 60 seconds (or for 15 seconds and the result multiplied by four) and the rate recorded on the temperature record just after the temperature, the pulse rhythm and volume are observed.

The pulse normally has a regular rhythm; that is, the beats are of uniform force and are separated by equal periods of time (Fig. 21-4).

An irregular pulse is one in which the beats are separated by unequal periods of time or are of unequal force or both (Fig. 21-5).

Then the pulse volume is observed. If the blood volume is normal, the pulse will be full and large as shown in Fig. 21-4.

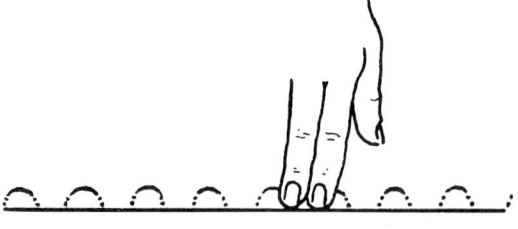

Fig. 21-4. Regular pulse.

However, if the blood volume is decreased either by hemorrhage or by a failing force in the heart (heart failure), the pulse will become weak, feeble, and thready (Fig. 21-6). The beats will be almost indistinguishable.

The observations of the pulse rhythm and volume are recorded on the temperature record along with the pulse rate.

FACTORS AFFECTING PULSE RATE

The pulse rate is a measure of the heartbeat. Therefore anything that affects the heart will also affect the pulse rate. Some of these factors are as follows:

1. Exercise increases the need of the body cells for blood and oxygen. Therefore exercise will increase heartbeat and pulse rate.
2. Fever increases heartbeat and pulse rate because the body speeds up all its activities to fight the disease. This is much the same mechanism as that in exercise (item 1).
3. A failing heart beats faster and faster, but each beat accomplishes less and less. Nevertheless, the heart beats more quickly in an attempt to accomplish the work of pumping the blood around the body. Therefore a failing heart causes an increasing pulse rate.
4. If hemorrhage or loss of blood occurs, the heart tries to do its work with the lessened amount of blood by pumping it around oftener. Therefore hemorrhage or blood loss causes an increased heartbeat and an increased pulse rate but a weaker pulse.
5. Fear or worry creates a problem to the body. The heart, which is under the control of the involuntary nervous system, speeds up its functioning to prepare the body to fight the feared object or to run away from it. This preparation to fight or flee includes an increased blood supply to the arms and legs. Therefore heartbeat and pulse rate are increased.
6. Pain increases heartbeat and pulse rate in the same way as does fear.
7. Brain injuries that damage or compress the circulatory center in the brain slow the heartbeat.

THE NORMAL PULSE RATE

The normal pulse rate (taken with the body at rest) varies from 60 to 70 beats per minute for men and 70 to 80 for women. It is regular in rhythm and full in volume.

During exercise, the pulse rate increases rapidly, but it decreases to its normal rate when the exercise ceases.

The pulse is affected by any condition that affects the body, such as fever, pain, fear, exercise, and worry. The pulse, which is under the control of the involuntary nervous system, speeds up in all these conditions to help the body meet the threat.

Since the pulse increases and slows with body activities, there may be a wide variation in the normal pulse range. However, pulse rates that are under 60 and those that

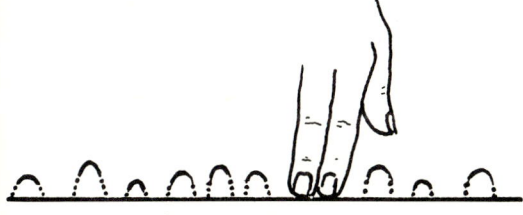

Fig. 21-5. Irregular pulse.

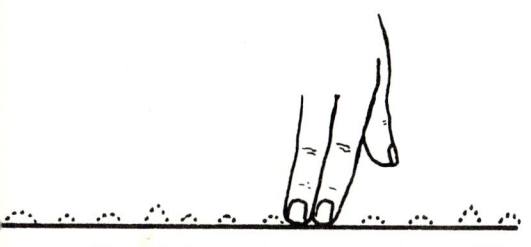

Fig. 21-6. Weak, thready pulse.

are over 120 are considered abnormal and should be reported to the nurse along with abnormal temperatures (those above 98.6° and those below 97.6° F.).

SUMMARY

The pulse is really a measure of heartbeat. Any condition (such as exercise, fear, pain, or fever) that increases the need for blood and oxygen in the cells will increase the heartbeat and the pulse rate.

The heart tries to maintain life as long as it can. It does this by increasing the number of heartbeats when failure occurs. Thus, it attempts to do its job by beating oftener even though each beat is weaker and accomplishes less than it should.

If hemorrhage (blood loss) occurs, the heart attempts to make the remaining blood do the work that all the blood once did by sending it around the body oftener. Therefore the pulse becomes rapid and weaker in the patient who is hemorrhaging.

The pulse is a good clue to the condition of the body. When body activities increase, so does the pulse; when life is threatened by a failing heart or a severe hemorrhage, the pulse gets faster and faster and weaker and weaker. Brain injuries involving the circulatory center or its message-sending nerves cause a slowing of the pulse. The pulse may become so slow that the flow of blood around the body is inadequate to support life, and death may occur.

DISCUSSION QUESTIONS

1 Observe your patient's temperature, pulse, and respiration records. Do you notice that the patient's pulse rises as his temperature rises? Why?
2 Take the patient's pulse at the radial artery. Now press down firmly on the artery with your fingers. Do you feel the pulse better? If not, why not?
3 Do a brief experiment on the accuracy of 15-second pulse observations. Take the pulse on three different patients for 15 seconds. Multiply the result of each count by four and record the pulse rates on a sheet of paper. Now retake the same three patients' pulses for a full minute. Compare the results. Are 15-second pulse determinations accurate?
4 Under what condition would a 15-second record of a pulse observation differ greatly from that of an observation for a minute?
5 Under what circumstances would you take the pulse for 1 full minute?
6 How would pulse observations give you a clue to the pain or stress that a patient is suffering?
7 Why does the pulse rate increase in such conditions as hemorrhage?
8 What pulse rates are abnormal and should be reported to the nurse?

VOCABULARY

artery Blood vessel that takes oxygen-full blood away from the heart to the body cells.
blood pressure The force exerted by the heart to pump the blood around the body.
carotid artery Artery that can be felt on either side of the neck below the earlobes.
dorsalis pedis artery Artery that can be felt on the instep of the foot.
posterior tibial artery Artery that can be felt on the inner side of the foot just below the ankle.
pulse Heartbeat.
radial artery Artery that can be felt about 1 inch above the base of the thumb.
temporal artery Artery that can be felt on either side of the head just above the outer edge of the eyebrow.

SOURCES OF ADDITIONAL INFORMATION

1 Book: Phibbs, Brendan. The human heart, ed. 2, St. Louis, 1971, The C. V. Mosby Co. *(Chap. 4 illustrates pumping action of the heart.)*
2 Film: Hemo the magnificent; may be obtained from local Bell Telephone Co. or American Telephone and Telegraph Co., 195 Broadway, Room 510A, New York, N. Y. 10007. *(Presents story of blood and circulatory system. Shows beating of human heart.)*

22/Counting the patient's respirations

STUDY QUESTIONS

1. What is respiration?
2. Why does the patient breathe?
3. How does the patient know when to breathe?
4. What is the normal respiratory rate?
5. Why are the respirations counted when the patient is at rest?
6. What body activities speed up the respiratory rate?
7. What disease conditions speed up the respiratory rate?
8. What disease conditions slow down the respiratory rate?
9. How do you count the respiratory rate?
10. What observations (other than counting the rate) should be taken when you count the respiratory rate?
11. What observations about the patient's respirations should you report to the nurse?
12. What is cyanosis? Why does it occur?

WHY THE PATIENT BREATHES

Respiration is defined as the process of inhaling air into the lungs and exhaling carbon dioxide from the lungs. The purpose of this process (commonly known as breathing) is to get oxygen into the blood and to remove carbon dioxide from the blood. This internal respiration occurs in the lungs in the following way:

1. The air is inhaled into the lungs through the nose and mouth.
2. The air passes down the trachea and into the lungs through the bronchi and the bronchioles.
3. The air finally passes into one of the little alveoli at the end of each bronchiole. Here at the alveoli the gaseous exchanges take place. Oxygen from the air passes through the alveolar wall and goes into the bloodstream, and carbon dioxide is given up by the blood and passes through the alveolar wall and into the alveoli. Then it is breathed out of the lungs with the next exhalation.

This movement of gas into the blood and from the blood into the alveoli occurs because of the gas pressures. Nature likes equality and tries to obtain it. You know that your automobile tire can be pumped up to an air pressure of 28 pounds. However, when a hole is punched in the tire, air (a gas) flows out until the air pressure in the tire is the same as the air pressure around the tire. Of course, the tire becomes flat. In the same way, gases (oxygen and carbon dioxide) flow in and out of the alveoli.

The alveoli are filled with oxygen-loaded air and therefore have a greater oxygen pressure than the blood, so oxygen flows into the blood through the alveolar wall. The blood is filled with carbon dioxide, so the pressure of carbon dioxide in the blood is greater than that in the alveoli, and carbon dioxide flows into the alveoli through the alveolar wall.

However, these gases flow into or out of the blood only until the gas pressures are equalized. Therefore much of the carbon dioxide, but not all of it, moves out of the blood, and much of the oxygen, but not all, flows into the blood. As will be discussed later, the air we breathe in is about 20% oxygen, and the air we breathe out is about 16% oxygen. This is an important fact to remember because of its relation to administering mouth-to-mouth resuscitation (artificial respiration with expired air) (discussed in Chapter 37).

CONTROL OF RESPIRATION

Respiration is controlled by the respiratory center in the brain. When the blood that flows through this center has a high concentration of carbon dioxide and a low concentration of oxygen, the center sends the message, by means of the involuntary nervous system, to the chest muscles to breathe. The breathing muscles contract (shorten), pulling downward and outward, thus enlarging the chest space. The lungs enlarge to fill up this space. As the lungs get larger, the air pressure in them is less than that outside the body, and so air is pushed into them through the nose (and mouth) until equality of pressure is again achieved. Inspiration or breathing in occurs. Then the chest muscles relax their pull and return to a resting position. As they do, they snap up and in (much like a stretched elastic band returns to its usual state). The chest space gets smaller, and

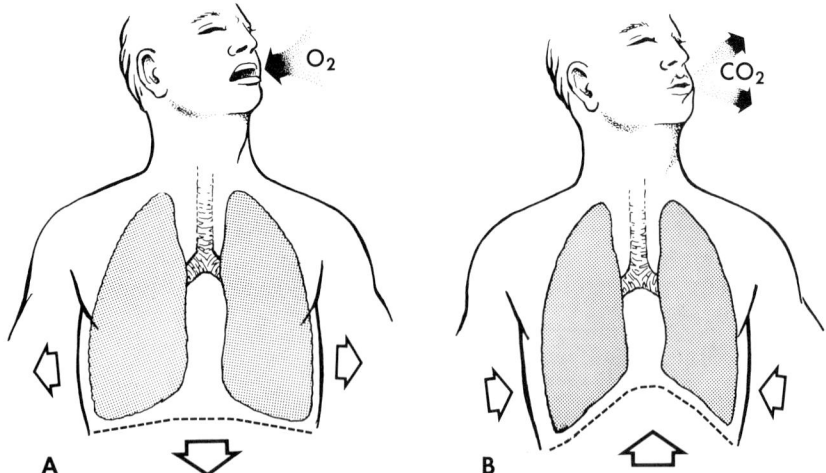

Fig. 22-1. A shows the chest and the lungs enlarging with inspiration. **B** shows the chest muscles returning to their resting phase. The lung space is getting smaller, and expiration is occurring.

the lungs are squeezed (by the muscles) into this smaller space. As they are compressed (reduced in size) the air in them is under greater pressure than that outside the body so breathing out or expiration occurs (Fig. 22-1).

Later in Chapter 38 you will learn that the problem of giving the patient artificial respiration is one of getting the air in—making the muscles of inspiration work. Expiration, the snapping back of the muscles in relaxation, occurs automatically.

Respiration is somewhat under the control of the will. You can breathe or you can hold your breath. However, it is impossible for you to hold your breath too long because the involuntary nervous system control of the lungs will not let you.

When the patient is in severe respiratory distress, he activates his voluntary muscles (those under the control of his will) to help him breathe because the usual mechanisms of breathing are inadequate. This is the type of patient who cannot sleep because when he does the voluntary muscles stop helping him breathe. Then the involuntary control of breathing is inadequate for life and the patient reawakens quickly with breathlessness and the need to breathe more oxygen quickly.

You can see this assist to breathing provided by the voluntary muscles and nervous systems by observing what happens when you participate in strenuous exercise for a short period of time (for example, running). As your muscles work hard to let you run, they utilize more food and oxygen to get the necessary energy. Therefore you will need to breathe in more oxygen. Notice how the muscles of your shoulders and arms assist breathing by working to pull your chest out and push it in. (This is why a patient with breathing difficulty is unable to work with his arms—he needs the arm muscles to help him breathe.)

NORMAL RESPIRATIONS

Normally, the respirations number about 20 per minute when the body is at rest, and they are accomplished effortlessly and soundlessly. Respirations are increased when body activities are increased. Therefore respirations would normally increase under the following circumstances:

1. With exercise, the cells in the muscles need more oxygen to convert the food to energy. As more food is converted to energy, more waste (which includes carbon dioxide) is produced. Therefore exhalation and inhalation are increased.
2. Fear, pain, worry, anger, etc. threaten the body. The involuntary nervous system activates the muscles, the heart, and the lungs to prepare for flight or fight. Therefore more oxygen is needed and more carbon dioxide is produced, so inhalation and exhalation are increased.

Respirations decrease, normally, when body activities decrease and when strong emotional states are avoided. Therefore you could expect the patient's respirations to be at their lowest at night when he is sleeping.

CONDITIONS THAT AFFECT THE RESPIRATORY RATE

Disease conditions can influence the respiratory rate by increasing or decreasing it. Those that increase the rate are as follows:

1. Conditions that take up space in the lungs (There is decreased remaining lung space for bringing in oxygen, so the body attempts to overcome this by increasing the respiratory rate.)
2. Conditions in which the blood supply in the body is lessened (In blood loss, or hemorrhage, there is less blood to carry the oxygen around to the cells of the body. The respiratory center in the brain needs more oxygen and so it sends the message, via the involuntary nervous system, to the lungs to breathe oftener, thus increasing the respiratory rate.)
3. Conditions that cause fever (The body increases its activities and fights

the germs causing the body infection. This increased body activity creates a need for more oxygen in much the same way as the need is created by exercise.)
4. Conditions that create strong emotional states such as pain, worry, fear, etc. (Oxygen need is increased as muscular activity is increased.)

Conditions that slow the respiratory rate include the following:
1. Conditions in the brain that interfere with the normal operation of the respiratory center (for example, the presence of a brain tumor)
2. Conditions (such as disease or injury) that destroy the nerve that carries the messages from the brain to the breathing muscles of the chest and diaphragm (big thick muscle just below the lungs)
3. Conditions in which drugs must be given for pain or for inducing sleep (Morphine and barbiturates slow down brain activity.)

The conditions just described can slow the respiratory rate, but they can also stop it altogether.

COUNTING THE PATIENT'S RESPIRATIONS

Respirations are counted routinely along with the temperature and the pulse. The patient must be at rest when both the pulse and the respirations are counted. Since respirations are somewhat under the control of the patient, he may alter them (unintentionally) if he knows that you are counting them. Therefore after you take the patient's pulse, loosen your fingers, but keep them on the patient's wrist. Now watch his chest movements. Count an inspiration and an expiration as one respiration. Continue counting for 15 seconds. Multiply the result (mentally) by four and remember that amount or jot it down, and recount the respirations for 15 more seconds to check yourself. If the two results are the same, the count is probably correct. Write the respiratory rate on the temperature record along with the pulse and the temperature. However, if the two results are different, count the respirations for 1 full minute. When the respirations are irregular, the full-minute count is essential.

If you have difficulty seeing the patient's chest move, observe his upper abdomen. The muscles of breathing are the chest muscles and the diaphragm. Men usually use the diaphragm muscle more than the chest muscles in breathing. Therefore you may see breathing movement just below the chest in the upper abdomen. Count the respirations, then, by watching the abdomen just below the ribs. Because women wear girdles and corsets, their abdominal movement is somewhat suppressed. They therefore use their chest muscles for breathing.

After you count the patient's respirations, listen to them for a few moments and watch the patient's face. If the patient's breathing is noisy or if he breathes with difficulty, record this on your record and notify the nurse. Snoring-type sounds may indicate that the trachea is obstructed by the tongue, which has fallen back into the throat and is blocking off the breathing space there. Gurgling-type respiration indicates that saliva from the mouth is being sucked down into the lungs with the air and that the patient may be drowning. Gurgling and snoring respirations are cries for help.

Report to the nurse any of the following observations that you make about the patient's respirations:
1. Respiratory rates above 28 or below 12
2. Noisy respirations
3. Irregular respiratory patterns
4. Labored or difficult respirations
5. Inadequate respirations to meet body oxygen needs (This condition will be demonstrated in the patient by a bluish discoloration of his fingernail beds, the tip of his nose, his lips, or

his earlobes. This bluish discoloration or sign of inadequate oxygen in the body is called cyanosis.)

SUMMARY

Breathing is the body process that brings air into the lungs so that the blood can be supplied with oxygen and that expels the carbon dioxide coming from the blood to the outside of the body. The two phases of respiration are inhalation and exhalation.

The respiratory rate is taken routinely when the temperatures and pulses are taken. However, special observation of the respiratory rate may be necessary in some patients.

The respiratory rate is affected by all body activities. It increases as body activities increase and it slows as body activities slow.

DISCUSSION QUESTIONS

1. Count the respirations on both male and female patients. Observe whether breathing movements occur in the chest or in the upper abdomen.
2. Find a patient who is breathing with a great deal of noise. Turn him over on his side. Did this lessen the noise? Why?
3. Observe your patients with elevated temperatures. Are the respiratory rates also elevated? Why?
4. Why would a patient who is short of breath have even greater difficulty breathing when you roll him over and massage his back?
5. Do your patients with breathing difficulty sleep all night? Why? Why not?
6. Why should the breathing rate of a patient with a head injury be checked every 15 minutes?
7. Why would a nurse ask you to check the patient's respiratory rate before she gives a medication to relieve pain?
8. How could you increase the patient's respiratory rate by failing to give an adequate explanation about a test he is scheduled to have done?
9. Observe how frightened a patient becomes when he cannot breathe. Why? (Think about the brain and how it supplies body needs when you give your answer.)
10. Do any of your patients have noisy respirations? If so, why?

VOCABULARY

alveoli Tiny air sacs at the end of the air tubes. Each alveolus or air sac is surrounded by a blood vessel.
bronchi Air tubes from the end of the trachea to the lungs.
carbon dioxide Gas in the blood that is a waste product of cell metabolism.
cyanosis Bluish color caused by inadequate oxygen in the body.
diaphragm Strong muscle just below the lungs.
dyspnea Difficult breathing.
exhalation Breathing out.
inhalation Breathing in.
oxygen Gas in the air needed to support life.
respiration Act of breathing, including inhalation and exhalation.
respiratory center That part of the brain that regulates breathing.
trachea Windpipe.

SOURCES OF ADDITIONAL INFORMATION

1. Film: Mechanism of breathing; may be obtained from Central Office Film Library, Veterans Administration, Vermont Ave. & H St. N.W., Washington, D. C. 20025. (*Illustrates the mechanisms of respiration through the use of animated drawing.*)
2. Film: Vital signs; part I: Cardinal symptoms; may be obtained from Director, Medical Film Library, United States Naval Medical Center, Bethesda, Md. 20014. (*This film explains how the temperature, pulse, respiration, and blood pressure show the condition of the body.*)
3. Film: Vital signs; part II: Taking temperature, pulse and respiration; may be obtained from Director, Medical Film Library, United States Naval Medical Center, Bethesda, Md. 20014. (*This film shows how these vital signs are taken. It also shows normal and abnormal vital signs and how to chart them.*)

23/Taking the patient's blood pressure

STUDY QUESTIONS

1. What is blood pressure?
2. How is the pressure of the blood measured?
3. What is the normal blood pressure of a healthy young adult?
4. What happens to the blood pressure during the aging process?
5. What is hypertension? Hypotension?
6. What does the blood pressure reading tell you about the patient's body?
7. What body structures are involved in a blood pressure change?
8. What are the dangers in hypertension?
9. How does hypertension affect the body?
10. What is the Trendelenburg or shock position?
11. Why is the blood pressure taken so frequently when the patient is receiving a drug such as Levophed, Aramine, or Wyamine?
12. Why must you observe an intravenous infusion carefully when drugs such as Levophed are being administered?
13. How can you determine whether or not an intravenous infusion is infiltrating?

BLOOD PRESSURE

Blood pressure is the force exerted by the heart on the blood to pump it through the arteries and round the body. Blood pressure is maintained and regulated by the brain and the involuntary nervous system. When the blood pressure in the arteries gets too high, a nerve automatically (without control of the will) sends this message from the large arteries to the brain. The brain receives the message, slows down the pumping action of the heart (heartbeat), widens the small arteries close to the surface of the body, and thus lowers the blood pressure.

Notice that your patients with high blood pressure have a slow pulse rate and throbbing arteries just under the skin in the neck and temple areas. When the blood pressure falls too low, a nerve automatically carries this message to the brain, and the brain increases the pumping action of the heart and narrows the arteries close to the surface of the body in an effort to raise the blood pressure. Observe that your patients with low blood pressure have a rapid pulse rate.

Blood pressure, then, is concerned with the (1) heart, (2) blood vessels (arteries), (3) blood, and (4) brain. Changes in any one of these four will show up as changes in the blood pressure.

NORMAL BLOOD PRESSURE

Like the pulse, the blood pressure has two phases. In the pulse these two phases might be the pulse beat and the rest. In blood pressure these two phases are the systole and the diastole.

The systole is the period when the heart pumps the blood out into the arteries. This is the period of greatest blood pressure. It is the pulse period when the beat can be felt.

The diastole is the phase during which the heart is filling with blood in preparation for the next pumping action. This is the period of the lowest blood pressure, since it is the period when the heart is relaxed. This would be the pulse period when you could not feel a beat.

The normal blood pressure reading for a young, healthy adult is approximately 120 mm. of mercury, systolic pressure, and 80 mm. of mercury, diastolic pressure. It is written 120/80. The first pressure, the greater pressure, is the systolic and is written over the second or lesser pressure, which is the diastolic.

As we grow older, arteriosclerosis occurs. Arteriosclerosis (hardening of the arteries) changes the elastic walls of the arteries so that they become firm and hard. The arteries do not widen as the heart pumps blood into them. Therefore the pressure in the arteries increases. We notice that blood pressure increases with age because hardening of the arteries (arteriosclerosis) is a disease that occurs with aging. The blood pressure in the older patient is considered to be within the normal aspects of this aging process if the systolic pressure reading is 100 plus the patient's age. The diastolic pressure remains about the same during aging because it is the pressure during the resting phase of the heart.

It is difficult to know what the patient's usual blood pressure is because of these changes that occur with aging. However, each patient's blood pressure should be taken and charted when he is admitted.

Further observations of the blood pressure may then be ordered by the doctor if he suspects disease associated with the heart, blood vessels, or brain, or with loss of blood (hemorrhage).

However, the blood pressure that is taken on admission is important, even when the doctor has no immediate need for blood pressure observation, because it can serve as the standard with which to compare future blood pressure readings. Normally, the blood pressure remains approximately the same. Changes in the blood pressure indicate serious changes in the patient's body.

CONDITIONS THAT AFFECT THE BLOOD PRESSURE

Conditions in the body that increase the blood pressure are those that involve the heart, the blood, the blood vessels, or the brain in the following ways:

1. Arteriosclerosis (hardening and narrowing of the arteries) occurs.
2. Strong emotion such as pain, fear, and worry activate the sympathetic section of the involuntary nervous system. The body is prepared to fight or run away from the threat responsible for the emotion. The heartbeat is increased, and the blood vessels close to the surface of the body are narrowed.
3. Pressure on the blood pressure–regulating center in the brain (vasomotor center) by brain injuries, tumors, or swellings causes an interruption in the blood supply to the brain area (much like the pressure of the bed causes interruption in blood supply to the back). The blood pressure rises higher and higher as the body attempts to get more blood to this damaged brain area.
4. Increased secretions of adrenocortical hormones or sex hormones increase the pumping action of the heart and increase the blood volume, thereby raising the blood pressure.

Another factor that causes the blood pressure to rise is kidney disease. However, the mechanism by which it does this is not clearly understood at this time.

Conditions in the body that lower blood pressure are those that affect the heart, the blood, the blood vessels, or the brain in the following ways:
1. Heart failure, or ineffective pumping action by the heart, can cause a decrease in blood pressure.
2. Hemorrhage (loss of circulating blood, usually through an opening in a blood vessel) causes a decreasing blood volume.
3. Relief of strong emotional tones such as those in fear, worry, and pain will lower blood pressure to within its normal range.

IMPLICATIONS OF HIGH AND LOW BLOOD PRESSURE

High blood pressure (hypertension) increases the load on the heart and increases the tension on the arterial walls. Two things may happen as a result of hypertension:
1. The heart may enlarge (hypertrophy), as does any muscle with an increased load, to do the increased job of pumping the blood around the body through these narrowed arteries. Eventually, a point will be reached at which the load of pumping the blood is too great even for the enlarged heart, and heart failure occurs.
2. The pressure of the blood on the narrowed arteries continually increases until one of the arteries develops a weakened wall from the pressure and ruptures (as a balloon ruptures when you keep blowing air into it until the pressure becomes too much for the rubber wall to hold). Usually, the artery that ruptures is one of the small but important ones in the brain. When this occurs, the patient has a stroke.

In order to avoid these serious complications, patients with high blood pressure (hypertension) are admitted to the hospital and are given treatments and drugs to reduce the blood pressure. The doctor will prescribe these drugs for the patient until his blood pressure drops to a desirable level. Before the nurse can give these medications, she will need to know what the patient's blood pressure is; therefore she may ask you to take it. Take the patient's blood pressure carefully, recheck it, and then report it to the nurse. Remember, the patient is receiving treatments and medications on the basis of your blood pressure readings. Tranquilizers are the drugs most commonly used to reduce the patient's blood pressure.

Low blood pressure or hypotension decreases the blood supply to the cells of the body. This decreased blood supply, in turn, leads to the following deficiencies:
1. Inadequate food supply
2. Inadequate oxygen supply
3. Inadequate removal of waste materials, including urea, water, and carbon dioxide
4. Inadequate utilization of medicine given
5. Inadequate water supply

Soon the cells of the body cease to function because of the decreased blood supply, and unconsciousness and even death may occur. Therefore the doctor considers a severe hypotensive episode an emergency, and he institutes immediate treatment to raise the blood pressure. The brain functions only a short time if it has an interruption in its blood supply, and so the doctor orders that the patient be placed in a Trendelenburg or shock position. You can place him in this position by taking the pillows from under his head and placing them under his feet. In this way, you lower the head and raise the feet so that gravity can help the blood run downhill from the patient's feet to his head. Then the blood supply to the brain improves.

After the patient is properly positioned, the doctor starts an intravenous infusion (to increase the volume of fluid in the blood vessels), and he adds a drug like Levophed, Aramine, or Wyamine to the infusion. These drugs cause the blood vessels to narrow, and this narrowing helps the blood pressure rise. The increased blood pressure then improves the circulation. The doctor writes the order for the flow of intravenous infusion to be speeded up when the blood pressure falls or to be slowed down when the blood pressure rises. This means that you will be assigned to stay with the patient and to take blood pressure readings every 5, 10, or 15 minutes. You will need to keep the nurse informed of each blood pressure change. While you are caring for the patient who is receiving an intravenous infusion, observe that fluid is dripping at the correct speed, that the patient is breathing quietly, and that the needle is in the vein. You can be sure that the needle is in the vein by the following methods:

1. Observe the patient's arm for swollen areas developing around the needle. If the needle is in the vein, the intravenous fluid will be carried away from the injection site with the blood. If the needle slips out of the vein but is still under the skin, the injection fluid accumulates around the needle under the skin, and the patient's arm swells.
2. Lower the intravenous bottle below the level of the patient's arm. If the needle is in the vein, blood returns from the arm through the needle and into the glass connector where you can see it.

When you are watching an intravenous infusion that contains Levophed, Aramine, or Wyamine, you must be sure that the needle remains in the vein. If it slips out of the vein and the fluid containing the drug is permitted to run under the skin in the patient's arm, the tiny blood vessels in the skin will be so narrowed that they will be shut off. The patient will then develop a necrotic area (area of dead tissue) that will look much like the necrotic spot of a bedsore.

Observing the hypotensive patient who is receiving an infusion of fluid containing one of the drugs mentioned previously might include:

1. Checking the blood pressure at intervals designated by the nurse (usually every 5, 10, or 15 minutes)
2. Keeping a record of the blood pressure readings and the rate of the intravenous drip
3. Checking the infusion site frequently for infiltration (fluid going under the skin instead of into the vein)
4. Keeping the nurse informed of any changes in the patient's condition or any changes in the blood pressure

TAKING BLOOD PRESSURE

Blood pressure readings are obtained by using a sphygmomanometer and a stethoscope to measure the force exerted by the blood on an artery in the arm. This is done in the following way:

1. Collect your equipment, which includes a sphygmomanometer and a stethoscope; obtain a pencil and paper for recording the blood pressure readings.
2. Go to the patient's bedside and explain that you are going to take his blood pressure reading.
3. Place the patient in a comfortable position lying in bed or sitting in a chair.
4. Have the patient place his right arm (with the palm up) on the bed or on the bedside stand. Be sure that the artery (which is felt in the arm just above the inner side of the elbow) is on the same level as the patient's heart.
5. Place the sphygmomanometer on the patient's bedside stand.
6. Position the cuff of the sphygmomanometer on the patient's arm in such a way that the tube to the bulb is on the side of his arm closest to his body and the tube to the blood

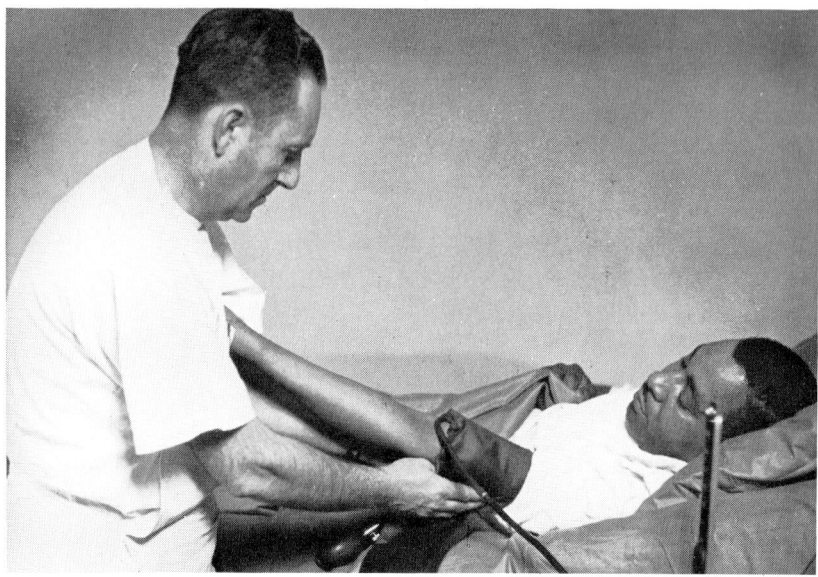

Fig. 23-1. The nursing assistant positions the sphygmomanometer cuff on the patient's arm. Note that the patient's arm is maintained in an elevated position while the cuff is placed on it by the nursing assistant, who holds it between his arm and his body.

pressure apparatus is on the other side of his arm away from his body (Fig. 23-1). Place the cuff on the arm so that the bottom of the cuff is about 1 inch above the bend in the elbow.

7. Wrap the rest of the cuff around the patient's arm and tuck the end into one of the cuff folds.
8. Sit down, if possible, so that your eye is on a level with the scale on the blood pressure apparatus (sphygmomanometer).
9. Palpate the patient's pulse at the inner aspect of the arm just above the bend of the elbow.
10. Keep your fingers on this pulse and pump up the cuff by pumping on the rubber bulb. If the cuff loosens or bulges awkwardly, remove it and rewrap it around the arm. If a hissing sound is heard, tighten the valve just above the rubber bulb.
11. Pump up the cuff until the pulse disappears; then pump it up about thirty more points.
12. Loosen the valve on the pump slightly (with the same hand used for pumping) and *try* to feel the pulse as the pressure decreases.
13. Tighten the valve immediately to stop the pressure drop when you feel the pulse.
14. Read the scale on the blood pressure apparatus. This is the systolic pressure.
15. Loosen the valve and permit the cuff to deflate completely.
16. Place the earpieces of the stethoscope in your ear (with the earpieces directed up) and position the bell of the stethoscope over the space where you felt the pulse. The stethoscope magnifies sound, so avoid any contact between the stethoscope and the cuff or your clothing. If contact occurs, you will hear interfering sounds.
17. Hold the stethoscope bell snugly in

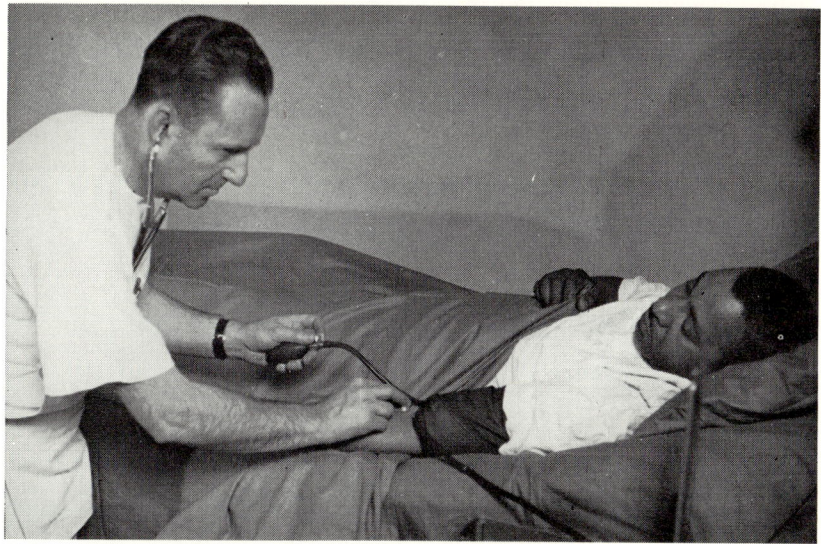

Fig. 23-2. Taking the blood pressure reading. Note the nursing assistant's fingers on the pressure release valve on the pump. This position permits him to shut the valve off immediately to obtain the blood pressure reading at the appearance of the first beat and at the disappearance of the last beat.

position over the pulse at the elbow with one hand while you pump up the cuff with the other. Pump until the mercury in the scale of the blood pressure apparatus is about thirty points above the systolic pressure you obtained previously by feeling the pulse.

18. Loosen the valve slightly and permit the pressure to drop slowly as you listen carefully for the blood pressure sound. (In taking the pulse, you *felt* the beat; now you will *hear* the beat.) Soon you will hear a definite beat, but it will be quite faint. If you missed it or are not quite sure where it started, pump once more and listen again. At the first sound of a beat, close off the valve on the pump, and read the pressure on the scale of the blood pressure apparatus. This is the systolic pressure (Fig. 23-2).

19. Loosen the valve again and listen for the beat to stop as the cuff continues to deflate. At first, the faint beat becomes louder and louder. Then it begins to soften, and finally it disappears. As soon as the beat disappears, close off the valve and read the pressure scale on the blood pressure apparatus. This reading is the diastolic pressure.

20. Open the valve completely and permit the cuff to deflate.

21. Repeat the entire procedure and check the blood pressure reading.

22. Take the patient's pulse. This gives you another clue about the patient's condition. The pulse rate should be taken and recorded each time that you take the blood pressure reading.

23. Remove the cuff. Make the patient comfortable. Chart the blood pressure reading and return the equipment you used to its proper place or proceed with the other blood pressure readings that you are assigned to take.

If you have difficulty getting the blood pressure reading, you are probably opening the valve so wide that the pressure is dropping too rapidly or you are expecting too loud a sound. Remember, you hear now only what you felt before in the pulse beat.

BECOME FAMILIAR WITH YOUR EQUIPMENT

Before you attempt to take the patient's blood pressure, become familiar with the equipment and how it works. Look at the scale on the blood pressure apparatus and learn to read it. Count the small lines between any two numbers and figure out how much each line represents. Remember, too, that you must pump up the cuff until the pressure reading is greater than the blood pressure, and then you permit the pressure to drop. This means that you will be reading the blood pressure scale downward rather than upward (that is, you will be going from larger to smaller numbers). Now place the earpieces of the stethoscope in your ears. Rub the bell of the stethoscope lightly with your fingers. Notice how the sound is magnified. Some stethoscopes have a double bell with a small lever on the top that directs the sound into one part or the other. If you have such a stethoscope, push the lever forward and tap the front bell piece. Now push it back and tap the second bell piece as you listen. Do this until you are sure which lever position directs the sound into which bell piece.

Take a classmate's blood pressure reading and let him take yours. Now you know why you must understand your equipment and the procedure before you can take the patient's blood pressure reading. The cuff is really a tourniquet, and if the blood pressure procedure takes too long, the patient will have an odd sensation in his arm as the circulation is stopped.

SPECIAL NOTE

The nursing service in your hospital will determine the ways in which they need you to assist in the care of patients. Taking the patient's blood pressure may or may not be one of these ways. Check your job description carefully and perform accordingly.

The inclusion of blood pressure taking skill in this book was motivated by the value of this procedure in the observation of patients and not by the authority to identify it among nursing assistant activities.

SUMMARY

The blood pressure is the force exerted by the heart on the blood to pump it around the body. The blood pressure is regulated by the brain through the involuntary nervous system. Normally blood pressure remains relatively stable. Therefore blood pressure changes indicate serious changes in the body that are due to changing conditions in any one of the following: (1) the brain, (2) the heart, (3) the blood, or (4) the blood vessels.

Hypertension or high blood pressure may result in heart failure or a stroke. Hypotension or low blood pressure may result in unconsciousness and death if the blood supply to the brain is interrupted for even a short period.

Blood pressure determinations give a significant clue to the condition of the body. Therefore the blood pressure reading must be taken accurately. Inaccurate information is worse than no information.

When the nurse asks you to take a patient's blood pressure reading every 15 minutes, it is essential that you know what change in the blood pressure she expects and what readings she wants reported to her. Unless you know this, you are not adequately prepared to observe the patient closely.

The pulse, like the blood pressure, gives the doctor a great deal of information about the patient's heart. Therefore the pulse rate should be taken and recorded each time that the blood pressure reading is taken.

DISCUSSION QUESTIONS

1. Since blood pressures are observed for changes, how are they charted on your ward so that changes will be immediately obvious to an observer?
2. Study a blood pressure record on your ward. What values do the large lines on the left-hand side of the record represent? Where are the date and time of the blood pressure reading put on the record?
3. Chart the following blood pressure readings on the proper form from your ward so that you can familiarize yourself with the record. Ask the head nurse or team leader to check your recordings.

    | 1/4/72 | 10 A.M. | 126/84 |
    | 1/4/72 | 2 P.M. | 140/96 |
    | 1/4/72 | 6 P.M. | 146/96 |

4. Which patients on your ward have blood pressure readings taken regularly? Why? What change are you expecting and what will this change indicate when it occurs?
5. Observe a patient with a severe hypotensive episode (shock). What are his blood pressure, pulse, and respiratory rates? How does his skin feel? Why does his skin feel this way?
6. Why does the blood pressure drop while the pulse rises when the patient is hemorrhaging?
7. Observe a patient with hypertension. Why is his face flushed? Why is the pulse on his forehead (near the surface) throbbing?
8. Why does a patient with pressure on the brain develop an increasing blood pressure? Is this a good sign?
9. Take several patients' blood pressure readings. Ask the head nurse or team leader to check them.
10. Observe a patient receiving an intravenous infusion. Count the rate of flow. Check the needle site. Is the needle in the vein or is the intravenous fluid infiltrating? Lower the intravenous bottle to check your observations.

VOCABULARY

arteriosclerosis Hardening of the arteries.
B/P Blood pressure.
diastole Blood pressure period during the resting phase of the heart.
hypertension High blood pressure.
hypertrophy Enlargement.
hypotension Low blood pressure.
sphygmomanometer Blood pressure apparatus.
stethoscope Instrument to magnify sound.
systole Blood pressure period during the beating phase of the heart.

SOURCES OF ADDITIONAL INFORMATION

1. Book: Phibbs, Brendan: The human heart, ed. 2, St. Louis, 1971, The C. V. Mosby Co., chaps. 13 and 14.
2. Film: Vital signs; part III: Taking blood pressure; may be obtained from Director, Medical Film Library, United States Naval Medical School, National Naval Medical Center, Bethesda, Md. 20014. (*Shows, with demonstration and sound effects, how blood pressure readings are taken and recorded.*)
3. Film: Intravenous administration of fluids; may be obtained from Director, Medical Film Library, United States Naval Medical School, National Naval Medical Center, Bethesda, Md. 20014. (*Depicts navy corpsmen preparing a patient for, and assisting the doctor with, an intravenous infusion.*)
4. Pamphlet: Clinical measurement of blood pressure may be obtained from W. A. Baum, Inc., Copaigue, N. Y.

24/Observing the patient's level of consciousness

STUDY QUESTIONS

1 What is consciousness?
2 How can you tell if a patient is conscious?
3 What are the levels of consciousness?
4 How can you differentiate between a stuporous state and a comatose state?
5 What does a changing level of consciousness indicate?
6 Why should extreme restlessness in a patient be identified and reported to the nurse?
7 How do drugs affect the level of consciousness?
8 Why is the use of hypnotics avoided in a patient who has had brain surgery?
9 How can you differentiate between sleep and coma?
10 What causes coma?

CONSCIOUSNESS

The level of consciousness is the fifth vital sign, and it is observed each time you check the other four signs (temperature, pulse, respiration, and blood pressure). Consciousness is the ability to observe, understand, and respond to the environment in an appropriate way. The patient who is conscious sees what we see, hears what we hear, answers when we speak to him, knows what his body needs, and requests the facilities to care for these needs. This means that the patient will ask for toilet facilities and fluids, that he will complain of discomfort and pain, and that he will put on his bedclothes when he feels cold or throw them off when he feels too warm.

Consciousness is controlled and regulated by the brain and the involuntary nervous system.

LEVELS OF CONSCIOUSNESS

There are four levels of consciousness: alertness, restlessness, stupor, and coma.

The alert patient is well aware of what is going on and reacts to the factors in his environment appropriately. He requests the facilities to supply his body needs, such as a urinal or bedpan, medication for pain, or a drink of water.

The restless patient is extremely sensitive to the factors in his environment, and he exaggerates them. He screams out with his pain, he calls for the urinal or bedpan but is unable to wait until it arrives, he wants constant attention, etc. He moves about in his bed constantly and thrashes about from side to side. His restless hands pull at the bedclothes, at his dressings, and even at his own body.

The stuporous patient lies quietly in bed and seems to be sleeping. He requests nothing. He may be awakened but he returns to this sleeplike state quickly. He is difficult to feed because he cannot stay awake. He may be incontinent.

The degree of stupor is determined by the stimuli required to awaken the patient. If he can be awakened by your voice, the level of consciousness would be described as light stupor. If he can be awakened only by pressure, for example, by tapping him lightly on the side of the face or by applying pressure above the eyes on the supraorbital ridges or on the sternum (middle of the front chest) or by a strong sensation such as severe pain, the level would be described as deep stupor.

The patient in a coma lies quietly in bed and appears to be sleeping. He cannot be awakened. He does not ask for drinks or for a urinal or bedpan. He cannot swallow, so he cannot eat or drink. He may be incontinent or he may retain (hold in) urine. Pressure above the eyes on the supraorbital ridges or on the sternum and strong sensations do not awaken him. He does not awaken when you call his name.

WHAT THE LEVELS OF CONSCIOUSNESS MEAN

The alert patient is one whose brain is functioning adequately.

The restless patient's brain is extremely active in its attempt to meet the body's needs. Restlessness is commonly observed in the following patients:
1. In the hemorrhaging patient because the brain is receiving a lessened and an inadequate blood supply
2. In the patient with a head injury or brain tumor, if the increased pressure on the brain is cutting off the blood supply to a part of the brain
3. In the patient who has suffered a heart attack because the weakened heart is not pumping enough blood around the body and to the brain
4. In the patient in shock whose blood pressure is so low that there is an insufficient force to pump blood to the brain
5. In the patient who is frightened or worried because the brain is hyperactive in preparing the body to fight or flee

Restlessness is an early sign of the preceding conditions. When the brain is unable to correct the conditions causing restlessness, this state will quickly be replaced by stupor, coma, and death.

The patient in stupor is one whose brain is not able to function adequately. There is interference in its function that may be due to one or more of the following:
1. Increased pressure on the brain
2. Decreased blood supply to the brain
3. Decreased oxygen supply to the brain
4. Decreased food supply to the brain

Because the brain also controls the other four vital signs, there will be some changes in these also, and these changes will help to give you a clue as to which problem is causing the stupor.

The brain of the comatose patient is functioning poorly and may even stop functioning at any time. This state is caused by the same conditions that produce stupor. However, the conditions may have continued for some time without relief, so that the patient's brain is beginning to deteriorate (lose the ability to function). The other vital signs will give some clues as to which condition is causing the coma.

OBSERVING THE LEVEL OF CONSCIOUSNESS

The significant factor in the observation of the levels of consciousness is change. Therefore in your first contact with the patient you must determine what his level of consciousness is and chart it accurately. This might be done at the time of the patient's admission or on your first rounds after you report on duty. You can observe the patient's level of consciousness by asking him how he feels and listening to his answer. This can then be charted as follows: "Level of consciousness—patient responds to questioning appropriately."

If you go to check the patient's level of consciousness 15 minutes later and find that he seems to be sleeping and does not answer your questions, speak louder. Then apply pressure above the eyes on the supraorbital ridges or on the sternum with your fingers. If the patient responds to your loud voice, report: "Level of consciousness—patient appears to be asleep, responds to a loud voice, answers questions asked, and promptly lapses into sleep again."

If the patient responds to the pressure and not to the loud voice, report: "Level of consciousness—patient responds only to painful pressures on supraorbital ridge and/or on sternum. He opens his eyes, answers yes or no to questions, and promptly lapses into deep sleep again."

If the patient fails to respond, chart: "Level of consciousness—patient does not respond to voice or pressure."

Notify the nurse immediately if you observe that a change in the level of consciousness has occurred. Remember that the patient in a stupor or coma appears to be sleeping but is really having a serious interference with brain functioning. Observation of the level of consciousness means, then, that the sleeping patient must be awakened, regardless of whether it is in the middle of the day or the middle of the night, so that you can observe whether he really is sleeping or whether he is in stupor or coma.

EFFECT OF DRUGS ON THE LEVEL OF CONSCIOUSNESS

Drugs that are given to the patient to help him sleep or reduce his pain may achieve the desired end by lessening or blocking the brain's ability to receive messages from the body about its needs and by lessening or blocking the brain's ability to send the messages activating the body functions to satisfy these needs. Therefore these drugs interfere with brain functioning and they may change the level of consciousness.

An overdose of or an allergic reaction to these drugs will produce a severe interruption in the brain functioning that will be evidenced by the patient's changed vital signs. He may become comatose, and he may develop a low blood pressure, a slowed pulse, and slowed respirations. He may die as the brain loses its ability to make the heart beat and the lungs breathe. Drugs that depress (lessen) the ability of the brain to receive messages of the body needs and send messages to activate body functions to satisfy these needs include the following:

1. Analgesics (pain-reducing drugs such as morphine, Demerol [meperidine hydrochloride], and codeine)*
2. Hypnotics (sleep-producing drugs such as paraldehyde, barbiturates, and bromides)
3. General anesthetics (drugs producing insensibility to pain and unconsciousness, such as ether, cyclopropane, and Pentothal sodium [thiopental sodium])
4. Nonanalgesics—alcohols (preparations that produce sleep and stupor, such as whiskey and gin)

The patient who is being constantly ob-

---

*These drugs are narcotics with addicting properties. Like all addicting drugs, they permit escape from the here and now by inducing changes in the levels of consciousness. These changes are of therapeutic value when they are used to dull the patient's pain. However, the nonmedical use of narcotics is dangerous not only because of their addicting properties, but also because of their effect on consciousness. Narcotics such as heroin dull and constrict the consciousness whereas other such as LSD expand it into the world of the unreal. The LSD trip, then, is really an hallucinatory experience.

served for changes in level of consciousness cannot receive any of the drugs just listed because they may conceal significant changes in his consciousness by their brain-depressing actions. It also means that you should observe your patient closely to be sure that the drug the nurse gave is doing exactly what it is expected to do. Be alert to changes in your patient's conditions. Know what the nurse expects the medicine to do and know also what she would consider an allergic reaction or an undesirable effect from it. Look for these undesirable reactions as you care for the patient.

These drugs, especially the analgesics, also affect the patient's blood pressure or respiratory rate or both. Therefore the nurse may ask you to check these vital signs before she gives the patient a drug to reduce his ability to feel pain.

CHARTING THE LEVEL OF CONSCIOUSNESS

The level of consciousness should be charted on the vital sign record along with the other vital signs. It is usually charted by writing alert, restless, stupor, or coma, as indicated by the patient's condition, on the record.

OBSERVATIONS OF LEVEL OF CONSCIOUSNESS DURING PATIENT ROUNDS

Observe your patients closely when you make rounds after the lights are turned out. Be aware of the fact that a patient may appear to be sleeping when he is really unconscious. Remember, too, that all vital signs change when the patient's condition changes. Therefore the patient who is lying too still, who is breathing noisily, or who has an increase or decrease in pulse rate may be unconscious. Ask the nurse to check this patient.

DISCUSSION QUESTIONS

1 How does an overdose of sleeping pills cause death? Do you think this might be why so many people have used them to commit suicide?
2 Why does the pharmacy dispense sleeping pills only with a prescription?
3 Why would observations of the patient's level of consciousness be taken every 15 minutes when he returns to the ward after undergoing brain surgery?
4 Do you have an unconscious patient on your ward? What are the measurements of his other vital signs?
5 Discuss your unconscious patients with the nurse and find out what is responsible for their coma.
6 What patients on your ward are receiving analgesics or hypnotics? What observations does the nurse want you to make on these patients?
7 What does a changing level of consciousness indicate?

VOCABULARY

allergy Sensitivity to a substance not usually known to cause difficulty in most persons.
analgesics Pain-relieving drugs.
barbiturates Drugs that depress or slow down brain activity.
coma A sleeplike state from which the patient cannot be awakened by any means.
consciousness The ability to know what is happening around you and to react appropriately to these happenings.
Demerol Pain-relieving narcotic.
general anesthetics Drugs that so depress brain activity that the patient becomes unconscious and insensible to pain.
hypnotics Sleep-producing drugs.
morphine Pain-relieving narcotic.
paraldehyde Drug that produces sleep.
reaction Response.
restlessness A state in which the patient moves about constantly, thrashing about the bed and picking at himself or his bedclothes.
sternum Breastbone.
stupor A sleeplike state in which the patient is unaware of his surroundings. However, he can be awakened by such stimuli as a loud voice, a firm pressure over the eyelids or on the sternum, or a strong sensation such as severe pain.

SOURCE OF ADDITIONAL INFORMATION

1 Film: Nursing care: the neurosurgical patient; may be obtained from Director, Film Library, United States Naval Medical School, National Naval Medical Center, Bethesda, Md. 20014. (*Illustrates the corpsman's constant observation and determination of level of consciousness in a patient suffering from a brain concussion.*)

25/Charting temperature, pulse, and respiration

STUDY QUESTIONS

1 What is a graph?
2 Why are vital signs charted on a graph?
3 How are the vital signs charted on a graph?
4 Who charts on the graph?

WHY TEMPERATURE, PULSE, AND RESPIRATION ARE CHARTED

The patient's temperature, pulse, and respiration give the doctor a great deal of information. Because of this, these vital signs are recorded on the patient's chart in a very prominent place, usually on the first sheet. During rounds, the doctor checks the record of the patient's vital signs first, and then he does his daily evaluation of the patient. This evaluation is not done blindly. The temperature record shows whether the patient's infection is getting better or worse. The pulse record shows how the patient's heart is functioning and meeting the body's increased need for blood during illness. The respiration record shows how the lungs are meeting the body's increased need for oxygen. Knowing these things, the doctor examines the patient's body to find out why these conditions or body reactions are occurring. He knows what is occurring from his observations of the vital signs, and his physical examination is done to determine why.

HOW VITAL SIGNS ARE RECORDED

The temperature gives information about the patient's infection. However, pulse and respiration determinations are needed to understand how the body is meeting the extra load imposed upon it by infection. Since the information given by all vital signs is essential to an understanding of the condition of the whole body, all the vital signs may be charted on one record.

As the condition of the patient's body changes, the vital signs also change. Therefore the record on which these signs are charted is one that will permit the doctor, nurse, and nursing assistant to easily identify changes at a glance. Since the nurse's record will not permit this easy identification of change because the recordings are inserted between accounts of the patient's treatments, medications, and reactions, a graph is used.

THE TEMPERATURE, PULSE, AND RESPIRATION GRAPH

The value of plotting temperature, pulse, and respiration determinations on a graph is that any changes up or down can be identified easily. Another value might be that any significant changes occurring in the body from a specific medication or treatment could be demonstrated clearly merely by writing in the therapy on the vital sign record.

At first, it may seem difficult to read and to chart information on a graph, but soon you will become quite familiar with it if you follow these directions:

1. Graphing is just like writing on any other sheet of paper. Writing and graphing are done from the left side of the paper or graph toward the right.
2. The graph has lines and numbers on the left-hand side. These are the values (numbers) to be charted. The numbers speak for themselves. The lines, like the lines on a thermometer, represent values between the numbers. In the example shown in Fig. 25-1, each line represents .2 of a degree. (Observe the graph on your unit. Figure out what the small lines mean.) Each small line between the numbers represents the same amount. Therefore count these lines (five in Fig. 25-1) from 98 to 99. Now observe the numbers on the chart and determine what value is represented by these five small lines: 99 − 98 = 1°. Now divide this value (1°) by the number of lines (5) and you will get the value of each line: 1 ÷ 5 = ⅕ of a degree. You learned previously that ⅕ is like ⅕ of a dollar or $.20. You learned also that the zero is usually dropped and this ⅕ is written as .2.
3. At either the top or the bottom of the graph are shown the dates and the times that these vital signs were taken.
4. Charting on the graph is done by placing a dot (.) or a zero (0), depending on hospital policy, in the correct place on the graph. First lo-

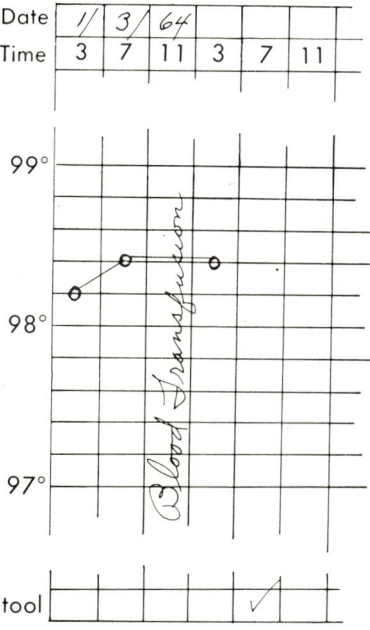

Fig. 25-1. Part of a vital sign graph. Temperatures are charted as follows: 3 A.M., 98.2°; 7 A.M., 98.4°; 3 P.M., 98.4°. Note that the patient's defecations are charted at the bottom of the chart.

cate on the left-hand side of the graph the number of the vital sign reading that you wish to chart. Now follow this line (at the number you wish to chart) across to the right until you locate the date and the time at which you wish to chart it. A temperature of 98.4° F. at 3 p.m. on 1/3/72 would be charted as shown in Fig. 25-1.

5. The graph has similar facilities to those just described for charting the pulse and the respiration. Follow the same procedure used for charting temperature to chart pulse and respiration readings in the proper places on the graph.
6. There may be space at the bottom of the graph for recording defecations, intake and output, and blood pressure. Be sure to chart these correctly under the proper date and time. Blood pressure readings may also be charted on a separate graph. The graph is developed in much the same way as the temperature graph. The level of consciousness is charted as described in Chapter 24.

The patient's response to blood transfusions, antibiotics, or other medications and treatments may be clearly demonstrated by writing in the name of the drug or treatment in a space on the graph under the date and time that it was administered. Your hospital may have a policy about how this is done (Fig. 25-1).

The patient's chart is a legal document; therefore recordings on it must be made in ink, and erasures are not permitted. Chart carefully. If you have any doubt about the recordings, check with the nurse first. Study the vital sign records on your patient's chart. Try to understand how these recordings were done. Ask the nurse to help you with your recordings the first time you chart information. After that, charting and graphing will be just like writing.

DISCUSSION QUESTIONS

1 Study the graph on a patient's chart on which the temperature, pulse, and respirations are charted. Can you understand the graph now? If not, ask the head nurse or team leader to explain it to you.
2 Ask the head nurse or team leader to help you chart those vital signs that you took on your patients today.
3 Where is the temperature, pulse, and respiration record kept on your patients' charts? Why?
4 At what times are the vital signs routinely taken on your unit? Why?
5 Discuss whether or not a graph makes it easy to see changes in the vital signs.

SOURCES OF ADDITIONAL INFORMATION

1 Film: Vital signs; part I: Cardinal symptoms; may be obtained from Director, Medical Film Library, United States Naval Medical School, National Naval Medical Center, Bethesda, Md. 20014. (*Explains, by live action, animation, and art work, how vital signs indicate the condition of the body.*)
2 Film: Vital signs; part II: Taking temperatures, pulse, and respiration; may be obtained from Director, Medical Film Library, United States Naval Medical School, National Naval Medical Center, Bethesda, Md. 20014. (*Demonstrates how temperature, pulse, and respirations are taken. It demonstrates also the equipment used, the disinfection of thermometers, and the techniques of charting.*)
3 Film: Vital signs and their interrelation; may be obtained from Loma Linda University Motion Picture Library, Audio-Visual Center, Loma Linda, Calif. (*Describes the physiology involved in the temperature, pulse, respiration, and blood pressure. It also demonstrates how to take and record these vital signs.*)

26/Collecting specimens from the patient

STUDY QUESTIONS

1. What is a specimen?
2. Why are specimens examined by the laboratory?
3. How many different kinds of specimens can you obtain from the patient?
4. Are all specimens examined for the same thing?
5. Why are there so many different departments in the laboratory?
6. What is a culture?
7. What is a smear?
8. Why do patients receive routine urine examinations?
9. How can you obtain a sterile voided specimen for a culture from a male patient?
10. Why must specimens for culture be taken to the laboratory as soon as they are collected?
11. Why should the specimen container be labeled before the specimen is collected?
12. Why does the nursing assistant on night duty have so much difficulty collecting feces specimens?

THE SPECIMEN AS A DIAGNOSTIC MEASURE

The vital signs give a great deal of information about the condition of the patient's body. However, they do not give the physician any information about the cause of this condition. An elevated temperature indicates that germs have invaded the body and are attacking it. However, the temperature gives no indication of where these germs may be in the body, nor does it tell what kind of germs they are. In the same way, a falling blood pressure and a rising pulse rate indicate that hemorrhage is occurring, but they give no clues as to the site of hemorrhage. Therefore the doctor will need to employ many other techniques to help him locate the condition so that he can make a diagnosis.

The techniques employed by the doctor will include your observations of how the patient's body functions and the collection of specimens from the part of the body that seems to be functioning inadequately. For example, you may observe a patient who is running an elevated temperature and who has a hacking cough. The doctor will examine the patient's chest and listen to his breath sounds carefully through the stethoscope. He may decide that there are some unusual breath sounds indicating that germs have invaded the body in this area. Then he will ask you to obtain a sputum specimen from the patient and to take it to the laboratory for an examination. The laboratory will study this specimen and will identify the germs present. Then the laboratory will notify the doctor that the patient's sputum contains tuberculosis or pneumonia germs. With this information, the doctor is able to diagnose the patient's condition as tuberculosis or as pneumonia (depending on the germs found in the specimen) and to start the correct treatment.

A specimen is defined as that part of something that is exactly the same as all the other parts of it. In the preceding example in which the doctor ordered that a sputum specimen be collected and sent to the laboratory, the patient coughed, brought up the secretions from his lungs, and expectorated them into a specimen container. The sputum that he coughed up was like all the other sputum in his lungs and therefore was a specimen (or a part) of all the sputum in his lungs. The doctor knows that anything found in the sputum specimen will also be found in the sputum in the patient's lungs.

KINDS OF SPECIMENS

Specimens of any body excretion such as urine, feces, or sputum can be obtained. Specimens of internal body fluids can also be obtained by inserting a needle into that body part and by aspirating (sucking out) some of the contents. Specimens obtained by needle aspiration include the following:
1. Specimens of blood obtained from a vein, an artery, or the heart
2. Specimens of spinal fluid obtained from the spinal canal
3. Specimens of fluid obtained from the pleural space (space around the lungs) or from a joint
4. Specimens of pus obtained by aspirating an abscess or an infected (pus-producing) area
5. Specimens of body cells obtained by aspirating the sternum, the liver, or the kidney (Specimens of body cells are called biopsies.)

Specimens can also be obtained by cutting off (resecting) a small piece of body tissue. These small tissue specimens are also called biopsies. Biopsies are usually taken from an abnormal growth in the body and are sent to the laboratory for the examination that will tell the doctor whether or not the growth is cancerous.

Smears can be obtained when a larger specimen cannot. Smears, which are usually taken from the inside of the nose, from the throat, or from a wound, are obtained by touching the area to be smeared with a sterile applicator and then quickly placing the applicator in a sterile test tube and sending it to the laboratory. A smear may look very small in the sterile test tube. However, the applicator will contain hundreds of germs if there were any on the body part from which the smear was taken. In the laboratory, the germs on this applicator will be placed under the proper conditions to help them grow and multiply. Then they will be studied and, finally, identified by name. The doctor will then receive the report naming the germs that are causing the sore throat, the infected nose, or the painful, draining wound.

HOW GERMS ARE IDENTIFIED IN THE LABORATORY

When the doctor wants the laboratory to study a specimen and identify the germs in it, he orders a culture. Just as cultured pearls are those made to grow in oysters by creating the right conditions (placing an irritant inside the shell), or as cultured orchids are those grown by man under special conditions, so too is a germ culture one grown by man under special laboratory conditions. The laboratory places these germs on a glass plate in a culture medium (a round dish containing a suitable kind of food). Then this plate is placed in an incubator in which the oxygen and heat supplies are ideal for the growth of germs.

Soon the germs grow and multiply. The laboratory then studies what conditions made them grow, what conditions slowed their growth, what food they liked, and what waste products they gave off. The laboratory determines how the different antibiotics affect the growth of the germs. After about 3 days, the laboratory is able to give the doctor a report naming the germ and also the antibiotic that stops its growth.

Because the laboratory report requires 3 days, the laboratory technician usually places a few germs on a slide and examines them under a microscope. In a few hours he sends a quick report to the physician, describing what the germ looks like. This quick report is of limited value, since many germs look alike. However, the quick report might state that the germ found was one of the following types:
1. Cocci (round-shaped germs)
2. Diplococci (round-shaped germs that occur in pairs)
3. Streptococci (round-shaped germs that occur in chains)
4. Staphylococci (round-shaped germs that appear in grapelike clusters)
5. Spirochetes (screw-shaped germs)
6. Bacilli (rod-shaped germs)

The disadvantage of the quick report is that there are many germs that have the same appearance. The diplococci of pneumonia and the diplococci of gonorrhea look very much alike. The spirochete of syphilis and the one causing the mouth infection called Vincent's angina also look alike. In the staphylococci group, there are about eighty-two varieties of germs that look alike. This report based on the microscopic examination that describes only how the germs look is therefore of limited value to the doctor in making his diagnosis.

The laboratory needs to examine the germ further to discover its true identity and what drug kills it. Then it can report to the doctor that the diplococci are really pneumococci (cocci causing pneumonia) and that they are killed by penicillin.

In order to identify the germs correctly, the laboratory must have specimens or smears for culturing collected in such a way that the only germs in the specimen container are those from the specimen or the smear. These specimens must be collected in sterile (bacteria-free) specimen containers and collected in such a way that bacteria from your hands or from the air are kept out. Since bacteria (animals that are so small that they cannot be seen by the naked eye) are everywhere, collecting cultures necessitates the use of autoclaved (sterilized) containers and special handling techniques.

WHAT INFORMATION THE SPECIMENS GIVE

A specimen can be examined for many different things. Just as doctors specialize in patient care, so do laboratory personnel specialize in laboratory skills. Therefore just as there are surgical wards, medical wards, and psychiatric wards in the hospital, so too will there be a bacteriology section, a chemistry section, a hematology section, and a pathology section in the hospital laboratory. Each laboratory section specializes in a type of specimen examination, just as the doctor specializes in a particular aspect of patient care. Therefore when you take a specimen to the laboratory, be sure that it is labeled with the patient's name and that it has an examination request attached. Usually the name of the appropriate laboratory section for making the desired test is printed at the bottom of the examination request. If the laboratory section is not specified on the form, find out from the nurse exactly where you are to take the specimen.

The names of the laboratory sections will give you some clues as to what kind of information they give.
1. The bacteriology section examines specimens for bacteria. This section

also identifies the bacteria and the drugs that control or kill them.
2. The chemistry section examines specimens for their chemical elements. This section would examine blood for sugar, proteins, urea, etc. It would also examine any body fluids or excretion for chemical elements.
3. The pathology section examines specimens for changes that are produced by disease. Biopsies would be handled here.
4. The hematology section examines blood to determine what has happened to its normal components. This laboratory does white cell counts, red cell counts, blood-typing, cross matching, etc.

Various specimens may be sent to the laboratory for many different types of examinations.

Feces specimen:
1. Germs
2. The presence of blood
3. The presence of digestive juices such as bile.
4. The presence of the chemical elements of food breakdown

The patient with diarrhea may have feces cultures taken to determine what germs are causing the diarrhea. The patient with suspected ulcers may have feces specimens sent to the laboratory to be examined for the presence of blood.

Urine specimen:
1. Germs
2. The presence of chemical elements such as sugar, proteins (albumin), acetone, calcium, and many other chemicals
3. The presence of cell destruction and disease in the urinary system as evidenced by cells, blood, casts, and pus in the urine
4. The presence of excessive or decreased amounts of water in the urine

Blood specimen:
1. Germs
2. The presence of chemical elements in the blood, such as sugar, proteins, electrolytes
3. For a measurement of various blood parts (for example, white blood cell count, red blood cell count)
4. For blood-typing
5. For cross matching in preparation for a transfusion

Sputum specimen:
1. Germs
2. Cancer cells

Spinal fluid specimen:
1. Germs
2. The abnormal presence of body elements such as cells, blood, or pus
3. The presence of chemical elements such as proteins or sugars

Biopsies:
1. To identify changes in body cells brought about by a disease so that the doctor can attempt to discover what disease the patient has

The examination of specimens gives the following information to aid the doctor in making the diagnosis:
1. Examination of feces specimens shows how the gastrointestinal tract (from the mouth to the rectum) is functioning.
2. Examination of urine specimens shows how the urinary tract (from the kidneys to the urinary orifice) is functioning.
3. Sputum specimen examinations show the presence or absence of infections (or cancer) in the respiratory tract from the mouth to the lungs.
4. Examinations of blood specimens show how the blood is performing its functions of carrying around food and oxygen and of removing waste from the cells.
5. Biopsies indicate the presence or absence of disease.
6. Spinal fluid specimens show the presence or absence of infections (as evidenced by germs) and of injuries (as

evidence by blood) in the brain and spinal cord.

7. Cultures show the presence of germs.

COLLECTING SPECIMENS FROM THE PATIENT

The doctor will order only those specimen examinations that will help him verify his guesses about the patient's condition and aid him in making the diagnosis. However, because the urine gives such a quick clue as to how the body is functioning, each patient usually has a routine urine specimen collected and sent to the laboratory for examination immediately after his admission. In many hospitals an examination of the urine for sugar and acetone is done by the nursing assistant on the floor as part of the admission procedure.

Usually, a specimen is ordered by the doctor the day before it is collected. This gives the nursing assistant an opportunity to explain to the patient that the specimen is to be collected and what he will need to do to help. Explain that the urine specimen (if one is to be collected) is to be taken from the first urine he voids that day. This is done so that a concentrated specimen is obtained. If all the patient's urine is to be collected for a 24-hour period, explain this to him. Label his bed with the sign "Collect all urine 6 A.M. Jan. 4, 1972, to 6 A.M. Jan. 5, 1972. Place it in the bottle in the utility room." Prepare and label the bottle to receive the urine.

Explain to the patient the night before when a feces specimen is to be collected. Remember, most people have a bowel movement after breakfast.

The patient who has an infection in his lungs will have a great deal of sputum to expectorate when he awakens. This is due to the fact that the secretions accumulate in the lungs during sleep. Therefore it is essential that the patient be informed that he is to have a sputum specimen collected in the morning.

The nursing assistant on evening duty should explain to the patient about the specimens that are to be collected the following morning. Then he should prepare and label the specimen containers.

The nursing assistant on night duty should distribute these specimen containers early in the morning when he awakens the patients for their morning care. When a urine specimen is to be collected, give the patient a urinal or bedpan. If a sputum specimen is to be collected, give the patient the container and ask him to try to cough so that he can bring up the sputum from his lungs. Sometimes a concentrated specimen is to be obtained by collecting all the patient's sputum over a 24-hour, 48-hour, or 72-hour period. Explain this thoroughly to the patient. Wrap a paper towel around the sputum container (if it is glass) and hold the towel in place with an elastic band. This makes the specimen bottle more presentable for the patient and his visitors. On the patient's Kardex note the time when the specimen that is being collected will be completed and should be picked up and sent to the laboratory.

The patient may have been unable to defecate upon awakening, in which case the nursing assistant on night duty will have failed to collect his specimen. However, you will be able to obtain the specimen easily after the patient eats his breakfast. Visit him, offer him a bedpan, assist him onto it, and explain that you need the bowel movement for a specimen. After the patient defecates, take the bedpan and specimen container to the utility room. Place the bedpan on a stand, remove about one tablespoonful of feces (with a tongue blade), and place it in the container. Attach the examination request slip, and send or take the specimen to the appropriate laboratory.

If the patient is unable to move his bowels, consult with the nurse. Remember that the doctor is waiting for the results of the specimen examination to help him diagnose and treat the patient.

COLLECTING A SPECIMEN FOR CULTURING

The only excreta that you might collect for a culture are sputum, urine, and feces. A voided specimen for a urine culture is collected from a male patient in the following way:

1. Explain to the patient that you want to collect a urine specimen from him. Ask him to call you when he needs to void.
2. Prepare your specimen container and equipment (Fig. 26-1).
    a. Obtain a sterile voided specimen collection tray from Central Service.
    b. Label the specimen container in the tray with the patient's name.
    c. Add solutions—sterile water and antiseptic soap solution.
3. Take the equipment and the specimen container to the patient's bedside when he tells you that he needs to void.
4. Get a urinal or a bedpan and take it to the bedside.
5. Position the patient. He may be placed in a sitting position by cranking up the head of the bed or by having him sit on the side of the bed, or he may stand at the side of the bed. The position of the patient will depend on his physical ability and on the nurse's instructions.
6. Place a towel under the patient's genital area (if he is in a sitting position), and set the emesis basin on the towel. Wash your hands.
7. Instruct the patient to hold the urinal in readiness.
8. Place two sterile 4-inch-square compresses in the soap solution.
9. Grasp the patient's penis with your left hand and pull back the foreskin.
10. Pick up a soap-soaked compress in your right hand and carefully wash the end of the penis.

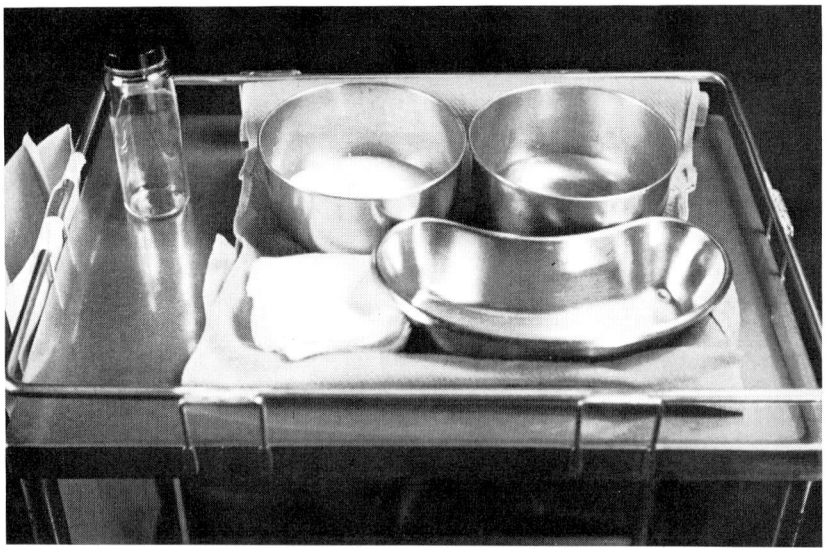

Fig. 26-1. A sterile tray used to collect a sterile voided specimen of urine from a male patient. The tray contains a basin of antiseptic soap solution, a basin of sterile water, some 4-inch-square compresses, and a sterile emesis basin. A sterile urine specimen bottle is on the table but not on the tray, because the outside of this bottle is not sterile.

11. Repeat step 10 with the second compress.
12. Pour some sterile water over the penis (into the emesis basin) to rinse off the soap. Continue to hold the penis with your left hand.
13. Loosen the cap on the specimen container with your right hand and hold it in readiness.
14. Instruct the patient to void into the urinal, which he holds about 3 or 4 inches below the penis.
15. Insert the specimen container into the urinary stream and collect the specimen. Cap the container immediately.
16. Permit the patient to complete his voiding in the usual manner.
17. Collect all the equipment and the specimen and take them to the utility room.
18. Attach an examination request to the specimen and send or take it to the appropriate laboratory immediately.
19. Make the patient comfortable and then clean up the equipment.

A specimen for a urine culture can also be obtained by catheterizing the male patient. The only way a urine specimen for a culture can be obtained from a female patient is by catheterization.

A feces specimen can be obtained for culture in the following way:

1. Prepare the patient by explaining to him that you are to get a special feces specimen and that he should call you when he needs to defecate. Instruct him that he is not to void or to put toilet paper in the bedpan with the feces.
2. Select a bedpan, clean it thoroughly, and then sterilize it in the bedpan sterilizer or autoclave. Cover it with a sterile towel. If you wait to do this until the patient informs you that he needs to defecate, the bedpan will be so hot that he cannot comfortably sit on it.
3. Obtain a sterile container and label it.
4. Take the specially prepared bedpan to the patient and assist him on it when he needs to defecate.
5. Give the patient a paper bag in which to discard toilet paper.
6. Remove the bedpan immediately after the patient is finished, cover it with a sterile towel, and take it to the utility room.
7. Remove about one tablespoonful of feces with a sterile tongue blade and place it in the specimen container.
8. Attach the laboratory examination request to the specimen container and send it or take it to the laboratory immediately.
9. Clean up your equipment in the utility room and then make the patient comfortable.

When a sputum specimen is to be taken from the patient for culturing, explain to him that the bottle is to be kept covered until he is ready to expectorate into it. Then demonstrate how he should remove the cap (without touching the inside), expectorate into the bottle, and quickly replace the cap.

Because many germs die at room temperature, cultures must be taken to the laboratory as soon as they are collected so that they can be put into the incubator.

Remember that inaccurate information is worse than none; collect specimens correctly and label them accurately.

SUMMARY

A specimen is a small part of something exactly the same as all the other parts. The doctor sends specimens of the patient's excretions or body fluids to the laboratory for examinations, knowing that anything found in that specimen can also be found in all other parts of that excreta or body fluid in the patient.

The vital signs give the doctor information about the condition of the patient's body, but examinations of specimens give the doctor information about the cause of the condition.

Specimens must be collected carefully, labeled accurately, and sent to the laboratory promptly so that the doctor will get the information he needs to diagnose and treat the patient.

DISCUSSION QUESTIONS

1. Is it a policy in the hospital in which you work to send urine specimens from all newly admitted patients to the laboratory for examination?
2. Who tells the patients about the specimens that are scheduled to be collected from them?
3. When are urine specimens collected on your ward? Why?
4. How much difficulty do you have collecting feces specimens? Why?
5. Do you feel if would be easier to collect feces specimens after breakfast or before?
6. What specimens did you collect from your patients today? Ask the nurse why they were collected.
7. How does the nurse on your ward know whether the urine or feces specimen was obtained from the patient and sent to the laboratory?
8. Visit the hospital laboratory. Ask the laboratory personnel if there is any way in which you could improve the delivery of specimens.
9. Ask the laboratory technician to show you a culture plate. Ask her to show you some bacteria under the microscope.
10. Take a smear of the material under your fingernails and send it to the laboratory. Ask the head nurse or team leader to help you. After you get the report from this study, discuss whether or not it is important to wash your hands thoroughly after caring for each patient and to keep your fingernails short.

VOCABULARY

bacteria Small living animals that exist everywhere. Bacteria cannot be seen by the naked eye but can be seen under a microscope.

biopsy A piece of a body part that is sent to the laboratory for examination. The results of this examination are of value in assisting the doctor in making a diagnosis.

culture A specimen that is sent to the laboratory for the identification of the germ that is causing the patient's illness.

germs Disease-producing bacteria.

specimen A small amount of body excretion or body fluid that is sent to the laboratory for examination. The results of the examination assist the doctor in making a diagnosis.

sterile Specially treated so that all bacteria are destroyed. Common methods of sterilizing are boiling and autoclaving.

SOURCE OF ADDITIONAL INFORMATION

1. Film: Basic care of patients; part VII: Sterile technique; may be obtained from United States Army (direct request to Commanding General, Attention: Surgeon of the army area in which you reside). (*Depicts practice of sterile technique, emphasizing the three rules of using only sterile equipment, keeping equipment sterile while in use, and keeping the area sterile.*)
2. Film: Hospital sepsis; may be obtained from the American Medical Association, 535 N. Dearborn St., Chicago, Ill. 60610. (*Shows the collection of cultures, the growth of bacteria on culture media, and how bacteria spread.*)
3. Film: Nursing care: the diabetic patients; may be obtained from Director, Film Library, United States Naval Medical School, National Naval Medical Center, Bethesda, Md. 20014. (*Illustrates care of the diabetic patient, including the testing of urine, by the hospital corpsman.*)

27/Giving the patient an enema

STUDY QUESTIONS

1. What is an enema?
2. What is the difference between a cleansing enema and a retention enema in relation to
   a. the purpose for which they are given?
   b. the amount of fluid given?
3. How does a cleansing enema clean the bowel?
4. How does a retention enema fail to excite or stimulate a defecation?
5. How many kinds of cleansing enemas are there?
6. How does a Fleet enema bring about a defecation?
7. How far is the rectal tube inserted when an enema is given?
8. In what direction is the rectal tube inserted? Why?
9. How long should a patient retain an oil retention enema? Why?
10. How can you get the fluid to return if the patient fails to expel the cleansing enema?
11. What causes a patient to fail to expel the cleansing enema?
12. What is a suppository?
13. How is a suppository inserted?
14. What is a barium enema? How is a patient prepared for it?
15. What is a proctoscopic examination?

TYPES OF ENEMAS

An enema is an injection of fluid into the rectum. There are two types of enemas: the cleansing enema and the retention enema.

In a cleansing enema, the fluid is expelled after 5 minutes. In the retention enema, the fluid may be retained in the rectum for periods as long as 4 hours and then expelled, or it is retained until it is absorbed into the blood and thus is never expelled from the rectum.

The enema to be expelled in 5 minutes (cleansing enema)

The enema to be expelled in 5 minutes is given to clean out the rectum, the sigmoid, and the descending colon (large bowel). It cleans them out by stimulating the patient to defecate or have a bowel movement.

In Chapter 8 you learned that the food taken into the body goes through a process of digestion, that the body then absorbs (takes into the bloodstream) what it needs, and that the remainder (waste) travels on down through the small and large intestines and is stored in the rectum. This unwanted food that remains after the process of digestion, together with the juices from the stomach and the intestines, collects in the rectum until a sufficient amount is stored there to stretch the rectal wall. Then the nerve from the rectum sends the message to the brain that the wall is stretched and that this stretch is causing discomfort. The brain automatically sends down another message telling the anal muscle to let go and telling the colon (large bowel) muscles to squeeze down and evacuate (empty) the rectum. However, toilet training has taught the person to send down an additional message telling the anal muscle to hold tight until the proper toilet facilities are obtained.

The cleansing enema activates the mechanism of defecation in the patient by filling the rectum with water and so stretching the rectal wall that the message goes to the brain that the rectum needs to be emptied. Therefore a sufficient amount of fluid must be injected into the rectum by the cleansing enema to stretch the rectal walls sufficiently to activate this mechanism of defecation. This amount of fluid (in the normal bowel) is approximately 2,000 ml. or 2 quarts. The patient receiving the cleansing enema will usually take the first 1,000 ml. of fluid easily. However, the second 1,000 ml. begins to stretch the rectal wall, and the patient feels the rectal pressure and receives the message to defecate. Therefore he will need to exert considerable effort to keep the anal sphincter (circular muscle at the end of the rectum) tightly closed in order to hold the enema fluid.

Another method of giving a cleansing enema is to inject into the rectum a small amount (usually 4 ounces) of a special fluid that so excites the rectal wall that it sends the message to the brain that the rectum needs to empty. Such a special fluid is contained in the many prepackaged enema units available commercially. One of these prepackaged enema units is the ready-to-use, disposable Fleet enema.

Use of the cleansing enema is indicated as follows:

1. In the patient who is constipated. The bedridden patient may fail to have a bowel movement for 3 days because the lying-down position slows down the movement of feces through the bowel and the muscles used in defecation are too weakened and sluggish to evacuate the rectum. The patient on intensive drug therapy for pain may have the complication of sloweddown peristalsis (muscle movements in the intestines) with resulting constipation due to the pain-relieving drugs he is receiving.

2. In the patient who is unable to defecate because of poor muscle tone. The patient may have diseased or injured nerves that are unable to carry the message to the brain that the rectum is full, or he may have paralyzed or weakened muscles that are unable to clamp down and empty the rectum.

3. In the patient who defecates automatically (is incontinent). The patient may have nerve or brain disease that prevents him from getting the message that the rectum is full or from sending down the message to hold the feces until the proper toilet facilities are obtained. The enema is used in this case to help the patient retrain his bowel to empty at certain specific times.

4. In the patient who is being prepared for an operation. The descending colon, sigmoid, and rectum, are emptied preoperatively by the enema so that the surgeon will have more space inside the abdomen in which to work during the operation and so that the newly operated upon muscles of the abdomen will be spared the job of squeezing down to empty the rectum until they are healed.

5. The patient who is being prepared for an operation or a diagnostic procedure (such as proctoscopy) upon the rectum and sigmoid colon receives cleansing enemas—usually three—until the return is clear. (The fluid returns as clear as it was when it was injected.) This procedure is done to ensure the surgeon a clean operating area.

The patient who is having an instrument

passed through the anus and into the rectum so that the doctor may look through it to determine the condition of the rectum, sigmoid, or descending colon may also have enemas until clear. These are given to remove all the feces so that the doctor is able to see the body structures clearly.

Enemas until clear may be given to those patients having barium enemas also. In this case they are given to clean the rectum, sigmoid, and descending colon of all feces so that a retention enema of barium can be given to fill these structures completely in preparation for an x-ray study.

6. In the patient who has an irritating substance, such as a food that does not agree with him or a spoiled food, in the colon. Such a patient will develop severe diarrhea. This diarrhea is an attempt by the colon to rid itself of the irritant. The lining of the colon does this by secreting water to dilute the irritant and to move it along the anus for excretion out of the body. Such watery stools are known as diarrhea. Therefore a cleansing enema may be given to help the colon by speeding up the removal of the irritating substances.

The following are the solutions and fluids most frequently used in cleansing enemas:

1. Soapsuds* and water—usually 1 ounce of mild soap solution, such as Ivory or castile soap, mixed in 2 quarts of water
2. Normal saline (salt) solution (called normal because it is the same kind of salt solution as that which is in our body fluids)—can be prepared by adding 2 teaspoonfuls of table salt to every quart of water used
3. Tap water—water as it comes from the spigot with nothing added
4. Prepackaged disposable enema units containing special drug mixtures

---
*All soap solutions are irritating to the lining of the bowel.

The enema to be retained (retention enema)

The retention enema must avoid the activation of the defecation urge (1) by consisting of such a small amount of fluid that the rectal wall fails to be stretched and (2) by consisting of a fluid so soothing to the rectum that it fails to irritate or excite the rectal wall.

The amount of fluid usually administered in the retention enema is limited to between 4 and 6 ounces.

The enema to be retained for a period of time up to 4 hours. The retention enema to be retained up to 4 hours is usually given to treat diseases and disorders of the rectum. The solution used is the one that acts upon the condition. The solution is injected into the rectum and left there for the period of time designated by the nurse. Actually the rectum and its contents are soaked in this solution. After the treatment time has elapsed the retention enema is expelled, either by the conscious effort of the patient to defecate or by the stimulation of the bowel with a cleansing enema. This type of enema is given to the following patients:

1. The patient who has a fecal impaction. The fecal mass in the rectum has become so large and so hard that the patient is unable to expel it. An oil retention enema is then given to soften and lubricate (grease) the fecal mass. After the enema has been retained for a designated period of time, the patient is given a cleansing enema to help him evacuate the mass.
2. The patient who has an irritated rectum and sigmoid colon. In the patient who is having frequent bowel movements, the anus may be raw and irritated. A starch enema is given and retained to coat and soothe and quiet the irritated rectum. After the treatment time has elapsed, the patient usually expels the enema by a conscious effort to evacuate.

The following solutions are used for

enemas that are retained for periods up to 4 hours:
1. Prepackaged disposal oil retention enemas containing 4 ounces of oil
2. Olive oil, 4 ounces
3. Starch solution, made by dissolving about 1 teaspoonful of starch (cooking) in about 1 ounce of cold water and then adding about 6 ounces of boiling hot water and stirring well. (This must be cooled to a temperature of between 100° and 105° F. before it can be given to the patient in an enema.)

The enema to be retained and never expelled. The enema to be retained and never expelled is usually used to give the patient a drug or a medicine that he needs when it cannot be given in any other way.* As discussed previously (Chapter 8), the colon (large bowel) is able to absorb (take into the bloodstream) water. Therefore the colon can also permit watery solutions of medication to pass through its lining and into the bloodstream. The bloodstream then carries these medications around the body in the same way as it would if the drug had been taken by mouth and absorbed into the blood from the small intestine.

A cleansing enema must be given about an hour before the medication enema is administered. The cleansing enema will empty the rectum of all feces. Then the medication enema will come in close contact with the walls of the rectum, and it will be able to pass through these rectal walls and into the bloodstream.

In order for it to be absorbed into the bloodstream, the medication-containing retention enema should be given as follows:
1. The enema should be administered about 1 hour after the rectum is emptied by a cleansing enema.
2. The enema should consist of a watery solution with the drug thoroughly dissolved in it. Drug-containing solutions usually given in a medication enema include the following:
    a. Aspirin tablets dissolved in about 3 ounces of warm tap water
    b. Paraldehyde (amount ordered by the doctor) added to about 3 ounces of starch solution (prepared as for a starch enema, and added because paraldehyde irritates the rectum)
    c. Ether (given by the anesthetist)
    d. Antibiotics like neomycin dissolved in about 3 ounces of water

WHEN THE DOCTOR DECIDES THAT THE PATIENT IS TO GET AN ENEMA

The doctor decides that the patient should have a cleansing enema and writes the order for it on his chart. The doctor may have made this decision as a result of the information you gave him about the patient's constipation or incontinence. In his order for the enema, the doctor will specify if it is to be a cleansing enema prepared with water and soap or a prepackaged special fluid type like the Fleet enema. He will also specify any special directions required in the administration of the enema. Some examples of this might be as follows:
1. The doctor may order a small soapsuds enema if the patient is recovering from surgery on the rectum and the doctor does not want the rectal wall stretched too much because he is afraid it might rupture at the operation site.*

---

*Medication can also be given by rectum in the form of a suppository. Suppositories are cone shaped, and they contain a drug dissolved in some soothing substance like glycerin or cocoa butter. They are a solid at room temperature, but when they are inserted into the rectum, the glycerin or cocoa butter melts and the drug is released. The drug is then absorbed through the rectal walls into the bloodstream.

---

*Since all soap is irritating to the lining of the bowel, it should be added to the enema only when the physician so specifies in his order for the enema.

2. The doctor may specify a low tap-water enema for a patient who has had surgery on the sigmoid or descending colon because he wants the enema given with such low pressure that the fluid will not go up high enough to enter the area of the operation.

The patient is placed in position

The best position of the patient for the enema is the left side-lying position because this so positions the rectum and sigmoid that the enema fluid runs downhill (Fig. 27-1). However, if the patient is unable to hold the enema fluid during the procedure, the side-lying position is undesirable because the escaping fluid may run all over the patient and the bed. In such a patient the second best position or the back-lying position with the patient on the bedpan throughout the entire procedure is really the most desirable one. With the patient in this position, the rectum and sigmoid are on a level plane so that the fluid runs on a straight line.

Undesirable enema positions are the right side-lying and the sitting positions. These are undesirable because the rectum and sigmoid are so elevated that the fluid must run uphill to enter them (Figs. 27-2 and 27-3). The extra force needed to push the fluid in so irritates the rectal wall that it stimulates the urge to defecate at the very beginning of the enema. Then, too, the fluid in the rectum lies right on top of the anal muscle (at the bottom of the hill) and creates such pressure on it that the patient has difficulty keeping the rectum closed in order to retain the enema fluid.

The temperature of the fluid

Rectal temperature is normally about 99.6° F. The temperature of any rectal injection should be this temperature (99.6° F.) when it enters the rectum. When a cleansing enema is given with such equipment that the fluid runs through about 6 feet of tubing between the fluid container and the rectum, the fluid is prepared at a temperature of 105° F. This allows for the five degrees of cooling that occurs during the procedure. However, when a small enema (such as a retention enema) is given with equipment close to the rectum, the fluid is prepared at a temperature of 100° F. So little cooling occurs that very little temperaure allowance is made for it.

Giving a cleansing enema

When the nurse assigns you to give a cleansing enema, she will also give you

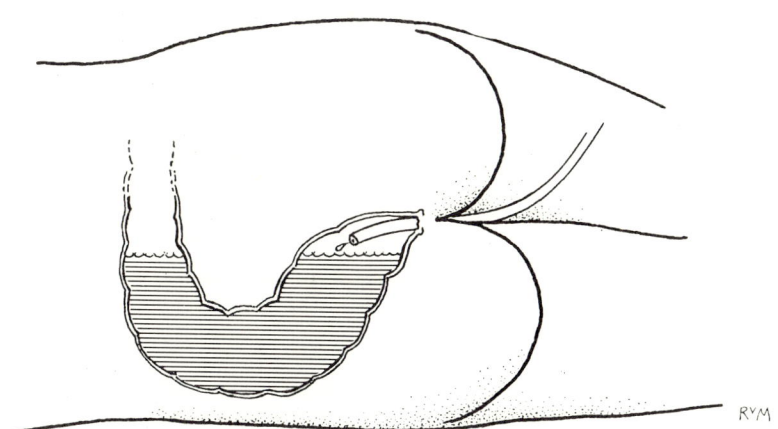

Fig. 27-1. Drawing showing a patient receiving an enema in a left side-lying position.

214   Nursing assistant meets patient's particular needs

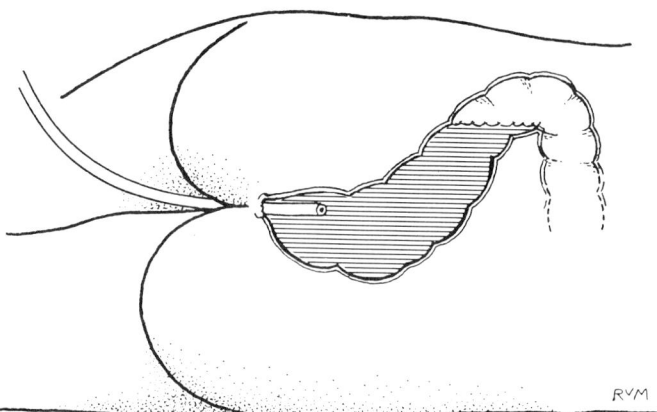

Fig. 27-2. Drawing showing a patient receiving an enema in the *incorrect* right side-lying position. Note that the enema fluid must run uphill, requiring more force to be exerted on the fluid and causing the patient to suffer more distress.

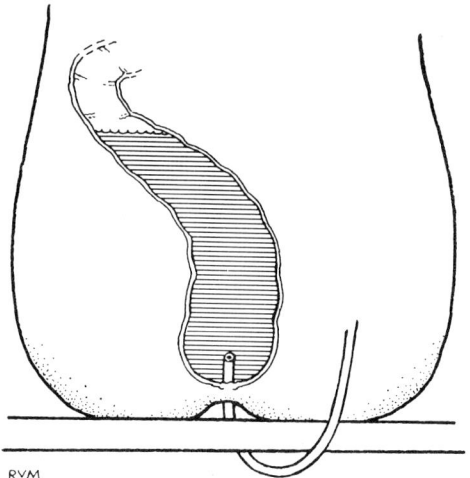

Fig. 27-3. Drawing showing a patient receiving an enema in the *incorrect* sitting position. This position will cause the fluid to remain in the rectum and result in so much pressure on the anus and so much stretching of the rectal walls that the patient will be able to hold only a very small amount. Therefore the enema will be ineffective.

any special instructions about its administration that the doctor ordered. The cleansing enema is given in the following way:

1. Collect the necessary linens, which include a treatment or bath blanket, a drawsheet, and a rubber sheet.
2. Take the collected linens to the patient's bedside.
3. Explain to the patient that he is going to receive a cleansing enema.
   a. Ask him if he ever had a cleansing enema before. If he has not, explain the procedure to him. Remember, you will need his cooperation, since he must work hard to hold the fluid after the first quart is injected.
   b. Explain that you are going to inject enough fluid into the rectum to so stretch the rectal wall that the entire colon will be stimulated to empty itself.
   c. Explain to the patient that he will feel some pressure but that you will warn him when it is coming so that he can be prepared to clamp down with his muscles in order to hold the fluid.
   d. Try to explain so that the patient

will not be frightened or worried. The emotions of fear and worry interfere with bowel functioning.
4. Prepare the bed for the enema procedure as follows:
   a. Fanfold the top covers to the foot of the bed while you cover the patient with the treatment blanket.
   b. Place the bed protection (rubber sheet covered by the drawsheet) under the patient from the middle of his back to the middle of his thighs.
5. Observe the patient carefully while you are explaining the procedure and preparing the bed. Try to find answers to the following questions:
   a. What is the probable condition of the patient's bowel muscle? An answer to this question is found by looking at his other muscles. If the patient is old and feeble, so are his bowel muscles. If the patient is half paralyzed, so are his bowel muscles. If the patient is strong and healthy, so are his bowel muscles.
   b. Will he be able to hold the enema fluid? If your answer to the preceding question was that his bowel muscles are strong and healthy, the answer is probably *yes*. If your answer was that his bowel muscles are weak or paralyzed, the answer is probably *no*.
6. Position a treatment pole at the patient's bedside. Adjust the pole height to that level which will permit the enema bag to hang about 1½ feet above the patient's hips.
7. Take the patient's bedpan out of his bedside stand and place it in an easily accessible spot on the bed. Obtain a bedside commode, if one is to be used, or prepare the patient's toilet area if he is to go there to expel the enema.
8. Return to the utility room and prepare your equipment as follows:
   a. Obtain a disposable enema setup from Central Service.
   b. Prepare 2 quarts of solution (tap water, soapsuds, or normal saline, as specified by the nurse) in a pitcher at a temperature of 105° F. Measure the solution temperature with a bath thermometer to be sure that it is 105° F.
   c. Attach a rectal tube to the connector on the tubing (if unattached).
   d. Close the clamp on the enema tubing and pour the water from the pitcher into the enema bag.
   e. Loosen the clamp on the tubing and permit enough fluid (about 1 ounce) to flow through to push all the air out of the tubing. Close the clamp again.
9. Take the filled bag and lubricant to the bedside.
10. Hang the enema bag on the treatment pole at the patient's bedside. Be sure that the clamp on the tubing is closed.
11. Lubricate the rectal tube well. Squirt the lubricant out of the tube and onto a piece of toilet paper. Place the rectal tube in the toilet paper containing the lubricant and rotate it sufficiently to lubricate it thoroughly.
12. Have the patient lie on his left side. Assist him to assume this position.
13. Separate the patient's buttocks with the thumb and fingers of your right hand while you insert the well-lubricated rectal tube 3 inches into the rectum with the left hand. Direct the tube toward the umbilicus as you insert it.
   a. If the patient has several large or painful hemorrhoids (varicose veins of the rectum), he will be so fearful that you might hurt him when you insert the tube that he will keep his anal muscles

clamped down tightly. Do not try to force the rectal tube in. Wait a few moments and then ask the patient to squeeze down as if he were going to have a bowel movement. This action will open the anus and you will be able to insert the well-lubricated rectal tube easily.
   b. If you meet resistance after you have inserted the rectal tube about 1½ inches, stop. Do not force the tube. Forcing or pushing may cause the rectal tube to go through the wall of the bowel. This resistance means that the muscle of the anal canal is tight and is blocking the entrance of the tube. Permit some enema fluid to flow in. This warm fluid will relax the muscle, and you will be able to insert the rectal tube the second 1½ inches.
14. Prepare to administer the fluid if you think that the patient is able to hold it. If you believe that he is not, place the bedpan in position under the patient and place him on it by turning him toward you and onto his back. Be sure that the enema tubing is between his legs and is not pinched off by being caught between his buttocks and the bedpan.
15. Hold the rectal tube in the rectum with your left hand.
    a. Hold it close to the rectum or it will come out. Remember that you lubricated it well and it can therefore slip out as easily as it slipped in.
    b. If the patient is in a back-lying position, put your hand between his legs and hold the rectal tube in position.
16. Loosen the clamp on the enema tubing.
17. Talk to the patient while you are giving him the enema. This will occupy his mind so that it will not be so alert to receive and answer the first message it gets that the rectal wall is stretching. Give the patient progress reports such as the following throughout the procedure: "You're doing well; you've taken nearly one third of the fluid." "You're about half through, but remember, the second half gives you the pressure feelings," "You're nearly through, you've got just a few more ounces to go." Continue until only 1 ounce of fluid remains in the enema bag.
18. If he fails to hold the enema fluid at any time during the procedure, close the clamp (stop the flow of fluid) and place the patient in a back-lying position on the bedpan.
    a. Each time the patient who is receiving the enema in a back-lying position on the bedpan expels some enema fluid, pinch off the enema tubing to stop the fluid flow into the rectum. Do not remove the rectal tube. When the patient ceases to expel the fluid, release the pinch on the tubing and permit the enema fluid to flow into the rectum again.
19. Pinch off the tubing. Then close off the clamp.
20. Withdraw the rectal tube from the rectum with one quick motion and place it in the bag.
21. Assist the patient onto the bedpan if he received the enema in the side-lying position, or assist him out of bed onto the bedside commode or out of bed into the bathroom, whichever is permitted.
22. Position the patient on the bedpan in a sitting position so that gravity can assist him to empty his bowel. This can be done by cranking up the bed. Place his call bell within reaching distance, give him the toilet paper, and leave him, thus giving

him privacy for his bowel movement.
   a. If the patient is sitting on a bedside commode or on the toilet in the bathroom, be sure that he has ample toilet paper and that the call bell is within easy reach.
23. Discard the disposable enema bag and tubing in the appropriate receptacle. Return the treatment pole to its proper place in the unit.
24. Check the patient frequently. Sometimes he becomes exhausted or develops signs of shock (cold, moist skin, rapid but weak pulse, low blood pressure, light-headedness). If the patient shows any signs of shock, send for the nurse immediately and return the patient to as flat-lying a position as possible as you wait for the nurse to arrive.
25. Remove the bedpan or the bedside commode as soon as the patient is finished. If the patient is expelling the enema in the bathroom, instruct him not to flush the toilet so you can see the results obtained from the enema.
26. Position the patient comfortably by lowering the head of the bed and by removing the treatment blanket as you replace the top covers. Leave the rubber-covered drawsheet under the patient for about 1 hour, since he may have several more bowel movements. However, if it is soiled, replace it with a clean one.
27. Give the patient a basin of water, a bar of soap, a washcloth, and a towel so that he can wash his hands.
28. Take the bedpan to the utility room.
   a. Inspect its contents carefully so that you can chart the results of the enema.
   b. If there is anything unusual about the contents of the bedpan, cover the bedpan and get the nurse to come in and see it.
   c. Observe the results of the enema—color, odor, consistency, and amount.
      (1) Color: *black* usually indicates the presence of blood that has gone through the process of digestion; *red* usually indicates bleeding in the rectum, sigmoid, or descending colon; *light yellow* usually means that the flow of the bile into the small intestine is blocked; and *white* usually indicates barium in the bowel from an x-ray study.
      (2) Odor: *foul odor* usually indicates that there are large amounts of bacteria, whereas *absence of odor* usually means that the patient has received such extensive antibiotic treatment that most of the intestinal bacteria have been killed.
      (3) Consistency: *hard formed stools* indicate constipation; *soft formed stools* are normal, and *liquid stools* are a sign of bowel irritation.
      (4) Amount: *large, small,* or *average.*
29. Place the bedpan in the flusher. Flush it thoroughly with cold water and then steam sterilize it.
30. Wash your hands thoroughly, remove the bedpan from the flusher, and place it in its proper place.
31. Chart the enema and the results obtained in the nurse's record on the patient's chart. This may be done as follows: "9:30 A.M.: soapsuds enema (2,000 ml.) given. Results: large amount of dark brown, hard-formed stool was expelled. The patient felt better." (M. Smith, N.A.)

Special note. Reusable enema equipment (can and tubing) rather than the disposable type may be in use in your hospital or nursing home (Fig. 27-4). However, if it is, the thorough cleaning and sterilizing of equipment after use is essential if the nursing assistant is to avoid giving hepatitis with the enema.

Failure of the patient to expel the fluid. Failure of the patient to expel the fluid may be due to one of the following conditions:
1. The patient is so tense that the anal muscle is clamped tightly closed.
2. A hard mass of fecal material is blocking the exit of the fluid.
3. The bowel has ruptured and the fluid has run out into the abdomen (much as air runs out of a tire when it has a hole in it).
4. The nerves that open the anus and stimulate the colon to empty are not functioning.

After the patient tries to expel the enema

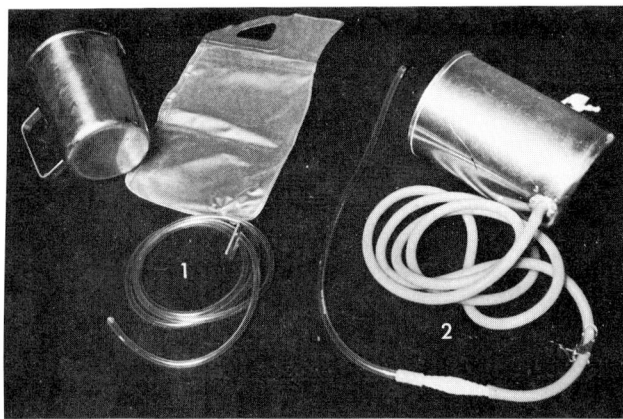

Fig. 27-4. Enema equipment: **1,** disposable enema unit; **2,** reusable enema can and tubing.

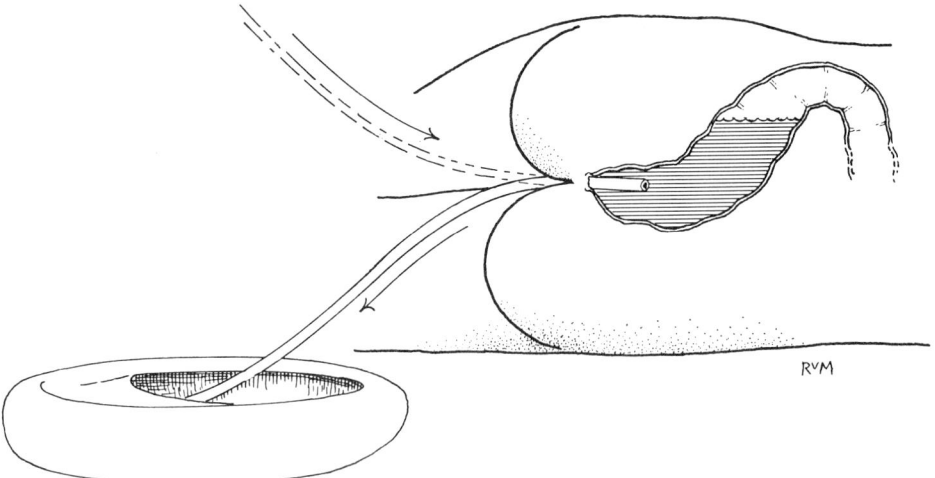

Fig. 27-5. Drawing showing the patient placed in a right side-lying position and the rectal tube reinserted in order to siphon the enema fluid back. The right side-lying position utilizes gravity to help siphon the fluid back. (Invert the picture and note that this position is just the opposite of the left side-lying position used in giving the patient the enema.)

for 30 minutes or so with no success, get an emesis basin, a rectal tube, some toilet tissue, and lubricant and return to his room. Lubricate the rectal tube well and insert it 3 inches into the rectum with the patient lying on his right side. Place the other end of the rectal tube in the bedpan (Fig. 27-5).

The rectal tube will open the tight anal muscle or push away the hard fecal mass and permit the water to run out of the rectum downhill into the bedpan. Siphon back all the fluid. Note the contents of the bedpan and report to the nurse that the patient could not expel the enema and that you siphoned the enema fluid back. Describe the return that you obtained.

Record the entire procedure and your results on the chart. The nurse will report this to the doctor, and he will examine the patient's rectum to determine why the patient failed to expel the fluid. However, if you are unable to siphon any fluid back, something serious may have happened; for example, the rectum may have been perforated (a hole was poked through it). Report this to the nurse immediately. She will notify the doctor and he will examine the patient thoroughly. Perhaps an operation may be done immediately to repair the rectum.

Emotions and bowel movements. It was noted previously that the extremely tense patient may have difficulty relaxing his anal muscle and expelling the enema. Emotions play a great part in bowel activity. The patient who remains frightened over a long period of time has such slowed peristalsis that he is constantly troubled with constipation. On the other hand, the patient who is worried about himself, who is mad at the world because of his illness, or who is constantly apprehensive about what will be done to him next is very likely to have such increased peristalsis that he has abdominal cramps and diarrhea.

Giving the cleansing enema with the prepackaged unit

The prepackaged enema comes already prepared with the fluid (approximately 4 ounces) and all the equipment needed to give it. The enema units can be stored at room temperature and can be given to the patient at this temperature without any special warming.

There are two types of prepackaged enema units: the plastic bottle with a 3-inch firm plastic rectal tube attached (Fleet) and the sealed plastic bag with a 12- to 14-inch flexible plastic rectal tube (Travad). The advantages of the second one over the first include (1) ease in giving and (2) safety of the softer, more pliable rectal tube (Fig. 27-6).

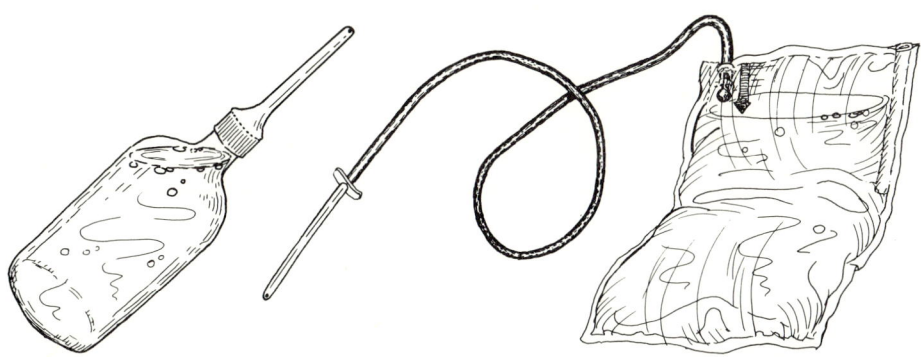

Fig. 27-6. Disposable cleansing enema units. Fleet on the left and Travad on the right.

The procedure is explained to the patient by telling him that 4 ounces of fluid will be injected into his rectum, that he will be required to hold this fluid for about 5 minutes or until he has the urge to defecate, and that he can then expel it by defecating.

The bed is prepared by fanfolding the top bedding to the foot of the bed and covering the patient with a treatment blanket. The rubber-covered drawsheet is usually unnecessary, since the patient can easily hold the 4 ounces.

Get a prepackaged enema unit, a bedpan, and some toilet paper and return to the patient's room. Turn the patient on his left side. Remove the cover from the rectal tube (if the plastic bottle type) or pull out the tube (if the bag type). Insert the already lubricated rectal tube about 3 inches into the rectum in the direction of the umbilicus. Inject the fluid by squeezing the plastic bottle or by flicking the red plug out of the bag outflow tube and holding the bag above the patient's hips. Remove the rectal tube with one quick motion. Then, if the patient is ambulatory, permit him to go to the bathroom. If he is not ambulatory, place him on the bedpan. Crank up the top of the bed until he is in a sitting position on the bedpan. The patient usually defecates in about 5 to 10 minutes. The prepackaged unit is then discarded.

Remove the bedpan, observe its contents, and chart the results as described previously.

Giving the retention enema

Visit the patient, sit down with him, and explain thoroughly that you are going to inject a *small* amount of *medicated* fluid into his rectum. Tell him that he may feel the urge to move his bowels and expel the fluid but that this urge will leave him in a few minutes. Instruct him that this fluid is a treatment for his bowel condition and that he is to hold it in. After you are sure that the patient understands, proceed as follows:

1. Collect the necessary linen, which consists of a rubber sheet and a drawsheet.
2. Take the linen to the bedside and place the rubber sheet covered by the drawsheet under the patient.
3. Work slowly and calmly. Avoid getting the patient so worried and apprehensive that peristalsis will be stimulated.
4. If a Fleet oil retention enema is to be given, get the prepackaged unit. No additional preparation is required. If you are going to prepare your own oil enema, do as follows:
   a. Pour 4 ounces of olive oil into a container.
   b. Set the container of oil in a basin of water (110° F.) to warm it.
   c. Check the temperature of the oil with an oral thermometer. When it reaches 100° F., remove it from the water bath and prepare to give it.
   d. Take the container of oil and put it on a tray containing (1) a Robinson catheter (size 18), (2) a small funnel, (3) an adequate supply of toilet paper, and (4) an emesis basin.
5. Take the Fleet oil retention enema or the tray of equipment and the container of oil you prepared to the patient's bedside.
6. Turn the patient onto his left side. Keep the bed flat.
7. Fold in the top covers at the side to expose the patient's rectum.
8. Give the Fleet oil retention enema exactly as described for the Fleet cleansing enema, or give the oil retention enema you prepared in the following way:
   a. Lubricate the catheter by dipping it in the oil.
   b. Separate the buttocks and insert

the Robinson catheter about 3 inches up into the rectum.
   c. Attach the funnel to the other end of the catheter.
   d. Pour the oil into the funnel and permit it to run into the rectum. Continue until all the oil is given.
9. Remove the Fleet rectal tube or the Robinson catheter with one quick movement and at the same time apply pressure to the rectum with a large wad of toilet paper as you squeeze the buttocks together.
10. Remain with the patient and continue this pressure on his anus until his urge to defecate passes.
11. Roll the patient toward you into a back-lying position.
12. Straighten the bedclothes and make the patient comfortable.
13. Avoid talking about defecation. Do not bring a bedpan into the area where the enema is given. Do not leave a bedpan in the patient's room. Do not put the patient into the sitting position, since this increases pressure on the anus.
14. Wash your hands.
15. Chart the date and time and kind of retention enema that you gave on the nurse's record on the patient's chart.

Remember that an oil retention enema is usually followed (in several hours) by a cleansing enema. Therefore you can leave the rubber sheet and drawsheet in place under the patient until the cleansing enema is given. The patient who receives an oil retention enema usually soils the bed with seepage of oil from the rectum. This is why the rubber sheet and drawsheet are used.

A medicated retention enema would be given in the same way as the oil retention enema. The medication to be administered is also warmed by setting the container of medicated solution in a warm water bath until it reaches the temperature of 100° F.

It differs from the oil enema in two ways:
1. The oil enema is followed by a cleansing enema, but a cleansing enema is given before a medicated retention enema.
2. The oil enema is expelled after a time lapse, but the medicated retention enema is never expelled, since it is absorbed into the blood.

Order for enemas until clear

When the doctor orders enemas until the return flow is clear, the following procedure is followed:
1. The patient is given a cleansing enema of 2,000 ml. of fluid (type of solution specified by the doctor). The enema return is observed. If it is clear, no additional enemas are given, If it contains feces or is highly colored, a second enema is given.*
2. The patient is given a second enema of 2,000 ml. of fluid (type of solution specified by the doctor). The enema return is observed. If the return is clear, no additional enemas are given. If the return is highly colored or contains feces, a third enema is given.
3. The patient is given a third enema of 2,000 ml. of fluid (type of solution specified by the doctor). The enema return is observed. If the return is clear, no further action is indicated. If the return contains fecal material or is highly colored, the nurse is notified; she will contact the doctor. No more enemas are given (even though the return was not clear) until the doctor gives further directions.

In summary, then, when the doctor orders enemas until clear, three enemas may be given. However, if the return is not clear after three enemas, the doctor is notified. Further action depends on his directions.

---

*Keep disposable enema unit until all three enemas are given. Dispose only after patient is adequately prepared and the total procedure is complete.

Enemas until clear are indicated in the patient who is to have the anal canal, rectum, and sigmoid studied because the doctor believes they are diseased. Therefore these diseased structures are filled up and stretched three times with three enemas. How safe it is to fill and stretch the rectum again must be determined by the doctor, who knows the condition of the patient's body, before another enema can be given.

The doctor may believe that examination of the rectum is so essential that he may ask you to give another enema. Usually, however, he decides that no more enemas are to be given until he reexamines the rectum.

Patients frequently become quite weak after receiving two or three enemas. Therefore it is advisable to keep such patients in bed and let them use the bedpan to expel the enema. In this way you can avoid their becoming dizzy or weak and fainting or falling on the floor. Remember to return the patient to the flat-lying position in bed if he develops signs of shock.

Sometimes the patient receiving enemas until clear will start to bleed. This is usually because the disease process in his bowel is irritated and not because of something you did. Notify the nurse immediately if bleeding occurs.

The barium enema

An x-ray film of the lower bowel and rectum will not show anything. Therefore the bowel and rectum are thoroughly cleaned of all feces (through enemas) and the patient is sent to the x-ray department. The x-ray technician will then give the patient an enema of barium that will fill up the anal canal, rectum, sigmoid, and part of the descending colon. Then an x-ray film is made. The barium shows up on the x-ray film; therefore the outline of all these structures is obtained. Any blurring or changes in the outline indicate a blockage in the flow of barium at that point and suggest to the doctor that the patient has a tumor or disease process.

Preparation for a barium enema. The anal canal, rectum, sigmoid, and descending colon must be free of fecal material before a barium enema can be given. Therefore the doctor may order one of the following:

1. Cleansing enemas until clear
2. Cathartic (drug to cause defecation—commonly called a physic) the night before the study and a prepackaged cleansing enema the morning of the study
3. Cathartic the night before and a suppository the morning of the study.

All of these methods of cleansing the bowel are equally effective. However, some doctors prefer one method, whereas other doctors prefer another. Find out which method the doctor prefers and follow that one. The important thing is that you clean the intestinal tract thoroughly by carrying out the method correctly.

After the barium enema. The patient returns from the x-ray department with most of the barium still in the rectum and colon. The barium will become a hard, caked, cementlike mass that will block the bowel if it is not removed. Even though the patient received cathartics, enemas, and/or suppositories and had many bowel movements before the study, he must have something to help him expel the barium after the study. The doctor usually orders a cleansing enema for this purpose. However, if the patient is not given an enema, remind the team leader or head nurse that the patient did not get one.

Cleansing enemas preceding proctoscopic or sigmoidoscopic examination

Cleansing enemas are ordered for the patient who is to have a proctoscopic or sigmoidoscopic examination. After the rectum has been thoroughly cleansed of feces (as for a barium enema), the doctor will perform the examination.

In a proctoscopy, he will insert a proctoscope (an instrument with mirror and lights) into the rectum to examine it. He looks through the proctoscope (much as the sailor in a submarine looks through a periscope) and sees the inside of the rectum.

The sigmoidoscopic examination is much like the proctoscopic examination except that the sigmoidoscope is longer and goes past the rectum and up into the sigmoid portion of the bowel. The doctor examines the sigmoid colon by looking at it through the sigmoidoscope.

Orders for an enema for the patient who is not eating

You may be quite surprised when the doctor orders an enema for a patient who is not eating. However, this is not so strange as it seems at first. The solid part of the feces is made up of bacteria (33⅓%), food (33⅓%), and juices and cells from the gastrointestinal tract (33⅓%).

Therefore the patient who is not eating will still have bacteria and juices and cells in the gastrointestinal tract and so he will still expel feces. He will have about one-third less feces than he would if he were eating, but he will still have feces.

Distention of the intestines with gas

Gas gets into the intestines in three different ways:
1. It is swallowed.
2. It is formed by the action of the bacteria in the intestines.
3. It passes from the blood into the intestines. This gas is mostly carbon dioxide.

When the gastrointestinal tract is functioning normally, much of the gas that has entered the intestines is absorbed into the blood from the large intestine and about a pint is expelled from the rectum. However, when the intestines have been handled during surgery or have been operated upon, they do not function normally. The gas forms in the same way, but it is not moved along the bowel to the rectum and expelled, nor is it absorbed through the lining of the large bowel. Instead, it remains in the intestines and collects until the intestines are blown up like a balloon and the abdomen is distended. The patient complains of much discomfort and pain. The doctor usually prescribes a drug to stimulate peristalsis and move the gas through the intestines and out of the rectum. An example of such a drug is neostigmine. When the nurse gives this drug to the patient, she will ask you to insert a rectal tube into the rectum to make it easier for the gas to leave the patient's body. The end of the rectal tube that is not in the patient should be taped into a small 4-ounce bottle or onto an abdominal pad to catch any liquid feces leaving the body with the gas.

If this method is not effective, the doctor may prescribe a low enema for the patient. Remember, the entire intestinal tract is not working because it has been injured or hurt, and it is already blown up with gas. Therefore a small enema of about 500 ml. of fluid (soapsuds, tap water, or saline, as ordered by the doctor) is given slowly, with the enema can held about 1½ feet above the level of the patient's hips. After the enema is expelled, the rectal tube may be reinserted (if ordered by the doctor) to make it easier for the gas to be expelled.

The small enema may be repeated frequently until the intestines regain their ability to move (peristalsis) and expel the gas. These small frequent enemas act very much like a warm soak to the injured colon, soothing the colon muscles much as a foot soak soothes a sprained ankle.

The results of these enemas would be charted not in terms of feces expelled, since there would be none, but in terms of gas expelled and decrease in abdominal distention. You will hear the gas being expelled; you will know the distention is decreased if the patient tells you that he feels better.

Use of the suppository to stimulate defecation

In those patients who have constipation or fecal incontinence because of muscle or nerve disease (such as the patient with a stroke, with a spinal cord injury, or with multiple sclerosis), the suppository is frequently used to stimulate defecation at a specific time and thus is used to retrain the bowel.

The suppository is inserted into the anus with a glove-covered finger and pushed up from 2 to 3 inches through the anal canal into the rectum. This means that the nursing assistant inserting the suppository will need to insert his entire index finger into the rectum to push up the suppository.

This suppository stimulates defecation in much the same way as the prepackaged cleansing enema. It excites and stimulates the rectal wall so that it sends a message to the brain that the rectum is full and needs to empty. The most frequently used suppositories are those prepared from glycerin, which have little or no effect, and those containing bisacodyl (Dulcolax), which are very effective.

When the suppository is given daily to retrain the bowel, it should be given before breakfast. Then the natural tendency of the bowel to empty after eating will help it act. Since the suppository acts by irritating the rectal wall, it must be inserted 2 or 3 inches up into the rectum and it must also be pushed against the rectal wall. If it is pushed into a fecal mass, it cannot stimulate the rectal wall.

Immediately after breakfast the patient should be put in a sitting position on a bedpan in bed, on a bedside commode, or on the bathroom toilet. Usually he will defecate in 30 minutes.

SUMMARY

An enema is an injection of fluid into the rectum. There are two types: cleansing enemas and retention enemas.

The cleansing enema works by filling the rectum so that the stretched rectal walls notify the brain of its need to empty. Then the normal mechanism of defecation is activated; that is, the brain stimulates the anus to open and the rectum, sigmoid, and descending colon to squeeze down and empty. A prepackaged disposable enema containing four ounces of a special solution can also be used to give a cleansing enema. This enema stimulates the urge to defecate by exciting and stimulating the rectal walls so that the defecation mechanism is activated. The suppository to aid defecation acts in the same way.

The retention enema is given to treat some condition in or of the rectum. The oil retention enema is given to soften and lubricate the hard fecal mass (impaction) that cannot be expelled through the rectum. The starch retention enema is given to soothe the irritated rectal walls.

The medicated retention enema is a method of giving drugs by rectum. This watery solution containing the drug passes through the walls of the colon and goes into the bloodstream.

The retention enema must meet two criteria if it is to be retained:

1. It must contain an amount of solution that is too small to fill the rectum and stretch the rectal walls.
2. It must be nonirritating to the rectal walls.

Medicated suppositories are also given by rectum. However, the medicated suppository or the medication enema must come in direct contact with the rectal walls if it is to be absorbed. Therefore a cleansing enema should be given to clean out the rectum before medication can be given rectally.

DISCUSSION QUESTIONS

1 Find out when one of your patients is scheduled for a proctoscopic or sigmoidoscopic examination. Ask the nurse if you can prepare the patient for the examination and if you can accompany him to the examination. Ask the doctor how well the patient is prepared. Ask the

doctor to let you see the inside of the rectum or sigmoid colon.
2 How many of your patients failed to have a bowel movement in the last 3 days? Did you report this to the nurse? What action was taken?
3 How do you know if your unconscious or confused patients had a bowel movement in the past 24 hours?
4 Discuss the value of putting a bowel movement record on a clipboard at the bottom of the bed of the unconscious patient so that the nursing assistant taking the bedpan or cleaning the patient could chart it there.
5 How many of your patients have fecal incontinence? Discuss this at your team meeting or at your morning conference. Ask the nurse to help you develop a plan for bowel training these patients.
6 How many of your patients received a barium enema this week? Ask your nurse if you may accompany a patient to the x-ray department and observe a barium study.
7 Develop a plan for explaining a barium enema to the next patient who is scheduled for one.
8 Ask the nurse to assign you to give the next enema that the doctor orders for one of your patients. Ask the nurse to help you chart the results.
9 Why is a right side-lying position the best one for siphoning back an enema that the patient failed to expel?
10 Why is it impossible to give the patient an enema when he is sitting on the toilet?
11 Why should a cleansing enema be given after a barium enema?

VOCABULARY

catheter A soft rubber tube smaller in diameter than the rectal tube. It is frequently used for giving retention enemas.
colon Another name for the large bowel or the large intestine.
defecation Act of having a bowel movement.
enema Injection of fluid into the rectum.
Fleet enema A prepackaged disposable enema unit containing 4 ounces of medicated solution.
neostigmine A drug to stimulate peristalsis.
proctoscope An instrument inserted into the rectum to enable the physician to actually see and examine it.
rectal tube A large soft rubber or plastic tube used for giving enemas.
rectum That part of the large bowel in which feces are stored until the rectal wall is stretched and the mechanism of defecation is activated.
retention enema An injection of fluid retained in the rectum for 4 hours or until it is absorbed into the bloodstream.
sigmoidoscope An instrument much like the proctoscope but longer. It permits the doctor to examine the sigmoid colon.
suppository Medication dissolved in a base such as glycerin or cocoa butter. This suppository is a solid at room temperature but melts at body temperature, thus releasing the medication. Then the medication can be absorbed by the body.

SOURCE OF ADDITIONAL INFORMATION

1 Film: Basic care of patients; part VI: The enema; may be obtained from United States Army (direct request to Commanding General, Attention Surgeon of the Army area in which you reside).

28/Caring for the patient with a colostomy

STUDY QUESTIONS

1. What is a colostomy?
2. Why does a patient have a colostomy?
3. What effect does a colostomy have on
   a. the way the patient expels feces?
   b. the control the patient has over expelling feces?
4. What is a sigmoid colostomy?
5. What is a transverse colostomy?
6. How does a sigmoid colostomy differ from a transverse colostomy?
7. Why should you know whether the colostomy is a sigmoid or a transverse one?
8. What is a double-barreled colostomy?
9. In a double-barreled colostomy, which is the proximal loop and which is the distal loop? Why should you know the proximal from the distal loop?
10. What is a colostomy bag? Why is it used?
11. Why are colostomies irrigated?
12. How do you irrigate a colostomy?
13. Why should the patient help you irrigate his colostomy?
14. Why should dressings be avoided around the colostomy?
15. What is the desired temperature for the solution used in irrigating the colostomy?
16. Why does the head nurse refer the patient with a colostomy to the local visiting nurse association when he is discharged?

THE COLOSTOMY

The word colostomy comes from the word *colon*, meaning large bowel, and the ending *-ostomy*, meaning opening into for drainage. A colostomy then is an operation in which an opening is made into a large bowel to drain the fecal material from the body, and it is done in those patients who are unable to expel feces through the rectum. When the physician operates on the patient and makes a colostomy, he actually disconnects the large bowel from the rectum and brings it to the outside of the patient's body through an opening in the abdomen. Therefore a colostomy is a surgically made anus.

Because the colon is disconnected from the rectum, the colostomy creates some problems for the patient. These problems are due to the following:

1. The patient no longer has a storage place for feces. Before the colostomy was performed, feces moved along the large bowel (colon) and were stored in the rectum. When enough feces collected there (once or twice a day), the rectal wall stretched, the nerves from the rectum informed the brain of the need to defecate, the patient sought the necessary facilities, and the brain sent down messages that activated the bowel muscles and relaxed the anus so that the patient defecated. After a colostomy the storage place (the

rectum) is no longer used. Fecal material moves along the large bowel and drains out of the colostomy opening constantly.

2. The patient no longer has a muscle around the end of that part of the bowel that expels the feces. Before the colostomy, the anal muscle at the end of the rectum remained tightly closed and held the feces in the rectum until the patient decided to defecate. The colostomy opening contains no such muscle and is open constantly.

3. The patient no longer gets the message that he needs to defecate. Before the colostomy, the patient had nerve connections between the rectum and the brain. When the rectum was so filled that the rectal walls were stretched, a nerve took this message to the brain and the patient knew that he needed to defecate. Now there is no such nerve connection between the colostomy opening and the brain to tell the patient that fecal material is coming along the bowel and needs to be expelled. The patient knows that fecal material is expelled only after it is expelled and he feels it on his skin.

WHY THE PATIENT HAS A COLOSTOMY

The surgeon performs a colostomy on the patient who is unable to expel fecal material through the rectum. The colostomy may be a temporary one in which the colon will later be reconnected, or it may be a permanent one that the patient will have the rest of his life.

A temporary colostomy may be performed on a patient who has a tumor or an injury such as a perforation (hole) in the rectum or large bowel. The surgeon operates and removes the tumor or sews up the hole. Then he makes an opening (colostomy) above the operative area so that the feces will leave the body through this opening and will not drain down over the operation. In this way the bowel that has recently been operated upon gets a rest and a chance to heal. Infection of the operative area is also avoided. Just as a cut on the finger fails to heal if it is constantly being moved and placed in water, so too will the bowel fail to heal if it has to keep working and if feces are constantly moving over the injured or operated upon area.

A permanent colostomy may be performed in a patient who has cancer of the rectum or an inflammatory process such as diverticulitis. In this operation the surgeon removes the entire diseased rectum to prevent spread of the disease and to save the patient's life. This patient will undergo two operations while he is in the operating room.

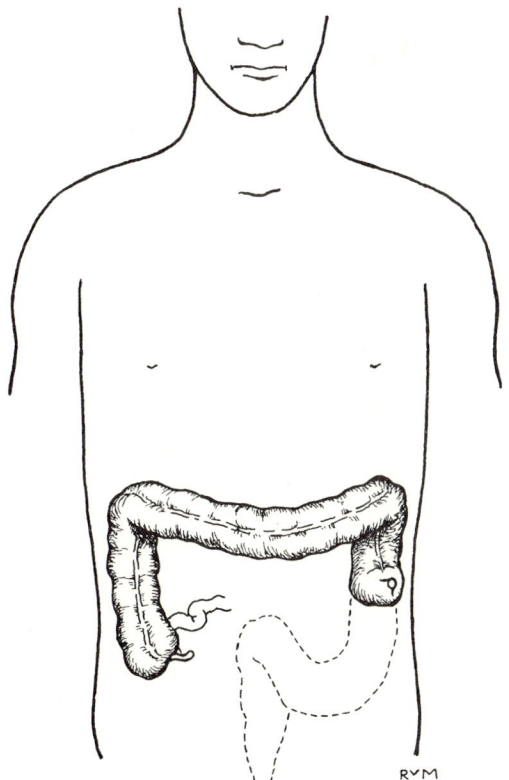

Fig. 28-1. An abdominoperineal resection. The entire rectum has been removed, and the descending colon has been opened out onto the abdomen to form a single-barreled or one-loop colostomy.

One incision will be made around the rectum (in the perineum) and the rectum will be removed. The other incision will be made in the abdomen to make the colostomy by bringing the disconnected loop of colon out here. This operation is called an abdominoperineal (*abdomino-*, pertaining to the abdomen; *perineal*, pertaining to the body area between the rectum and the genitals) resection (cutting out). Therefore an abdominoperineal resection is an extensive operation in which the rectal structures are removed through an operation in this area and in which a colostomy is made through an abdominal incision. This colostomy is always a single-barreled or one-loop colostomy (Fig. 28-1).

DOUBLE-BARRELED TEMPORARY COLOSTOMY

The temporary colostomy is always a double-barreled colostomy, which means that two loops of the colon are brought out onto the abdomen (Fig. 28-2).

The temporary colostomy may be reconnected after the operated upon colon or rectum below it has thoroughly healed. This may be done at any time from 4 weeks to 4 months after the original operation. The colostomy is reconnected in the operating room simply by sewing the two ends of the colon together again.

PERMANENT COLOSTOMY

A permanent colostomy may be performed on a patient for the following reasons:

1. A cancer or an inflammatory process in the descending colon, sigmoid, or rectum. The surgeon operates on the patient and removes some or all of these structures in order to get rid of all of the cancer or disease. Since the rectum is removed, the colon can never be reconnected to it. The colostomy is therefore permanent.

2. Cancer of the colon or rectum that

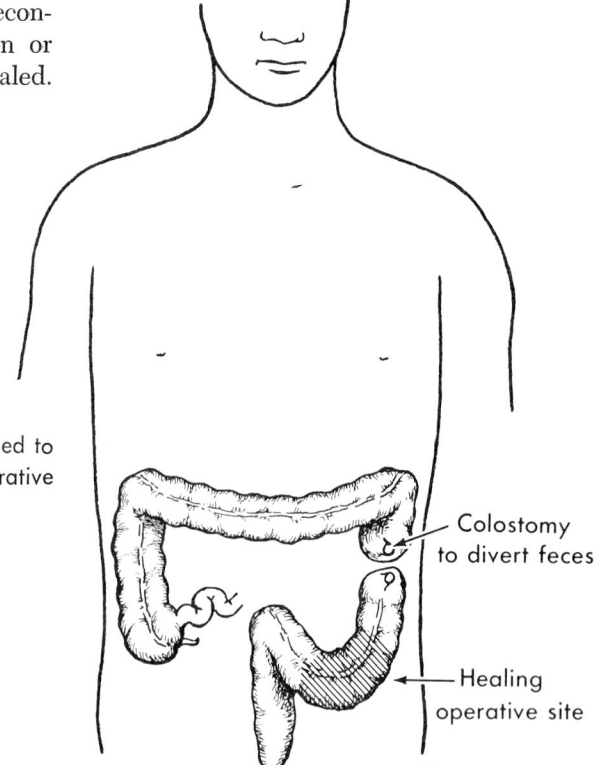

Fig. 28-2. A temporary colostomy performed to divert the feces away from a healing operative site.

has spread so much that the surgeon cannot remove it. However, he can and does make a colostomy above the cancer so that the patient can expel fecal waste from the body. Although the surgeon is unable, in such a case, to remove the cancer and cure the patient, symptoms caused by the blocked (obstructed) colon are relieved and the patient is made more comfortable. In this way the surgeon enables the patient to live for a longer time. This palliative colostomy (one that relieves the symptoms but does not cure the disease) is always a double-barreled one.

TYPES OF COLOSTOMIES

Colostomies are named in such a way as to describe them. Therefore they may be named as follows:

1. By the section of the colon in which the colostomy is made (Fig. 28-3)
   a. Ascending colostomy
   b. Transverse colostomy
   c. Descending colostomy
   d. Sigmoid colostomy
2. By the number of loops the colostomy has
   a. Double-barreled or two-loop colostomy
   b. Single-barreled or one-loop colostomy
3. By the effect the colostomy has on the patient
   a. Curative colostomy (disease removed)
   b. Palliative colostomy (disease remains but patient's symptoms are relieved)
4. By the future plan for the colostomy
   a. Temporary colostomy (one that is to be reconnected in the future)
   b. Permanent colostomy (one that is to remain throughout the patient's life)

SIGNIFICANCE OF THE TYPE OF COLOSTOMY IN PATIENT CARE

You must know what type of colostomy a patient has in order to care for him effectively. The name describing the location of the colostomy will give you many clues about the patient's care. In Chapter 8 the functions of the large bowel or colon were described as the absorption of water into the bloodstream as well as the carrying of fecal material to the rectum. This information tells you that the closer the colostomy is to the small intestine, the more liquid will be the feces and the more frequent the expulsion of feces. Therefore liquid feces will be expelled frequently from a colostomy in the ascending colon. In a transverse colostomy, feces the consistency of toothpaste will be expelled quite frequently, whereas in the sigmoid colostomy, formed feces (similar to that from the rectum) will be expelled much less often.

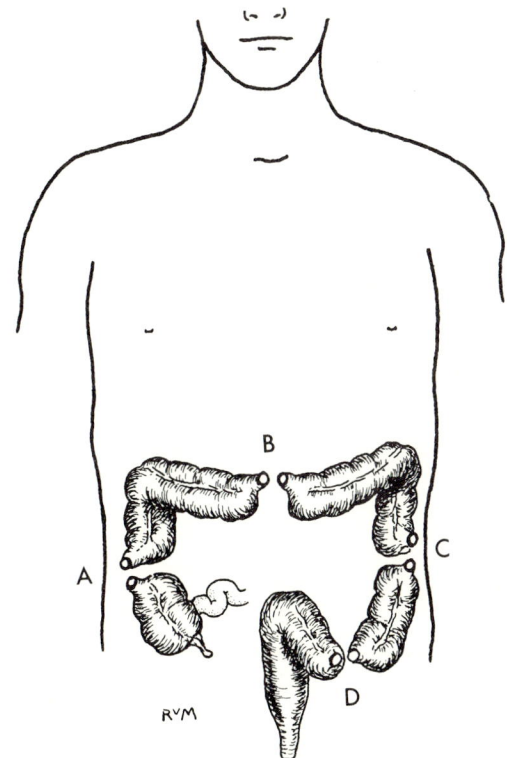

Fig. 28-3. Types of colostomy. **A,** Ascending colostomy. **B,** Transverse colostomy. **C,** Descending colostomy. **D,** Sigmoid colostomy.

This knowledge also gives you clues for patient care because the patient with an ascending colostomy will need more fluid to drink and he will need more frequent emptying of his colostomy bag than will the patient with a sigmoid colostomy.

The name describing the location of the colostomy will also tell you how the tube is to be inserted when it is irrigated.

The name of the colostomy describing the number of loops it has gives you the clue that you will need to know which loop is still connected to the intestinal tract and which loop is the disconnected one that goes to the rectum before you can irrigate the double-barreled colostomy correctly. The loop connected to the intestinal tract is called the proximal loop, whereas the one that is disconnected from the intestinal tract and goes from the abdomen to the rectum is called the distal loop. The proximal loop (the one connected to the intestinal tract) is usually the one placed closest to the midline of the body when both loops are located side by side on the patient's body or the one that is closest to the mouth when one loop is located under the other on the patient's body.

However, it is not always possible to identify the proximal and distal loops by their position. Therefore it is important for you to find out from the nurse which is the proximal loop (the one to be irrigated) and which is the disconnected distal loop. Jot this information down on the Kardex so that the entire ward staff will know it.

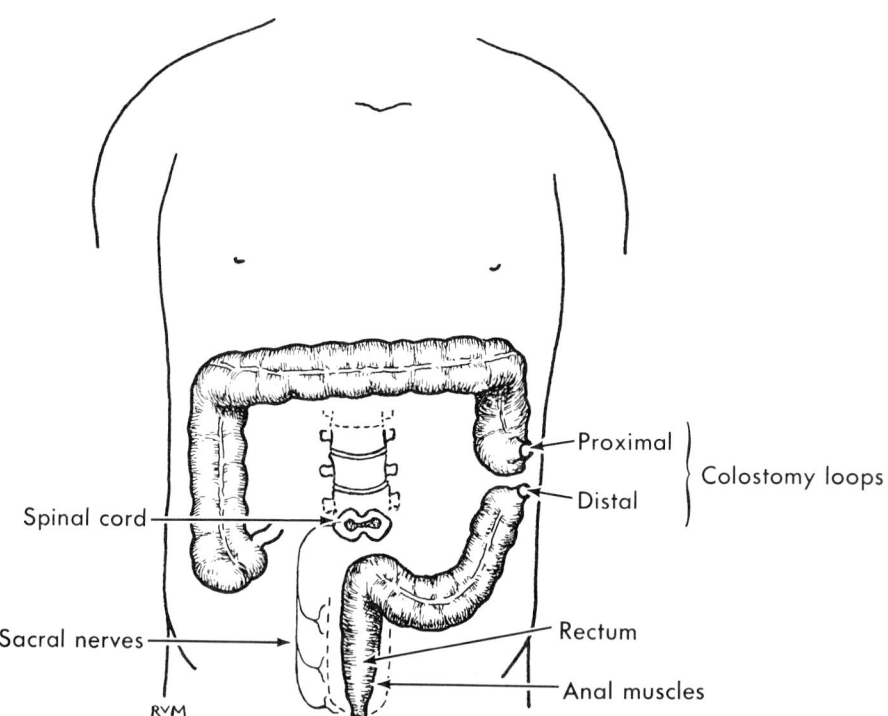

Fig. 28-4. The colostomy opening (surgically made anus) is disconnected from the controlling nerve supply to the rectum. Therefore the patient gets no message of the need to expel feces through the colostomy opening. (*Note:* The sacral nerves are actually embedded in the rectal wall. However, the illustration shows these nerves as they would appear when stimulated by the distended rectal walls.)

The name referring to the effect of the colostomy on the patient will help you to understand why the patient with a palliative colostomy continues to have pain, whereas the patient with a curative colostomy has none after the operative wound has healed.

The name temporary or permanent will help you to understand the patient's depression and fear of living with this body over which he has lost control. Usually the patient with a temporary colostomy is well able to tolerate the changes because he knows that they will last only for a short time, but the patient with a permanent colostomy believes that his life is ruined, that he is a messy, smelly person, and that no one will want him around (Fig. 28-4).

CARING FOR THE PATIENT WITH A COLOSTOMY

After the patient is operated on, he will go from the operating room to the recovery room, where he will be cared for until his vital signs indicate that his body is sufficiently recovered from the effects of the surgery to carry on the essential activities of living effectively (pumping the blood, breathing, etc.). Then he will be returned to his unit. The patient who has had an abdominoperineal resection may be so acutely ill and may require so many blood transfusions that he will be sent from the recovery room to the intensive care unit for specialized medical and nursing care. However, after he has recovered sufficiently from the effects of the operation, he will be returned to his unit.

When you check the patient carefully on his return to his unit, you will probably find that his abdomen is covered with many dressings. These dressings will not need to be changed because the colostomy will not yet be opened. The surgeon will "keep" the colostomy closed for about 3 days to permit the operative incision to heal sufficiently so that it will not be contaminated by feces. He does this in one of two ways:

1. He pulls a loop of the colon through an incision (surgical cut) in the abdomen, but he does not open this loop of colon (Fig. 28-5). This loop of colon remains on the abdomen. The surgeon usually places a glass rod under this loop to keep it from slipping back inside the abdomen. After 3 days the colon is usually cut in half, thereby opening it and making two loops with an electric cautery (cutting instrument) (Fig. 28-6).
2. He makes the colostomy but places a clamp on the proximal loop (the one connected to the intestinal tract) to prevent the drainage of feces. After 3 days when the incision has healed sufficiently, he will remove this clamp (Fig. 28-7).

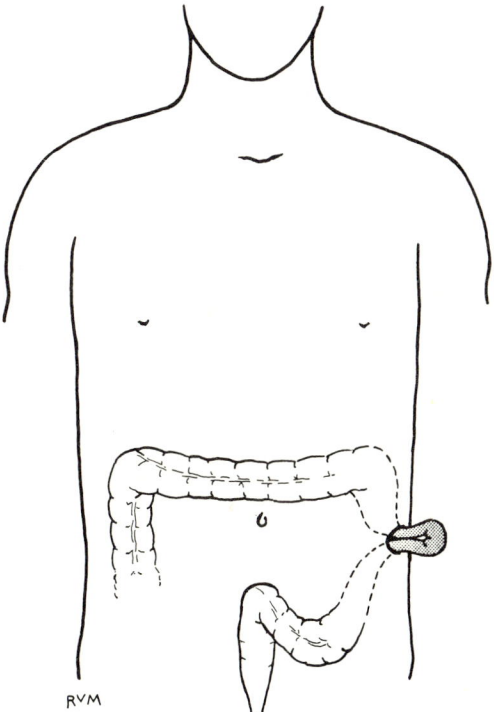

Fig. 28-5. An unopened colostomy.

Sometimes the patient's colon is so filled with feces because it has been blocked for such a long time that the doctor has to drain the feces out before the incision is sufficiently healed. He usually does this in the first 3 days after the operation while the incision is healing by placing a drainage tube in the colon, which is then connected by long rubber tubing to a bottle on the floor. This technique permits feces to drain out of the colon through the tube by gravity and at the same time keeps the operative site clean and free of fecal drainage.

However, when the colostomy is opened after 3 days, the patient will have constant fecal drainage from the colostomy. If dressings such as 4-inch-square compresses and abdominal pads are used to collect this drainage, they will be filled with feces every 2 hours and will require changes every 2 hours. Soon too, the skin around

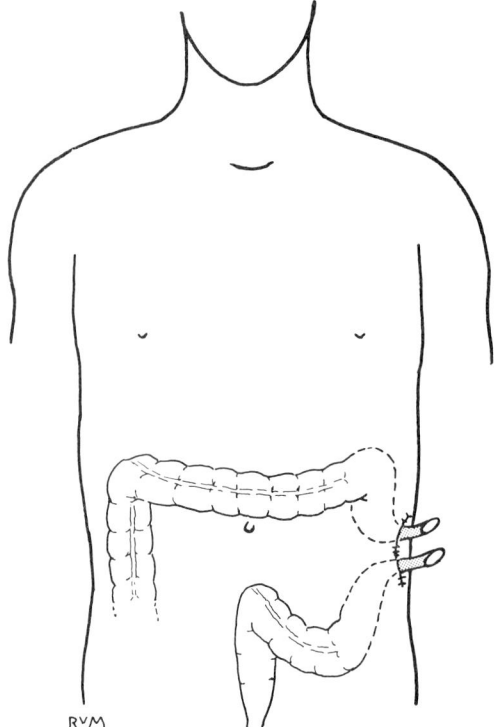

Fig. 28-6. Colostomy that has been opened with an electric cautery.

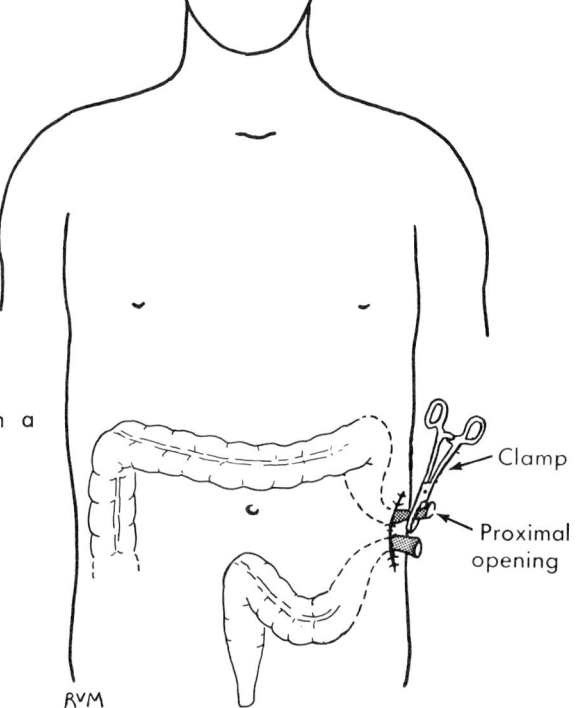

Fig. 28-7. Recently made colostomy with a clamp on the proximal colostomy loop.

the colostomy will become red, raw, and excoriated from the constant fecal drainage that the dressings keep plastered against the skin. In a few days the skin will look as sore as the skin on a baby's buttocks does when his mother keeps him in soiled diapers. The patient will become frightened and disgusted with the constant fecal drainage and the dressing changes every 2 hours. He will be certain that he is condemned to a hospital bed and the constant care of the medical staff because of this messy, smelly colostomy. A feeling that life is not worth living will overtake him.

Most of these problems can be avoided by replacing the dressings with a colostomy bag as soon as the colostomy is opened (Fig. 28-8). This bag has an adhesive surface that is applied to the skin around the colostomy, and the fecal material then drains away from the skin and into the bag. The 2-hour dressing changes are replaced with the simple task of emptying the colostomy bag. The patient then sees how simple it is to empty the bag. His skin is kept free of irritation, and mental depression usually disappears.

Applying the disposable colostomy bag

Demonstrate and discuss every step of applying the colostomy bag with the patient as you do it. Prepare the skin around the colostomy by washing it well with soap and water and then rinsing it thoroughly and patting it dry. Avoid wetting any of the dressings on the patient's abdomen.

Paint an area about 2 inches in diameter around the colostomy opening (stoma) with tincture of benzoin. This will help the bag adhere (stick) to the skin. Check to see that the bag opening is large enough to fit over the stoma (that part of the large bowel brought out onto the abdomen by the colostomy). Enlarge the opening in the

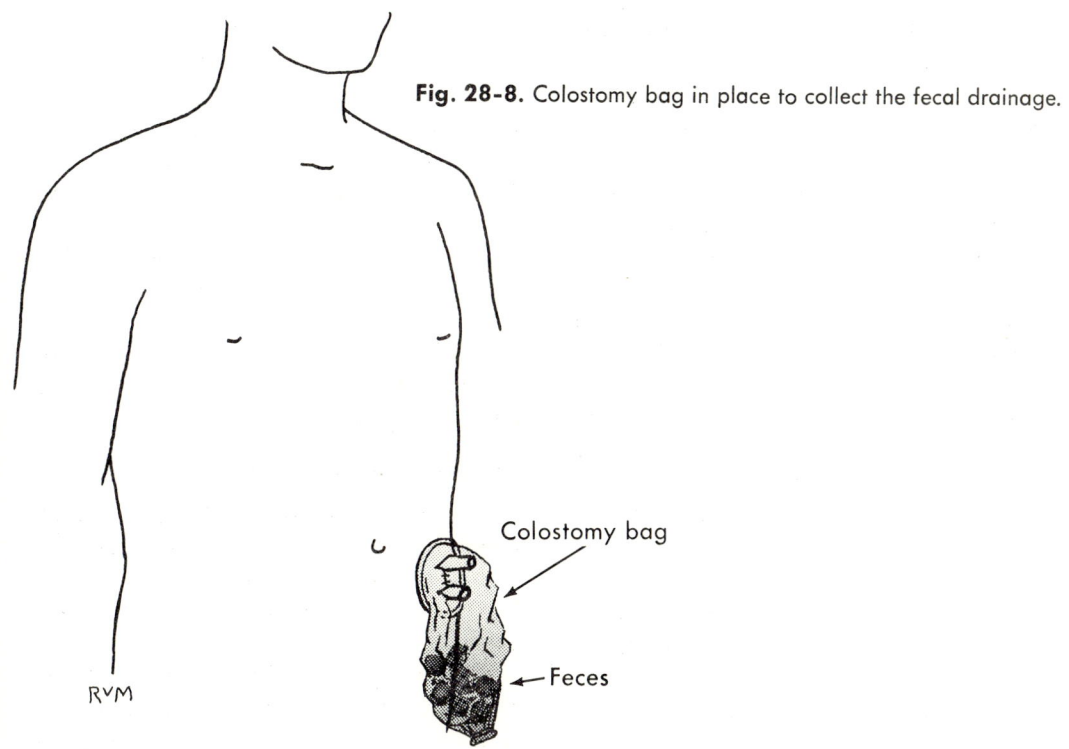

Fig. 28-8. Colostomy bag in place to collect the fecal drainage.

bag with your scissors as necessary. When the benzoin is thoroughly dried, remove the covering over the adhesive portion on the bag. Place your hand through the opening in the bottom of the bag and up inside the bag. Grasp the inside of the top of the bag firmly and guide it into place over the stoma. Now press the adhesive surface of the bag firmly against the skin around the stoma that has been painted with tincture of benzoin. Be sure that the entire surface of the bag is stuck to the skin. Remove your hand from the inside of the bag.

Close the bottom of the bag by rolling it on itself a few times and then folding it in from the sides. Place a rubber band around the bottom of the bag to keep it closed. Remember to put the bag on the patient so that the bottom of the bag is pointing downhill. This will permit gravity to help the feces run into it.

Emptying of the disposable colostomy bag

The colostomy bag will usually function adequately on the colostomy for 24 hours if you have it firmly adhered to the skin. However, the newly opened colostomy will drain such large amounts of fecal material that the bag will need to be emptied every 2 hours. The bag is emptied by removing the rubber band from the bottom and by unrolling the bag. Then the opened ends are placed in an emesis basin. An Asepto syringe (rubber-bulbed syringe) full of tepid tap water can be squirted into the bottom of the bag to rinse out the feces and to keep the patient free of odor.* Then the bag is closed again by the previously described method of rolling up the bottom and putting a rubber band around the folds. Demonstrate and discuss every step of the procedure with the patient as you do it.

There are two sizes of colostomy bags: one with an average-sized opening for single-barreled colostomies and one with a large opening for double-barreled colostomies. Ask the nurse to obtain a supply of the right bags for your patient.

Colostomy control

Any time after the fifth postoperative day, the doctor may order colostomy irrigations for the patient with a colostomy. The purposes of these irrigations are as follows:
1. To empty the colon at the time of irrigation
2. To train the bowel to empty only at the time of irrigations, which are given at regular intervals, or to empty only when the patient irrigates the colostomy (wants the colon to empty), thus reestablishing fecal control
3. To keep the patient clean (free of fecal drainage from the colostomy) between irrigations

Fecal control through irrigations is easily attained in the patient with a descending or sigmoid colon colostomy; it is a little more difficult to attain in the patient with a transverse colostomy and impossible in the patient with an ascending type of colostomy. Therefore the patient with an ascending or transverse colostomy is usually fitted with a permanent type of bag. The patient with a descending or sigmoid colostomy usually wears a temporary type of bag until control is established (2 to 6 weeks after irrigations start), and then he wears nothing but a 4-inch-square compress, lubricated with some water-soluble lubricant over the stoma to protect it from irritation by his clothing.

The colostomy irrigation

The doctor orders colostomy irrigations when he feels that the bowel has sufficiently healed after the operation. He specifies the amount and kind of solution to be used.

Since the patient will continue to irrigate the colostomy in order to attain fecal continence all the rest of his life, a colostomy

---

*Placing an aspirin tablet in the bag also helps to control odor.

irrigator is ordered and delivered to him while he is still in the hospital. The patient's own irrigator should then be used for the irrigation.

The doctor usually irrigates the colostomy the first time to be sure that it is well made and that it functions correctly. Then he will give you (in his medical orders) the following information:

1. Which loop is the proximal one (the one that is hooked up to the intestinal tract and the one that you are to irrigate)
2. The amount of solution to be used in the irrigation (usually 1,000 to 2,000 ml.)
3. The type of solution to be used (usually tap water or normal saline, which is prepared by adding 2 teaspoonfuls of salt to every quart of water used)

The head nurse or team leader will then study the patient's normal pattern of living in order to determine the best time for this irrigation. The irrigation usually takes about 1 hour. Therefore the nurse will try to find the hour that is free to use for irrigating in the patient's normal living pattern and the hour that permits him to use the family bathroom in privacy for that long a period. Then she will tell you what time the irrigations are to be given.

The colostomy irrigations that are given to train the bowel must be done in the hospital at the same hour that the patient is going to continue to do them at home. If you help the patient to train his colostomy to empty at 10 A.M. because that is a convenient time for you to help to irrigate, the colostomy will empty at 10 A.M. However, when the patient goes home and has to change the time of irrigations to the early morning or late evening because he works from 7 A.M. to 4 P.M., the colostomy will lose control and drain feces frequently throughout the 24-hour period. The entire procedure of training the colostomy will then have to be started all over again. The patient will have to remain away from his job during this retraining period because of the unpredictable eruptions of feces from the colostomy. Therefore it is important for you to irrigate the patient's colostomy at the time that the head nurse instructs you to do it. She will also tell you the location of the colostomy in the colon and give you instructions on how to insert the catheter. The colostomy can be irrigated in the following way:

1. Explain the procedure to the patient. Have him watch as you do each step. Have him assist as much as possible. Remember that he must learn how to do this irrigation by himself before he can go home. Do the irrigation just as the patient will do it at home.
2. Prepare the environment:
   a. Bedpatient. Protect the bed in the same way as you do when you give an enema.
   b. Bathroom. Select private bathroom facilities. Hang an "in use" sign on the door.
3. Position the patient:
   a. Bedpatient. Place him in one of the following positions that his physical condition permits:
      (1) Side-lying position. (If the patient has a right-sided colostomy, he lies on his right side. If he has a left-sided colostomy, he lies on his left side.)
      (2) Sitting position in the bed or on the side of the bed.
   b. Out-of-bed patient. Assist patient out of bed, dress him, and take him to private bathroom facilities (Fig. 28-9).
4. Collect the equipment you will need:
   a. When the hospital equipment is used:
      (1) Disposable enema setup
      (2) Intravenous pole or treatment standard
      (3) Robinson rubber catheter

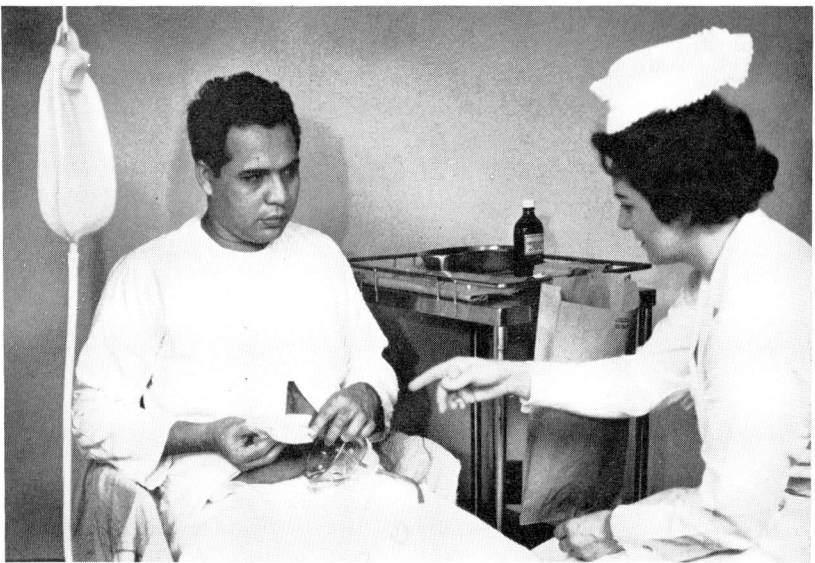

Fig. 28-9. The patient is positioned on the bedside commode and is preparing to do his own colostomy irrigation with the assistance of the nurse. The patient's own equipment is being used for this irrigation.

(usually no. 22) attached to enema tubing
(4) Water-soluble lubricant such as Lubrifax
(5) Solution thermometer
(6) Solution ordered by the doctor warmed to a temperature of 105° F., or a pitcher in which to prepare the solution
(7) A bedpan (if the patient is in bed) and toilet tissue
(8) Temporary ostomy bag, bottle of tincture of benzoin, and a few applicators
b. When the patient's own personal equipment is used:
(1) Intravenous pole or treatment standard
(2) Solution thermometer
(3) Solution ordered by the doctor warmed to a temperature of 105° F., or a pitcher in which to prepare the solution
(4) A bedpan (if the patient is in bed) and toilet tissues
(5) Temporary ostomy bag, bottle of tincture of benzoin, and a few applicators
5. Place the equipment on the top of the movable table. Place the bedpan on the bottom. Push the table and pull the standard with you to the patient's treatment area. (Patient's bedside for bed patients or bathroom for out-of-bed patients.)
6. Prepare the solution in the pitcher at 105° F. Prepare it in the patient's room. (Tap water or normal saline—add 2 teaspoons of salt to a quart of tap water.) The doctor usually directs the patient to irrigate with one of these solutions after discharge so he should know how to prepare it. Let the patient immerse his whole hand in the prepared solution so that he will begin to be aware of the desired temperature for the solution. Work slowly and quietly but efficiently so that you will dispel any fear or worry the patient has about

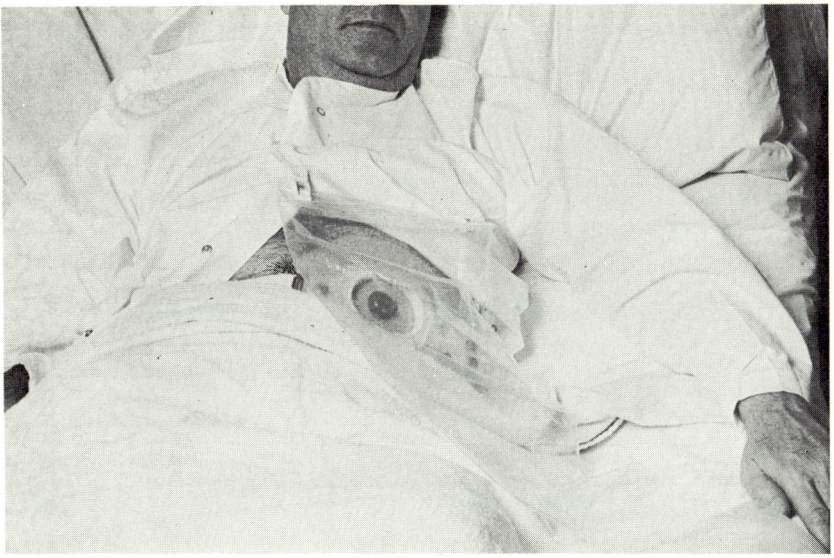

Fig. 28-10. The irrigating shield is positioned over the colostomy of the bed patient.

the procedure. (If the patient becomes upset, frightened, or worried, the colon and the stoma, which is part of the colon, will squeeze down tightly, and you will be unable to get the catheter in and/or the irrigation fluid out.)
7. Assemble the equipment:
   a. Pour the solution into the irrigating bag.
      (1) Be sure the clamp on the tubing is closed.
   b. Hang bag (the patient's irrigator or enema bag) on the standard.
      (1) The bottom of the irrigator can be no higher than 18 inches above the stoma.
      (2) Use a length of bandage to lower the irrigator, if necessary.
   c. Expel the air in the tubing.
      (1) Open the clamp on the tubing and permit about 1 ounce of water to flow through. Close the clamp.
   d. Get the irrigating shield ready.
      (1) Connect an irrigating sheath to the cup, if one is used, and fix it in place with a rubber band.
      (2) Place the belt around the patient and get the irrigating sheath in readiness to attach as soon as you remove the temporary bag (Figs. 28-10 to 28-12) or
      (3) Prepare to irrigate through the temporary ostomy bag if the patient's set does not contain an irrigating shield.
         (a) Empty the temporary ostomy bag.
         (b) Rinse it out thoroughly. (Squirt water into the bottom of the bag. Use an Asepto syringe.)
         (c) Make a small slitlike opening in the top of the colostomy bag with your

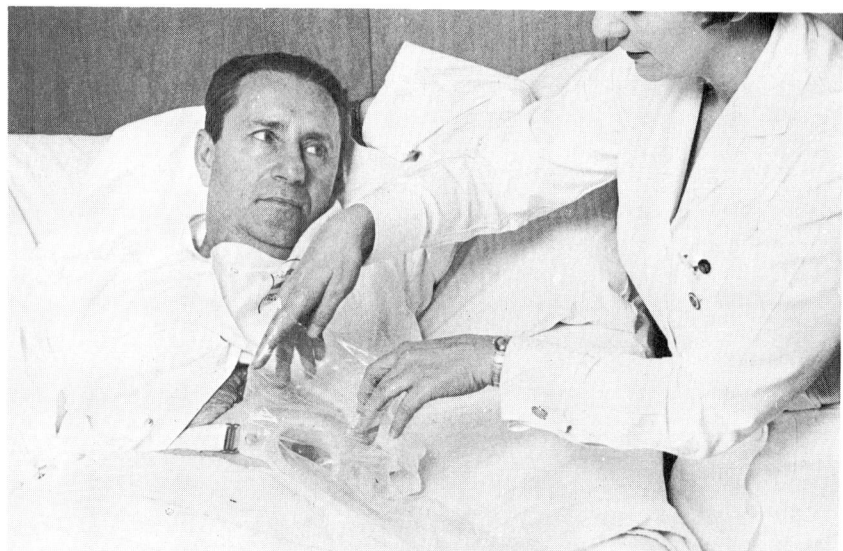

Fig. 28-11. The nurse is folding down the irrigating shield to expose the stoma. Note how she demonstrates and teaches the patient as she does the procedure.

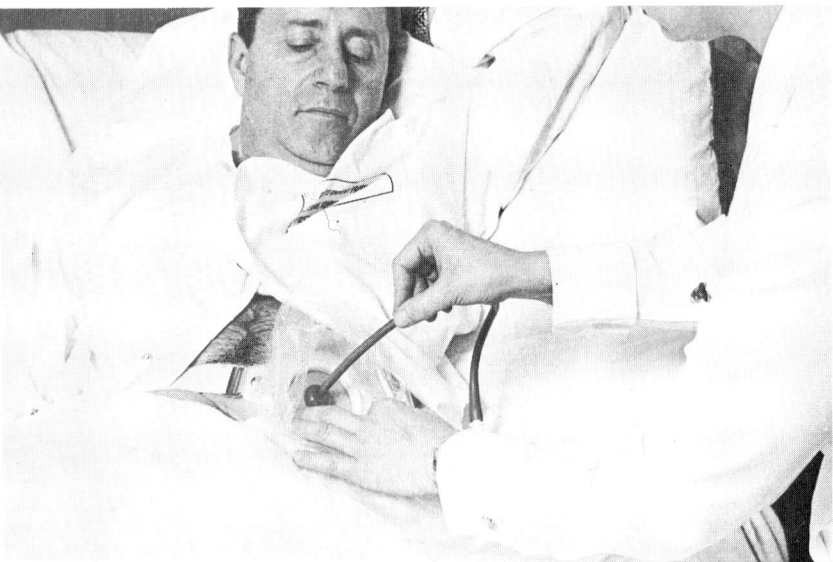

Fig. 28-12. The nurse is inserting the catheter into the stoma through the top of the irrigating shield. Note how the patient watches and learns.

Caring for the patient with a colostomy 239

scissors (the bag that the patient is wearing).
8. Prepare to irrigate the patient:
   a. Through the bag if he has no irrigating shield:
      (1) Lubricate the catheter well with a water-soluble lubricant.
      (2) Insert the Robinson catheter through the slitlike opening you made in the bag and 3 or 4 inches into the colostomy opening (proximal loop) with a gentle rotary motion (Figs. 28-13 to 28-15).
   b. Through the irrigating shield:
      (1) Remove the colostomy bag and clean the area around the stoma with moistened toilet paper or cleansing tissue.
      (2) When the cup type is used (Deddish):
         (a) Insert the catheter through the window of the cup.
         (b) Lubricate the catheter well (Fig. 28-16).
         (c) Insert the catheter (which is through the window of the cup) from 3 to 4 inches into the colostomy opening by using a gentle rotary motion (Figs. 28-13 to 28-15).
         (d) Attach the shield to the

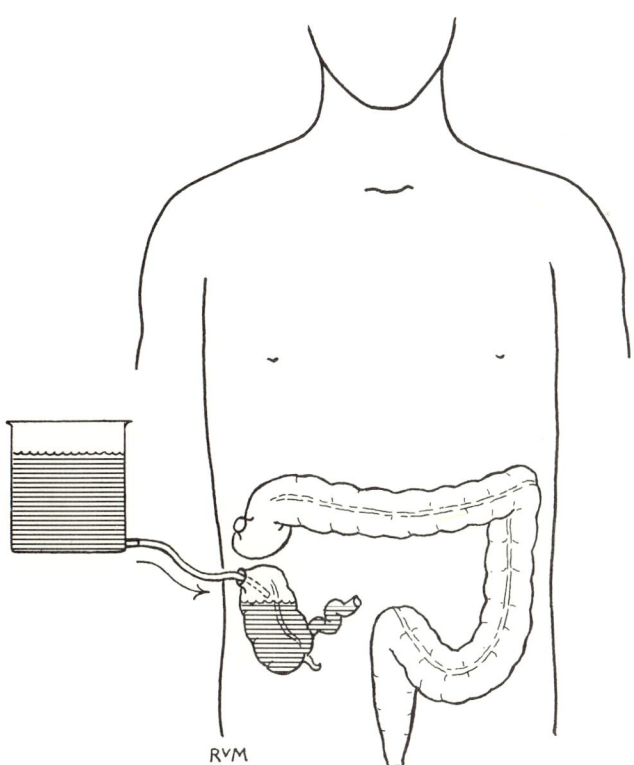

Fig. 28-13. In an ascending colostomy, the catheter is directed down toward the patient's feet.

240 Nursing assistant meets patient's particular needs

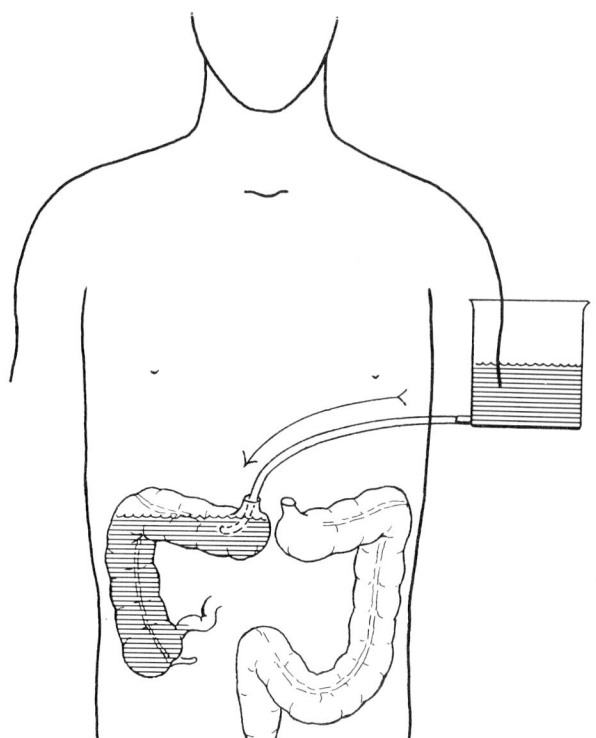

Fig. 28-14. In a transverse colostomy, the catheter is directed toward the right side of the patient.

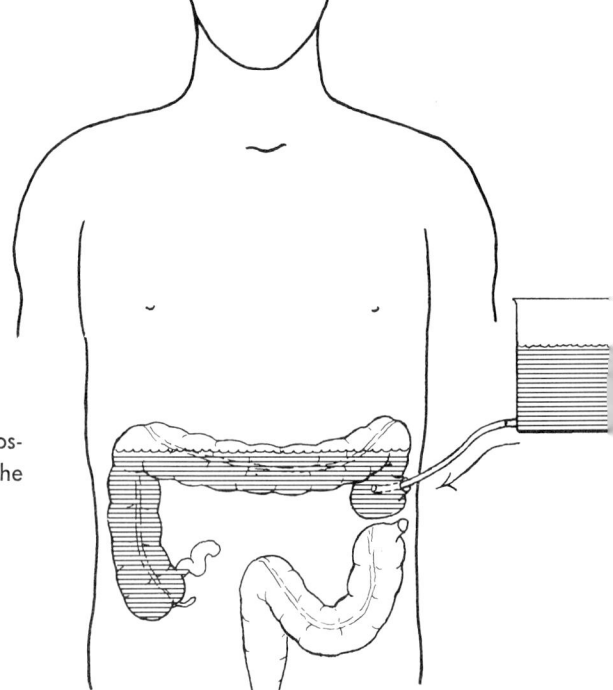

Fig. 28-15. In a descending or sigmoid colostomy, the catheter is directed up toward the patient's head.

Caring for the patient with a colostomy 241

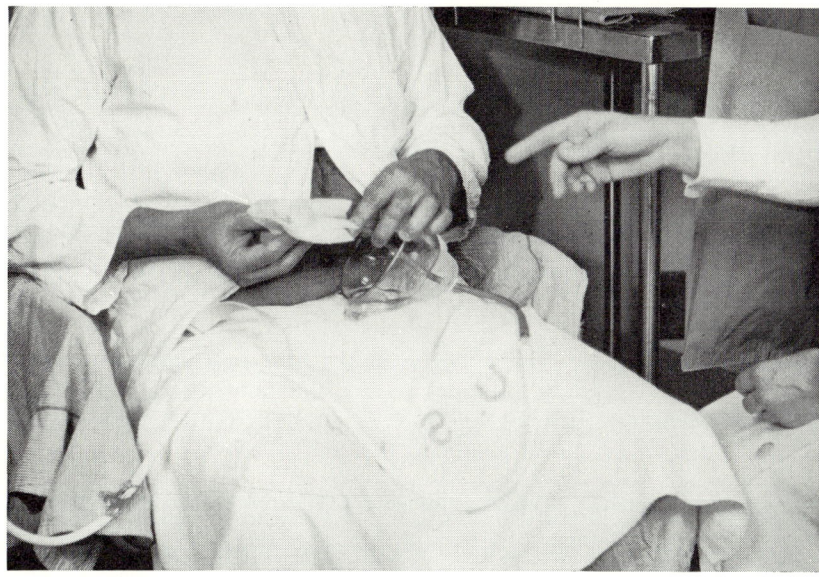

Fig. 28-16. The catheter has been inserted through the window of the irrigator and is now being lubricated well. After this step, the irrigator will be attached to the patient's belt and the catheter will be inserted into the colostomy.

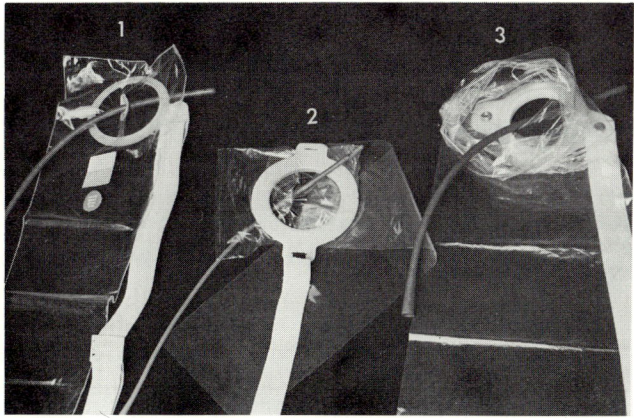

Fig. 28-17. Catheter insertions with various irrigating sheaths: **1,** insertion of catheter through sponge-encircled opening in the Hollister sheath; **2,** insertion of catheter through opening in Marsan's irrigating sheath—note that a plastic tab closes off the opening during the fecal return; **3,** insertion of catheter through the folded-down top of the Greer irrigating sheath.

patient's body by hooking it to the belt, around the patient's waist.
        (3) When a baglike shield is used (Davol, Greer):
            (a) Attach the shield to the patient's body by hooking it to the belt around the patient's waist.
            (b) Lubricate the catheter.
            (c) Insert the catheter through the opened top of the shield and into the stoma (Fig. 28-17).
 9. Direct the opened end of the ostomy bag or irrigating shield into the toilet bowl (between the patient's legs) or into a bedpan (if a bed patient).
10. Irrigate the colostomy by opening the clamp on the tubing and by permitting the solution to flow into the proximal loop of the stoma.
11. Insert the catheter, using the same gentle rotary motion, 3 to 4 inches farther into the colostomy. The flowing solution will relax the colon muscles and permit the catheter to go in easily.
12. Continue the irrigation in the following manner:
    a. Permit the solution to flow into the colostomy. However, if fluid begins to return, clamp off the tubing to shut off the solution in flow. Do not remove the catheter from the colostomy when the solution is returning, but hold it firmly or it will slip out.
    b. Open the clamp and again permit solution to flow into the colostomy when the return flow ceases.
    c. Continue the irrigation (as described) until the prescribed amount of solution is given or until the return flow is clear.
13. Terminate the irrigation:
    a. Clamp off the tubing.
    b. Remove the catheter from the stoma and place it in the emesis basin on the tray or in the bag.
    c. Close the irrigating sheath or patch the slit in the colostomy bag with a piece of adhesive.
14. Permit the patient to evacuate his bowel:
    a. Encourage the patient to move from right to left, to stretch or to bend backward and forward. This stimulates peristalsis and encourages defecation.
    b. Close off the bottom of the irrigation bag and permit the patient to ambulate, if desired.
    c. Permit the patient to have at least an hour of privacy for his bowel evacuation.
15. Clean up the equipment:
    a. Clean the equipment in the patient's room after the entire procedure is finished. (Have patient observe.)
    b. Wash bag, cup, and sheath as well as all tubing in warm soapy water, rinse well, and dry.
    c. Replace in patient's bedside stand.
    d. Keep the disposable enema equipment for reuse. Place it in patient's bedside stand.

Applying the temporary ostomy bag

After the patient has evacuated his bowel, which usually takes about an hour, return to his room and apply the temporary ostomy bag over his stoma. This is usually done in the following way:
1. Remove the irrigating shield or colostomy bag (if one was used). Discard the bag or the disposable part of the irrigating shield into a paper bag or newspaper.
2. Wash the skin around the stoma with soap and water, rinse it well, and pat it dry. Do not rub, since rubbing will irritate the skin.

3. Apply one coat of tincture of benzoin to the skin around the stoma (Fig. 28-18). Fan it dry. Apply a second coat. Fan it dry. Be sure that the benzoin-painted skin is dry before you apply the colostomy bag. Cut an opening in the bag large enough to fit over the stoma. Place the bag over the stoma and press it firmly to the benzoin-painted skin so that it will adhere well (Fig. 28-19). Fold the bag closed. Keep it closed by placing a rubber band around the folds in the bottom.
4. Make the patient comfortable. If he is in bed, remove the linen-covered drawsheet, replace the bath or treatment blanket with the top covers, and assist the patient into a comfortable position. If he is out of bed, assist him back into bed, or help him bathe and dress.
5. Clean the rest of the equipment. Discard the temporary colostomy bag filled with feces in a covered can for disposal of body wastes or flush it down the toilet. Empty the bedpan. Wash the patient's irrigating bag and shield and replace them in the bedside stand.
6. Chart the colostomy irrigation and the results you obtained on the patient's chart in the nurse's record.

The patient assists with the colostomy irrigation

The next time you irrigate the colostomy (which will probably be the next day), encourage the patient to do more of the irrigation for himself. If he is acutely ill, he may be able to do only a very little, but do have him help (Fig. 28-20). As his condition improves, let him do more and more of the irrigation until he is doing it all and you are just standing by giving advice.

Patient teaching material

Good patient teaching material will be included in the container with the pa-

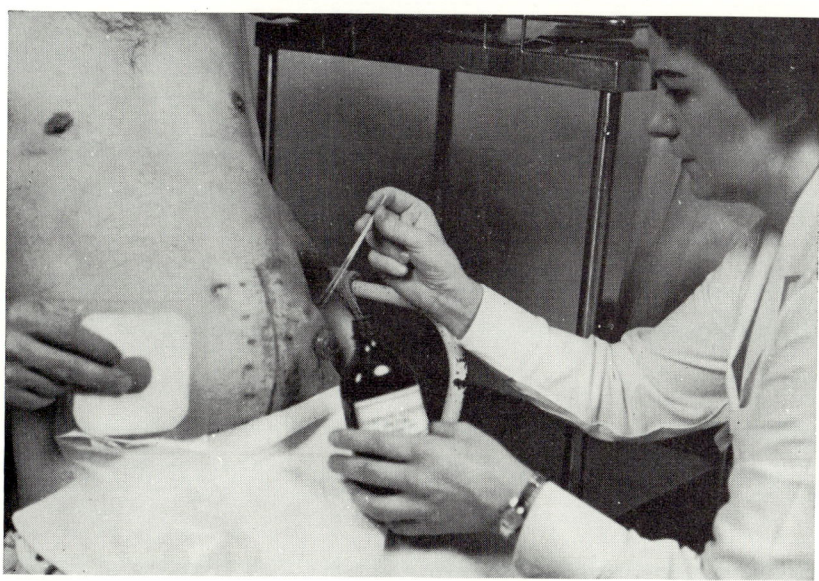

Fig. 28-18. The nurse applying a coat of tincture of benzoin to the area around the stoma. When this is dry, a second coat is applied.

244 Nursing assistant meets patient's particular needs

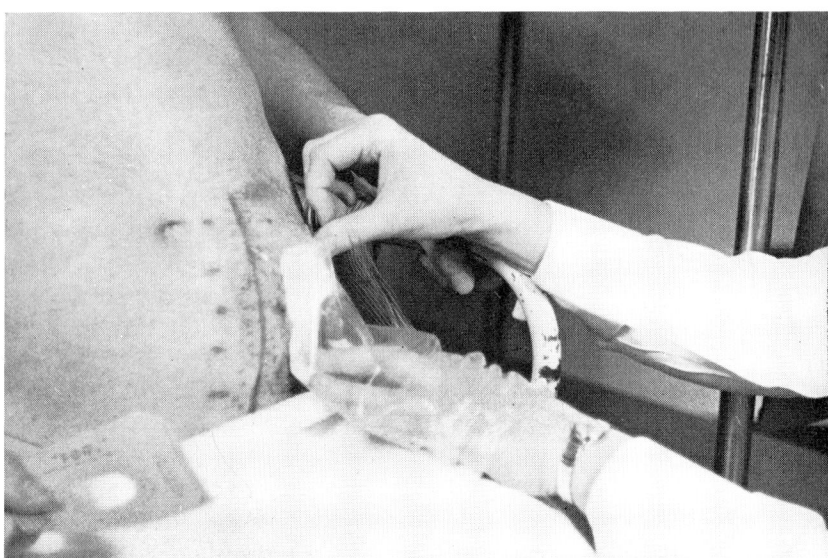

Fig. 28-19. The opening in the colostomy bag has been enlarged. The nurse has placed her hand up through the bottom of the bag and is guiding it into place over the stoma and onto the skin prepared with tincture of benzoin. Note how the nurse is pressing the adhesive surface of the bag firmly against the skin so that it will adhere well.

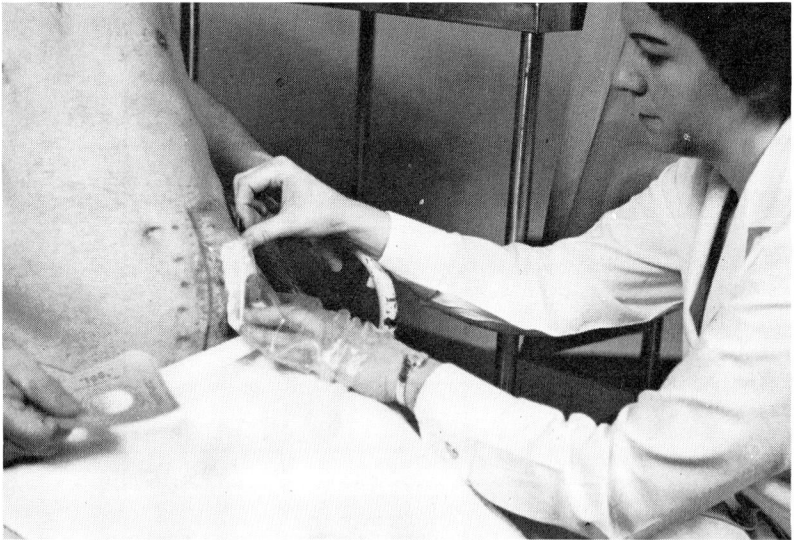

Fig. 28-20. This patient is too weak to care for his own colostomy. Note, however, that the nurse is letting him help by having him hold the covering removed from the adhesive surface of the bag.

tient's personal irrigating bag and shield. Have the patient read this. Answer his questions if you can. Refer the questions you cannot answer to the doctor or to the nurse.

Your local cancer society has a pamphlet on colostomy care. Obtain some of these for your patients. Find out if your community has a local colostomy association and call them to find out what teaching information for patients they can send you. The colostomy association also sends recovered colostomates (persons who have a colostomy and are living effectively) to visit colostomy patients in the hospital to help them with their problems. A visit from a colostomate usually makes the patient feel that he will be able to live again with his changed body.

Keep a record on your Kardex of what the patient has been taught and what he is able to do.

Find out from the head nurse or team leader just how much you are to show the patient about his care, what part of the irrigation you are to do, and how much the patient is to help. Find out what answers you are to give to the patient's questions. Remember that you are not to give the patient any confidential medical information.

The head nurse will probably refer this patient to the local visiting nurse association for help at home with his irrigation after he is discharged from the hospital.

Care of the permanent type colostomy bag

The permanent type colostomy bag may be obtained for the patient who is too ill or too feeble to irrigate and achieve control. This prosthesis (artificial body replacement—in this instance rectum-storage or collection place for feces) usually consists of a metal or plastic rim and reusable rubber or disposable plastic bags. The bag slips over the rim and is held in place with a metal clamp or rubber band. Then the rim holding the bag attaches to a belt which the patient wears around his waist to keep the bag in place over the colostomy. Every permanent colostomy bag comes from the manufacturer with a list of instructions for its care and application. You and the patient should read these together. Then apply the bag, demonstrating and explaining each step of the procedure to the patient as you go along. Remember that the patient needs to learn how to care for his changed body and its altered way of defecating.

The permanent colostomy appliance with reusable rubber bags (usually two come with each appliance) are usually more economical for the patient to maintain than is the one with the disposable bags. However, it also requires more care and is repulsive to the patient, since the bags must be emptied and washed.

Remove the reusable rubber bag when it is about one third full and apply the fresh one. Empty the used bag into the toilet. Rinse with cold water to remove all feces. Wash the bag thoroughly in warm soapy water, rinse well, and dry. Turn the bag inside out and expose to the air to remove or prevent odors.

Empty the bag in the patient's toilet and wash it in his room. Permit the patient to observe as you clean the bag. Explain what you are doing and why. After you clean the bag, leave it in the patient's room turned inside out and exposed to the air.

Assist the patient to open the disposable plastic bag (if one is used on the permanent appliance) at the bottom. Empty it into the toilet (if the patient is out of bed) or into a bedpan (if he is not). Assist the patient to rinse out the inside of the bag by squirting an Asepto syringe full of tepid water into the bottom of the bag (as in the disposable bag, p. 234). Close the bottom of the bag.

Replace the disposable bag with a fresh one when the bag is quite soiled or when an odor develops (every 24 to 72 hours). Remove the rubber band or metal clip that is fixing the bag to the rim, and slip off the bag. Replace with a fresh one.

A cement-on type of permanent appliance (Chapter 29) is worn by a patient with a right-sided (ascending) colostomy.

Usually the patient wears temporary colostomy bags after his colostomy is opened and until his permanent appliance is obtained from a supply company or until he develops bowel control.

Role of the nursing assistant in colostomy care

The patient's ability to continue living after a colostomy is made possible only by helping him to regain continence or fecal control. Nurses know this. Therefore the nursing service in your hospital may define colostomy care and control as a professional nursing responsibility. Check your job description carefully and perform accordingly.

SUMMARY

A colostomy is an artificial anus created surgically in the colon because the patient is no longer able to expel feces through the rectum.

The new anus or colostomy opening creates problems for the patient because he loses the ability to control the evacuation of feces from the body.

The colostomy can be controlled, in many instances, by retraining it through irrigations to empty each day at the same time.

An irrigation differs from an enema in the following ways:
1. An enema is an injection of fluid into the rectum. The patient holds this injected fluid and then expels it when he wants to.
2. An irrigation is also an injection of fluid, but in an irrigation the fluid is injected into the colon. The patient is unable to hold this fluid. Therefore the irrigating fluid runs in and out of the colon without the patient's controlling its flow in any way. The patient with a permanent colostomy must be taught how to care for himself and control his colostomy before he may return home.

DISCUSSION QUESTIONS

1 In what direction is the catheter inserted into a transverse colostomy? Into an ascending colostomy?
2 Why are dressings a source of irritation to the colostomy patient?
3 What method of collecting fecal drainage is better than that of using dressings?
4 How is a colostomy bag applied? Ask the head nurse to demonstrate the procedure for you.
5 Attend a meeting of the local colostomy association and report on it at the next ward conference.
6 Why should it be extremely distressing to the colostomy patient to receive a cathartic?
7 How is a colostomy irrigation done? Ask the head nurse to demonstrate this for you.
8 Why should a patient with a colostomy learn to irrigate it and apply his own colostomy bag before he is discharged?
9 How do you feel about caring for the patient with a colostomy? Do you think this attitude helps or hinders your patients? Why?

VOCABULARY

abdomen That area of the body from the breasts to the genital area.
abdominoperineal resection A double operation, the first part of which consists of opening the abdomen (near the umbilicus) and freeing the colon and rectum from their attachments in the body. Then the perineum is opened and the rectum and colon are removed through the perineal opening. That part of the colon that is disconnected from the diseased colon and rectum is brought out onto the abdomen as a colostomy.
anus Opening from the rectum to the outside of the body.
colon Large intestine; also called the large bowel.
colostomate A person who has a colostomy.
colostomy bag A plastic bag with an adhesive attachment that is placed on the skin around the stoma. The bag opens at the bottom to permit emptying.
irrigation Injecting fluid into a cavity without interrupting its return.
irrigator Equipment used to irrigate. The irrigator used by the colostomy patient consists of (1) a rubber irrigating bag and tubing and (2) an irrigating shield that consists of an irrigating sheath attached to a plastic cuplike dome or a plastic baglike sheath. These shields are placed

over the colostomy during the irrigation to catch and direct the return into the toilet bowl or the bedpan.

palliative That which relieves the patient's symptoms without actually curing the disease.

perineum That area of the body between the genitals and the rectum.

permanent colostomy A colostomy that will remain for the rest of the patient's life.

permanent colostomy bag A collecting bag held in place over the stoma by a reusable belt and rim attachment. The bags themselves may be of the reusable rubber or the disposable plastic type.

stoma The part of the colon that is out on the abdomen when the patient has a colostomy; sometimes called a rosebud.

temporary colostomy A colostomy that will be eliminated by reconnecting the colon after a period of time.

temporary colostomy bag A colostomy bag used for 24 hours and then discarded.

SOURCES OF ADDITIONAL INFORMATION

1 Contact the national office of the United Ostomy Association to learn if there is a local chapter in your community. The address is United Ostomy Association, 3915 Harding Ave., Cincinnati, Ohio.

2 Pamphlet; Care of your colostomy, may be obtained from the local cancer society. *(Use the pamphlet for your own information so that you will be able to help the patient more effectively.)*

3 Film: Postoperative management of a colostomy; may be obtained from United States Public Health Service, Communicable Disease Center, Atlanta, Ga. (Attention: Public Health Service, Audio-visual Facility).

29/Caring for the patient with an ileostomy, a "wet" ileostomy, or ureterostomies

STUDY QUESTIONS

1. What is colitis?
2. What is an ileostomy?
3. Why does a patient have an ileostomy?
4. Why does the patient have to wear a bag over his ileostomy stoma constantly?
5. How do you apply a temporary ileostomy bag?
6. How do you apply a permanent ileostomy bag?
7. What are electrolytes?
8. What are the patient's symptoms when he has an excessive loss of electrolytes?
9. Why do patients with an ileostomy develop postoperative depression?
10. How can you help the patient overcome postoperative depression?
11. What is a rectal bladder?
12. Why is removal of the urinary bladder (cystectomy) performed?
13. What are some of the possible reactions of the male patient toward voiding through the rectum?
14. What is a "wet" ileostomy?
15. What is a ureterostomy?
16. How is the urinary drainage collected when the patient has ureterostomy?
17. Why is it important to keep an accurate record of the intake and output of the patient with an ileostomy or urinary diversion.

THE ILEOSTOMY

The patient who will need to wear an ileostomy-type bag constantly is the one who has had his urine-storing bladder or feces-storing colon and rectum removed by an operation. After such an operation, the waste material from his body can no longer be stored until the bladder or rectum stretches and the patient decides to empty it; instead, urine or feces drain constantly from the ileostomy opening. The patient has lost all control over his bladder or his bowels.

This control can be regained through the use of an artificial bladder or rectum in the form of a rubber bag. This bag is cemented to the skin over the ileostomy opening, and it collects and stores the urine or feces until the patient decides to empty the bag. However, the bag, which is attached to the outside of the patient's body, does not function as well as the patient's own bladder or rectum, and the patient will therefore need your help in learning how to take care of his changed body.

WHY THE PATIENT HAS AN ILEOSTOMY

The patient who must have an ileostomy is usually a young adult with colitis whose colon and rectum must be removed because they are filled with ulcers and abscesses. He has probably suffered from bloody diarrhea, abdominal pain, and severe cramps for some time. He is in pain and is thin, weak, and thoroughly discouraged. The doctor explains to him that the ileostomy operation means that the rectum will be removed and the feces will drain through an opening in the abdomen (Figs. 29-1 and 29-2).

He is taken to the operating room and his entire large bowel, including his rectum, is removed by an abdominoperineal resection. Then the loop of the small bowel, which has been disconnected from the large bowel, is brought to the outside of the patient's body through the abdomen. A temporary ileostomy bag is applied over the ileostomy opening into the small intestine, and the patient is returned to the recovery room or to his unit.

UNDERSTANDING THE ILEOSTOMY

The small intestine receives food from the stomach and digests and absorbs a large part of it. The remaining food is moved along through the small intestine by the constant peristaltic action of the small bowel and is emptied into the large bowel. However, after the entire large bowel has been removed by a colectomy (*col-*, large bowel; *-ectomy*, removal of), the liquid feces cannot empty into it. Instead, the feces are expelled to the outside of the body through the ileostomy stoma on the abdomen. Since the small intestine has almost constant peristaltic movement, the liquid feces will be expelled frequently in spurts.

Therefore for the first 3 weeks after the

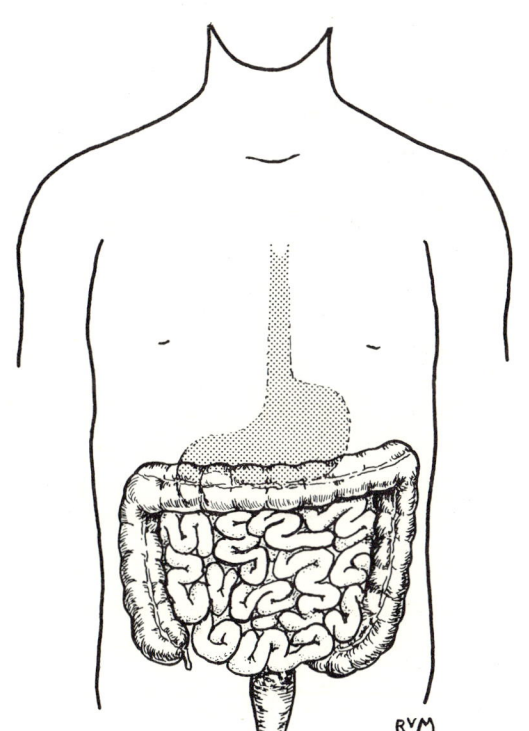

Fig. 29-1. The normal intestinal tract.

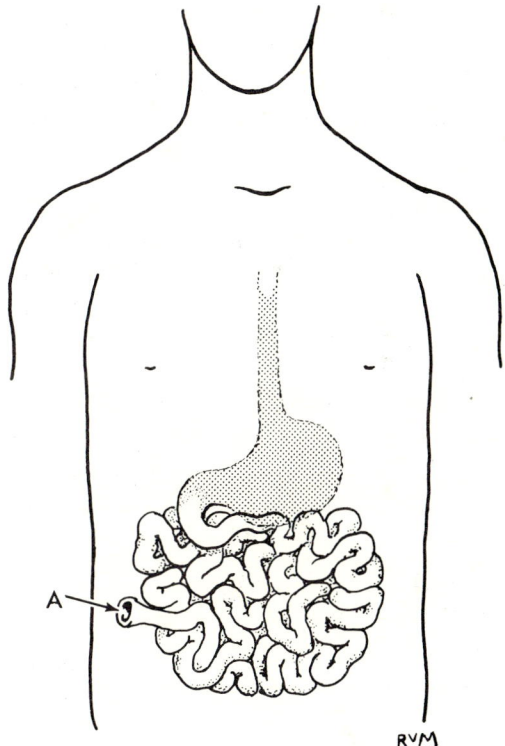

Fig. 29-2. The entire large bowel has been removed (colectomy), and the small intestine has been opened onto the abdomen at the ileum. The patient has an ileostomy at **A**.

operation, the patient with an ileostomy will have an almost constant spurting of liquid feces from the stoma. After this period, the ileum (third section of the small intestine) usually takes over some of the job of the missing large bowel and absorbs some water. Then the feces becomes less watery and more like a paste (similar to the consistency of toothpaste).

FACTORS TO REMEMBER IN CARING FOR THE PATIENT WITH AN ILEOSTOMY

The nursing care of the patient with an ileostomy revolves around the following factors:

1. The patient usually becomes depressed after his operation when he sees the stoma constantly spurting feces. He believes that he has exchanged his preoperative problems of pain and diarrhea for this worse one of an unpredictable stoma. He dislikes the sight, the sound, and the smell of the feces, and he is sure that he is so different and so strange that people will think he is a freak and will avoid him.

2. The patient's skin becomes irritated and excoriated very quickly when the feces, which contain large amounts of digestive juices, are permitted to flow over it or lie on it. Then, too, the liquid content of the feces indicates that the patient is not absorbing the fluids he needs.

3. The patient will have his ileostomy the rest of his life. How effectively he will be able to go on living will depend to a great extent on how he learns to accept and care for the ileostomy.

CARING FOR THE PATIENT WITH AN ILEOSTOMY

You can help the patient overcome his feelings of depression and strangeness by helping him learn how to manage his ileostomy. Words mean nothing to the patient. How can he believe you when you tell him that he can stay clean by using an ileostomy bag if he is constantly dirty in the hospital? You must show him that it is possible for him to go on living by making this living possible. Making it possible means helping the patient regain control of his unpredictable stoma. The patient will be unable to leave his home, will be unable to work, will be unable to go out on dates, and will be unable to live until he is sure that he can stay clean.

Visit the patient as soon as he returns to his unit from the recovery room and inspect his abdomen. If a temporary bag has been applied, check its contents. Empty the bag into an emesis basin as necessary by releasing the rubber band on the bottom and opening the bag. Rinse out the bag through the bottom with a bulb syringe and enough tepid water to clean out all the feces and to limit the amount of fecal odor. Wipe the end of the bag dry with a paper towel, refold it closed, and apply the rubber band to keep it closed.

Return to see the patient at 2-hour intervals. Check his vital signs and empty his ileostomy bag. When you are emptying the bag, avoid any facial expression that reflects distaste because of an odor. The patient will be watching you carefully to see how you react toward this strange way to defecate, and he will believe that everyone on the ward and perhaps even the whole world feels as you do. Therefore a calm, quiet, interested, and efficient manner on your part will help the patient accept his ileostomy and his job of learning how to take care of it.

Keep an accurate record of the patient's intake and output. Encourage the patient to take as much fluid by mouth as he can as soon as oral fluids are permitted (usually on the third day). Chart all the fluids the patient takes. Record all output, including the liquid fecal drainage from the ileostomy bag. The liquid feces contain not only water but also the minerals (electrolytes) that are so necessary for proper body functioning. The doctor will order intravenous fluids to replace those lost in the feces, and he will add sodium and potassium chloride to these intravenous fluids to replace the lost electrolytes. Therefore you must keep the intake and output record accurately so that the doctor will know how much fluid and electrolytes to replace.

Observe the patient carefully for any signs of excess electrolyte loss. The electrolytes are those minerals of the body that carry the positive and negatives charges required to make the electrical current that the nerves use to carry messages between the brain and the muscles of the body. Signs of excessive electrolyte loss, then, would be irritated nerves and weak muscles. The symptoms the patient might present are extreme restlessness, irritable personality, weak body muscles, and a weak heart muscle (slow, irregular pulse). Usually the doctor will prescribe juices* for the ileostomy patient to drink between meals (after he is on oral feedings) because juices are filled with electrolytes and will help to replace those that the patient is losing. Be sure that the patient drinks these juices. Keep the nurse informed of any changes in the patient's personality, pulse changes, or signs of increasing weakness.

Change the patient's temporary ileostomy bag every day when you give him a bath. Explain to him what you are doing and show him how you are doing it. As soon as he has sufficiently recovered from his operation and has enough physical strength, have him help you. When he knows how to change the bag, let him do it for himself. Stand by to give advice or help when he needs it.

About a month after the operation, the ileostomy stoma will have shrunk all that it is going to. At this time the doctor will order a permanent type of ileostomy bag for the patient. The patient may have been discharged from the hospital by this time. However, if he is still in the hospital, you must help him learn how to apply and care for his permanent bag, which will be the type of bag that he will wear for the rest of his life.

---

*Cranberry, Gatorade, or tolerated fruit juices such as apricot, apple, pear, or grape.

Application of the temporary bag

1. Collect all the necessary equipment for applying a temporary ileostomy bag. This consists of the following:
    a. Ostomy bag (temporary)
    b. Solvent and an eyedropper
    c. Gauze pads, 4-inch squares or 2-inch squares
    d. Appliance cement
    e. Scissors
    f. Tongue blades
    g. Karaya gum powder or karaya ring.
    h. Paper bag or newspapers
2. Place all the equipment on a tray and take it to the patient's bedside.
3. Fold down the bedclothes and expose the patient's abdomen.
4. Cover the patient's abdomen below the stoma with a bath towel.
5. Apply the solvent with the eyedropper to the area between the bag and the patient's skin. Allow the solvent to seep between the skin and the bag. Ease off the bag as it loosens. Discard it in the paper bag.
6. Clean the skin with a gauze pad saturated with the solvent. Rinse the skin off with water and pat it dry.
7. Cover the stoma with a small piece of toilet tissue or cleansing tissue (to catch the drainage).
8. Measure the stoma. Prepare the ostomy bag by cutting a circular hole in the disk (adhesive square that attaches the bag to the body) about one-eighth inch larger than the stoma.
    a. The stoma can be measured with a quarter or half dollar, and a circle can be drawn on the disk.
    b. Do not make the hole so small that it irritates the stoma.
    c. Do not make the hole too large. Skin around the stoma will then be exposed to the digestive juices.
    d. Place your hand inside the bag when you cut out the hole in the disk. This will help you to avoid

cutting through to the opposite side of the bag.
9. Remove the backing from the adhesive disk.
10. Apply two coats of appliance cement to the adhesive disk as follows*:
    a. Apply a thin coat of cement to the disk and spread it over the entire disk with the tongue blade.
    b. Permit the cement to dry well (usually takes about 2 minutes).
    c. Apply the second coat of cement to the adhesive disk.
    d. Set the disk aside to dry.
11. Replace the toilet tissue or cleansing tissue covering the stoma with a fresh piece.
12. Dust the skin with karaya gum powder and brush off the excess.
13. Apply two coats of cement to the skin around the stoma in the following way*:
    a. Apply one coat of cement and spread it with a tongue blade.
    b. Permit the cement to dry.
    c. Apply the second coat.
    d. Permit the second coat of cement to dry well.
14. Place your hand up through the bottom of the bag and grasp the inside of the disk.
15. Center the opening of the bag over the stoma and press the adhesive disk down over the entire cemented section of the skin for several minutes so that it will adhere tightly and form a good seal (Fig. 28-19).
16. Close the bottom of the bag as follows:
    a. Fold it up twice from the bottom.
    b. Bring the sides together by making several pleatlike folds.
    c. Seal the bottom with a rubber band.
17. Sprinkle talcum powder around the adhesive disk to keep the excess cement from adhering to the patient's clothing.

The important point to remember in applying the ileostomy bag is that the liquid feces may seep between the skin and the bag and loosen it. Therefore the bag should be sealed to the body with appliance cement. The liquid feces are full of the digestive juices, which can irritate and excoriate the skin. Therefore as little skin as possible should be left exposed around the stoma and thus be permitted to come in contact with these juices. The exposed skin should be protected from the digestive juices by covering it with karaya gum powder.

The ileostomy bag should be applied in such a way that the liquid feces will run downhill into the bag and not flow back over the stoma. You can do this by putting the bag on the patient in such a way that the bottom of the bag points to the patient's feet if he is allowed out of bed or to the side of the bed if he is a bed patient.

Empty the ileostomy bag frequently. Even the most carefully applied bag will become full enough to leak back over the stoma if it is not emptied frequently. Plan to change the ileostomy bag at a time when the stoma is relatively quiet. Ask the patient to determine the best time for the change. Normally the stoma is most active the 1 or 2 hours after meals. Encourage the patient to participate in his care. Remember that he is going home alone with this stoma. Therefore he will be unable to go home until he can care for the ileostomy by himself.

Application of the permanent bag

1. Collect all the necessary equipment for applying a permanent bag. This includes the following:
    a. Clean appliance
    b. Solvent and eyedropper
    c. Appliance cement

---

*Steps 10 and 13 may be eliminated when a karaya ring or washer is used both to protect the skin and to adhere the bag to the body.

d. Karaya gum powder
e. Toilet tissue or cleansing tissue
f. Small gauze squares (4 × 4)
g. Emesis basin
2. Place the equipment on a tray and take it to the patient's bedside. (It is quite convenient to keep an ileostomy change tray set up on your ward ready for use at any time.)
3. Apply two thin coats of cement* to the disk on the clean appliance.
  a. Be sure to let the first coat dry thoroughly before you apply the second coat.
  b. Set the appliance aside to let the second coat dry.
4. Apply solvent to the area between the bag and the skin. Permit the solvent to seep under the disk that is holding the bag to the patient's abdomen. Ease the disk off. Place the removed bag in the emesis basin.
5. Remove any adhesive remaining on the abdomen with a gauze pad saturated with solvent. Do not rub. Pat the solvent on the patient's abdomen to avoid irritating the skin.
6. Wash the skin around the stoma with soap and water, rinse well, and pat it dry.
7. Wrap a piece of toilet tissue or cleansing tissue around the stoma to catch any fecal drainage.
8. Sprinkle karaya gum powder on the skin. Brush off any excess.
9. Apply two coats of cement to the skin around the stoma. Be certain that the first coat is completely dry before you apply the second.
  a. Each coat of cement should be thinly and evenly applied. Use a tongue blade to spread it.
  b. The cement will not injure the stoma, so apply it as close to the stoma as possible.
10. Separate the sides of the clean bag (without touching the cement-coated disk) to pull in a little air.
11. Hold the appliance near the belt hooks. Position it over the stoma correctly so that the hooks on the bag will be in alignment with the belt.
12. Ease the appliance over the stoma. Hold it level and apply the top and bottom of the disk to the skin at the same time.
13. Hold the disk firmly in place and attach the belt to the hooks on the side of the bag. Hold the disk in place for about 5 minutes to be sure that the cement has set.
14. Close the bottom of the bag by folding up the spout end. (Fold the spout in thirds, the first part over and the second part under.)
15. Wrap a heavy rubber band around the folded spout to keep it closed.
16. Make the patient comfortable and then clean the bag that you removed. Empty the fecal contents from the bag into the toilet bowl. Rinse the bag well with cold water. Remove the old cement from the disk on the bag with a gauze pad soaked in solvent. Place the bag in a basin of warm soapy water. Scrub it thoroughly (inside and outside) with a stiff brush and rinse it. Take it back to the patient's area and hang it (somewhere in his unit) upside down. This will dry and deodorize the bag.
17. Collect the equipment you used and clean it. Reset the tray and return it to the proper place.

Be careful that you do not tear the permanent appliance (Fig. 29-3) when you clean it, and be sure that you return it to the patient's area for safekeeping after you clean it. Always clean the bag as soon as you remove it so that it will be ready for the next change.

The patient usually wears the well-applied permanent ileostomy bag for as long

---
*Double-faced adhesive disk or a karaya ring may be used instead of cement.

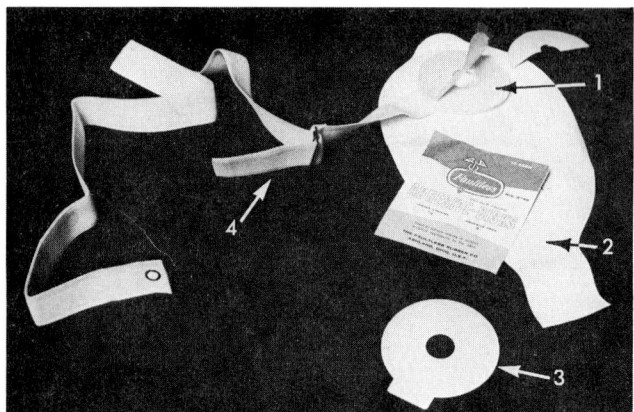

Fig. 29-3. Permanent appliance for a patient with an ileostomy: **1**, face plate being covered with a double-faced adhesive disk; **2**, emptying spout; **3**, double-faced adhesive disk; **4**, belt.

as 3 to 7 days. However, if the patient has any sensation of pain around the stoma, excessive itching around the stoma, or a feeling of fecal drainage on the skin, the appliance should be removed, even if it has just been in place for 2 hours, and the skin should be checked. It is much easier to prevent skin irritation than to cure it. However, when irritation does occur, the skin must be well protected with karaya gum powder or a karaya gum seal (circlet of karaya gum) before a disk (holding plate for an appliance) can be cemented on.

WHY THE PATIENT HAS A RECTAL BLADDER, A "WET" ILEOSTOMY, OR URETEROSTOMIES

The patient who must have a rectal bladder or a ureterostomy is usually a middle-aged man with cancer of the bladder who went to see his family doctor because he was voiding bloody urine (hematuria). The doctor became quite concerned about this and arranged for the patient to be admitted to the hospital for further studies.

The patient is admitted to the hospital with the symptoms of hematuria, frequency (voiding oftener than usual), urgency (need to void as soon as the brain sends a message that there is urine in the bladder), and dysuria (*dys*, painful; *uria*, urine—painful urination). He does not feel sick and is very anxious to get the studies done so that he can get back to work.

However, when the physician passes a cystoscope (*cyst*, bladder; *scope*, instrument with mirror and light that permits the doctor to look inside the body) into the bladder, he sees a tumor. The surgeon cuts a piece off the tumor through the cystoscope and sends this specimen of the tumor to the laboratory. Soon a report is returned to the doctor with the information that the patient's bladder tumor is cancerous.

The doctor explains to the patient that his bladder must be removed.

The patient with cancer of the bladder is taken to the operating room for removal of the bladder (cystectomy). However, cystectomy is done only when the patient is curable. If the doctor believes that the cancer has spread so much that the patient cannot be cured, there is little purpose in doing this type of operation.

After the bladder is removed, there is no storage place for urine in the body. The surgeon may attach the ureters to the rec-

Caring for the patient with an ileostomy, a "wet" ileostomy, or ureterostomies

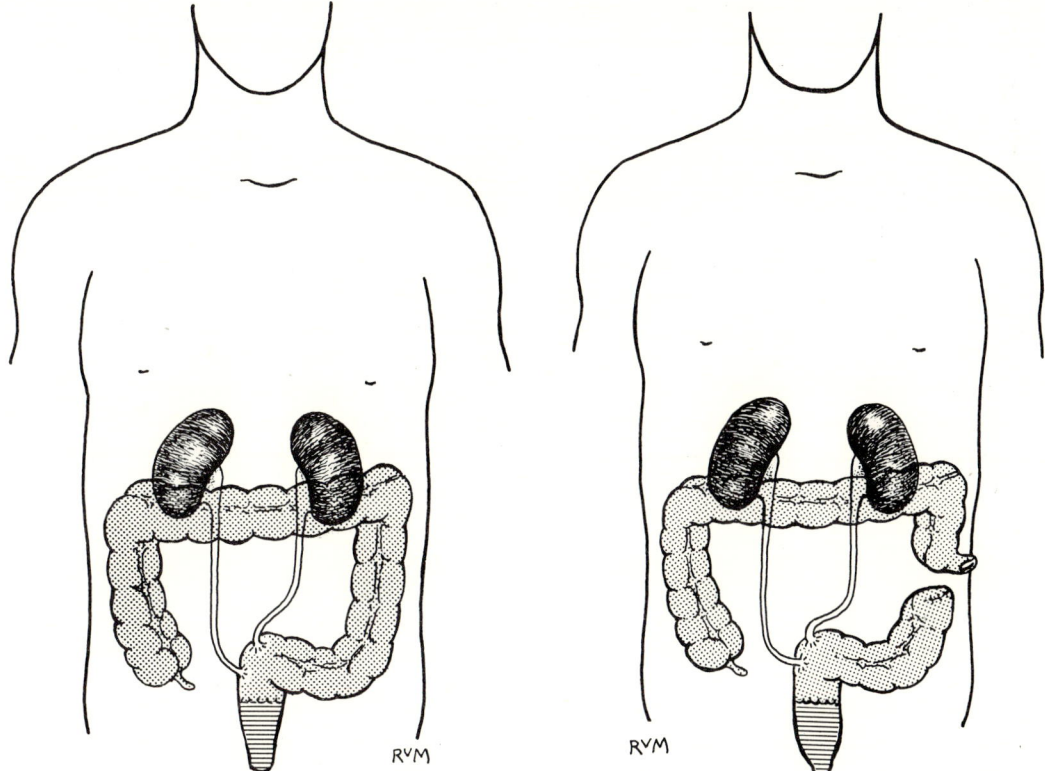

Fig. 29-4. The patient's urinary bladder has been removed and the ureters are attached to the rectum. Now the rectum will be used as a storage place for urine and feces. Compare this illustration with the one showing the normal urinary system (Fig. 11-3).

Fig. 29-5. The patient's bladder has been removed and the ureters are attached to the rectum. The rectum is now used as a substitute for the removed bladder. A colostomy has also been done to divert the feces away from the rectum and the ureters in an attempt to avoid infection of the ureters and kidneys.

tum, he may use parts of the small bowel to make a bladder for the patient, or he may bring the ureters to the outside of the patient's body on the abdomen. Then the patient returns to the recovery room or to his unit.

UNDERSTANDING THE URINARY DIVERSION
Rectal bladder

The urine may be diverted into the rectum for storage (Fig. 29-4). The patient who has a ureterorectal anastomosis (ureters joined to the rectum) usually returns to the ward with a rectal tube in the rectum. The rectal tube is connected by tubing to a drainage bottle on the floor. After 24 hours, urine drains through this tube to the drainage bottle. In approximately 10 days the rectal tube is removed and the patient learns to cope with the rectum made to function also as a bladder. At first he feels strange pressures in the rectum as it fills with urine, but soon he learns to tell the difference between urine and feces in the rectum.

The bowel movements will be liquid after the tube is removed, but in a few

256 Nursing assistant meets patient's particular needs

weeks they will become soft and pastelike in consistency. However, the patient must always void by sitting down and going through the motions of having a bowel movement. This alteration in function bothers the male patient a great deal, perhaps making him feel like a woman instead of a man. He feels that he is different. He hopes that other people cannot see his strangeness, but he is certain that they do, so he keeps to himself.

Rectal bladder and colostomy

The urine may be diverted into the rectum as just described, and the feces may be diverted to the outside of the body through a colostomy (Fig. 29-5) to prevent it from coming in contact with the ureters and infecting them. The patient will void from the rectum after this type of operation too, but he will expel feces through a colostomy. The colostomy will be cared for in exactly the same way as described for all colostomies (Chapter 28).

"Wet" ileostomy (ileal bladder)

The urine may be diverted into a piece of the ileum that is made into a bladder (Fig. 29-6). A piece of the ileum (third section of the small intestine) is cut off from the rest of the small intestine and sewed closed on one end. The other end is then

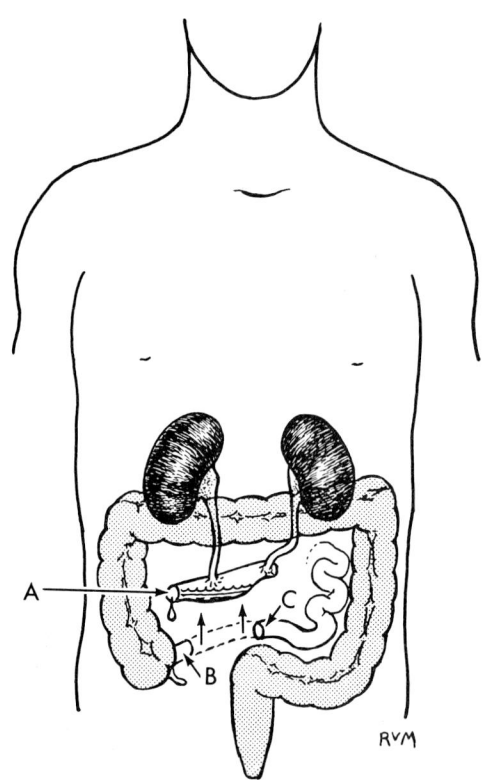

Fig. 29-6. A piece of ileum (small bowel) has been removed between **B** and **C** and has been made into a urinary bladder, **A**. The small bowel has been reconnected by joining **B** with **C**. The ileum-made bladder (ileobladder) opens to the outside of the body at **A**.

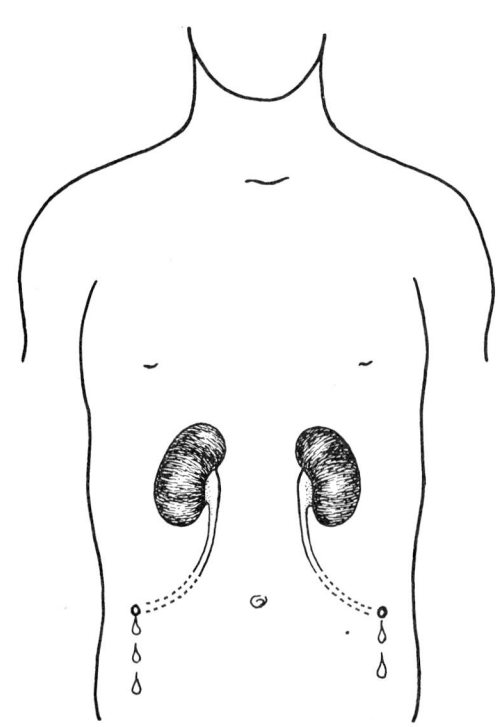

Fig. 29-7. The bladder has been removed and the ureters have been opened out onto the abdomen. The patient now has two urine-draining openings on the abdomen.

opened out onto the abdomen like the usual ileostomy. However, this ileostomy is called a "wet" ileostomy because it drains urine instead of feces, as in the usual type.

The patient with a "wet" ileostomy moves his bowels in the usual way, and he drains urine constantly from the one opening on the abdomen. However, he does not need to sit down to void. Psychologically this is better for the patient.

Ureterostomies

The urine may be brought out directly onto the abdomen through ureterostomies (Fig. 29-7). The patient thus has two openings on the abdomen through which urine drains constantly.

CARING FOR THE PATIENT WITH A RECTAL BLADDER

After the patient recovers from his operation (usually in about 5 days), he may become depressed as he realizes how his body is changed. He becomes embarrassed at having to sit down to void and wonders if everyone can see his strangeness. He avoids the other patients and keeps to himself.

You must listen carefully to the assignment the team leader or head nurse gives you. Ask her any questions, for you will need to know all about this patient when you go in to care for him.

The thoughtless question "Is that urine coming out of your rectal tube?" is enough to convince the patient that even you think he is strange, and his depression deepens. However, a calm, accepting, concerned attitude about the patient, coupled with frequent visits to give him the care he needs, will help to dispel the depression.

Encourage the patient to drink as much fluid as he can (usually after the third or fourth postoperative day) so that his kidneys will keep working and his ureters will be flushed out well. Keep an accurate record of the patient's intake and output. Watch him for signs of electrolyte imbalance. Remember that the large bowel absorbs water and now that the patient is using the rectum as a bladder he may reabsorb waste material from the urine. The signs of electrolyte disturbance are the same as those discussed earlier in this chapter.

Offer the patient a bedpan every 2 hours (after the drainage tube is out of the rectum) and encourage him to void. The patient usually is too embarrassed to ask for a bedpan. Do not make jokes.

CARING FOR THE PATIENT WITH AN ILEAL BLADDER OR WITH URETEROSTOMIES

The patient with an ileal bladder or with ureterostomies will have a temporary ileostomy-type bag applied over the abdominal opening through which urine drains until he is fitted with a permanent bag (Fig. 29-8).

The temporary ileostomy-type bag is applied in the same way as it is for a patient with an ileostomy, with the following exceptions:

1. Karaya gum powder is used to protect the skin under the cement when

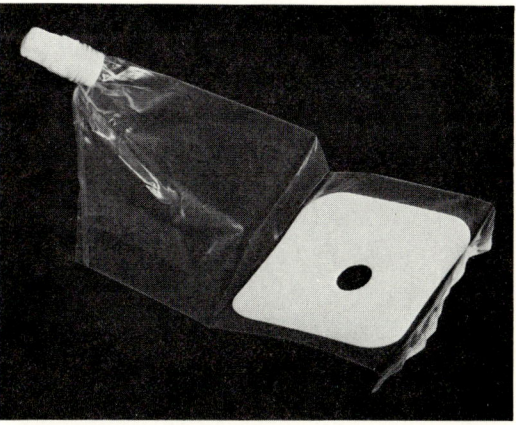

Fig. 29-8. A disposable ileobladder bag. Note the screw-in plug at the bottom, which is removed in emptying the bag or in attaching it to a urinary drainage tube at night.

the bag is kept on for a period longer than 24 hours.
2. Cement is not used to apply the bag unless it is kept on for more than 24 hours.
3. Tincture of benzoin is painted on the skin (instead of cement and karaya gum powder) to protect it and to make the bag adhere.

Be sure that you place a piece of cleansing tissue or toilet tissue on the abdominal opening to absorb the urine during a bag change. If the skin gets wet, the bag will not adhere.

When the patient is able to stand up, have him do so while the bag is being changed. This will smooth the wrinkles out of his abdomen and permit the bag to adhere better.

The permanent type of bag is applied to the "wet" ileostomy or to the ureterostomy in the same way that it is applied to the "fecal" ileostomy. However, the urinary ileostomy bag differs from the others in that the spout on the bottom is closed with a screw-in type plug instead of being folded up and closed with a rubber band. At night, a urinary drainage tube is attached to the spout and connected to a drainage bottle on the floor, and the plug is removed. This is necessary because the kidneys secrete about 60 ml. of urine each hour (½ pint every 4 hours), and the weight of this urine may very easily pull the bag loose at night.

The patient with a permanent ileostomy should receive large amounts of liquids, and accurate recordings of his intake and output should be made. He should be observed carefully for electrolyte disturbances.

The removed permanent "wet" ileostomy bag is cleaned in the same way as is the "fecal" ileostomy bag, except that it is soaked for 30 minutes in vinegar solution (4 tablespoonsful of vinegar to 1 pint of cool water) after it is cleaned. Then it is rinsed well in cold water, dried, and hung in the patient's room.

The enterostomatist

Enterostomatists are technicians employed and trained by hospitals or surgeons to help ostomy patients learn how to care for their stomas.

Role of the nursing assistant

The nursing service in your hospital may identify ostomy care as a professional nursing responsibility because of the need for teaching the patient self-care. The patient's ability to continue living depends on his learning the skills to care for his stoma.

Check your job description carefully, identify your patient care activities, and perform accordingly.

SUMMARY

The patient with an ulcerated and bleeding colon may have it removed. Then the small bowel is brought out onto the abdomen and the patient has an ileostomy. Since the fluid is no longer absorbed from the fecal contents (the colon does this), the ileostomy will drain liquid feces. Eventually, the small bowel will begin to absorb some fluid and the feces will become less liquid. However, the ileostomy will always be unpredictable in its spurting of soft pastelike feces. Therefore the ileostomy patient must wear a bag over the stoma constantly.

The patient with cancer of the bladder may have the entire urinary bladder removed. The ureters (tubes bringing urine from the kidneys) may be planted in the rectum, or they may be brought out through openings in the abdomen. However, these two draining ureterostomies can be made into a single opening by the surgeon. He does this by cutting off a piece of small intestine (the ileum, to be more specific) and by planting the ureters in it. Then one end is sewed shut and the other end is brought out onto the abdomen as a "wet" ileostomy. The ileostomy, the "wet" ileostomy, and the ureterostomy drain constantly. Therefore the skin around these draining openings must be carefully cared for and protected, or it will become raw, irritated, and infected. It is much easier to prevent than to cure a skin problem.

DISCUSSION QUESTIONS

1. Ask the nurse to arrange to have a member of an "ileostomy club" visit the unit and demonstrate the care of an ileostomy.
2. Attend a meeting of the local "ileostomy club." Discuss your observations of the meeting at the next team conference.
3. Ask the supply service in the hospital to send a temporary ileostomy bag to the ward. Inspect it carefully. Discuss possible uses for this bag on the patient who has a draining wound.
4. Ask the nurse to demonstrate (a) the application of a temporary ileostomy bag and (b) the application of a permanent ileostomy bag.
5. Which patients on the unit are losing a great deal of digestive juices from the intestines or from a draining wound?
6. What are electrolytes?
7. Ask the doctor or nurse if the patients referred to in question 5 are losing electrolytes. If they are, what observations would you make on these patients in order to identify electrolyte imbalance?
8. Why should a patient with an infection or operation involving the urinary tract receive an increased amount of fluid?
9. Ask the doctor how he feels about the intake and output records on the ward. How could you improve their accuracy?
10. How does an ileostomy differ from a colostomy?

VOCABULARY

anastomosis Joining together by surgery.
colitis Disease of the large intestine that causes irritation, ulceration, and inflammation.
cystectomy Surgical removal of the bladder.
cystoscope An instrument that is passed into the bladder and through which the doctor can see to examine the bladder.
diversion Change in the direction of flow of a body discharge. A urinary diversion would be a change in the direction of the flow of urine from the bladder to the rectum or to the outside of the body.
ileal bladder Urinary bladder formed from a piece of the small intestine (ileum). The ileal bladder opens out onto the abdomen through an ileostomy.
ileostomy Opening of the ileum (third portion of the small intestine) onto the abdomen.
permanent bag A rubber or plastic bag applied to an ileostomy opening for a period ranging from 3 to 7 days. The bag is then removed, cleaned, and reused. This bag is held on the patient's body by cement and a belt.
rectal bladder Diversion of urine from the bladder to the rectum.
temporary bag A plastic bag that is applied to an ileostomy opening for a short period of time (24 to 48 hours) and then removed and discarded.
ureterostomy Opening of the ureters onto the patient's abdomen.
"wet" ileostomy Ileostomy through which urine drains.

SOURCES OF ADDITIONAL INFORMATION

1. Pamphlet: The ABC of ileostomy; may be obtained for $2 from Custom Service, 1770 Andrews Ave., Bronx, N. Y. 10543.
2. Slides: Changing the permanent appliance; may be obtained from the United Surgical Supply Company. Arrangements can be made for these through your supply department or the local ostomy association.
3. The manual for ileostomy patients; may be obtained for $2 from QT, Inc., c/o The Medical Foundation, 227 Commonwealth Ave., Boston, Mass. 02100.

30/Applying heat to the patient's body in the presence of infection

STUDY QUESTIONS

1. What are the signs of infection in a part of the body that you can see, such as a leg?
2. What are the signs of infection in a part of the body that you cannot see, such as the lungs?
3. Why does a swelling occur at the site of infection?
4. How do those body cells that are injured by bacteria tell the body that they need help?
5. How does the body help?
6. How does an application of heat help the infected part of the body?
7. How is a foot soak given?
8. What is the correct temperature for a foot soak?
9. Why is the application of excessive heat to an infected part of the body dangerous?
10. How is a medicated bath given?
11. What is the correct temperature for a medicated bath?
12. Why should an infected part of the body be elevated?
13. How high should an infected body part be elevated?
14. At what temperature is a hot-water bottle prepared?
15. Who prescribes heat applications for the patient?

THE BODY NEEDS HELP IN THE PRESENCE OF INFECTION

When the body cells are injured, they notify the blood vessels of their need for help by secreting a special fluid and by releasing this fluid into the blood. The blood vessels help by dilating (widening) quickly and bringing in more blood. This increased blood supply helps the injured cells as follows:

1. By bringing in more food and oxygen so that the body cells will have more energy for fighting the bacteria and repairing the injury (cut, bruise, etc.)
2. By bringing in more white blood cells (the "soldiers" of the body) to kill the germs and repair the injury
3. By removing the waste material from the cells
4. By removing the dead body cells and bacteria so that the functioning body cells and the white blood cells have more room to work

At first, the blood vessels are able to do the job well. They bring in the increased blood supply and they give the cells more food, more oxygen, and more white blood cells ("soldiers") in the watery fluid (serum) of the blood. Soon, however, the blood that gave up so much of its watery material becomes quite thick and has difficulty flowing through the blood vessels. Then the injured cells are in trouble because their supply of foodstuffs and "soldiers" is cut off and their waste material cannot be removed.

SIGNS OF INJURY OR INFECTION

Signs that you can observe at the site of difficulty in the patient's body (if the injury or infection involves a part of the body that you can see) are the following:
1. *Redness* brought about by the increased blood supply to the part
2. *Swelling* brought about by the increased amount of fluid sent from the blood to the part
3. *Heat* brought about by the increased blood supply to the part
4. *Pain* caused by pressure on the nerve by the swelling or from the effects of the injury or infection on the nerve itself
5. *Loss of function of the part* usually brought about voluntarily by the patient because movement further irritates the nerves and therefore increases the pain

Changes in the vital signs also occur as a result of injury or infection. Such changes include the following:
1. *Fever* caused by the reaction of the body to the bacteria
2. *Elevated pulse rate* caused by the increased need of the body for blood
3. *Elevated respiratory rate* caused by the increased need of the body for oxygen

In those areas of the body that you cannot see (for example, the lungs and the bladder), changes in the vital signs may be the only clues that the patient is being invaded by bacteria which are injuring his body.

One change in the blood count that the doctor will look for when the patient has an infection is an increased white blood cell count. Normally the white blood cell count is between 7,000 and 9,000. However, when the body is invaded by germs, it will manufacture more white blood cells ("soldiers") and send them into battle to kill the germs. Usually the severity of the infection is determined by the extent to which the white blood cells are increased.

The doctor will probably ask the laboratory to identify the germ responsible for the infection so that he can give the patient the right antibiotic. The doctor will do this by sending a specimen to the laboratory from the infected (germ-invaded) body area for a culture.

THE ROLE OF THE NURSING ASSISTANT IN THE PATIENT'S CARE

The most significant aspect of the nursing assistant's role in giving patient care is observing the patient's temperature each day for an elevation (fever) and reporting these elevations to the nurse promptly when they occur.

The head nurse or the team leader will plan the patient's care with the doctor. Then she will assign you to do those nursing care activities in the plan that you are able to do. Some of these activities and their purposes are given in Table 30-1.

THE AMOUNT OF HEAT APPLIED TO THE PATIENT'S BODY

Although moderate degrees of warmth may help the body overcome infection and stimulate healing by bringing in an increased blood supply and by making the cells work harder, excessive heat may cause further damage. It does this by making the cells (in the entire heated area) work so hard just to live that they have no time or energy left to fight the infection or to heal the body.

A clear understanding of the effect of excessive heat on the body can be obtained easily if you think about your entire body and the way it functions. On a cold day in winter your body functions poorly. Your toes and fingers are numb and stiff with cold, and your muscles shiver to help you heat your body. On an extremely hot day in summer your body also functions poorly.

Table 30-1. Nursing care for the patient with an infection

Activity	Purpose
Giving the patient fluids (water, juices, etc.) every waking hour; 8 ounces (1 glass) of fluid per hour between 6 A.M. and 10 P.M. provides an intake of 3,840 ml.	This increased fluid intake will keep the blood in a liquid state so that it will circulate easily. This is necessary because of the patient's increased loss of the fluid through sweating. The increased fluid intake also stimulates the kidneys to take more water out of the blood (in excess of body need), and with the excess fluid, the kidneys also take germs out of the body. In this way, the fluids that the patient drinks help to dilute and remove the infected (germ-laden) material from the body.
Applying heat to the affected part of the patient's body	This application of warmth dilates (widens) the blood vessels and increases the blood supply to and away from the affected part. This means that oxygen, food, and white blood cells ("soldiers") will be brought to the affected part much faster, and that waste material and dead germs and cells will be removed more quickly. Warm applications also speed up the activities in the body cells themselves.
Helping the patient to eat his meals and even supplying him with extra nourishment between meals	The carbohydrates and fats in the food provide the cells with the energy to fight the infection while the proteins and vitamins provide the building blocks for repairing the body and promoting healing.
Elevating the affected body part	Gravity helps the blood flow through the veins and back to the heart. This avoids stagnation of blood in the affected part and overloading of the veins. Then the cells in the affected part can dump their waste material into the veins quite easily. Speeding up the movement of waste-laden venous blood away from the part by gravity also permits the arteries to bring in more blood loaded with food and oxygen. It does this by making more space available for the arteries and thus permitting them to dilate, and at the same time it decreases the backflow pressure into them.
Keeping the patient at rest in bed	Limiting the patient's activities permits the body to divert all of its energies to the healing process.
Observing the patient's vital signs and body signs carefully to identify any worsening or improvement in the patient's condition	Reporting promptly to the nurse any significant changes in these signs.
Observing the patient's body carefully for signs of an undesirable reaction to the antibiotic he is receiving	Reactions such as nausea and vomiting, rashes, breathing difficulties, stomach pain, pain between the shoulders, and diarrhea may occur. The head nurse will tell you what undesirable reaction the drug that the patient is receiving may cause and which patient observations you are to make.

You perspire profusely, your muscles are weak, and breathing is difficult. You are exhausted just sitting down because all the body's energy is being used just to help you live. However, on a nice spring day you are full of pep. You work hard and you give little or no thought to the needs of the body.

Therefore it is desirable to apply warmth, not excessive heat, to the body. This warmth can be provided by soaks or wet dressings or both at a temperature just slightly above that of the skin. Skin temperature is normally about 92° F.

When warmth is applied to a large surface area of the body (as in a warm bath), the temperature of the solution should not be higher than 100° F. However, when warmth is applied to a small area of the body (as in a foot soak), the temperature of the solution can be as high as but not higher than 110° F. The reason for the bath temperature's being 100° F. is to prevent the general widening of the blood vessels throughout the body caused by this temperature from becoming so great that they take up all the blood and thereby rob the brain of its supply. In a warm application to a smaller body surface, this danger of depriving the brain of an adequate supply of blood does not exist, and so the solution temperature may be the higher one of 110° F.

When heat is applied by the use of a hot-water bottle, the temperature of the water in the bottle should be 115° F. By the time the heat travels through the rubber bottle and its cover, it will reach the patient's skin at the temperature of 110° F.

If heat is supplied by a lamp, the degree of heat reaching the skin must be tested with a thermometer (an ordinary bath thermometer will do this). A safe temperature is 110° F. or below. Heat above 110° F. may cause skin burns.

CARE OF THE PATIENT RECEIVING HEAT APPLICATIONS

As you apply heat to the patient's body, be sure to carry out the following safety measures:
1. Test the solution or the device that you are using and be sure that it is at the exact temperature that the doctor ordered or that the nurse instructed you to use. The following temperatures are guides only:
   a. Hot bath: 100° F.
   b. Warm bath: 95° F.
   c. Foot soak: 110° F.
   d. Hot wet dressing: 110° F.
   e. Heat lamp: 110° F.
   f. Hot-water bottle (water): 115° F.
2. Watch the patient's skin carefully for the excessive redness that may indicate that a burn is occurring.
3. Keep the application at the ordered temperature. If the solution cools, its effect on the patient will be the opposite of the one that is desired; that is, the blood vessels will narrow instead of dilate.
4. Keep the patient warm during the treatment. Since all the blood vessels in the affected area dilate (widen) when heat is applied to a part of the body, the patient will have more blood going to the surface of his body and therefore more blood being cooled. He is thus very likely to become chilled easily.
5. Apply heat for the specified time.
6. Keep the treated part warm after the heat application is removed in order to continue the effects of the treatment for as long as possible.
7. Put the patient in a comfortable position so that he will be able to continue the treatment for as long as it is ordered. Be sure that the position is a safe one. Avoid accidents such as those in which the patient falls or the soak spills.
8. Reheat the soak by first removing the patient's limb and then adding the hot water required to bring the solution temperature up to 110° F. or to the temperature ordered.
9. Reheat the hot bath by first removing the patient and then adding the hot water required to bring the temperature up to 100° F. or to the temperature ordered by the doctor.
10. Give a heat application only when the doctor prescribes it and the nurse instructs you to give it.

GIVING THE PATIENT A HOT-WATER BOTTLE

The head nurse or team leader will direct you to apply a hot-water bottle to a specific part of the patient's body. The hospital has probably established the temperature they consider to be the safe one to use for the water in hot-water bottles. Ask the head nurse what this temperature is (temperature usually used is 115° F.). Then prepare the hot-water bottle. You will need the following:

1. Hot-water bottle
2. Pitcher
3. Bath thermometer
4. Flannel cover for the hot-water bottle
5. Towel

Fill the pitcher with water heated to the ordered temperature. Use a temperature of 115° F. if a specific temperature is not specified. Test the temperature of the water with a bath thermometer. Pour the water, which is usually at the temperature of 115° F., into the hot-water bottle until it is about one-third full. Then place the hot-water bottle down on a flat surface and permit the water in it to flow near the top, thus expelling the air. This makes the hot-water bottle flatter and more manageable on the body surface. Put the top on the bottle and wipe off any spilled water. Enclose the bottle in the cover.

Take the hot-water bottle to the patient and apply it to the body area specified by the nurse. Be sure to test the hot-water bottle for leaks by squeezing the bottle and observing the top before you apply it to the patient. It is extremely important for you to remember to fill the hot-water bottle only one-third full. The weight of a full bottle would increase the patient's pain and the bulk would cause it to keep falling off his body.

Return to the patient in 15 minutes and check his skin for excessive redness and burning. Report any evidence of a burn to the nurse at once. Many lawsuits directed against hospitals are brought by patients who were burned by heat treatments.

Refill the hot-water bottle as often as necessary to keep it at the desired temperature. This will probably be at least every hour.

An easier and safer way to apply heat to a body part is by using the Aquamatic K-Pad. The Aquamatic K-Pad is a closed heat supplying system, and it consists of a hot water-bottle–like pad that is connected to an electrically heated water reservoir by two tubes. The advantages of this method of supplying heat to a patient are as follows:

1. The temperature desired is set with a key and is maintained constantly throughout the entire treatment.
2. The temperature setting is that one prescribed by the physician.

To operate the Aquamatic K-Pad simply follow these instructions:

1. Fill reservoir with distilled water.
2. Plug unit into AC circuit.
3. Set desired temperature with key.
4. Turn on. Refill reservoir to cap level. Replace cap, but loosen one-fourth turn.
5. Check periodically.
   a. Refill with distilled water.
   b. Identify that temperature setting is the desired one.

GIVING THE PATIENT A SITZ BATH

The head nurse or team leader may tell you to give the patient a sitz bath. She will also tell you the correct temperature for the bath and the duration of the treatment. The usual temperature of the sitz bath is 110° F. Use this one if you have no other directions. A sitz bath is one in which the patient sits in a tub of water one-sixth full in order to apply a warm soak to the rectal area. It is frequently ordered by the doctor for those patients who have had hemorrhoids removed (hemorrhoidectomy) or the rectum removed (abdominoperineal resection).

The sitz bath can be given in a special sitz tub, in the usual bathtub, or even in any basin large enough for the patient to sit in. It is usually given in the bathroom. However, if it is given in a large basin, it may be done in the patient's room. You can give the patient a sitz bath in the following way.

Collect the necessary equipment, which includes the following:
1. Bath thermometer
2. Bath blanket
3. Two towels, one to dry the patient and the other for him to sit on in the tub
4. Bathtub cleaning equipment such as a disinfectant, a can of cleanser, some cleaning cloths, and a brush
5. Basin, armchair, and footstool (if the sitz bath is to be given in a large basin)

Take the equipment to the bathroom and fill the tub with 6 to 8 inches of water at 110° F., or at the temperature specified by the nurse. Go to the patient. Assist him out of bed and into a wheelchair. Take him to the bathroom. Help him to undress and assist him into the bathtub or sitz tub. Drape the bath blanket around his shoulders to keep him warm.

When a basin is used, half fill it with water at the correct temperature. Place it with the other equipment on a movable table and take it to the patient's bedside. Place the basin of water on an armchair. Assist the patient out of bed; then help him step on a footstool, turn around, and sit down in the basin of water. Support the patient's feet on the footstool and cover his entire body with the bath blanket. Instruct the patient to support himself on the arms of the chair and on the footstool to stabilize his position. Tell him not to get up without your assistance.

Continue the treatment as directed, usually for about 20 or 30 minutes. Check the temperature of the water after 10 minutes. If it is 5° or more below the treatment temperature, remove the patient from the tub and add enough hot water to raise the bath temperature to the desired one. Check the patient frequently for any signs of weakness, dizziness, or shock. Remove the patient from the sitz bath at once if any such signs occur. Wrap him in the bath blanket, sit him in the wheelchair, and return him to bed promptly, even if the treatment time is not yet up.

At the end of the treatment, assist the patient out of the tub and help him to dry and dress. Help him into the wheelchair and return him to bed. Make him comfortable, and then return to the bathroom. Discard the bath blanket and the used towels in the linen hamper. Pour about a quart of disinfecting solution into the tub. Use the brush to wash the bottom and sides of the tub thoroughly with this disinfectant (germ killer). Drain out the disinfectant. Scour the tub with the cleanser and rinse it well. Now the tub will be ready for the next patient.

When the patient has the sitz bath in a large basin, clean the basin by autoclaving it for 20 minutes at 250° F. and then by scouring it and rinsing it well. If an autoclave is not available, disinfecting solution can be used.

Check with the pharmacy to determine what disinfecting solution you can use in your hospital.

GIVING THE PATIENT A MEDICATED BATH

The head nurse or team leader may tell you to give the patient a medicated bath. She will instruct you as to the temperature of the water (usually 100° F.) and the duration of the treatment (usually from 20 to 30 minutes). She will also prepare and add the medications to the bath water. The most commonly used medicated baths are prepared in the following way:
1. *Starch bath.* One pound of cornstarch is mixed with about 4 ounces of cold water. A quart of boiling water is

added to the mixture. The mixture is boiled until it is thick and then it is added to the water in the bathtub.

2. *Oatmeal bath.* Two or three cups of oatmeal are cooked in the usual way. The oatmeal is then poured into a double layer of gauze that is about a foot square. The ends of the square are brought together and tied securely. This oatmeal bag is then used as a washing sponge.
3. *Saline bath.* One pound of table salt is added to every 6 gallons of water in the tub.
4. *Sulfur bath.* A sulfur compound ordered specifically by the doctor is added to the bath.

These baths are given in much the same way as the sitz bath. However, they differ in that the tub must be about two-thirds full of water. Since the purpose of these baths is to soothe the patient's irritated skin, no rubbing should be done during or after the bath. The patient's skin is patted dry. This patting not only lessens irritation, but it also permits a layer of the medication to remain on the skin and continue soothing it.

Clean the bathtub as you did after the sitz bath.

GIVING THE PATIENT AN ARM SOAK OR FOOT SOAK

The head nurse or team leader will tell you to give the patient an arm soak or a foot soak. She will also specify the temperature of the solution (usually 110° F.) and the duration of the treatment (from 20 to 30 minutes). The most frequently used solutions are saline (1 teaspoonful of table salt to 1 pint of water), potassium permanganate (at a strength of 1 to 5,000), and Epsom salts (magnesium sulfate, 1 tablespoonful to 1 gallon of water).

Prepare the patient's bed (if he is to have the soak in bed) by placing a rubber sheet on it. Collect the equipment, which consists of the following:

1. Arm basin or foot basin
2. Bath thermometer
3. Pitcher
4. Towels

For an arm soak, prepare the solution at 110° F. Ask the nurse to add any medication ordered by the doctor. Take the basin containing the solution to the patient's bedside. Place the basin on the bed on top of the rubber sheet. Position the patient's arm in the basin. When the patient is in a room or ward where there is a water supply, it is much easier to take the basin to the patient's bed and position it. Water can then be obtained in the pitcher (at the correct temperature) and added to the already positioned basin. When a sufficient supply of solution is in the basin, the patient's arm can be comfortably positioned in it. This method usually avoids spilling. However, if some solution is spilled, wipe it up off the rubber sheet at once.

The foot soak is done in the same way, except that the patient usually sits on the side of the bed and places his foot in the basin, which is positioned on a footstool at the side of the bed. Be sure to keep the patient warmly covered with a bath blanket during the arm soak or foot soak.

When the soak is completed, remove the limb from the basin and place it on a towel. Remove the basin from the bed or footstool and place it in a more convenient place where it is less likely to spill. If there is a sink in the patient's area, empty the basin. Pat the limb dry. Remember that it is painful. Then cover it well to keep it warm and return the patient to a comfortable position.

GIVING THE PATIENT CONTINUOUS WARM WET SOAKS

The head nurse or team leader will tell you to give the patient continuous warm wet soaks on dressings. She will also tell you what solution to use (usually saline solution or Epsom salt solution) and at what temperature (usually 110° F.) you are to use it. Collect the following equipment:

1. Flannel cloths long enough to cover the area to be soaked (If flannel cloths are not available, bath towels can be used.)
2. Bath or treatment blanket
3. Rubber or plastic sheet (large enough to enclose the entire body part to be treated)
4. Several strips of gauze bandage
5. Basin
6. Pitcher
7. Bath thermometer

In the utility room, prepare the solution at a temperature of 100° F. The nurse will add the medications to the solution. Place all the equipment and linens, as well as the basin of solution, on a movable table and take it to the patient's bedside.

Lift the limb to be soaked; place the bath blanket and then the rubber sheet under it. Dip the flannel cloths or bath towels in the solution. Wring them out well and place them on the limb in such a way so as to enclose it completely (Fig. 30-1). Next, wrap the rubber sheet and then the bath blanket around the limb and tie them securely in position with the gauze bandages.

The limb itself will give off heat and keep the wet dressing warm. Since wet dressings or wet soaks do not hold heat, it is necessary to wrap the bath blanket and the rubber sheet securely around the dressings to trap the body heat and prevent it from being lost into the air. It is unnecessary to apply such external heating devices as hot-water bottles or heating pads to these wet soaks.

Position the patient comfortably. Remove the table and the excess equipment to the utility room. Clean the solution basin and return it to the proper place.

Return to the patient's bedside every 2 hours. Dampen the flannel cloths or bath towels and rewrap the limb.

Continuous hot wet soaks to a flat surface of the body such as the chest or abdomen are somewhat more difficult to do.

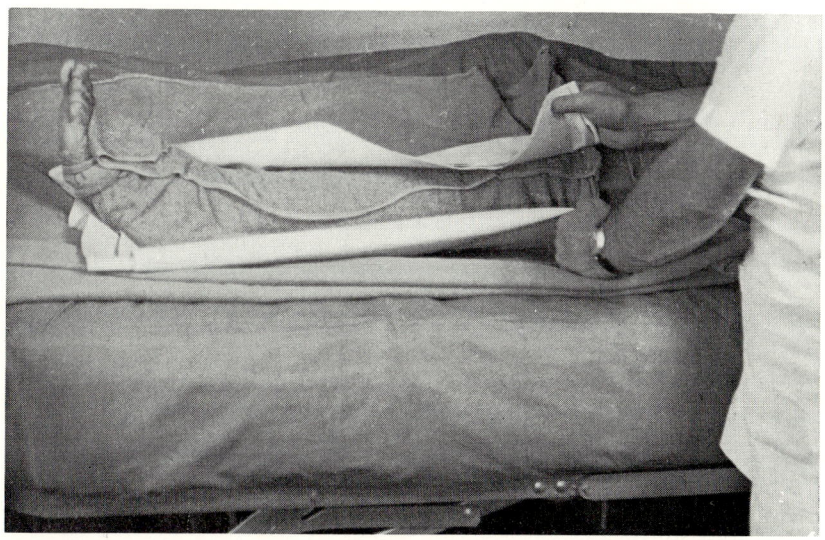

Fig. 30-1. Patient's leg enclosed in warm, wet towels. The nursing assistant is preparing to wrap the leg first in a rubber sheet and then in a bath blanket to trap the body heat in order to keep the towels warm.

However, the solution-dampened flannel cloth can be applied and covered with a small piece of rubber or plastic and held in place with a binder. This slows but does not stop the heat loss; therefore the doctor may order the application of a hot-water bottle or heating pad.

A hot-water bottle is applied only on the specific order of the doctor. Therefore do not apply a hot-water bottle unless the nurse instructs you to do so.

GIVING THE PATIENT HEAT APPLICATIONS WITH A LAMP

The head nurse or team leader will tell you to apply heat with a lamp. She will also tell you what lamp to use, what area of the body to treat, and how long to continue the treatment.

Collect the equipment, which will consist of the following:
1. Heat lamp
2. Bath blanket
3. Bath thermometer

Take the equipment to the patient's bedside. Position the patient comfortably and expose the area of the body that is to be treated with the heat lamp. Drape the bath blanket around the patient to keep the rest of his body warm. Position the lamp over the body part to be treated. Be sure that the lamp is at least 1 foot away from the patient's body. Test the amount of heat that the patient is receiving by placing a bath thermometer under the lamp on the patient's skin. If the thermometer registers a temperature greater than 110° F., raise the lamp until the heat that the patient is receiving is only 110° F. In order to prevent fires, do not cover the lamp, and keep bed linen and paper away from it.

After the treatment is completed, pat the body part dry. Then apply a skin lubricant or body oil and cover the patient well to prevent chilling.

Gentle heat can be applied to a denuded area (draining body part such as a decubitus ulcer or a skin graft site) safely and effectively with a small hand-type hair dryer. The same precautions necessary with the use of the heat lamp apply (Fig. 30-2).

ELEVATING THE LIMB IN THE PRESENCE OF INFECTION

The nurse will instruct you to elevate the limb and describe how you are to do it. Remember that elevating a limb means it is to be higher than the heart. The feet can be elevated by raising the foot of the bed,

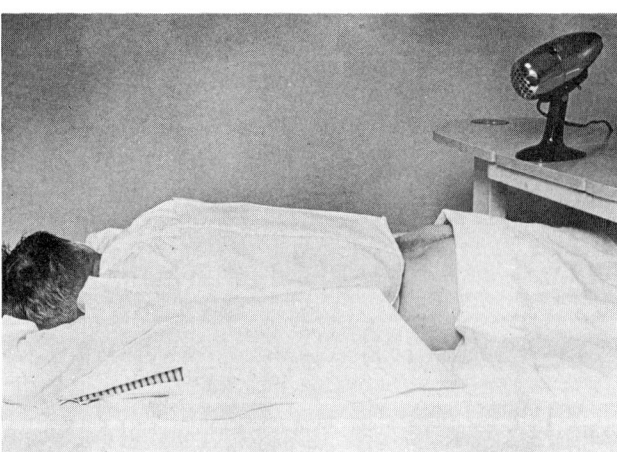

Fig. 30-2. Gentle drying heat is applied with a hair dryer to an oozing area.

by cranking up the bed frame to elevate the mattress, or by putting several firm pillows under the feet.

The arm can be elevated by placing several pillows under it, by placing it on a high table alongside the bed (overbed table can be positioned alongside the bed and cranked up), or by placing a glove on the hand and tying this glove to a treatment standard or intravenous pole. Visit the patient frequently and help him adjust to his position. If you fail to do this, he will move himself about and the elevated limb will soon be out of the correct position.

CARE OF THE PATIENT'S ENTIRE BODY IN THE PRESENCE OF INFECTION

Your treatment of the infected part will not be effective in helping the patient to get well unless you also give his whole body the care it needs. This means that you must visit the patient at mealtimes and encourage him to eat. It means also that you must bring him fluids each hour and encourage him to drink them. Keep an accurate record of his intake and output; the doctor will want to see it each day. Take the patient's vital signs frequently and promptly report any changes to the nurse.

SUMMARY

When an infection or injury occurs, the cells of the body notify the blood that they need help. The blood vessels widen and the blood supply to the part is increased. However, this blood supply is soon cut off because the blood gives the cells so much of its liquids that the blood becomes too thick to circulate easily. The injured part becomes hot, red, swollen, and painful.

External applications of heat correct this problem in the blood by dilating (widening) the blood vessels and speeding up the work of the cells, which is to fight germs and repair body damage.

Gravity will help the blood drain from the infected or injured part if the part is elevated above the level of the heart. As the stagnation of the blood in the veins of the infected part is corrected, the arteries can bring in more food-laden blood to help the infected body part.

Warmth assists the body but excessive heat damages it. Therefore the temperatures of all applications of heat to the body must be tested by a thermometer to be sure that they are safe. Applications of heat to a large surface of the body (for example, a bath) must be at a temperature not greater than 100° F. Applications of heat to a small area of the body may be at the higher temperature of 110° F.

Heat is applied to a patient's body only when a doctor orders such treatment and when the nurse directs its use.

DISCUSSION QUESTIONS

1 Did any of your patients have an elevated temperature today? Did you report it to the nurse?
2 Discuss with the nurse those patients who have elevated temperatures. Ask her what further patient observations you can make to help discover the site of the infection.
3 In the hospital in which you work, what is the temperature of the water used to fill hot-water bottles?
4 Are heat lamp treatments used for decubitus ulcers in the hospital in which you work? Why is the heat used?
5 Are intake and output recordings being kept on all your patients with fevers? Why?
6 Ask the nurse to demonstrate the procedure for continuous warm wet soaks or dressings.
7 What is the safe temperature for a medicated bath?
8 How do you elevate a leg?
9 Lie in bed with your leg elevated in the way you described in the answer to question 8. Is it comfortable? How can you make this position more comfortable?
10 Take a very warm bath. Remain in the tub for 30 minutes. How do you feel? Why?

VOCABULARY

disinfectant Chemical that kills germs.
hemorrhoidectomy Removal of the varicose veins in the rectum.
hemorrhoids Varicose veins of the rectum.
infection Invasion of the body by germs.
inflammation Reaction of the body to infection or

injury. It is characterized by redness, heat, pain, and swelling at the site.

sitz bath A warm soak to the rectum given by having the patient sit in a tub about one-sixth full of water. The temperature of the sitz bath is usually 110° F.

warm applications Applications to the body at a temperature above 92° F.

SOURCES OF ADDITIONAL INFORMATION

1 Film: Therapeutic uses of heat and cold; part 1: Administering hot applications; may be obtained from Public Health Service Audiovisual Facility, Chamblee, Ga. 3005, Attention: Film Distribution. *(Describes basis for and methods of applying heat to the body.)*

2 Film: The enemy bacteria; may be obtained from Public Health Service Audiovisual Facility also. *(Shows by animation the entry of bacteria and the resultant effects on the patient.)*

31/Reducing the patient's temperature

STUDY QUESTIONS

1. How does the body maintain a normal temperature on a hot day in summer and on a cold day in winter?
2. How much fever is too much?
3. At what temperature should fever-reducing techniques be started on the patient?
4. How is fever reduced?
5. What is a chill? What is the purpose of a chill?
6. Why is it dangerous to apply heat to the leg of a patient with arteriosclerosis?
7. Why are cold applications used on a sprained ankle or an injured eye?
8. How is an alcohol sponge bath given?
9. How is a cold wet pack given?
10. How do cold baths reduce body temperature?
11. What is the hypothermia-hyperthermia machine? How does it work?
12. How are cold applications used on the eye?
13. What is the danger from continuous cold applications?

HOW THE BRAIN CONTROLS BODY TEMPERATURE

The brain has a thermostat that regulates body temperature, and it does this in much the same way as you control the temperature in your home. When your home is too cold, you speed up the furnace to produce more heat; when it is too warm, you slow down the furnace and open the windows to get rid of the excess heat. The brain controls body temperature in a similar way. Heat is produced by the cells inside the body. These cells are insulated from the outside by the skin. Therefore when the body is too cold, the brain makes the cells work harder to produce more heat. The brain also retains this heat in the body by keeping the flow of blood to the skin at a minimum. On the other hand, when the body is too hot, the brain slows down the work of the body cells, and less heat is produced. The brain also gets rid of the excess heat by dilating the blood vessels in the skin and sending large amounts of blood to the surface of the body to be cooled. Therefore your skin is pale when you are too cold, and it is flushed or quite red when you are too warm.

FEVER

Fever occurs when the thermostat in the brain is set at a temperature above 98.6° F. Such resetting of the thermostat in the brain

can occur as a result of one of the following:
1. Invasion of the body by bacteria
2. Brain injury
3. Destruction of the body tissue (for example, by decubitus ulcers or an extensive burn)
4. Lack of fluid in the body
5. Altered operation of the brain due to drugs

The brain resets the thermostat and produces the fever in an attempt to help the body kill the bacteria or overcome the problem. The high temperature and the hard work of the cells kill the bacteria or speed up the decay and removal of the destroyed tissue. The thermostat, which is reset at a high temperature, prevents body cooling through perspiration and prevents further fluid loss at a time when the body is already too short of fluids (dehydrated).

In the injured or drugged brain, the thermostatic center is also injured or drugged and functions poorly. Therefore the fever that occurs in this case helps the body only in that it tells you that the brain is in trouble.

CHILLS

When bacteria enter the body, a nerve takes this message to the brain immediately. The brain suddenly resets its thermostat at a temperature high enough to make the cells work hard to try and kill the bacteria or overcome the problem they cause. Then the brain brings the body temperature up to this new level as follows:
1. The brain stimulates all the muscles of the body to work hard and produce more heat. The patient shivers, and the shivering muscles produce three or four times their usual amount of heat by this process.
2. The brain causes the blood vessels close to the surface of the body in the skin to narrow. Therefore the blood is not cooled and body heat is saved. The skin feels cold because of the limited blood supply to the surface of the body.

The process of bringing the body temperature up to a higher level is called a chill. As soon as the thermostat is set at a higher level, the patient feels cold. He shivers and shivers. When the high temperature is reached, the patient loses his feeling of chillness and feels comfortable, even though his temperature may be as high as 103° or 104° F.

EFFECT OF EXCESS HEAT ON THE BODY

Every time the body temperature goes up one degree, the cells of the body must work 7% harder. When the body temperature goes up ten degrees, the cells have to work 70% harder. Therefore the temperature level of the body at which cell damage occurs really depends on the condition of the body. If a patient has such a severe heart condition that his pulse rate is 120 weak beats per minute when his temperature is 98° F. and he is on complete bed rest, how will the pulse be able to speed up to a rate of 144 when his temperature goes up to 101° F? If the patient has such diseased lungs that he is cyanotic and short of breath when his temperature is 98.6° F., how will his lungs be able to work hard enough when his temperature goes up to 100° F.? These are the kinds of questions the doctor answers for himself when he decides what temperature is too high for a particular patient. Therefore the temperature that the doctor decides is too high and must be lowered may differ from patient to patient and depends more on the condition of the patient's body than on the actual temperature.

Generally speaking, however, the body temperature that is too high for everyone is 106° F. At temperatures of 106° F. and over, the body cells are unable to work hard enough to keep on living at this rapid pace, and they die. Therefore the amount of heat that is too much may be a matter of degrees, but it is more often a matter of what the condition of the patient's body is.

CONDITIONS IN WHICH SLIGHT ELEVATIONS IN TEMPERATURES ARE DANGEROUS TO THE PATIENT'S BODY

The patient whose body is weakened by disease or worn out by old age cannot tolerate even a slight elevation of temperature for very long because his body cells are already working at capacity to support life. Therefore when the temperature is elevated only a few degrees (101° F.), the old patient becomes weak, helpless, and confused. The patient with severe heart disease develops the rapid pulse, swelling feet, and blue lips characteristics of heart failure, whereas the patient with lung disease lies motionless in bed, using all his energy to breathe. Because of this, the doctor will prescribe fever-reducing treatments for these patients when they have a very slight fever.

Another patient whose body may be damaged by a slightly elevated temperature is the one who has a brain injury or has had brain surgery. Here the thermostat is injured or damaged and works poorly. Usually the damaged thermostat resets itself at a body temperature that is higher than normal, and this forces the injured brain to work harder in controlling and regulating body activities. However, the injured brain is unable to do the extra work required, and the patient soon lapses into unconsciousness with a slowing pulse and a falling respiratory rate as the temperature rises and death approaches. Therefore the doctor will maintain a close check on the temperature of patients with brain injuries or brain surgery, and as soon as the doctor observes that a fever is developing, he will prescribe fever-reducing treatments.

Since all patients suffer damage to the body when the temperature reaches or goes above 106° F., the doctor will prescribe fever-reducing treatments to keep the temperature from reaching this level in all patients.

CONDITIONS IN WHICH APPLICATIONS OF HEAT ARE DANGEROUS TO THE BODY

When the cells of a part of the body are already working at full capacity to do their job, more heat will cause difficulty. Therefore if heat is applied to an infected foot in which blood vessels are narrowed and rigid with old age or disease (arteriosclerosis), the cells of the foot will speed up their activities. However, the blood vessels will be unable to widen in order to bring in more blood carrying food and oxygen for these cells. The cells in the foot will soon die from starvation, and gangrene of the foot will occur.

It is interesting to note that the cells in the foot were living adequately with a poor blood supply and that their food supply became inadequate and death occurred only when living was speeded up by the application of heat. This may be compared to the way we are able to live adequately and comfortably on our salary until a family member becomes ill. Then the extra costs for medical attention, drugs, and special foods make our expenses so high that our salary becomes inadequate and we must go into debt. In the same way, the cells of the infected foot are forced to work harder without being able to get more food and oxygen because of the arteriosclerotic blood vessels. Soon they are in food and oxygen debt. When this debt continues for even so short a period as 2 or 3 hours, death of the cells may occur and gangrene will result.

Heat must also be avoided when an increased blood supply to the body part will cause damage. Examples of such situations include the following:

1. A blood vessel bursts and hemorrhage occurs. Heat applications would increase the blood supply to the body part and would therefore increase the bleeding.

2. An ankle is sprained. Heat applica-

tions to the recently sprained ankle will increase the blood supply, the tendency to bleed (if a blood vessel is injured or torn), and the amount of swelling.

3. An infection occurs, but it is unsafe to organize the body's fighting defenses at the site of the infection. For example, an infected appendix will be swollen and its walls will be taut. Heat will increase the blood supply to the appendix, and the taut walls may rupture. Another example might be an infected tooth. Swelling has already squeezed the nerves in the jaw and caused pain. Heat and an increased blood supply will cause more pressure and more pain. Therefore, in the two instances just described, the doctor will usually prescribe cold applications rather than hot ones. In the case of a sprained ankle, however, the doctor will usually prescribe cold applications for the first 24 hours, and then, when the danger of bleeding is over, he will prescribe heat.

HOW THE BODY COOLS ITSELF

You know that heat is lost from the skin. Therefore in the summer you expose as much of your skin to the air as is decently possible in order to increase heat loss, whereas, in the winter you keep as much of your skin covered as you can in order to conserve and retain body heat.

You know also that wind cools the body, so you avoid it in the winter, but you buy fans to make breezes in the summertime. You know, too, that water cools your body, so you wear boots to keep you feet dry and warm in the winter, and you go swimming to cool yourself in the summer. However, an understanding of how the skin, the wind, and the water cool the body will give you many clues as to how you can help to reduce a patient's fever. The skin cools the body as follows:

1. The skin gives off rays of heat to the cooler air around it. The greater the surface area of the body exposed to the air, the greater will be the loss of heat. However, when the air around the body reaches the same temperature as the body, no further heat loss will occur. When the temperature of the air is higher than that of the body, the body actually absorbs or picks up heat from the air. This explains why you are so uncomfortable on those hot summer days when the temperature of the air is higher than that of the skin (above 92° F.).

2. The skin gives off heat to objects in contact with the body. However, when an object reaches skin temperature, no further heat will be lost to it. This explains why you feel so chilled when you sit on a cold automobile seat (increased body heat loss) and why you again feel comfortable when the seat is finally warmed (no further heat loss occurs).

3. The skin cools the body through perspiration. Water absorbs more heat than air does. The body produces perspiration to take up its excess heat. The heated perspiration then passes from the surface of the body and into the air and removes body heat as it does so. However, on a humid day the air is loaded with water vapor; the air cannot take in any more water and so the perspiration remains on the body. Heat loss is therefore decreased. This explains why you feel so hot and uncomfortable on a humid day, even though the temperature is lower than the skin temperature of 92° F., and so very distressed on the humid days when the temperature is over 92° F.

At such times the brain regulates the body temperature by increasing or decreasing the heat-producing activities of the cells in the body and by increasing or decreasing the amount of blood sent to the skin for cooling.

REDUCING THE TEMPERATURE THAT IS TOO HIGH

The doctor will decide when the patient's temperature is too high, and he will prescribe the method to be used in reducing it. This prescription may include such techniques as exposure to air, increased air circulation, alcohol sponge bath, cold sponge bath, cool wet packs alone or with a fan, and application of ice by bath, pack, or icecap.

Exposing the patient's body to air

The head nurse or team leader will assign you to expose the patient's body to the air. You can do this by:
1. Removing all the patient's clothing
2. Covering his genital area with a hand towel
3. Turning the patient onto his side

In this way you expose the patient's entire skin surface (except for the side on which he is lying) to the air and permit it to give off heat. Air will be trapped under the side on which the patient is lying, and when this trapped air warms, no further heat loss will occur here. This is why you placed the patient in a side-lying position rather than a back-lying position, which would have left a larger area of the body surface unexposed.

Check the patient's temperature every 15 minutes to see if it is rising or falling. Keep the nurse informed.

Increasing the air circulation around the body

The head nurse or team leader will instruct you to increase the air circulation around the patient's body. You can do it by the following:
1. Exposing as much of the patient's skin surface as possible (described previously)
2. Turning on a fan in the patient's room and being sure that the fan is not blowing directly on the patient. This fan will move the heated air away from the patient's body and permit the cool air to move toward it. In this way the temperature of the air around the patient's body will always be lower than the body temperature, and the body will continue to give off heat to the cooler air.

Check the patient's temperature every 15 minutes. Keep the nurse informed of changes.

Giving an alcohol sponge bath

The nurse will assign you to give the patient an alcohol sponge bath and to report the results to her immediately. You can do this in the following way:
1. Collect the equipment, which consists of the following:
   a. Supply of alcohol, 1½ quarts per gallon of water or 3 quarts per gallon of water, as directed by the nurse (The amount if alcohol used depends on the strength of the alcohol.)
   b. Large bath basin
   c. Two washcloths
   d. Towel
   e. Large rubber sheet
   f. Two bath blankets
   g. Rectal thermometer, lubricant, and thermometer wipes
   h. Bottle of rubbing alcohol
   i. Hot-water bottle (if directed by the nurse)
2. Prepare the solution; use cool water from the faucet (60° F.) and add the alcohol.
3. Fill the hot-water bottle with water at a temperature of 115° F. *Note:* Use the hot-water bottle only if specifically directed to do so by the nurse.
4. Place the linen and the equipment on a movable table and take it to the patient's bedside.
5. Fanfold the top bedding to the foot of the bed and, at the same time, cover the patient with the bath blanket.
6. Remove the patient's hospital clothing, such as his gown or pajamas.
7. Turn the patient onto his side and

place the large rubber sheet covered by a bath blanket under him.
8. Place a hot-water bottle at the patient's feet if the nurse specifically directs you to do so. The hot water prevents frostbite of the feet from occurring by keeping the small blood vessels of the feet and toes dilated.
9. Check the patient's temperature, pulse, and respiration. Watch the pulse throughout this procedure by checking it every 5 minutes. If the patient's pulse becomes rapid and weak or if his lips turn blue, stop the alcohol sponge bath immediately. Cover the patient and get the nurse.
10. Sponge the patient in the following way:
    a. Expose the part.
    b. Sponge for half the designated time.
    c. Rub part briskly to increase blood supply to the part.
    d. Sponge for remaining half of designated time.
    e. Blot dry and cover (Fig. 31-1).
11. Rub the patient's back vigorously (after sponging it for 5 minutes) with a solution of alcohol. Then cover the patient with the bath blanket.
12. Check the patient's temperature rectally and report it to the nurse. The nurse may do any of the following:
    a. If the patient's temperature has gone up, she may ask you to give the patient another sponge bath.
    b. If the patient's temperature remains the same, she may ask you to give him another sponge bath.
    c. If the patient's temperature has dropped, she may ask you to check his temperature every 15 minutes for an hour.
13. Repeat the sponge bath if the nurse directs you to do so, and watch the patient's pulse and lips carefully.
14. If the sponge bath is not to be repeated, remove the bath blanket and rubber sheet under the patient. Remove the bath blanket over the patient and cover the patient loosely with a sheet folded in half. Leave the patient's arms, chest, and legs exposed to the air. Give the patient a drink of ice water if it is permitted. Make him comfortable. Collect your equipment and return it to the utility room. Clean the equipment and put it away. Remember that the patient probably has an infection from germs that have invaded his body. Therefore wash the rubber sheet well in hot soapy water, rinse it, and dry it. Wash and scour the basin well. Autoclave it if it is possible to do so or

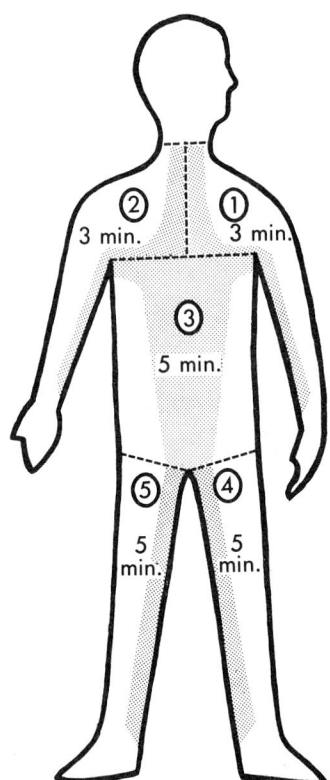

Fig. 31-1. Time and pattern of sponging body areas in the fever-reducing sponge bath.

rinse it out well with a disinfecting solution.
15. Return every 15 minutes and check the patient's temperature rectally. Report it to the nurse.
16. Give the patient fluids after you take his temperature. Chart these fluids on the intake and output record.

Friction is applied throughout the sponge bath to stimulate and increase the blood supply to the skin. Without stimulation, the blood vessels will narrow with the cold applications, and little blood will flow near enough to the skin to be cooled by the alcohol sponge bath.

Alcohol is used because it evaporates from the body at a lower temperature than water does. Therefore it will evaporate from the body quickly and will take heat away from the body at a rapid rate.

The alcohol sponge is a shock to the patient's hot body and will cause him to shiver. If this shivering continues, he will produce more heat than you can take away with the sponge, and he will develop a weak, rapid pulse and blue lips as his overworked heart fails. Therefore you should report to the nurse immediately if you observe any of the following signs:
1. Shivering that continues and becomes more severe
2. Rapid and weak pulse
3. Blue lips

The nurse will notify the doctor immediately, and he will give the patient a drug like promethazine hydrochloride or chlorpromazine hydrochloride to quiet the brain thermostat so that shivering will stop. Be sure that you leave as much of the patient's body as possible exposed to the air after the sponge bath is completed. This will permit the skin to go on giving off heat to the cool air around the body.

Giving a cold sponge bath

The head nurse or team leader will direct you to give the patient a cold sponge bath. You can do this in the same way that you give an alcohol sponge bath, except that you use plain cool water just as it comes from the faucet (temperature about 60° F.) instead of the alcohol and water mixture.

Applying cool wet packs

The head nurse or team leader will direct you to give cool wet packs. The procedure for giving such packs is as follows:
1. Collect the equipment, which includes the following:
   a. Large bath or foot basin or bucket
   b. Large rubber sheet
   c. Three linen sheets
   d. Hot-water bottle (if it is specifically ordered by the nurse)
   e. Two bath blankets
   f. Bottle of rubbing alcohol
   g. Rectal thermometer, lubricant and thermometer wipes
   h. Four ice caps
2. Half fill the basin or bucket with water at a temperature of 60° F.
3. Place all the equipment on a movable table and take it to the patient's bedside.
4. Prepare the patient as follows:
   a. Fanfold the top bedding to the foot of the bed as you cover the patient with a bath blanket.
   b. Turn the patient and put a large rubber sheet covered with a bath blanket under him.
5. Check the patient's vital signs and record them on a sheet of paper as follows: 2:30 P.M.: TPR—104.6-132-44.
6. Dip one of the sheets in the cool water, wring it out, and place it under the patient.
7. Return the patient to a back-lying position.
8. Dip another sheet in the cool water, wring it out, and place it over the patient. (Remove the bath blanket as you place the wet sheet on.)

9. Place the hot-water bottle at the patient's feet (if specifically ordered to do so).
10. Place the four ice caps in the axillary and inguinal (groin) areas.
11. Change the wet sheets every 5 minutes as follows:
    a. Dip the third sheet in the water and wring it out.
    b. Turn the patient.
    c. Remove the wet but warmed sheet under the patient.
    d. Place the cool, wet sheet under the patient.
    e. Return the patient to a back-lying position.
    f. Dip and wring out the sheet you just removed from the patient.
    g. Remove the warmed sheet on top of the patient.
    h. Replace the warmed sheet with the cool, wet sheet.
12. Watch the patient's pulse and lips carefully. If the pulse becomes weak or the lips turn blue, stop the treatment. Remove the wet sheets, cover the patient with the dry bath blanket, and summon the nurse.
13. Continue the treatment for 20 minutes if no complications occur.
14. Check the patient's temperature rectally. Report it to the nurse and ask for further directions.
15. Discontinue the treatment at the end of 20 minutes unless the nurse directs you to do otherwise.
16. Remove the wet sheets, rubber sheets, ice caps, and hot-water bottle.
17. Rub the patient's back briskly with alcohol.
18. Cover the patient with a sheet folded in half. Leave his arms, chest, and legs exposed to continue the heat loss.
19. Check the patient's temperature (rectally) every 15 minutes and report it to the nurse. Give the patient a drink of ice water (if permitted) after you take his temperature.

Using the fan with the cool wet pack

If a fan is to be used with the cool wet pack, the nurse will so direct you. This treatment is accomplished by applying the cool wet pack as described previously. Then, instead of replacing the warmed sheets with cool, wet ones, turn on a fan in the patient's room. The fan will circulate the air and move the wet air away from the wet sheets and the dry air toward them. This will permit rapid evaporation of water and quick cooling to occur. Every 5 minutes you must sprinkle the sheets well with water to keep them wet.

Watch the patient's pulse and lips closely. If no complications occur, continue the treatment for 20 minutes. Then check the patient's temperature rectally. Proceed as directed by the nurse. If you have no further directions, proceed as follows:

1. Continue the treatment for 10 more minutes (total of 30 minutes) if the temperature is the same or higher than it was when you started.
2. Check the temperature at the end of the 30-minute period. If it is falling, discontinue the treatment. If it is the same or higher than it was when you started, contact the doctor or nurse and ask for further directions. Do as directed. Discontinue the treatment by removing the wet packs, rubbing the patient's back well with alcohol, and covering the patient with a dry sheet folded in half. Watch the patient's temperature carefully by checking it every 15 minutes. Report temperature changes to the nurse promptly.

Ice water sponge baths or packs

Occasionally you may be directed to give a sponge bath or pack with ice water. This sponge bath or pack is given in the same way as those described previously, except that the solution used will have ice added to it. However, this iced solution usually is ineffective in reducing the patient's temperature because it causes him to shiver violently. Therefore you should report the shivering to the nurse promptly so that medications can be given to stop it. Then the patient can be cooled because his shivering muscles will not be manufacturing heat.

Occasionally you may see someone, who does not really understand how alcohol cools, adding ice to alcohol sponges. This does more harm than good. Alcohol cools the body because it evaporates quickly and not because of its temperature. Cooling is increased not by putting ice in the alcohol but by leaving the alcohol on the skin (not drying it) and increasing the air circulation around the body with a fan.

Applying an ice cap

If you are directed by the nurse to apply an ice cap, proceed as follows:
1. Collect the following equipment:
   a. Pan of ice chunks
   b. Ice cap
   c. Ice cap cover
2. Fill the ice caps with chunks of ice over the sink or over a basin. Discard the unused ice.
3. Dry the ice cap.
4. Cover the ice cap with a flannel ice cap cover.
5. Take the covered ice cap to the patient and place it on that body surface indicated by the nurse.

Return and check the patient's skin under the ice cap frequently (at least every 30 minutes). Report any signs of extreme whiteness or blueness to the nurse. These signs would indicate that frostbite is occurring. Refill the ice cap at least every 2 hours. Remember that the body gives off heat to those objects in contact with it, and it will warm the ice cap until it becomes a hot-water bottle.

Frequently, as was mentioned previously, four ice caps may be applied to those parts of the body with a good blood supply when the temperature is being reduced. These are the inguinal (groin) and the axillary areas.

THE HYPOTHERMIA-HYPERTHERMIA MACHINE

The hypothermia-hyperthermia machine consists of an electrically driven cooler and heater and a pump that is connected by tubing to two hollow plastic or rubber blankets. The machine cools or warms a solution, which it then circulates through the hollow blankets. The machine also contains a mechanical brain and a mechanical nerve (temperature-taking device). When the hypothermia-hyperthermia machine is to be used, proceed as follows:
1. Collect the following equipment:
   a. Hypothermia-hyperthermia machine filled with special alcoholic fluid
   b. Thermometer probe to be connected to the mechanical brain on the machine
   c. Two bath blankets (to cover the thermia blankets)
   d. Sheet (to cover the thermia blanket-enclosed patient)
   e. Hot-water bottle if specifically ordered by the doctor
2. Take the equipment to the patient's bedside.
3. Lubricate the thermometer probe, insert it into the patient's rectum, and plug the opposite end into the mechanical brain on the machine.
4. Plug the machine into the electrical outlet. Then set the mechanical brain at the desired temperature for the patient and the machine controls at the upper and lower limits of heating and cooling permitted. Turn on the machine by pushing in the button labeled "automatic."
5. Fanfold the top covers to the bottom of the bed, cover the patient with a

bath blanket, and then remove all of his clothing.
6. Turn the patient onto his side and place a hypothermia-hyperthermia blanket covered by a bath blanket under the patient.
7. Return him to a back-lying position and place the second hypothermia-hyperthermia blanket over him on top of a bath blanket. The patient's toes and fingers are kept free of the cooling blankets because their tiny blood vessels may be shut off easily by the cold permitting frostbite to occur.
8. Then cover the bed by the sheet (Fig. 31-2).

The patient's temperature will be taken by the probe and will register on the dial on the mechanical brain. The brain on the machine sets the heater in motion to warm the fluid and the pump in motion to pump the heated fluid through the blanket if the patient's temperature falls below the desired level. Or it activates the cooler to lower the temperature of the fluid and the pump to circulate the cooled fluid through the blankets if the patient's temperature rises above the desired level. When the patient's temperature is at the desired level, the mechanical brain shuts off the machine.

The hypothermia-hyperthermia machine warms the body when it is cold and cools and takes heat away from the body when it is too warm.

To care for the patient in the hypothermia-hyperthermia machine, proceed as follows:

1. Observe for shivering. If shivering occurs, notify the nurse at once. She may give the patient promethazine hydrochloride or chlorpromazine hydrochloride to quiet the brain thermostat and control the shivering. If shivering is permitted to continue, the patient's temperature will not fall, and his overloaded heart will soon start to fail. This will be noted by the rising pulse rate and the cyanotic lips.
2. Check the machine-recorded temper-

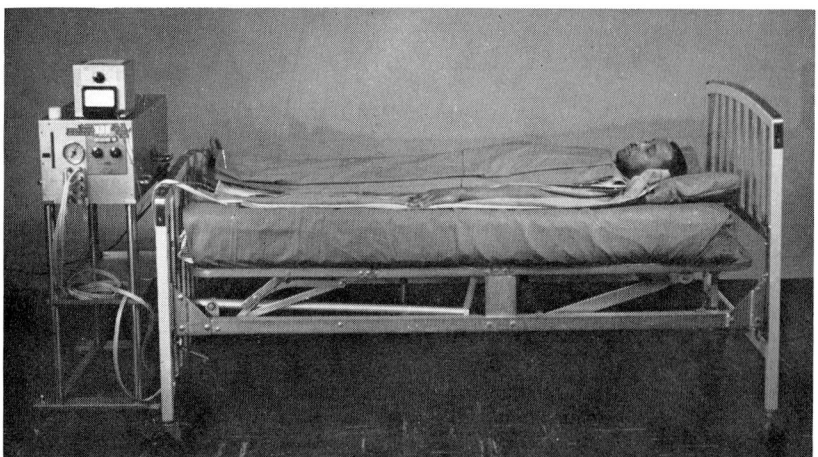

Fig. 31-2. The patient is enclosed in hypothermia-hyperthermia blankets. The bedclothes are folded back so that the hypothermia-hyperthermia blankets and the bath blankets covering them can be observed. Note the electrically driven cooler and heater (hypothermia-hyperthermia machine) at the foot of the bed. Note, too, the mechanical brain on the top of the machine that is connected to the patient by an electric rectal thermometer probe.

atures (those of the patient and the machine) every 15 minutes and also check the patient's pulse, respiration, and blood pressure every 15 minutes. Report to the nurse immediately any signs of heart failure, falling blood pressure, rising pulse, blueness of the lips, etc.
3. Check the patient's temperature rectally every 2 hours with a regular thermometer.
4. Replace the perspiration-soaked bath blankets under and over the patient with fresh, dry ones every 2 hours.
5. Give the patient as much fluid as he can take.
6. Turn the patient every 2 hours.
7. Clean the patient's mouth every 2 hours, since it is usually very dry.
8. Report any changes in the patient's condition to the nurse promptly.
9. Keep the patient's fingers and toes out from under the cooling blanket to avoid frostbite.

Use of the hypothermia-hyperthermia machine may be continued for as long as 3 days. However, the top blanket can usually be removed after the patient's temperature drops, and he can then be maintained at the lower temperature by the use of the one blanket under him. Be sure that the upper surface of the patient's body is left uncovered (except for a towel over the genital area) and exposed to the air so that it can continue to give off heat when the top blanket is removed.

EFFECT OF COLD APPLICATIONS TO THE BODY

The effects of cold on the body are exactly the opposite to those of heat. In other words:
1. The work in the cells is slowed down.
2. The blood supply to the body part is decreased because the blood vessels narrow. Therefore cold applications are applied to any part of the body that is injured and may bleed. The cold is applied to narrow the blood vessels and prevent hemorrhage. This is why cold applications are placed on an injured eye to keep it from getting black (ecchymosed from blood under the skin).

Cold applications are also indicated in patients with certain infections (for example, an infected appendix or abscessed tooth) to prevent swelling and the further damage that the swelling could cause. Therefore cold applications in the form of ice caps are frequently used after an operation in which bleeding is highly possible, after an injury (such as a blow to the eye or a sprained ankle) in which bleeding is possible, or in treating an infected area to prevent it from filling with blood and swelling.

Cold, in the form of cold compresses, is frequently applied to an inflamed (reddened) eye to reduce the blood flow to the eye and thereby reduce the bloodshot appearance and ease the pain caused by swelling. Compresses are applied as follows:
1. Collect the equipment, which includes:
    a. Four-inch-square compresses or eye pads
    b. Small basin (about 6 inches in diameter)
    c. Bath towel
    d. Paper bag
2. Place several large pieces of ice in the basin and add the prescribed solution, which is usually tap water, normal saline solution (1 teaspoonful of salt in 1 pint of water), or 2% boric acid solution.
3. Take the equipment to the patient's bedside.
4. Drape the patient with a bath towel.
5. Dip a compress in the solution, wring it out, and place it over the eye quickly.
6. Prepare the next compress. Remove

the one on the eye and replace it with the fresh cold one.
7. Repeat steps 5 and 6 for the duration of the treatment, usually from 15 to 30 minutes.
8. Use a fresh compress each time and discard the used one in a paper bag if the eye is infected. Use the same two compresses throughout the treatment if the eye is not infected.
9. Discontinue the treatment and make the patient comfortable.
10. Return the equipment to the utility room, clean it, and return it to its proper place.

EFFECTS OF EXCESSIVE OR PROLONGED COLD

Prolonged applications of cold or exposure to excessive cold causes death of the body cells. It does this by so narrowing the blood vessels that the blood supply to the body part is cut off. Then, even though the activities of the cells are slowed down, they die because they are unable to take in any food or oxygen and they cannot remove the waste material.

Therefore you must watch the body part receiving a cold application just as carefully as you watch the one receiving a hot application.

The hot application may produce a burn. Therefore you watch the body part carefully for the sign of burning—extreme redness. The cold application produces death of tissue from blood starvation, so you must watch for signs of this effect. Such signs include paleness, grayish white appearance, or cyanosis.

ROLE OF THE NURSING ASSISTANT

The nursing service in your hospital will determine those fever-reducing activities that you can do for patients. This determination must be made by the professional nurses who have diagnosed the patient's nursing needs and cannot be made without these clinical data. This book therefore does not attempt to identify activities that should or should not be included in your job description. It only attempts to teach those that are.

Check your job description and assignment. Perform accordingly.

SUMMARY

The brain controls body temperature by slowing down heat production and increasing heat loss when the body is too warm and speeding up heat production and slowing heat loss when the body is too cold. However, when bacteria invade the body or when the brain is injured, the brain thermostat is reset at a high temperature in an attempt to correct the problem. This new thermostat setting may produce a fever that will permanently injure the body, so the doctor orders fever-reducing treatments for the patient.

The body cools itself by sending large amounts of blood to the skin. The skin loses this heat by:
1. Giving it off to the air when the air is cooler than the body
2. Giving it off to cool objects in contact with the body until they are warmed to skin temperature
3. Giving off water (perspiration), which takes heat from the body and turns the perspiration into steam that passes off into the air as water vapor

The methods that the doctor prescribes make use of the preceding three principles of cooling. These methods are as follows:
1. Cold applications to the body
2. Movement of cool air around the body
3. Application of cool water or alcohol to the body

Cold applications slow down the workings of the body cells, and they also slow down the blood supply to the cells. Therefore continuous applications of cold or exposure to excessive cold may cause death of the tissue (gangrene).

DISCUSSION QUESTIONS

1 Why would you feel warmer after a cool shower on a hot day?
2 How does a fan help to cool your body?
3 How could you keep patients cool and comfortable on a hot summer day?
4 Observe the next patient who has a chill. Notice how his feeling of discomfort and coldness leaves him when his temperature is elevated to a high level. Why is this so? How could you make the patient who is having a chill comfortable? (Answers in terms of whether you would give him warm or cold applications.)
5 Why would you give a patient with a fever as much fluid as he could take?
6 What are the signs of frostbite?
7 Observe the mouth of each patient on the ward who has a fever? Why is it as it is? How can you correct this condition?
8 What would an increasing fever indicate in a patient with a brain injury?
9 Ask the nurse to demonstrate for you an alcohol sponge bath and a cold wet pack.
10 Why should patients wear hospital clothing that will permit them to expose their arms and legs to the air in the summertime?
11 How do you make the hospital beds in the winter? Do you make them the same way in the summer? If your answer is yes, explain.

VOCABULARY

alcohol sponge bath Sponge bath with a solution of alcohol and cool water. Alcohol evaporates from the body quickly and absorbs heat from the body in this process of evaporation.
brain thermostat Heat-regulating center in the brain.
chills Generalized muscular movement (shivering) to raise the body temperature to the new brain thermostat setting.
cold sponge bath Sponge bath with cool water. The body gives off heat to the cool water, and the patient's temperature is thereby reduced.
fever Elevation of body temperature above 98.6° F. orally, 99.6° F. rectally, or 97.6° F. axillary.
hyperthermia Temperature that is above normal. This term is usually used to indicate methods of applying increased warmth to the body in an attempt to raise body temperature.
hypothermia Temperature that is below normal. This term is usually used to indicate methods of cooling the body or reducing body temperature.

SOURCE OF ADDITIONAL INFORMATION

1 Film: Therapeutic uses of heat and cold; part 2: Administering cold applications; may be obtained from Public Health Service Audiovisual Facility, Chamblee, Ga. 30005. Attention: Film Distribution. *(Describes body response to and methods of applying cold.)*

32/Internal and external urinary drainage

STUDY QUESTIONS

1. What is catheterization?
2. Why is a patient catheterized?
3. What are some of the possible causes of difficulty in voiding?
4. Why does a postoperative patient frequently have difficulty voiding?
5. How does catheterization of the female patient differ from catheterization of the male patient?
6. How is a patient catheterized?
7. Why is catheterization a sterile procedure?
8. What is a catheter?
9. What are the dangers to the patient being catheterized?
10. What is a Foley catheter?
11. When is a Foley catheter used?
12. What is the procedure for disconnecting a catheter when the patient goes on an off-the-ward trip?
13. How is a urinary drainage tube connected?
14. Why is a catheter irrigated?
15. How is a catheter irrigated?
16. Why is it important to be sure that the irrigating solution returns?
17. What is an external urinary drainage set up?
18. Why is an external urinary drainage set up used more frequently than is the catheter?

THE PATIENT WITH A URINARY CONTROL PROBLEM

The patients with urinary control problems either have difficulty emptying their bladder (retention of urine) or difficulty in holding their urine until proper voiding facilities are obtained (incontinence of urine).

The patient with retention of urine (inability to empty the bladder) will need to have a catheter (tube) inserted into his bladder to remove the urine held there. This insertion of the drainage tube into the urinary bladder is called catheterization or internal urinary drainage. The procedure of catheterization is quite easy to do, and yet it is done only as a last resort after all other nursing measures to encourage the bladder to empty have failed. The reluctance to catheterize is based on the fact that each time a tube is put into the bladder germs are carried in with it. So the danger of infection arises each time that the patient is catheterized, and it exists for as long as the tube remains in the bladder (provides a freeway for germs to enter).

The patient with urinary incontinence needs a collecting device to catch and divert the urine flow into a urinal. This need can be met easily in the male patient by applying a condomlike attachment over the penis. The condom is connected to a tube that runs to a urine drainage bag attached to the side of the bed. This urine-catching device, which is applied over the penis, is called an external urinary drainage.

Since the external urinary drainage device goes over the penis and not into the bladder, it cannot carry germs into the body. Therefore it is safer than catheterizing the patient.

The external urinary drainage can be used only on male patients. The female patient who needs control of incontinence will need to be catheterized.

UNDERSTANDING THE URINARY SYSTEM

Urine is formed constantly by the kidneys from the waste material that they take from the blood. This urine is then sent down to the bladder through the ureters and is stored there normally. As the urine collects, the bladder muscles must stretch to enlarge the urine-holding capacity of the bladder. After 3 ounces of urine collects, there is sufficient stretch to the bladder muscles to stimulate them to send a message by way of a nerve to the brain that there is urine in the bladder. The brain then sends the bladder sphincter muscle (muscle at the entrance to the bladder) a message to keep tightly closed. The brain may activate the body to attain the proper facilities for voiding, or it may decide to wait until more urine is collected. Even though the brain is notified when there is as little as 3 ounces of urine stored, the bladder may hold as much as 8 ounces (½ pint) of urine quite easily and comfortably.

When the brain decides that it is necessary to empty the bladder, the brain activates the body to get the proper facilities. The brain then stimulates the bladder muscle to squeeze down to empty, and at the same time it notifies the bladder sphincter muscle to relax, so that urine flows to the outside of the body. This process reveals that there is a direct connection between the outside of the body and the blood. However, germs cannot get in (under ordinary circumstances) because the urine flows out and cleans the body tubes to the outside frequently. Therefore the entire system from the kidneys to the outside (including the urine) is sterile.

THE PATIENT WITH AN EXTERNAL URINARY DRAIN

Those male patients who may have an external urinary drain applied over their penis to collect the urine that is voided automatically include the following:

1. The patient who has a brain or nerve disease that prevents him from receiving or understanding the message from his bladder that it is full and from sending the message down to the bladder to hold his urine until the proper facilities can be obtained. Such a patient is usually incontinent because of the damage (caused by injury or disease) to the brain or spinal cord.

2. The patient who has weak-stiff bladder muscles. These muscles cannot stretch to enlarge the bladder enough to permit urine to collect there for at least 2 hours. Instead, the bladder remains small, urine cannot be stored, and so it dribbles out almost constantly. This deformity, like the others, is caused by muscle disease or disuse of the bladder-stretching muscles in the patient because of continual use of a retention catheter. Then when the catheter is removed the deformed bladder fails to function to hold urine.

APPLYING THE EXTERNAL URINARY DRAIN

You may use the external urinary drain to control the urinary incontinence of an unconscious, confused, or paralyzed patient. Avoid the assumption that this patient cannot or will not understand the procedure. Visit him. Explain what you are going to do and how it will help keep him dry and comfortable. Permit him to watch (if he is able) while you apply the drain. Try to eliminate fear or apprehension by your explanations and demonstration. This preparation of the patient may enable him to understand the value of the external urinary drain and the need to keep it on.

Check the patient's bed. Bathe him and change the bed linen if he is incontinent.

Collect the equipment needed to apply the external urinary drain. It consists of the following:
1. a. A Uro-Sheath (small, medium, or large) and a wide, rubber fitting device, *or*
   b. A condom, a 2-inch piece of rubber tubing and a narrow strip of adhesive tape—¾-inch wide strip of Elastoplast (adhesive elastic bandage)
2. Urinary drainage tubing.
3. Urinary collection bag and hanger.

Prepare the condom (if one is used) by attaching it to the tubing with a water-tight seal.
1. Put the small tube inside the condom. Unroll the condom over the tube. Hold the condom firmly around the tube. Wrap adhesive tape over the condom and around the side of the tube.
2. Cut condom to expose hole in rubber tubing.
3. Reverse condom and roll back over and away from the small rubber tube.
4. Fix the condom securely to the tube by wrapping the second piece of adhesive tape around the outside of the condom and over the tube.
5. Check the attachment of the condom to the tube. Pull on tube firmly (Fig. 32-1).

Take equipment to the patient's bedside. Fold in the bed clothing and expose the patient's penis. Place the Uro-Sheath or prepared condom over the penis and unroll it a few turns. Grasp the covered tip of the penis. Hold it firmly with one hand while you unroll the sheath or condom with the other. Fix the sheath in position by placing the rubber fitting device over it and around the penis. Button it (collar-type button in fitting device). Be sure that the button is on the top of the penis (urethra-urine outlet tube runs through the bottom of the penis and may be blocked by the pressure of the button) and that the fitting device is positioned as close to the body as possible.

Fix the prepared condom in position with the ¾-inch piece of Elastoplast (wrap it over the condom and around the penis in the same way as you do the rubber fitting device).

Apply the Elastoplast or rubber fitting device firmly but not tightly enough to cut off the circulation in the penis. Insert that end of the urinary drainage tubing with the connector into the rubber tube attached to the Uro-Sheath or prepared condom and the other into a urinary collection bag. Fix the bag to the side of the bed.

Caring for the patient with an external urinary drain

Visit the patient frequently and check the penis for swelling. Swelling indicates

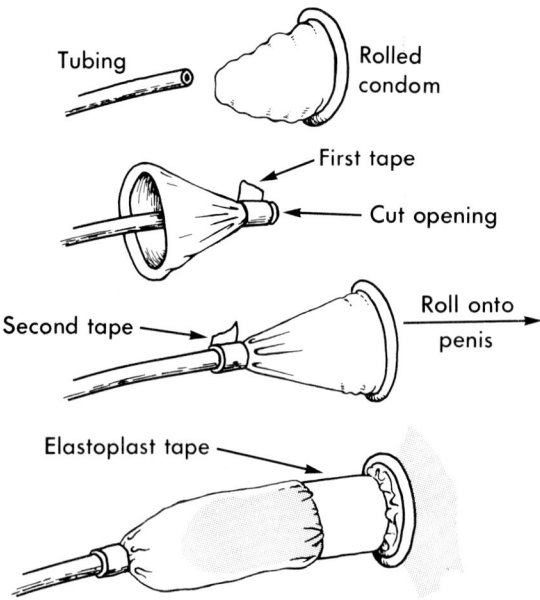

Fig. 32-1. An external urinary drain is made from a condom and a piece of rubber tubing.

that circulation is interrupted by the too tight application of the fixing rubber or Elastoplast. Loosen the fixing device if swelling occurs.

Remove the external urinary drain each day when you give the patient his bath. Bathe the penis well and powder it. Reapply the well-washed and dried external urinary drain in the same manner as was described previously.

The patient with an internal urinary drain

Those patients who may have a catheter (tube) inserted into the bladder to remove the urine stored there include the following:
1. The patient who has a nerve disease or nerve injury that makes it impossible for his body to send the message from the brain to the bladder to empty. Such patients are usually those who have back (spinal cord) injuries that paralyze them from the waist down (paraplegia) or from the neck down (quadriplegia).
2. The patient who has an injured bladder muscle that is unable to squeeze down and push the urine to the outside of the body. This usually occurs in those patients who have had operations in which the bladder was manipulated and pushed around.
3. The patient being prepared for surgery on or around the bladder. The surgeon will want the patient's bladder empty so that the operation can be done safely.
4. The patient having urine studies made. The catheter will be inserted into the bladder so that the specimens can be obtained at specified times.
5. The patient who has a disease blocking the tube that carries urine from the bladder to the outside of his body (urethra), such as occurs in male patients with disease of the prostate gland.

The patient who has a block in the urethra must be catheterized by the doctor because catheterization is usually such an extremely difficult procedure in this instance. However, the other patients just described may be catheterized by the nursing assistant if it is a procedure that is included in his job description and training program.

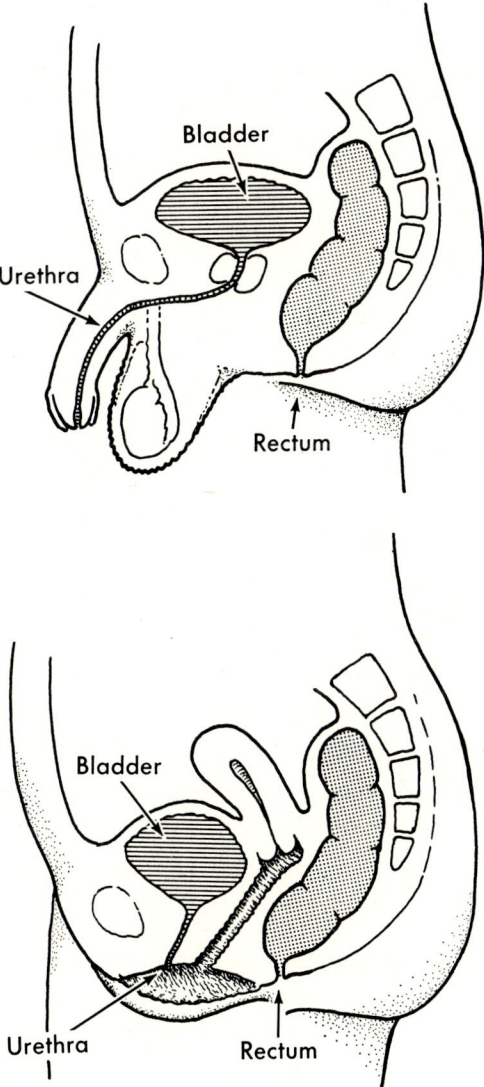

Fig. 32-2. Cross sections of the male pelvis and the female pelvis. Note that the male urethra is much longer than the female urethra.

THE APPROACH TO THE MALE AND FEMALE BLADDER FROM THE OUTSIDE OF THE BODY

The body structure that carries the urine from the bladder to the outside of the body is called the urethra. The urethra of the male patient differs greatly from that of the female (Fig. 32-2). Therefore the techniques of catheterizing a male patient differ from that of catheterizing a female patient.

Observation of the drawings in Fig. 32-2 reveals the following information:
1. The male urethra is longer than the female urethra.
   a. The male urethra is about 8 inches long.
   b. The female urethra is about 2 inches long.
2. The male urethra opens directly to the outside of the body, whereas the female urethra opens between the labia.
3. The male urethra is quite a distance away from the anus, but the female urethra is very near the anus.

These facts explain why the catheter must be inserted about 8 inches before it reaches the bladder in the male but only 2 inches in the female and why it is much easier to catheterize the male patient without contaminating the catheter than it is the female patient.

CATHETERIZING THE MALE PATIENT

Visit the patient and explain what you are going to do and why. This explanation must be thorough enough to enable the patient to understand the procedure and to eliminate any fears or apprehension that he may have about it.

The explanation must be given in a calm, quiet, but efficient manner so that the patient will have enough confidence in you that he can relax his muscles. Remember that fear and worry stimulate the patient's muscles to tighten (tense) and that if the muscles tighten, you will never be able to get the catheter into the bladder.

When the patient thoroughly understands the procedure and is no longer fearful of the pain that it may cause, you can leave his unit and collect your equipment. The standard equipment consists of the following:
1. Sterile disposable catheterization tray containing the following:
   a. Two solution basins
   b. Several gauze or cotton sponges
   c. Emesis basin
   d. Towel or drape
   e. Specimen container
2. Pair of sterile gloves
3. Tube of sterile lubricant
4. Sterile catheter, usually ranging from no. 16 to 26 (Robinson catheter)
5. Bath blanket, a small rubber sheet, and bath towel

If the catheter is to be kept in place in the bladder for a period of time (days or hours), a Foley catheterization tray is required. This tray differs from the one above in that it contains:
1. A retention catheter (Foley) instead of the Robinson catheter mentioned in item 4 above.
2. Equipment to inflate the rubber balloon at the end of the Foley catheter. This equipment may include:
   a. A 10-ml. syringe and a 20-gauge, 1½-inch needle or
   b. A 10-ml. syringe with a catheter adaptor
3. Connecting tip, urinary drainage tubing, and a drainage bottle
4. Jar of antiseptic solution (such as benzalkonium solution, 1 to 750 strength) containing a catheter plug

After the necessary equipment has been collected, prepare it for the catheterization as follows:
1. Place the tray on a movable table.
2. Place the bath blanket, rubber sheet, and bath towel on the bottom of the movable table.

Internal and external urinary drainage **289**

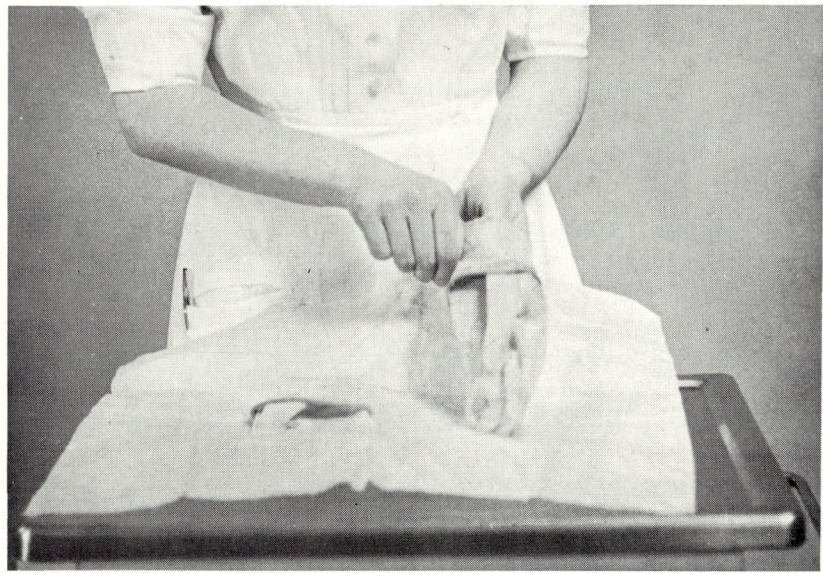

Fig. 32-3. The ungloved hand picks up and holds the sterile glove by the folded-down cuff (inside of the glove).

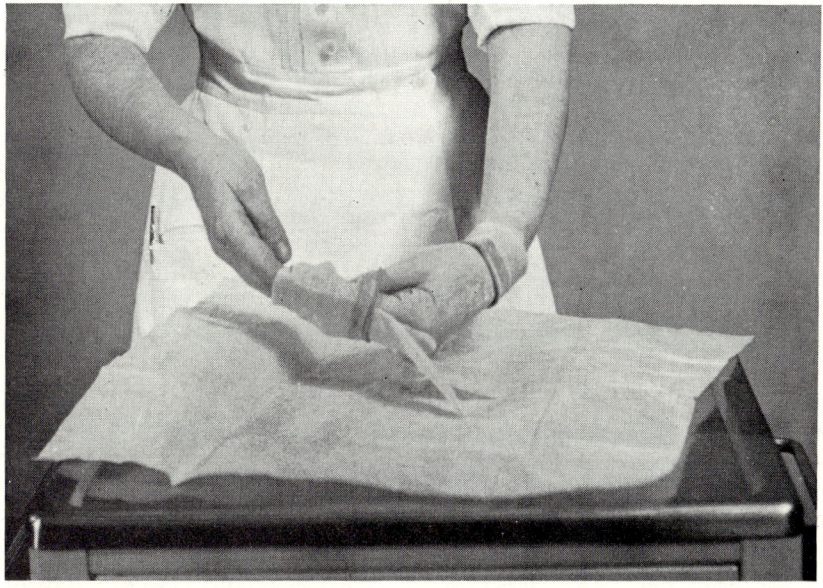

Fig. 32-4. The second glove is picked up and held by the gloved hand. Note that the gloved hand holds the glove under the folded-down cuff.

Take the movable table to the patient's bedside and prepare the patient as follows:
1. Fanfold the top covers to the foot of the bed while at the same time you cover the patient with the bath blanket.
2. Place the patient on his back. Ask him to bend his knees.
3. Place the small rubber sheet covered with the bath towel under the patient's hips. (Ask the patient to lift his hips if he is able to do so; if he is not able, roll him onto his side to position the bed protector.)
4. Expose the patient's penis but keep all the rest of his body covered. This can be done by pushing the bath blanket in from the side or by draping the patient in the same way as described previously for draping the female patient for a pelvic examination.

After the patient is prepared, wash your hands thoroughly, being sure to clean under the fingernails. Then proceed with the catheterization as follows:
1. Open the tray.
2. Pull the table as close to the patient's bedside as possible.
3. Put on the rubber gloves.
   a. Pick up the first glove by the folded-down cuff (avoid touching the outside of the glove).
   b. Hold the cuff firmly with the fingers of one hand while you slip the other hand into the glove (Fig. 32-3).
   c. Pick up the second glove with your gloved hand by placing your fingers *under* the cuff (Fig. 32-4).
   d. Hold the cuff firmly over your fingers and slip the ungloved hand into the glove.
   e. The rule for putting on gloves is this: *Never touch the outside of the glove with your bare hands.* The glove that is touched by bare hands has bacteria on it and is no longer sterile.
4. Grasp the penis with your left hand (stand at the patient's right side). Pull back the foreskin on the penis and hold it back.
5. Avoid touching the patient's body with your right gloved hand as you use it to complete the following steps of the procedure.
6. Dip a sponge in the soap solution and scrub off the end of the penis well. Discard the sponge and use another to repeat the cleansing procedure.
7. Dip a sponge in the saline solution or water and rinse off the end of the penis. Discard the sponge into the emesis basin and repeat this step.
8. Keep holding the penis with your left hand.
9. Reach for the towel on the tray with your right hand and place it under the penis.
10. Reach for the catheter on the tray and grasp it at least 8 inches from the tip. Do not touch the part of the catheter that is to be inserted inside the patient's body.
11. Dip the tip of the catheter into the lubricant.
12. Hold the penis erect with your left hand while you insert the catheter with your right (Fig. 32-5). This positioning straightens out the urethra.
13. Use gentle but steady pressure to insert the catheter. You may feel a slight resistance as you approach the bladder sphincter muscle, but gentle pressure will be sufficient to push the catheter past it. However, if you cannot insert the catheter with gentle pressure and you feel a firm resistance, stop and get the doctor or nurse. Never force the catheter. You may puncture the bladder if you do.
14. Insert the catheter until urine begins to flow (usually 7 to 8 inches).
15. Loosen your grasp on the penis and

Internal and external urinary drainage 291

position the emesis basin under the draining catheter.

16. Remove the catheter with one gentle tug when the urine stops draining or inflate the balloon on the Foley catheter by filling it with 5 ml. of water inserted through the balloon spout on the catheter.

17. Attach the urinary drainage tubing to the Foley (retention) catheter. Place the draining end of the tubing in a bottle or in a disposable urinary

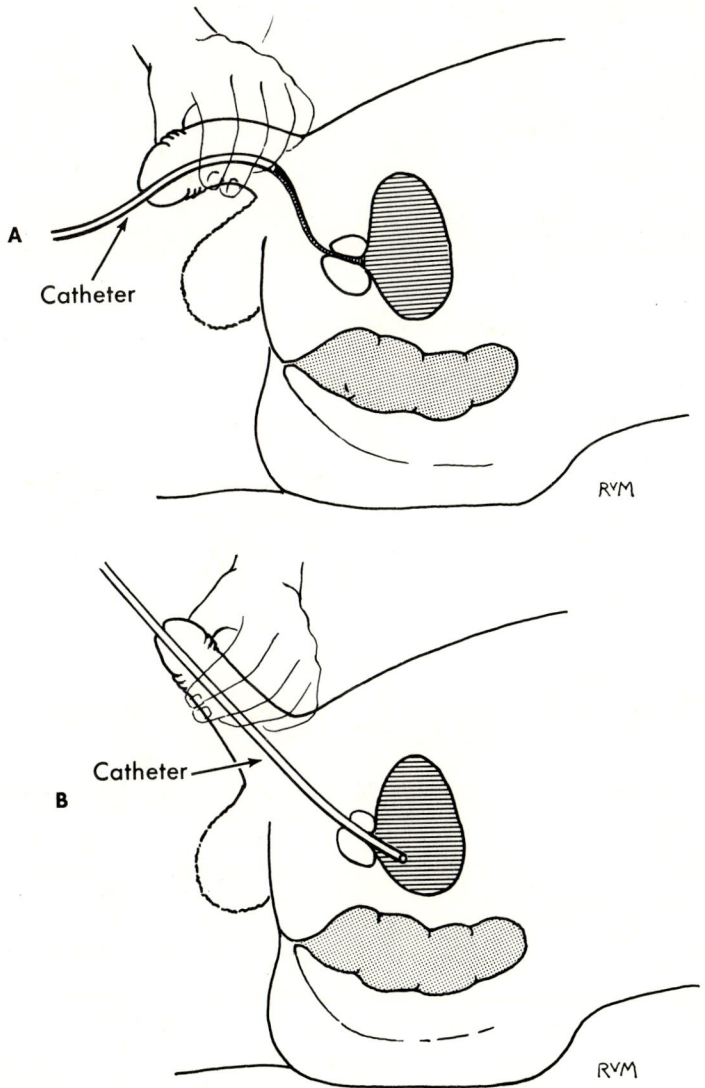

Fig. 32-5. A shows incorrect positioning of the penis for catheterization and the reasons for difficulty in inserting the catheter. **B** shows the penis held erect as the catheter is inserted. This position straightens the urethra and facilitates insertion of the catheter.

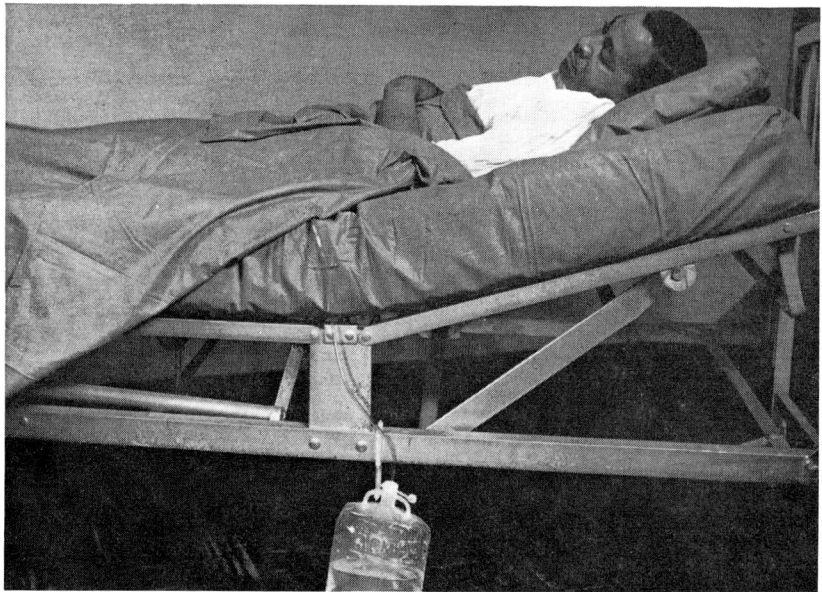

Fig. 32-6. Correctly positioned urinary drainage tubing. Note the safety pin on the bottom sheet at the side of the bed, which is maintaining the tubing in the correct position. Note that the urine runs downhill into the collecting bottle.

collection bag. Place the cap from the urinary tube in the jar of benzalkonium solution (1 to 750 strength).
18. Pull the foreskin back over the tip of the penis.
19. Remove the bed protector, position the patient comfortably, remove the bath or treatment blanket, and pull the top bedclothes into position over the patient.
20. Pin a safety pin to the bottom bed sheet at the side of the bed just above the drainage bottle and around the drainage tubing (Figs. 32-6 and 32-7). The pin holds the tubing in position above the drainage bottle and prevents urine seals from forming in the tubing.
21. Place the jar containing the catheter plug and tubing cap in the patient's bedside stand if a Foley catheter is left in place.
22. Take the used equipment to the utility room. Discard the used linen in the hamper. Discard the disposable tray.
23. Return in 30 minutes to check the patient to be sure of the following:
    a. That the urine is draining
    b. That the catheter is still in position
    c. That the foreskin is slipped over the tip of the penis (If the foreskin remains behind the top of the penis, it will cut off the blood supply to the penis and swelling will occur. If this swelling is not observed and relieved, gangrene of the penis will occur.)
24. Chart the patient's urinary output on the intake and output record. Chart the catheterization that you just did and the results that you obtained on the patient's chart in the nurse's record.

Internal and external urinary drainage 293

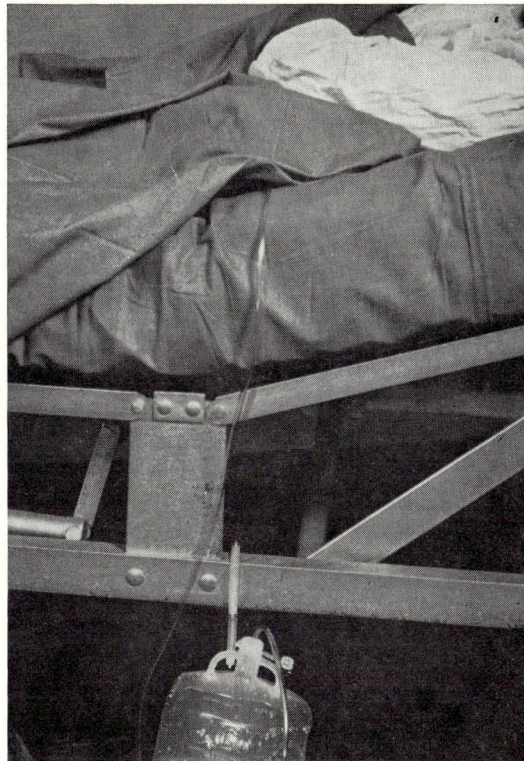

Fig. 32-7. Incorrectly positioned urinary drainage tubing. Note that the drainage tubing droops below the urine collection bottle. With the tubing in this position, the urine must run up a steep hill before it can get into the bottle. Of course, the urine cannot do this. Therefore, the incorrectly positioned tubing shuts off the flow of urine from the catheter.

CATHETERIZING THE FEMALE PATIENT

Both the equipment and the preparation for the catheterization of a female patient are the same as described previously for catheterization of the male patient. However, you will probably need a treatment lamp to give you some extra light. After the equipment is collected and the patient prepared, proceed with the catheterization as follows:

1. Separate the patient's vulva (lips of the vagina) with the thumb and index finger of your left hand. Keep your fingers positioned here.
2. Locate the opening to the vagina. Place a sponge halfway into it.
3. Look above the vaginal opening until you locate the urethral opening. This opening is a much smaller one than the vaginal opening.
4. Proceed to clean the area over the urethra well with a soapy sponge. Then rinse the area with the sponge soaked in saline solution or water.
5. Prepare the catheter (grasping it about 3 inches from the tip), lubricate it, and insert it into the bladder with a gentle steady pressure.
6. Continue the procedure as described for catheterization of the male patient.

A common error in catheterizing the female patient is to insert the catheter into the vagina. You can avoid this by:

1. Getting a good light so that you can see what you are doing.
2. Finding the vaginal opening first and inserting a sponge halfway into it. The sponge will keep you notified that this is not the right opening. However, if you do insert the catheter into the vagina, replace this catheter with a sterile one and start all over again. The vagina is not sterile as is the urethra.

THE DANGERS INVOLVED IN CATHETERIZING THE PATIENT

The following are the two dangers involved in catheterizing a patient:

1. The possibility of perforating (poking a hole through) the bladder with the catheter
2. The possibility of pushing germs into the bladder with or through the catheter

The danger of perforating the bladder can be eliminated if you learn to apply gentle pressure on the catheter when you are inserting it and to stop when and if you

294 Nursing assistant meets patient's particular needs

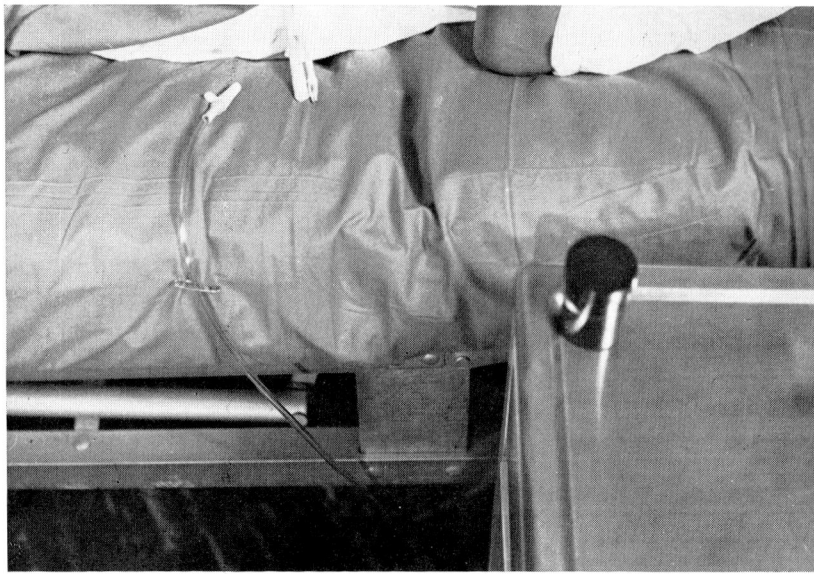

Fig. 32-8. The catheter is disconnected from the drainage tubing, and the ends of both tubes are kept sterile by plugging the catheter and capping the drainage tubing. Note the jar of benzalkonium solution used to hold the catheter plug and tubing cap.

meet resistance. No resistance can be overcome safely by exerting a great force. When the resistance is due to tightness of the muscle (for example, in a poorly prepared patient), the force will increase the irritation to the muscle and tighten it more. However, if the resistance is due to a block in the urethra, all the force can do is perforate the urethra.

The danger of infection can be minimized during catheterization if you clean the entrance to the urethra well, if you hold the catheter above the part going into the patient's body, and if you use the sterile equipment in the way described previously. However, the danger of infection will exist as long as the catheter is in the patient's bladder. Remember that the patient's urethra (passageway to the bladder) is kept open by the catheter. Therefore any time the catheter is disconnected from the drainage tubing, the germs have a wide-open tube from the outside of the body right into the bladder.

To prevent infection each time the cath-

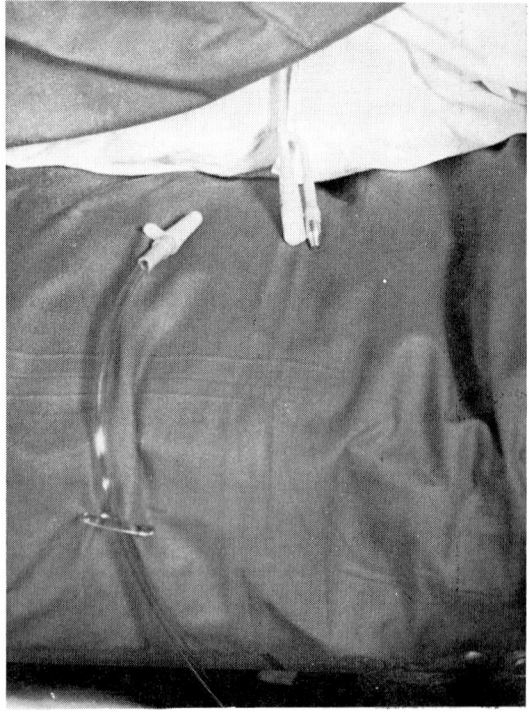

Fig. 32-9. Enlargement of view of capped tubing and plugged catheter.

eter is disconnected from the drainage tubing, the open end of the catheter and the top of the drainage tubing must be kept as sterile as possible. This can be done as follows:

1. Take the jar containing the catheter plug and the drainage tubing cap out of the patient's bedside stand.
2. Open the jar.
3. Disconnect the catheter from the tubing (Fig. 32-8). Hold both tubes (the catheter and the drainage tube) in your left hand.
4. Take the tubing cap and the catheter plug out of the jar.
5. Plug the catheter (Fig. 32-9).
6. Cap the drainage tubing (Fig. 32-9).

When the catheter is to be reconnected to the drainage tubing, simply remove the cap and plug and return them to the jar of benzalkonium solution. Then reconnect the catheter to the tubing. Clean and sterilize the benzalkonium jars weekly and refill them with fresh solution.

CATHETERIZE THE PATIENT ONLY AS A LAST RESORT

When the doctor has operated on the patient in the area around the bladder, the chart will contain an order to catheterize the patient after 8 to 12 hours if it is necessary (p.r.n.). Although it is quite easy to do (after you have had a little experience), catheterizing the patient must be avoided until all other means of helping him void have failed. Infection occurs so frequently after this procedure that a well-known surgeon once said he knows that the patient who develops a fever 3 days after an operation and 3 days after catheterization has this fever because of a bladder infection.

Methods that you can use to encourage the patient to void after an operation include the following:

1. Help the patient to relax. This is done by removing those factors that are making him tense. Find out what they are and, if possible, relieve them.
   a. If the patient has pain, notify the nurse. She will give him a medication to relieve it.
   b. If he is uncomfortable, make him comfortable. Change his position. If his mouth is dry, give him a drink. If he is cold, give him an extra blanket.
   c. If he is frightened and worried, sit down at the bedside until he is relaxed.
2. Gently massage the area over the bladder. This will increase the bladder pressures, and the brain will work with you on getting the bladder to empty. Be gentle.
3. Ask the patient to try to void while you turn on running water. The sound of running water sometimes stimulates the urge to void. If running water is not available, you may get the same effect by placing the patient's hands in a basin of warm water.
4. Elevate the patient's body. Gravity will cause the urine to press down harder on the bladder muscle. Sometimes the male patient will be helped to void by letting him sit on the side of the bed or by standing him on his feet at the side of the bed. However, you should do this only if the doctor or nurse so directs you.
5. Apply a hot-water bottle to the patient's body over the bladder area. This, too, is done only on specific directions from the doctor or nurse. The heat in the hot-water bottle sometimes soothes and relaxes the bladder muscle and permits voiding to occur.
6. Catheterize the patient only as a last resort and only on specific directions to do so from the doctor or nurse.

IRRIGATING THE CATHETER

The catheter is put into the bladder to drain out the urine. Therefore the catheter must be kept open and draining. The bladder (like the mouth, throat, and lungs) is lined with mucous membrane, and it secretes (makes) more mucus (similar to the mucus you spit up) when it is irritated by the retention catheter. This thick mucus will plug up the holes in the catheter unless it is washed out frequently. Therefore the doctor usually orders bladder irrigations to wash the mucus out of the tube.

Bladder irrigation is accomplished as follows:

1. Collect the following equipment:
   a. Sterile irrigating set consisting of an Asepto syringe, a bottle, and an emesis basin
   b. Flask of irrigating solution
2. Set up the equipment:
   a. Open the sterile irrigating set.
   b. Pour the irrigating solution (usually saline) into the bottle.
   c. Assemble the syringe by picking up the syringe barrel near the top, holding it, and picking up the rubber bulb (without touching the part that connects to the syringe). Moisten the tip that connects to the syringe in the sterile irrigating solution and attach the rubber bulb to the syringe barrel.
   d. Place the Asepto syringe in the bottle of irrigating solution.
3. Set up one irrigating bottle for each patient whose bladder is to be irrigated. (If several different irrigation solutions are used, label each irrigating bottle with the patient's name as you prepare it.)
4. Place the irrigating setup and the emesis basin on the movable table and take them to the patient's bedside (Fig. 32-10).
5. Fold back the patient's bedclothes to expose the area where the catheter is connected to the drainage tubing.
6. Get out the jar of benzalkonium solution containing the plug and cap. Open the jar and put it on the patient's bedside table.

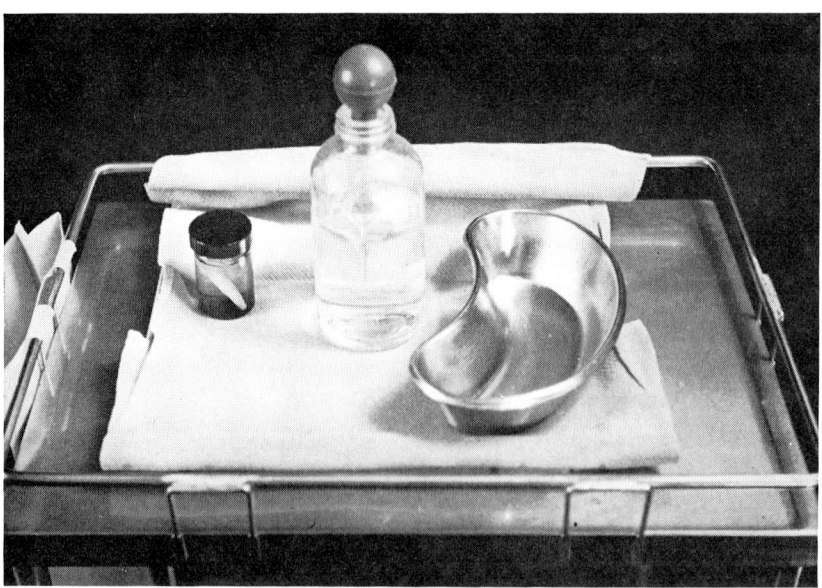

Fig. 32-10. The bladder irrigation setup.

Internal and external urinary drainage 297

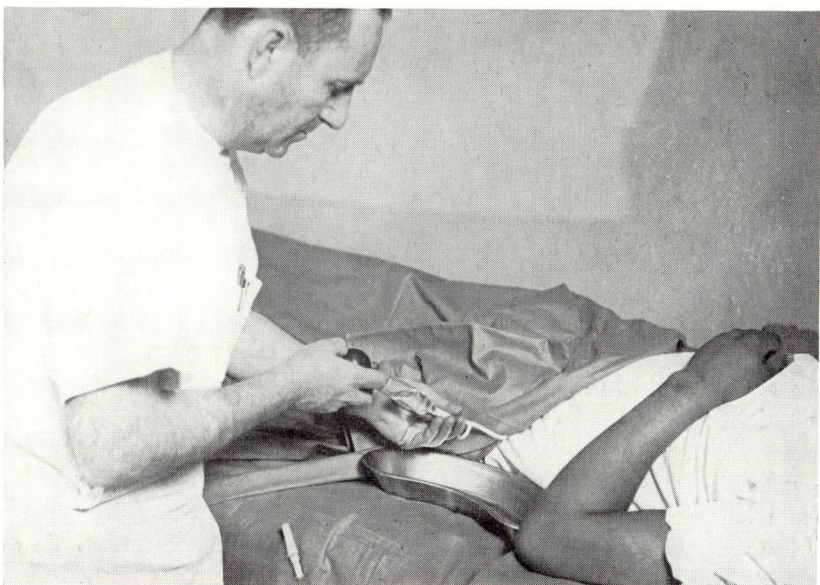

Fig. 32-11. The bulb is gently squeezed in order to inject the irrigating solution into the bladder. Note the capped urinary drainage tubing.

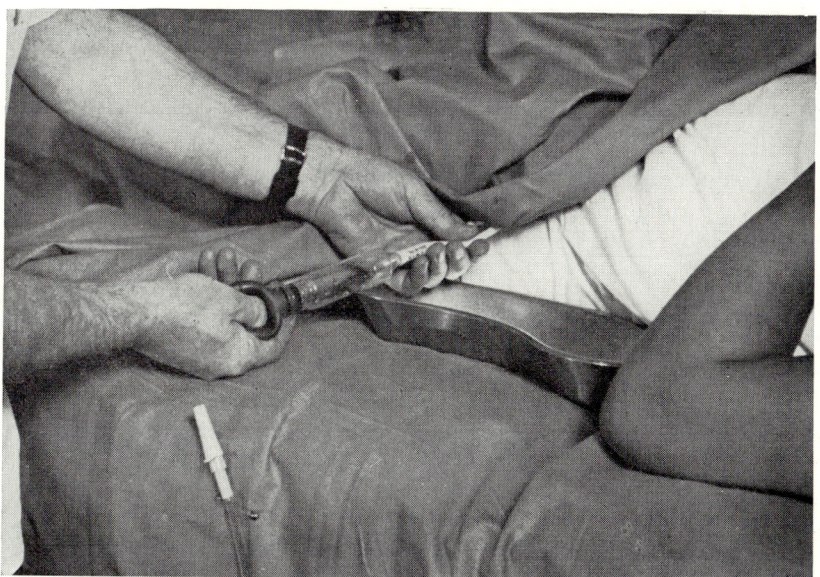

Fig. 32-12. Suction is applied to the catheter by reattaching the empty syringe with its bulb squeezed when the fluid does not return.

7. Disconnect the catheter from the drainage tubing. Hold both tubes in your left hand.
8. Remove the cap from the jar and place it on the drainage tubing. Put the drainage tubing down on the bed. (It will usually fall to the floor unless you tuck it under the patient's leg or under the safety pin.)
9. Continue to hold the catheter with your left hand.
10. Fill the irrigating syringe by squeezing the bulb.
11. Remove the irrigating syringe from the bottle, attach it to the catheter, and gently squeeze the bulb to inject the fluid into the bladder (Fig. 32-11).
12. Disconnect the syringe from the catheter (over the emesis basin) and hold the catheter over the basin with your left hand as you refill the syringe from the bottle with your right hand.
13. Observe the fluid returning through the catheter. If none returns, be sure that you are holding the catheter as close to the emesis basin as possible so that the urine can come out of the bladder by running downhill. If you do this and the fluid still does not return, empty the syringe and reattach it to the catheter with the bulb still squeezed (Fig. 32-12). This may create enough suction to pull out the blood or mucus blocking the catheter. However, if the fluid still does not return, fill the irrigating syringe with fluid once more and inject it into the bladder. Repeat the application of suction on the catheter with the use of the Asepto syringe with the bulb squeezed (Fig. 32-12). If the fluid still does not return, stop the procedure and summon the doctor or nurse.
14. Continue the irrigations (if the fluid returns) until the returned fluid is clear and free of mucous threads (long, white, stringlike pieces of mucus).
15. Stop the procedure anytime that the patient complains of pain, and summon the doctor or nurse immediately.
16. Complete the irrigation. Leave the sterile irrigating setup on the patient's bedside stand for further use. Collect the used irrigating set up from the patient's stand and put it and the used emesis basin on the bottom of the movable table.
17. Be sure that you reconnect the catheter to the drainage tubing and that you replace its cap in the jar of benzalkonium solution.
18. Make the patient comfortable.
19. Wash your hands.
20. Record your observations about the returned irrigation fluid on a paper so that you can chart it later.

Some of the reasons why the irrigating fluid may not return

Failure of the irrigating fluid to return indicates that something is wrong, and the doctor must inspect the catheter. A few of the possible causes for such failure are as follows:

1. The catheter may be plugged by a piece of mucus. This piece of mucus may act as a flap attached to the catheter near a hole. As the fluid enters the bladder, the flap is pushed away from the hole, but as the fluid tries to return, the flap is pushed back over the hole (much like a swinging door) and blocks the flow.
2. The catheter may be kinked in the bladder.
3. The catheter may have slipped out of the bladder.
4. The bladder may be perforated, so that the fluid that is inserted into the bladder runs out through the hole and into the abdomen.

Remember that any fluid you put into a hollow cavity like the rectum, the bladder, or the colostomy must come back. If it fails to return, notify the nurse immediately. The whereabouts of the fluid must be determined.

BLADDER EXERCISES

When a catheter is inserted into the patient's bladder, the bladder no longer can be used to store urine. Instead, the urine runs through the tube to the outside of the patient's body. Therefore the patient with a catheter will develop weak, stiff bladder muscles because of disuse, just as he would develop weak, stiff arm muscles if he kept his arm still for an extended period of time (for example, to receive an intravenous infusion). However, the arm muscles recover their use much more quickly than those of the bladder. After the catheter is removed, the weak, stiff bladder muscles will not stretch to hold the urine, and so the patient will dribble urine constantly. This can be prevented by bladder exercises. These exercises are ordered by the doctor and consist of the following.

1. *Bladder irrigations.* The bladder muscles are forced to stretch to hold the irrigating solution.
2. *Clamping the catheter.* The catheter is plugged for 2-hour periods throughout the day. During the periods when the catheter is plugged, the bladder muscles are stretched (exercised) by the urine stored there.

Bladder exercises such as irrigations or clamping the catheter are done only when the doctor or nurse directs you to do them. However, failing to do the exercises when they are ordered results in the patient's developing such weak bladder muscles that he is forced to have a catheter in place the rest of his life.

• • •

The nursing service in your hospital will determine the patient care activities that you can do to help them care for the patients safely. All, some, or none of the procedures included in this chapter may be in your job description. Check it carefully and perform accordingly.

This chapter attempted to teach the techniques for doing the procedures included here. It did not intend to identify these procedures as those that should or should not be done by nursing assistants.

SUMMARY

Bladder control problems either result in retention of urine or in urinary incontinence.

Urinary retention is relieved by catheterization. However, this procedure usually results in bladder infections so it is done only after all measures to encourage voiding fail. The retention catheter must be kept open and draining. This requires frequent sterile irrigations of the catheter.

The patient with urinary incontinence can be kept dry and comfortable with the use of an external urinary drain. This is safer than a catheter because it does not permit germs to enter the inside of the body. The external urinary drain can interfere with circulation in the penis if it is applied too tightly. This tourniquet-like action of the external urinary drain will result in swelling of the penis. Unrelieved swelling will progress to gangrene.

DISCUSSION QUESTIONS

1 Ask the head nurse to help you set up a catheterization tray.
2 What solutions are used in an irrigation setup? Why?
3 Observe the doctor catheterizing a patient. How did he prepare the skin area before he passed the catheter? Why did he do this?
4 What patients assigned to you have catheters in place? Why?
5 Why are catheters irrigated?
6 Observe the urinary drainage tubing connected to the catheters on the patients assigned to you. Are they correctly or incorrectly connected? How could you improve these urinary drainage tubes?

7 Why must the end of the catheter be kept sterile?
8 How can the end of the catheter be kept sterile?
9 What observations should you make on the postoperative patient in relation to his voiding?
10 What nursing measures could you use to encourage the patient to void?
11 Why is an external urinary drain safer than a catheter?
12 What is the care of a patient with an external urinary drain? Why?
13 Why do patients with indwelling catheters get elevated temperatures?

VOCABULARY

bladder That part of the body that stores the urine.

catheterization Insertion of a tube into the urinary bladder to remove the urine stored there.

Foley catheter Catheter that is inserted into the bladder and left there for a period of days or weeks. This type of catheter is frequently referred to as an indwelling or a retention catheter because it remains in the patient for a period of time. This catheter has a balloon on the inserted part and a connection to inflate this balloon on the other end. The purpose of the balloon is to prevent the Foley catheter from slipping out of the bladder.

irrigate To wash out by injecting a stream of water, saline solution, or an antiseptic solution.

penis Male organ that contains the urethra. The penis is also the male organ of copulation.

Robinson catheter Catheter that is inserted into the bladder to empty it and is then removed. It is a plain tube with several holes in the inserted end.

ureters Connections from the kidneys to the bladder.

urethra Connection from the bladder to the outside of the body.

urinary drainage tube Tube connected to the catheter and to a drainage bottle or a plastic bag attached to the bed frame. This arrangement permits the urine flowing out through the catheter to drain by gravity into the bottle or bag.

vagina That part of the body of a female that connects the outside of the body to the womb (uterus).

voiding Act of passing urine. This is also called urinating.

SOURCES OF ADDITIONAL INFORMATION

1 Film: Catheterizing the male patient; may be obtained from Director, Medical Film Library, United States Naval Medical School, National Naval Medical Center, Bethesda, Md. 20014.
2 Film: Work of the kidneys; may be obtained from Central Office Film Library, Veterans Administration, Vermont Ave. & H St., N. W., Washington, D. C. 20025. (*Describes the structure and function of the renal system.*)

THE NURSING ASSISTANT MEETS THE NEEDS OF SPECIAL PATIENTS IN THE HOSPITAL

SECTION IV

Chapter 33 Caring for the patient with a communicable disease
34 Caring for the patient in reverse isolation
35 Caring for the patient who is unable to cope with the problems in living
36 Caring for the preoperative patient
37 Caring for the postoperative patient
38 Caring for the patient who is breathless
39 Caring for the aged person with problems in living
40 Meeting the first-aid needs of the patient
41 Caring for the dying patient
42 Meeting the patient's need for comfort and safety on an off-ward trip
43 Assisting the patient to get ready to go home

33/Caring for the patient with a communicable disease

STUDY QUESTIONS

1. Why is the patient with a communicable disease isolated?
2. How is isolation accomplished in a busy hospital?
3. From what is the patient isolated?
4. What is the difference between isolation and solitary confinement?
5. How is an isolation unit set up?
6. Where is an isolation unit set up?
7. Are all communicable diseases spread in the same way?
8. How can you know what protective clothing to wear in caring for a patient with a communicable disease?
9. Why do you wear protective clothing when you care for a patient with a communicable disease?
10. How do you put on a gown?
11. How do you take off a gown?
12. How would you decontaminate an isolation unit after the patient is discharged?
13. How would you take a recovered patient out of isolation?
14. How would you protect the hospital staff when you take the isolation patient on an off-ward trip?

THE PATIENT IN ISOLATION

The patient with a communicable disease has the same needs and the same fears as any other sick person, but he differs in that he can give his illness to anyone who comes in close contact with him. Therefore the hospital puts him in a single room or in a closed-off section of the ward by himself. This arrangement is called isolation. The other hospital patients are prevented from coming in contact with the patient who has a communicable disease. The patient may give his disease to those hospital staff members who come in contact with him, so personnel caring for him have to use protective measures to prevent this from occurring.

The criminal who threatens our physical safety is isolated from the community by being put in jail, so the patient with a communicable disease who is a threat to public health is isolated from the hospital community by being kept in a hospital area by himself. However, the patient is different from the criminal in that he does not want to hurt people by giving them his disease. In fact, he does not want the disease himself. Hospital isolation also differs from confinement in jail in that the members of the nursing staff give the patient the same kind of good care that they give to other patients. Nursing personnel do not penalize or punish the patient who has a communicable disease. They recognize the loneliness and fear associated with being in isolation. The members of the nursing staff visit the patient frequently even when they have nothing to do for him, and they dilute his boredom and worry with their caring, their concern, and their presence.

If the nursing staff members are too busy or too frightened of "catching" the disease to visit the patient in isolation frequently, then the isolation really becomes a jail-like hospital sentence. The patient sentenced to this aloneness in a hospital room or sectioned-off part of the ward will become so frightened, so worried, and so lonely that he will be forced to come out of his isolated area and search for the companionship of another human being. Of course, when he comes out, he brings the danger of spreading his disease with him, and this usually causes all the members of the ward staff to become angry with the patient and to label him as uncooperative or difficult. However, the patient does not mean to be either of these. He comes out only to save his sanity by relieving his loneliness and the distortion of reality that it causes.

THE PROBLEM OF LONELINESS

The patient with a communicable disease must be kept separated from the other hospital patients. However, he does not need to be sentenced to absolute aloneness because of the nature of his illness. Your training will teach you how to use protective techniques that will permit you to stay well while you visit and care for the patient. However, you must have a clear understanding of the nature of communicable diseases, the way they are spread, and the adequacy of these protective techniques; otherwise, you will avoid the patient because of your own fear of "catching" the disease. This avoidance of the patient will condemn him to the worst punishment possible—solitary confinement. The only difference between isolation and solitary confinement for the patient is your caring presence.

Aloneness, particularly in the hospital, is frightening. Disturbing thoughts and worries creep into the patient's mind when he has nothing to occupy it. Soon his pains worsen, his fear of dying increases, and his imagination starts to play tricks on him. Soon he becomes disoriented and confused. He has imaginary visitors to talk or fight with, and he loses track of time and place. However, the patient may fight this loneliness by refusing to stay in his room or by ringing his bell constantly for you to come in.

You can understand the emotional distress associated with isolation if you just think about how you feel when your family goes out and leaves you home alone. Better still, think about how you felt when your family went away and left you alone for a few days and nights. Remember how loud the clock ticked at night and how many strange and frightening night sounds you heard to keep you awake and a little uneasy. Remember, too, how your thoughts spilled out and how you soon found that you were even talking to yourself.

The patient has the same experiences you have had when you were left alone. He hears the footsteps in the hall as people pass his door. He wonders why they do not stop. He imagines that you do not care about him, or that you believe he is going to die anyway so you do not want to waste your time on him, or that you know he has a disease much more horrible than he was told. He lies in bed, and these festering thoughts increase. Soon the patient is forced to come out of his room to escape from them, or he is forced to go off into a dreamworld where he rejects the thoughts by imagining he is at home. The patient will not need to come out of his room and spread his germs nor will he need to live in an imaginary dreamworld if you dilute the loneliness of isolation with your caring presence.

THE NATURE OF COMMUNICABLE DISEASE

So that you can care for the patient in isolation rather than condemn him to solitary confinement in the hospital, it is necessary for you to understand the nature of communicable disease and how to protect yourself from getting it.

Illness is caused by any disturbance in the functioning of the body that does not permit the patient to live comfortably. This disturbance may be due to many different causes, a few of which are as follows:

1. Toxic substances, such as alcohol, lead, or cigarettes
2. Injuries, such as broken legs or fractured skulls
3. Wearing out of body parts, such as heart disease or old age with its senility
4. Stress and strain of living, such as the fear and worry that cause mental illness
5. New growths, such as benign tumors or cancers
6. Improper food or the lack of food, as in vitamin deficiencies

Disease or illness resulting from the causative factors just listed cannot be spread from patient to patient, so these diseases are classified as noncommunicable, and isolation or protective techniques are not a required part of patient care. There is another cause of disease, however, that does make isolation and protective techniques an essential part of patient care. This cause is germs. The diseases that develop when the patient's body is invaded by germs are called communicable diseases because anyone who comes in contact with these germs may get the disease. In other words, the disease travels from the patient to any person who picks up a supply of germs from the patient. Therefore the hospital staff members who care for patients with communicable diseases must do the following three things:

1. Keep the germ-carrying patients with communicable diseases away from all other patients
2. Keep the germ-laden equipment (such as linen, thermometers, and trays) that was used in the care of patients with communicable diseases away from all other patients and the staff members until the germs on the equipment are killed
3. Set up protective techniques to prevent hospital workers from getting disease from the germ-carrying patients

The members of the hospital staff can do these three things by practicing the following procedures:

1. Putting the germ-carrying patient in isolation
2. Decontaminating (killing the germs on) everything that leaves the patient's room
3. Developing a technique of caring for the patient in isolation that prevents the germs from contaminating the workers and from getting out of the patient's area and being circulated about the hospital

GERMS

Germs are small living organisms that cause disease. The germs are too small to be seen by the naked eye, but they can easily be seen in the laboratory through a microscope. It would be a valuable experience to visit the laboratory and see the germs from a specimen taken from one of your patients who has a communicable disease. Once you do this, you can accept the fact that germs are present in the patient (even if you cannot see them with your naked eye), and you become more conscientious in carrying out the proper isolation technique. You will then be able to see the germs with your "mind's eye."

Since germs are small living organisms, they can do all the things you can. They eat, they move, they give off waste material, they reproduce (multiply), and they do all these things in the patient's body. These germs travel around in the patient's body, but they also leave his body in his excretions or in the drainage from a wound. When they do, they travel from the patient to other people, who then become infected with the disease.

In order to know how to protect yourself from the patient's disease, you must know how the germ leaves the patient's body, how it travels, and how it enters your body. Then you can protect yourself simply by preventing the germ from traveling and by blocking its entrance into your body.

PROTECTION OF THE NURSING ASSISTANT

The most important protective measure against contracting the patient's disease is to maintain your body in such a good state of health that your body is able to resist the disease. This means that your body is so strong and healthy that it is able to fight and kill the germs that invade it. Health practices that build up body resistance are the following:

1. *Eating a well-balanced diet.* This includes starting off the day with a good breakfast. Some people jump out of bed, gulp down a cup of coffee, and rush off to work. All morning they force their body machinery to do its hardest work of the day, even though it does not have the food in it to provide the energy to do the work. Then they come home at night, eat a big meal, and sit motionless, watching television. An automobile would absolutely refuse to work under these conditions. The body, too, soon has difficulty with this eating pattern.

2. *Getting enough sleep* (usually 8 hours). Sleep enables the body to rest and regain its ability to function effectively the next day.

3. *Meeting today's problems today.* This involves taking care of today and its problems so that you can start tomorrow with an eager, welcoming manner—free from the fears and worries and burdens of festering unsolved or unsettled issues. If problems are not solved on a daily basis, they accumulate and build up until the individual has so many problems that he feels it is worthless to get out of bed and face the new but miserable day. There is nothing that wears out the human body and lowers its resistance to disease as much as worry does. The way to avoid worry is to settle the problems of the day on the day that they occur and then forget about them.

4. *Enjoying life.* Recreation actually re-creates our ability to enjoy and appreciate the joys in living. Life without fun soon becomes full of problems and worries. This not only makes us a dull person, but it also lowers our resistance and increases our susceptibility to disease.

5. *Having a good friend.* A friend shares our joys and makes them worthwhile, but more important, he shares our problems. This sharing helps to dilute and minimize the problems so that they soon disappear.

Now think about the last time you contracted a cold. How did you lower your body resistance to the point where you were unable to fight off the germs so that you succumbed to the disease? Were you overburdened with fears or worries? Did you eat or sleep poorly? Were you bored and discouraged? You will probably discover that you developed the cold after a period of worry over bills or after a period of staying up late with a sick child or perhaps after a weekend of overeating, overdrinking, and undersleeping.

You are protected from communicable disease by other measures also. Some of these are as follows:

1. *Acquired immunity.* Some of the acquired immunities that you may have are those against poliomyelitis, smallpox and diphtheria. You may have acquired these immunities by receiving injections of germs that cause the disease when the germs were dead or too weak to cause it. After

you received the injection, your body notified your blood that it was invaded by germs. The blood immediately manufactured antibodies ("soldiers") to kill the germs. You still have a supply of these "soldiers" standing by in your body. If your body is invaded by the disease-producing germs that you are immunized against, the antibodies will attack and kill the germs immediately, and you will not get the disease.

2. *Natural immunity.* In this type of immunity, your body has developed antibodies that are now standing by just in case your body is invaded again by the germ that they have learned to fight and kill. However, this natural immunity was obtained by actually having the disease. Therefore once you have diseases such as measles, mumps, chickenpox, scarlet fever, or whooping cough you will probably never have them again.

3. *The skin.* The skin covering the body prevents germs from invading your body. However, when there are breaks in the skin, the germs may enter the body through the break. It is extremely important for you to take good care of your hands and to avoid chafing (cracks in the skin), nicks, cuts, and bruises.

4. *Body secretions.* The fluid in the eye as well as the secretions in the nose and throat wash away the germs that ride on dust particles and attempt to invade the body in these areas. The eye waters and washes out the eyes, and the sneeze or cough reflex is stimulated and clears out the nose and throat.

Even though you may have all the protective measures just listed, you may contract disease under the following circumstances:
1. If an excessively large number of germs (to which you have no specific immunity) enter your body
2. If your body resistance has been lowered
3. If repeated contact with the disease has permitted a large number of germs to accumulate in your body

There is no specific immunity for such diseases as tuberculosis, hepatitis, staphylococcal infections, and many others. Therefore the hospital must isolate the germ-carrying patient, and it must instruct you in the use of the proper protective technique to keep the patient's germs from entering your body. You must learn these techniques well, and you must use them each time you care for the patient with a communicable disease.

PROTECTIVE TECHNIQUES THAT PREVENT THE SPREAD OF COMMUNICABLE DISEASES

Although the patient with a communicable disease is isolated in the hospital, he is still cared for by the doctors, nurses, and nursing assistants. So they can care for the patient and at the same time protect themselves from contracting the disease, the medical and nursing personnel must use special protective techniques that are called isolation techniques. All isolation technique is not the same. It differs from disease to disease. The way that isolation technique should be carried out when you care for a patient depends on:
1. The location of the germs in the patient's body
2. How the germs leave the patient's body
3. How the germs travel from the patient to the hospital staff member
4. How the germs enter the body of the hospital staff member
5. How the port of entry in the hospital staff member can be blocked so that the germs cannot enter his body and make him sick

You will need to know these facts about the germs that infect your patient before you can safely protect yourself.

The nurse will give you these facts when she assigns you to care for the patient. The facts about a few of the most common com-

Table 33-1. Facts about some common communicable diseases

	Respiratory diseases (colds, pneumonia, tuberculosis, etc.)	Gastrointestinal diseases (hepatitis, dysentery, typhoid)	Staphylococcal infections (infected, pus-draining wounds)
Germs are:	In sputum	In saliva, in urine, and in feces in (hepatitis, also in blood)	In nose, in throat, in urine, in feces, and in pus
Germs leave the patient:	In sputum when patient coughs, sneezes, or expectorates (spits)	In saliva, in urine, in feces (in hepatitis infections, also in blood)	In sputum when patient coughs, sneezes, or expectorates; in urine, in feces, in wound drainage
Germs travel:	In spray from cough and sneeze; in air currents; on articles touched by patient's sputum; on unclean hands of hospital staff member who touched some sputum-contaminated article	On articles touched by patient's saliva, urine, and feces; on unclean hands of hospital staff member who touched some article contaminated by saliva, feces, or urine of patient; with hepatitis; also on articles that came in contact with patient's blood	In spray from patient's cough and sneeze; in air currents; on articles touched by patient's sputum, feces, urine, and/or pus; on unclean hands of hospital staff members who touched some articles contaminated with sputum, feces, urine, and/or pus
Germs get into your body:	Through your nose and throat when you breathe in patient's cough or sneeze; when you bring articles sprayed by patient's sputum up to your nose and mouth; when you touch your nose and mouth with your unwashed hands that have handled articles sprayed by patient's sputum	Through your mouth when you bring articles sprayed with patient's saliva, urine, and feces in contact with it; when you bring your unwashed hands to your mouth after they have been handling articles sprayed by feces, urine, or saliva from patient (germs from patient with hepatitis can also enter your body through breaks in your skin)	Through your mouth and nose when you breathe in patient's cough or sneeze or germ-full air currents; through a break in your skin that permits pus and germs to enter; through your nose and mouth when you bring articles sprayed by patient's sputum, feces, urine, or pus up to your face; when you touch your face with your unwashed hands that have handled articles sprayed by patient's sputum, pus, feces, or urine

municable diseases encountered in hospitals are found in Tables 33-1 and 33-2.

The information given in Tables 33-1 and 33-2 helps you to understand how to prevent the patient's germs from entering your body, but that is not enough to prevent the spread of a communicable disease. You must also prevent the germs from leaving the patient's room and spreading to the other hospital patients. Think for a few minutes about the many items that come out of the patient's room laden

Table 33-2. Facts about protection for common communicable diseases

	Respiratory isolation	Enteric precautions	Wound and skin precautions	Strict isolation
Protective Techniques that block entry of germs into your body:	Wear mask when entering room; wash hands on entering and leaving room	Wear gown and gloves; wash hands on entering and leaving room	Wear gown and gloves; wash hands on entering and leaving room	Wear gown, mask, and gloves; wash hands upon entering and leaving room

with germs. These items must be decontaminated (germs on them killed) immediately or they will carry germs to other hospital patients and workers.

Remember, too, that the patients and the hospital workers depend on you to decontaminate all germ-laden equipment and make it safe for them to handle or to label it contaminated so that they will know that they must use precaution in handling it. The kitchen maid who washes the dishes will not know that they are contaminated and need special handling unless you specifically label them as such. The laundry worker will not know that the linen came from a patient with a communicable disease unless you so specify. The central service personnel will depend on you to decontaminate all the equipment that you return to them, so they will take no special care in handling it.

In order to carry out the procedures that will prevent the spread of disease from the patient to you and to the other hospital staff members or to patients, the nurse will need to set up an isolation unit. This isolation unit should contain the following:

1. Protective devices that you will need to prevent germs from entering your body
2. Covered receptacles to receive all the contaminated material leaving the patient's room
3. Proper handwashing facilities
4. The best toilet facilities available (The patient's isolation unit should have private toilet facilities, or, when this is not possible, the isolation unit should be set up as close as possible to a utility room containing equipment for cleaning bedpans and urinals.)

THE ISOLATION UNIT

The isolation unit can be set up quite simply in a single room that contains running water and private bathroom facilities. However, when a room with a private bathroom and running water is not available, the isolation unit should be set up in an area of the ward as close as possible to running water and equipment for cleaning bedpans and urinals.

Set up the single room in the following way:

1. Collect the equipment which consists of the following:
   a. Isolation cart containing:
      (1) Protective clothing—gowns, masks, gloves.
      (2) Bags—plastic (to line and waterproof linen hamper and trash can).
         Bags—paper (to enclose patient articles that are to be decontaminated).
      (3) Linen hamper with cover (labeled *isolation linen*). Line with plastic bag.
      (4) Trash can with cover. Line with plastic bag.
   b. Patient care equipment and material:

(1) Bath and mouth care utensils (disposal set most desirable).
(2) Toilet equipment (bedpan, urinal).
(3) Solutions (mouthwash and massage lotion).
(4) Water utensils (pitcher and glass).
  c. Sign—*Isolation* or *Protection*.
  d. Thermometer and container:
(1) Half fill oral thermometer container with mouthwash, *or*
(2) Half fill rectal thermometer container with a disinfecting solution such as benzalkonium chloride solution 1:750 (1 part benzalkonium to 750 parts of water) or pHisoHex solution.
2. Prepare the patient area as follows:
  a. Place the patient care equipment in the patient's bedside table.
  b. Fill the patient's pitcher with ice water.
  c. Place the thermometer and thermometer container in the patient area on the bedside stand, or attach them to his bed, or place them in the patient's bathroom area.
  d. Position the isolation cart in the hall.
  e. Place an adequate supply of paper towels in the towel container over the patient's sink and ample soap in the soap dispenser; if the sink in the patient's room or bathroom does not have a soap dispenser and a closed towel rack, place an ample supply of soap and towels on the isolation cart.
3. Don a mask if the patient is on respiratory precautions or a gown and gloves if he has hepatitis, and move the patient into the prepared room.
4. Make the patient comfortable; explain to him what isolation means. Explain, too, that you will be caring for him but that you will need to wear this protective clothing when you do. Also explain the safety measures that he will be asked to carry out, such as covering his mouth and nose when he coughs or wearing a mask when he leaves the ward.
5. Stay with the patient until his apprehension subsides. Answer his questions. Assure him that you will visit him frequently to give the care he needs.
6. Remove your protective clothing (technique for doing this is outlined on pp. 314-315). Wash your hands.
7. Position the isolation cart in the corridor outside the patient's room. Screen it off from the patient's coughing, etc. if you need to position it inside his room.
8. If the patient is not placed in a single room, screen off that section of the ward in which he is placed and proceed to set up the unit as decribed previously. However, it is imperative that the unit be set up as close as possible to running water so that hospital personnel can wash their hands safely. The technique of putting a basin of water on a table and using it for washing the hands is unsafe. Antiseptics, too, are unsatisfactory because they dry out the skin on the hands and cause it to crack.
9. Label the area with the isolation or protection sign.

WEARING PROTECTIVE CLOTHING

You must wear protective clothing each time you come in contact with the germs that the patient is carrying. Indications for wearing such clothing are as follows:

In the patient on respiratory precautions:
1. You should wear a mask each time you enter the patient's room.

In the patient on enteric precautions:
1. You should wear a gown and gloves each time you have direct contact

(touching) with the patient or with any article contaminated with fecal material.
2. You can enter the room without a gown and gloves if you are visiting the patient or picking up a tray. However, if you are giving or taking away a bedpan or urinal you will need to wear the gown and gloves.

In the patient on wound and skin precautions:
1. You should wear a gown, mask, and gloves when you have direct contact (touching) with the patient.
2. You can enter the room to deliver things without wearing the gown, mask, and gloves, but when you give the patient personal care, they must be worn.

In the patient on strict isolation:
1. You must wear the gown, mask, and gloves each time you enter the patient's room. In this instance the patient has a constant flow of germs from the infected area into the room. Air currents will soon make the room too dangerous for you to enter it safely without protective clothing.

GETTING READY TO CARE FOR THE PATIENT IN ISOLATION

When the nurse assigns you to care for a patient in isolation, listen to the assignment carefully. Then review the isolation and precaution directions posted on the door of patient's room (Figs. 33-1 to 33-4). Since it is almost impossible to remember which precautions apply to any one pa-

---

Strict Isolation
Visitors—Report to Nurses' Station Before Entering Room

1. **Private Room**—*necessary*; door must be kept closed.
2. **Gowns**—must be worn by all persons entering room.
3. **Masks**—must be worn by all persons entering room.
4. **Hands**—must be washed on entering and leaving room.
5. **Gloves**—must be worn by all persons entering room.
6. **Articles**—must be discarded, or wrapped before being sent to Central Supply for disinfection or sterilization.

Fig. 33-1. Strict isolation card; color-coded yellow. (From Isolation technique for use in hospitals, PHS Publication no. 2054, Washington, D. C., Superintendent of Documents, U. S. Government Printing Office.)

Wound & Skin Precautions
Visitors—Report to Nurses' Station Before Entering Room

1. **Private Room**—desirable.
2. **Gowns**—must be worn by all persons having direct contact with patient.
3. **Masks**—not necessary except during dressing changes.
4. **Hands**—must be washed on entering and leaving room.
5. **Gloves**—must be worn by all persons having direct contact with infected area.
6. **Articles**—special precautions necessary for instruments, dressings, and linen.

NOTE: *See* manual for Special Dressing Techniques to be used when changing dressings.

Fig. 33-2. Wound and skin precautions card; color-coded green. (From Isolation technique for use in hospitals, PHS Publication no. 2054, Washington, D. C. Superintendent of Documents, U. S. Government Printing Office.)

Respiratory Isolation
Visitors—Report to Nurses' Station Before Entering Room

1. **Private Room**—*necessary*; door must be kept closed.
2. **Gowns**—not necessary.
3. **Masks**—must be worn by all persons entering room if susceptible to disease.
4. **Hands**—must be washed on entering and leaving room.
5. **Gloves**—not necessary.
6. **Articles**—those contaminated with secretions must be disinfected.
7. **Caution**—all persons susceptible to the specific disease should be excluded from patient area; if contact is necessary, susceptibles must wear masks.

Fig. 33-3. Respiratory isolation card; color-coded red. (From Isolation technique for use in hospitals, PHS Publication no. 2054, Washington, D. C., Superintendent of Documents, U. S. Government Printing Office.)

tient, the nurse will label the patient's room door with a list of the protective techniques required in caring for him as soon as it is determined that he has a communicable disease.

Now collect all the items you will need to give this care. Do not be in a hurry. Plan carefully. Once you have put on the gown and mask and have gone into the patient's room, you will not be able to come out and get what you need. If you have forgotten something, you will have to use the patient's signal light to summon other staff members to get the item that you need.

After you collect the equipment, which will include clean linen, mouthwash, a paper cup of rubbing alcohol or back massage lotion, and a bar of soap, take it to the cart outside the patient's room. Ask the patient (if he is conscious) if he needs anything. Ask him also if he has an adequate supply of soap and if his patient care utensils are in the bedside stand in his room. Get any additional equipment requested by the patient. If the patient's room is not equipped with running water, get a pitcher of bath water and put it on the cart outside the patient's room. Now check the hamper for contaminated linen. If the hamper is full, close the laundry bag and discard it in the laundry chute. Replace it with an empty one.

Don the protective clothing indicated by the patient's illness, and take the linen and patient care materials with you as you go into the patient's room. Proceed to care for the patient just as you care for a patient who is not in isolation. (If the patient's room does not have running water, get your bath water supply from the pitcher of water that you prepared and placed on the cart outside the room before you went into the

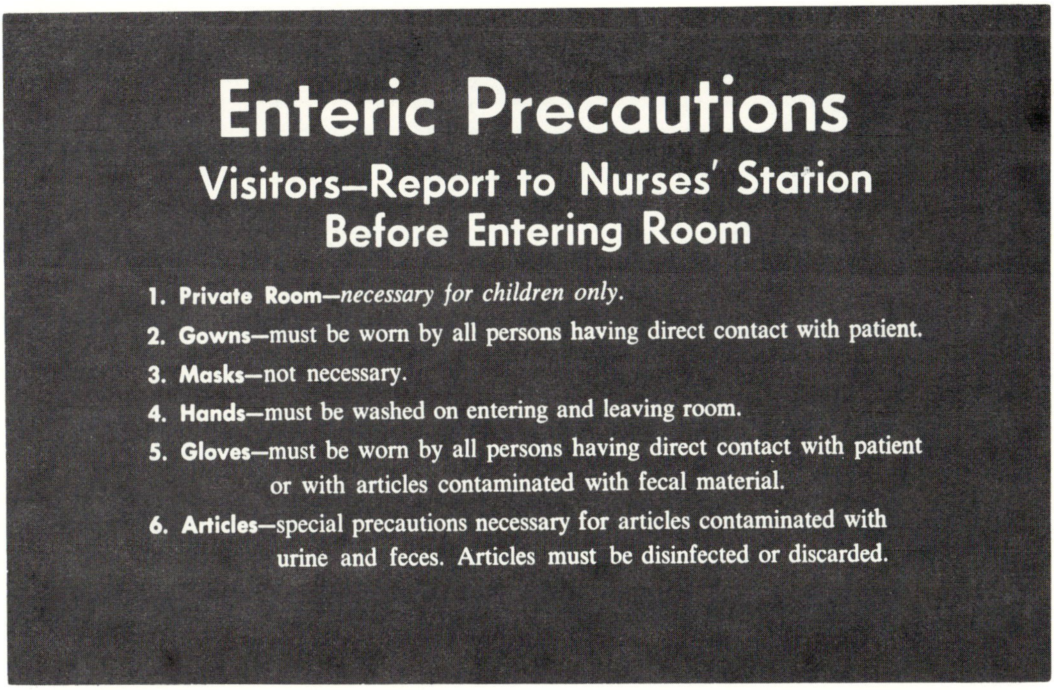

Enteric Precautions
Visitors—Report to Nurses' Station Before Entering Room

1. **Private Room**—*necessary for children only.*
2. **Gowns**—must be worn by all persons having direct contact with patient.
3. **Masks**—not necessary.
4. **Hands**—must be washed on entering and leaving room.
5. **Gloves**—must be worn by all persons having direct contact with patient or with articles contaminated with fecal material.
6. **Articles**—special precautions necessary for articles contaminated with urine and feces. Articles must be disinfected or discarded.

Fig. 33-4. Enteric precautions card; color-coded brown. (From Isolation technique for use in hospitals, PHS Publication no. 2054, Washington, D. C., Superintendent of Documents, U. S. Government Printing Office.)

room. Since your hands have been handling the patient and his equipment inside the room, you will need to grasp the handle on the pitcher, which is in the clean area outside the room, with a paper towel. Then take the pitcher into the patient's room, pour the water into the bath basin, and return the pitcher to the clean stand outside the door. Discard the towel in the covered trash can.)

PUTTING ON THE CAP,* GOWN, AND MASK

Remove your watch and rings and put them in your pocket. Then don your protective clothing just outside the patient's area.

1. *Select a cap* and put it on. This cap may be a disposable tam-type cap that simply slips on the head, or it may be a cloth cap with two ends that cross in the back and come around the head to tie in the front. The important thing in putting on the cap is to cover all the hair. A strand of hair that falls in your eyes will certainly bring your contaminated hand up to your face to brush it away.

2. *Select a mask* and put it on. This mask may be a disposable type made of paper that has two elastic cords that slip over the ears, or it may be a cloth mask that ties at the back of the head. It is important, however, that this mask cover the mouth and nose completely and that it be dry. The mask must be changed when it gets wet.

3. *Select a gown* and put it on as if you were putting a coat on backward. Tie it at the back of the neck. Grasp the sides of the gown in the area of the hips and wrap one end around your back. Now wrap the second end of the gown over the first. Hold the gown closed with the elbow while you grasp the strings on the gown and bring them around to your back. Cross the strings at the back, bring them to the front of the

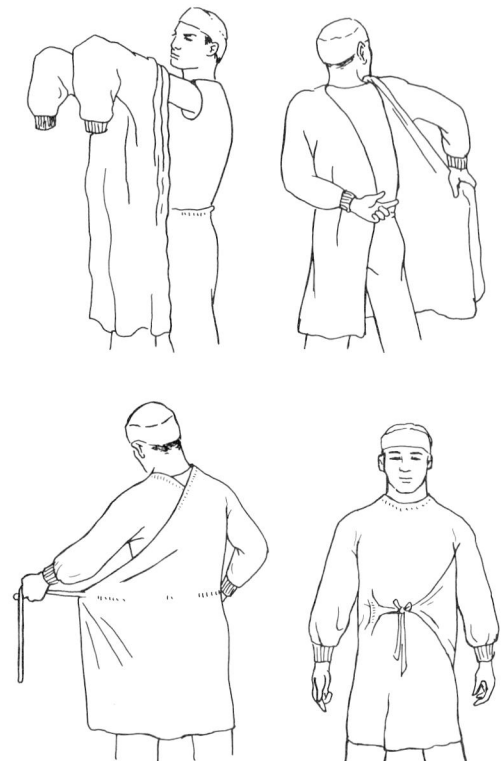

Fig. 33-5. Putting on the gown.

gown, and tie them. Pull up the sleeves to just above the wrists (to keep the sleeves dry) and go into the patient's room (Fig. 33-5).

REMOVING THE CAP, GOWN, AND MASK

After you have finished caring for the patient, discard the dirty linen in the linen hamper. Lift up the lid of the hamper by stepping on the foot pedal or by using a paper towel to cover your contaminated hand. Discard the bath water in the toilet. Clean the basins and replace them in the patient's stand. Take the patient's temperature.

Next, remove your cap, gown, and mask by the following method if the patient's area has running water:

1. Open the waist ties at the front of

---

*Cap will be worn when caring for the patient in protective isolation.

the gown. Make a slip knot in them if they are long so that they will not drag on the floor.
2. Wash your hands thoroughly in the patient's room at the sink. Pat your hands dry with a paper towel.
3. Turn off the faucet with your paper towel–covered hand.
4. Move to the protected area outside the room or in the screened-off portion of the patient's room near the clean stand.
5. Reach to the back of your neck and open the ties at the neck of the gown.
6. Hold the opened ties and pull the gown forward and loose around your shoulders.
7. Slide the thumb and forefinger of the left hand inside the cuff of the gown on the right arm.
8. Pinch the inside of the cuff (clean area) with the thumb and forefinger and pull the sleeve of the gown over the right hand but not off the arm entirely. Avoid touching the outside of the sleeve.
9. Cover the right hand with the right sleeve of the gown.
10. Grasp the outside of the left cuff with the sleeve-covered right hand and pull the left arm about two-thirds of the way out of the gown.
11. Slide both arms out of the sleeves to the inside of the gown. Grasp the gown on the inside and roll it up, being sure to fold the inside (clean area) of the gown over the outside (contaminated area). Touch only the inside of the gown.
12. Discard the rolled-up gown in the linen hamper.
13. Take off the mask by slipping the ends of it over the ears or by untying the ends. Swing the mask away from the face as you remove it. Remember that the outside of the mask may be contaminated. Because of this fact, a mask must be taken off completely. It can never be just slipped off and hung around the neck to be reapplied at a later time. Discard it in the trash can if it is disposable or in the linen hamper if it is reusable.
14. Take off the cap by slipping it from the front to the back if it is a tam-type cap or by untying the ends of the cloth cap and then slipping off the cap from the front to the back. Discard it in the trash can if it is disposable or in the linen hamper if it is reusable.
15. Wash your hands well, pat them dry, and apply hand lotion.

If the patient's area does not have running water, do not tie the gown at the back of the neck when you put it on. The procedure for removing the protective clothing is as follows:

1. Untie the gown at the front of the waist.
2. Grasp the outside of the sleeves of the gown and pull it off. Discard it in the linen hamper.
3. Keep the hands away from the uniform and from the face, since the hands are contaminated.
4. Go to an area with a sink.
5. Wash your hands thoroughly. Turn off the faucet with a towel-covered hand.
6. Return to the supply area in or near the patient's area.
7. Remove the mask and cap as described previously.
8. Wash your hands thoroughly, pat them dry, and apply hand lotion.

HANDWASHING

Every faucet in the hospital is considered contaminated, since everyone who washes his hands does so because they are dirty. Therefore always turn on the faucet with your dirty hands and regulate the temperature of the water. Wet your hands thoroughly; squirt some liquid soap preparation on them from the soap dispenser or pick up a bar of soap. Work up a good lather. Hold your hands downward over the sink as you wash them. Rub them well with the soapy lather around the wrists and in between the fingers. Clean the area under the fingernails with an orangewood stick. Rub the soapy lather around the fingertips. Rinse the hands under running water, keeping them pointed downward. Pat them dry. Turn off the faucet with a paper towel–covered hand. Apply hand lotion.

In handwashing, the rubbing loosens the germs and the soapy lather is mildly antiseptic—the lather is more significant because the germs stick to it, and the running water then rinses the lather and the germs off the hands. Handwashing facilities consist of the following:

1. Running water
2. Soap
3. Paper towels
4. Orangewood sticks in an antiseptic solution
5. Hand lotion
6. A covered trash receptacle

It is extremely desirable to have a foot-pedal sink and a foot-operated soap dispenser in the isolation unit. However, the ordinary faucet-controlled water supply is adequate. It is imperative, however, that handwashing be done under running water; no other method is adequate or safe.

CARING FOR THE PATIENT IN ISOLATION
Serving the patient's tray

When the patient needs to be positioned so that he can feed himself or when he needs you to feed him, bring the patient's tray to the clean stand outside his area. Prepare newspapers or a large paper bag to receive the used tray. Don the necessary protective clothing, as indicated by the patient's illness, and serve his tray. Position and/or feed the patient.

When he has eaten his meal, discard the solid portion of the uneaten food in the covered trash can, and discard the liquid portion in the toilet. Take the tray out of the patient's room and place it on the prepared newspapers or in the prepared paper bag. Make the patient comfortable. Offer him a bedpan or urinal. Be sure that his signal cord is within easy reach.

Remove your protective clothing in the prescribed manner. With clean hands, fold the bag closed or cover the tray with newspapers (thus completely enclosing it), put it on the tray-collecting cart, and return it to the ward kitchen.

Modern dishwashing machines adequately decontaminate dishes. Therefore there is no need for you to wash them on the ward. However, if the hospital in which you work still uses the old-fashioned pan method for dishwashing, it will be necessary to decontaminate the dishes. This can be done easily by asking the kitchen staff to send a metal pan to the ward on the tray-collection cart for the dishes of patients in isolation. Then you can place the patient's tray of dishes directly in this pan and return them to the kitchen at the same time as you do the other patient's trays. The kitchen staff can then add water to the pan of contaminated dishes and boil them for 20 minutes.

It is extremely important to label the patient's diet card with the words "isolation patient" so that his food will be served in utensils that can be boiled or decontaminated in the dishwasher. However, it is also important to have a plan for picking up the patient's dishes at the same time as you do all the others. If you do not collect the patient's tray at the same time, it is very likely to remain in his room until the next meal is served. Then he will truly feel as if he is in solitary confinement.

Removing the patient's bedpan or urinal

If you need to assist the patient off the bedpan or to empty the urinal, you must don protective clothing. The remainder of the procedure is as follows:

1. Discard the contents of the bedpan or urinal into the patient's toilet. Rinse out the bedpan or urinal with cold water. Then wash it out with soapy water. Rinse it again. Dry off the outside with a paper towel and return it to the patient's bedside stand.
2. If the patient does not have toilet facilities, follow this procedure:
   a. Place the removed bedpan or urinal on newspapers on the floor near the clean supply area.
   b. Remove the protective clothing in the prescribed manner.
   c. Take the covered bedpan or urinal to the utility room and place it in the flusher. Flush it and steam sterilize it. If your hands are needed to manipulate the flusher, cover them with paper towels.
   d. Wash your hands thoroughly.
   e. Remove the bedpan or urinal from the flusher and take it back to the patient area.

The nurse will have checked with the public health authorities in the town, and she will know whether or not it is safe to dispose of contaminated feces and urine directly into the sewerage system. If it is not safe, a chemical such as chlorinated lime may be added to the urinal and bedpan to kill the germs in the urine and feces before they are emptied into the flusher. The amount and kind of chemical to be added as well as the time required to decontaminate the excreta will be discussed with you by the head nurse. If you have additional questions, the bacteriology section of the laboratory will be able to answer them.

Giving the patient fresh ice water

To provide fresh ice water for the patient on isolation, fill a bag with ice. Don protective clothing as required. Take the bag of ice into the patient's area. Empty the water pitcher into the sink or toilet. Pour the ice from the bag into the pitcher. Add freshwater. If the patient does not have a supply of running water in his room or unit, you will need to place a pitcher of water on the clean supply stand outside the area before you put on the protective clothing. Proceed as just described. Then, instead of adding freshwater from the faucet, go to the clean area. With your towel-covered hand, grasp the handle of the clean pitcher and take it into the patient's area. Fill his water pitcher. Return the clean supply pitcher to the clean area.

Giving the patient a treatment

Use disposable equipment wherever possible in the care of this patient and discard it in the trash can after use. When reusable equipment is used to give the patient care, bring the treatment tray (fully set up) to the clean area outside the patient's room.

Prepare a paper bag or newspaper to receive the contaminated tray after the treatment is completed. Don protective clothing as required. Take into the patient's room only those articles on the tray that are absolutely essential for the treatment. Give the patient the treatment.

After the treatment is completed, place the contaminated equipment in the prepared paper bag or in the prepared newspaper on the clean supply stand. Remove your protective clothing as described previously. Take the paper-bagged or newspaper-wrapped contaminated equipment to the utility room. Decontaminate it by autoclaving it at 250° F. for 20 minutes or by boiling it for 20 minutes. Perhaps you can label the equipment contaminated and return it to Central Service in the bag if there is no ward autoclave. It can be decontaminated easily in Central Service.

If you have to resort to boiling in order to decontaminate the equipment you use, prepare a bucket or large basin on newspapers on the floor outside the patient's area instead of preparing the newspapers or bag as described previously. Then the contaminated equipment can be placed directly into the basin or bucket when it is removed from the patient's room. However, it is much more desirable to return contaminated equipment (safely bagged) to Central Service for decontamination by autoclaving than to have it boiled on the ward, and it is even safer still to use disposable equipment. After the equipment is decontaminated by autoclaving for 20 minutes at 250° F. or by boiling for 20 minutes, clean it thoroughly and return it to the proper place.

Equipment that is carrying germs should be handled only once, and then it should be decontaminated. After decontamination, when the germs on it are killed, the equipment should be cleaned. To summarize then, in giving the isolated patient a treatment, this procedure is followed:

1. The treatment is given.
2. Contaminated equipment is placed in a basin or paper bag.
3. Used equipment is then decontaminated (without further handling) by boiling or autoclaving.
4. The decontaminated equipment is cleaned.

Cleaning and handling of contaminated equipment can take place safely only when the germs on it are killed. Then the stuck finger or the splashed eye has little significance.

Escorting the patient off the ward

The patient with a communicable disease should stay in the isolated area. Sometimes, however, he may need to leave the isolation area in order to go to a diagnostic service such as x-ray or to a therapeutic service such as the operating room. Trips out of the isolated area should be kept at a minimum and should be limited to those absolutely essential to the patient's recovery. Each time the patient comes out of the isolation area and goes on an off-ward trip, the results are as follows:

1. He carries his germs off the ward with him.
2. He becomes a potential danger to everyone (patients and personnel) whom he passes on the trip.
3. He becomes a potential danger to all personnel at the diagnostic or therapeutic service.
4. He leaves his germs on everything he contacts.

Because of the possible hazards brought about by his leaving the isolated area, the patient must be prepared for an off-ward trip as follows:

1. Plan the trip so that the patient's contacts with other patients and personnel are kept at a minimum.
2. Protect the hospital patients and personnel whom he contacts by preventing the patient from giving off germs.
3. Keep the patient from coming in contact with and from leaving his germs on hospital equipment during his off-ward trip.

You can help protect other patients and the hospital personnel by planning the patient's off-ward trip with the personnel in the area to which the patient is to go. Call them and explain that the patient is in isolation. Ask for a specific appointment and eliminate any waiting time at the off-ward area. Usually the x-ray department or operating room will schedule this patient as the last one for the day. Perhaps the ward clerk can eliminate this need for special planning if she marks all study requests with the words "isolation patient."

As a further precautionary measure have the patient wear protective clothing. If he has a respiratory or staphylococcal infection have him wear a mask during his off-ward trip.

If the patient is not ambulatory, at the time of the scheduled appointment get the proper vehicle (stretcher or wheelchair) and drape it with a sheet. Then don protective clothing and take this vehicle into the patient's room. Assist the patient into the wheelchair or onto the stretcher. Give him a mask if he is to wear one. Give him an ample supply of cleansing tissue and a paper bag in which he can discard the used tissues. Push the wheelchair or stretcher out into the hall. Wash your hands and remove the protective clothing as described previously. Then enclose the patient in the sheet. Keep the outside area of the sheet clean (Fig. 33-6).

Take the patient to the proper therapeutic or diagnostic area. Be sure to keep him enclosed in the sheet at all times. If this is not possible (as will happen if he is being x-rayed), open the sheet and expose the patient, but keep the outside of the sheet clean. If the patient is to be moved onto an examining or treatment table, move him over in the sheet. Then expose him by opening the sheet.

After the examination or the treatment, again enclose the patient in the sheet. Move him back to the wheelchair or stretcher and return him to the ward. Assist him (still enclosed in the sheet) into bed. Remove the stretcher or wheelchair from the patient's room. Return to his room and don protective clothing. Then remove the sheet and mask and position the patient comfortably. Remove your protective clothing in the prescribed manner.

In order to keep the outside of the sheet clean and free from germs, enclose the patient in it by folding the sides up and over him. He can be exposed by peeling the sheet off and permitting it to hang down over the sides of the stretcher (much like a banana is peeled). The patient can be enclosed in the sheet by folding up the sides again in much the same manner as you would fold up the parts of the banana skin. If the outside of the sheet is kept clean (free from germs) the personnel who brush against the stretcher are safe from germs, as is any equipment that the patient lies on. However, if the outside is contaminated, personnel who brush against the stretcher are contaminated, as is any equipment that the patient lies on or uses.

Taking the patient's temperature, pulse, and respirations

Whenever possible, the patient's temperature should be taken by the route that minimizes your contact with the germs. Therefore rectal temperatures should be taken in patients with respiratory and staphylococcal diseases, and oral temperatures

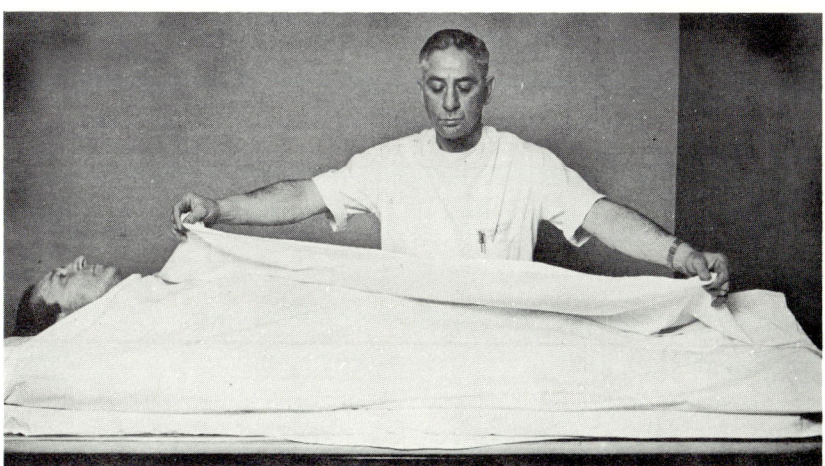

Fig. 33-6. The nursing assistant is enclosing the isolation patient with a sheet in preparation for an off-ward trip.

should be taken in patients with hepatitis.

Prepare to take the patient's temperature, pulse, and respirations by enclosing your watch in a disposable plastic bag or clear plastic-type container. Close the bag or plastic-type container. Place a newspaper on the clean stand. Don protective clothing as required by the patient's illness and proceed to check the temperature, pulse, and respirations. After you have finished, place the bag-covered watch on the prepared newspaper on the clean stand. Remove the protective clothing in the prescribed manner. Open the bag and shake the watch out of it and onto a clean area of the stand. Discard the bag and newspaper. Wash your hands thoroughly and put on the watch.

It may be unnecessary to wear protective clothing when you take the patient's temperature orally if he has hepatitis. Then, you can hold the watch in one clean hand while the other one handles the patient and becomes contaminated. After you take the patient's temperature, pulse, and respirations, return your watch to the clean stand and wash your hands. Then you can put on your watch.

THE PATIENT LEAVES THE ISOLATION UNIT

When the patient recovers and is no longer spreading germs, or if he dies, the isolation unit is decontaminated (freed from germs) and prepared for another patient. When the patient recovers, he is removed from the isolation ward as follows:
1. Prepare a stretcher or wheelchair as for an off-ward trip.
2. Prepare another unit on the ward for the patient.
3. Don protective clothing and give the patient a complete bath (bed bath, shower, or tub bath). Place a clean sheet under him and let it hang over the sides of the bed.
4. Remove your protective clothing in the prescribed manner.
5. Bring in the prepared stretcher and assist the patient onto it.
6. Take the patient to the clean unit.
7. If there is no clean unit available, fasten the stretcher straps and permit the patient to lie on the stretcher until you clean the unit.

Decontamination of patient's unit

After the patient has been removed, clean (decontaminate) the unit in the following way:
1. Prepare a receptacle outside the patient's room on a movable cart. This receptacle can be a large paper bag if you have access to an autoclave, or it can be a bucket or large basin if you have to decontaminate by boiling.
2. Prepare a small paper bag on the cart by opening it.
3. Don protective clothing as required.
4. Enter the isolation room or unit and remove all linen and equipment.
   a. Strip the bed and discard the linen, including the patient's towels and blankets, in the linen hamper.
   b. Put the patient's water pitcher and glass in the prepared receptacle outside the area.
   c. Put the thermometer container in the prepared receptacle.
   d. Place the patient's thermometer in the small paper bag.
5. Leave the unit and remove your protective clothing in the prescribed manner.
6. Close the bags.
7. Take the cart of equipment to the utility room.
8. Autoclave for 20 minutes at 250° F. all the equipment in the large bag, or boil the equipment in the basin or bucket for 20 minutes.
9. Label the bag containing the thermometer "contaminated" and return it to Central Service if they are re-

sponsible for cleaning the thermometers. If you are to clean the thermometer, place it in a small metal container with thermometer-cleaning solution and permit it to remain there for approximately 30 minutes. Then remove it and proceed to clean the thermometer as you do all other thermometers. *However,* if the patient has hepatitis, the thermometer should be discarded.
10. Notify the housekeeping department that you have an isolation unit to be decontaminated.
11. While you are waiting for housekeeping to clean the room with a disinfectant, break down the unit outside the patient's room as follows:
    a. Send the hamper of linen to the laundry.
    b. Empty the trash can.
    c. Wash the cart and return it to Central Service.
12. Wash your hands well. Pat them dry and apply hand lotion.

Decontamination of items used in patient care

The hospital in which you work has a method of decontaminating the material or the equipment used in caring for the patient in isolation. Ask the head nurse what these methods are. However, a few guides that you may use in carrying out decontamination procedures are as follows:
1. Hepatitis organisms are difficult to kill and impossible to see, so it is also impossible to tell when they are killed. Therefore patient care equipment coming in *direct contact* with the germ-carrying secretions or excreta should be (a) boiled for 30 minutes, (b) autoclaved for 30 minutes, or (c) discarded if neither boiling nor autoclaving is possible. Since the germs are in the patient's saliva, urine, feces, and blood, the thermometer and needles and syringes and the gastrointestinal tubes should be discarded.
2. Patient care items that can be boiled should be autoclaved or boiled for 20 minutes, except in the case of patients with hepatitis, where the time should be increased to 30 minutes.
3. Patient care items that cannot be boiled (items such as oxygen tents, stethoscopes, blood pressure apparatus, electrical equipment, etc.) should be washed thoroughly in hot soapy water, rinsed well, and dried.

When you care for a patient in isolation, it is imperative that you take into his room only the equipment you need and that you remove it from the room and decontaminate it as soon as it is no longer needed. In this way, the patient's room will not develop into a junk pile of equipment that will take hours to clean up after the patient is taken out of isolation. Then, too, limit the patient's personal belongings in the room. These will only gather germs, and on the patient's discharge from isolation, many of them may have to be discarded.

"PROTECTIVE CARE"

Isolation is an unpleasant word, and it frightens patients. Just imagine being in a strange hospital filled with pain and suffering and worry. Then imagine how you might feel if the nursing assistant came in and said that you were being "isolated." Perhaps it would be better to describe this arrangement to the patient as "protective care," since the purpose of isolation technique is certainly to protect the hospital patients and staff from communicable disease. If you describe the technique that way, the patient will feel that he is getting the care he needs rather than being condemned to painful aloneness by isolation.

SUMMARY

The germ-carrying patient with a communicable disease is placed in a protected area of the hospital. His germs are pre-

vented from spreading to other patients or to the hospital personnel as follows:
1. By keeping the patient separated from the other patients
2. By decontaminating all material and/or equipment that leaves the isolation unit
3. By protecting the staff members who care for the patient with such protective clothing as needed to prevent germs from entering their bodies
4. By stressing the fact that the agents most often responsible for the spread of germs are the contaminated hands of hospital personnel, by minimizing this danger by keeping handwashing areas equipped, and by carrying on a continuous campaign to keep the staff aware of the need to wash their hands after caring for each patient

Isolation is emotionally painful to the patient and becomes solitary confinement unless your caring presence dispels loneliness. You will need to plan your patient care activities in such a way that you have the time to visit the isolated patient frequently, even when you have nothing to do for him.

DISCUSSION QUESTIONS

1 Do you like to care for a patient in isolation? Explain your answer.
2 Select a patient on the ward who is in isolation. Give the patient a pencil and paper and ask him to record all the trips into his room made by hospital staff members. Ask him to record the purpose of their visit. Discuss your findings at your ward conference or team meeting in relation to whether the patient is in isolation or solitary confinement.
3 Ask the head nurse to demonstrate the technique for putting on or taking off a gown. Then you try it.
4 How do you prepare the patient in isolation for an off-ward trip? Do you feel that this method could be improved? How could it be improved?
5 How are the patient's dishes decontaminated? Discuss that at your ward conference. Determine ways in which the handling of dishes could be improved.
6 How do the hospital personnel know that a patient on the ward is on isolation precautions?
7 How would you decontaminate suction apparatus?
8 Why is the use of disinfectants dangerous in cleaning units?
9 How do you know what protective clothing to wear when you care for a patient in isolation? Is it outlined in the patient's Kardex?
10 How should you take the patient's temperature, pulse, and respirations when he has pneumonia? Would you need to wear a gown when you do this?
11 How do you decontaminate a thermometer used by a patient who has hepatitis?

VOCABULARY

acquired immunity Protection from a disease obtained through contact with weak or dead germs. This contact is obtained by a medical treatment or an injection such as a vaccination or an oral feeding. A common example is poliomyelitis immunity.
autoclave Piece of equipment that decontaminates material by subjecting it to steam (high temperature) and pressure.
boil Bringing liquid to a temperature of 212° F.
clean area Area that is free of germs or disease-producing material.
communicable disease Disease that can spread from one person to another.
contaminated Area that contains germs or disease-producing material.
decontamination Removing the contaminated material (germs) from an item used on or by a patient with a communicable disease. Autoclaving and boiling are the most common methods.
dirty Same as contaminated.
disinfectant Chemical used to kill germs.
enteric Pertaining to the intestines.
excreta Bowel movement or stool.
gastrointestinal diseases Diseases affecting the gastrointestinal system, which consists of the mouth, throat, esophagus, stomach, and large and small intestines.
germs Disease-producing organisms that are too small to be seen by the naked eye but that can be seen easily under a microscope.
hepatitis Infection of the liver caused by germs. The germs are found in the mouth, urine, feces, and blood.
isolation Placing the patient with a communicable disease in an area of the hospital where he is separated from all other patients. Hospital personnel who enter the room wear protective clothing, and material or equipment leaving the room is decontaminated before it is returned to general hospital use.

natural immunity Protection from a disease obtained through actually having the disease. An example of this might be immunity to measles.

pneumonia Invasion of the lungs with germs such as the pneumococcus.

protective care Caring for a patient with a communicable disease in such a way that the other patients and the staff are prevented from contracting the disease; commonly called isolation.

protective clothing Clothing worn to prevent germs from invading the body.

respiratory diseases Diseases affecting the respiratory (breathing) system, which consists of the nose, throat, windpipe, bronchi, and lungs.

staphylococcal infections Infections caused by staphylococcal germs and characterized by the production of pus.

SOURCES OF ADDITIONAL INFORMATION

1 Film: Handwashing in patient care; may be obtained from United States Public Health Service, Communicable Disease Center, Atlanta, Ga. 30322. Attention: Public Health Service, Audio-visual Facility.
2 Film: The nurse combats disease; may be obtained from United States Public Health Service, Communicable Disease Center, Atlanta, Ga. 30322. Attention: Public Health Service, Audio-visual Facility. *(Depicts the nurse's role in preventing the spread of disease.)*
3 Film: Isolation technique; may be obtained from Director, Medical Film Library, United States Naval Medical School, National Naval Medical Center, Bethesda, Md. 20014.
4 Pamphlet: Isolation technique for use in hospitals, PHS Publication no. 2054; may be obtained from Superintendent of Documents, U. S. Government Printing Office, Washington, D. C. 20402.

34/Caring for the patient in reverse isolation

STUDY QUESTIONS

1. What is reverse isolation?
2. Why are patients placed in reverse isolation?
3. Whom is the patient in reverse isolation protected from?
4. Can the staff give a patient with a low blood count an infection? How?
5. Can healthy staff members carry bacteria?
6. What causes a decreased white blood cell count in the patient?
7. What is the value of the white blood cells to the body?
8. Why does the nursing assistant limit his patient-care trips into a patient's room in reverse isolation?
9. What are the rejection phenomena?

THE PROBLEM OF STAFF HEALTH IN REVERSE ISOLATION

In Chapter 33 you learned that the hospital staff maintains a state of good health by isolating those patients who threaten it with communicable diseases. In this chapter, the situation is reversed. The patient with little or no resistance to illness is isolated to protect him from the diseases that he may get from the healthy staff members. Although the staff members are healthy, they do carry bacteria on their skin and in their mouths and noses. A disease-producing number of these bacteria do not develop in the staff members because their white blood cells constantly battle and kill them off. However, in the patient with a low white blood cell count these bacteria do grow unchecked and will develop in sufficient numbers to produce a life-threatening illness or disease. Therefore the patient with a low white cell count is susceptible to disease from the bacteria that live on and in the normally healthy person. This patient must be protected by isolating him from the healthy persons. This protection is accomplished not only by isolating the patient from the hospital community but also by preventing any bacteria from entering his room on patient care materials or equipment. The purpose of reverse isolation then is to prevent bacteria from entering the patient's room, and

you can keep them out in the following ways:
1. Keep the susceptible patient away from all other patients.
2. Use clean or sterile material and equipment when giving patient care.
3. Wear clothing that blocks the exit of bacteria from your body (barrier clothing).

THE PATIENT IN REVERSE ISOLATION

The leukopenic patient (one with a low white blood cell count) must live in an environment as germ free as the hospital can make it. The patient's ability to continue living depends on your skill in keeping bacteria away from him. The patients who will be protected by reverse isolation may include the following:
1. Those receiving treatment (such as radiation or perfusion) for cancer. These treatments destroy the cancer but they also reduce the patient's white blood cell count.
2. Those receiving drugs to lower the white blood cell count and so reduce the possibility of "rejection" of a transplanted organ (kidney or heart).
3. Those with leukemia (a form of cancer that attacks and destroys the white blood cells and the white blood cell producing glands).
4. Those with injuries (such as burns) that not only destroy the skin and provide a freeway for germs to enter the body, but that also decrease or lower the body's resistance to fight off the infection caused by these germs.
5. Those having surgical operations. When an incision (opening) is made into the body, germs can enter. These germs will grow and multiply, and postoperative infections will result. Therefore all surgical operations must be done in a germ-free environment by hospital personnel wearing barrier clothing (cap, mask, gown, gloves) to prevent bacteria from leaving their body and entering the patient's body.

THE REVERSE ISOLATION UNIT

The reverse isolation unit can be set up in a single room with running water and toilet facilities. Prepare the room for the patient as follows:
1. Clean the room with a disinfecting solution.
2. Attach the sign, "Reverse Isolation."

Ask your nurse if the patient needs a sterile environment or just a clean one. A sterile environment will mean that all linens, clothing barriers, and patient care equipment entering the room must be sterile. A clean one means that this equipment and material need not be sterile but that it must be clean.

Set up a sterile or clean unit as your nurse directs. You can do this in the following way:
1. Collect the equipment:
   a. Reverse isolation cart containing:
      (1) Supply of barrier clothing—caps, gowns, masks, gloves (sterile or clean as directed by the nurse).
      (2) Hand washing equipment (towels and soap). (Note that linen hampers and trash cans are unnecessary because the material *going in* presents the danger to the patient and that *coming out* presents none. Therefore all linen and trash from the room can be discarded into the usual ward receptacles.)
      (3) Supply of linen. Sterile (if sterile environment is to be provided) or clean (if a clean environment is sufficient).
   b. Personal hygiene equipment (disposable or thoroughly cleaned reusable basins, etc.).
   c. Solutions—mouthwash and massage lotions in covered containers.

d. Drinking water container (covered) and cup (thoroughly cleaned).
e. Stretcher to transfer patient to prepared room.
2. Prepare equipment and then place it on a movable table and take it to the patient's room.
   a. If sterile environment is to be established, prepare equipment in the following way:
      (1) Place reusable equipment in bag and autoclave for 20 minutes at 250° F., *or*
      (2) Select only packaged disposable equipment.
   b. If clean environment is desired, prepare the equipment in the following way:
      (1) Wash all equipment well (unless packaged disposables are used) before taking it into the patient's room.
3. Take the reverse isolation cart to the patient's room and position it in the hall outside his door.
4. Push the stretcher to the corridor area just outside the room being prepared for the patient.
5. Set up the patient's room.
   a. If sterile environment is desired:
      (1) Wash your hands.
      (2) Select packages of sterile linen. Take them into the patient's room, and place them on top of the bedside stand. Peel open the packages. (Use sterile technique. Do not touch the linen inside.)
      (3) Don sterile cap, gown, mask, and gloves.
      (4) Make up the bed with the sterile linen.
      (5) Drape the stretcher with a sterile sheet. Fold sides of sheet up and over the stretcher.
      (6) Place a patient's gown on the stretcher.
   b. If a clean environment is desired:
      (1) Wash your hands.
      (2) Don cap, gown, and mask.
      (3) Select the required linen.
      (4) Make the patient's bed.
      (5) Stock the bedside stand with the patient care equipment.
      (6) Drape the stretcher with a clean sheet (as described above).
6. Transfer the patient to the prepared room.
   a. If a sterile environment is desired:
      (1) Push the stretcher to the patient's area. Unfold the sheet on the stretcher.
      (2) Ask the patient to remove his gown.
      (3) Slide the patient onto the sterile sheet-covered stretcher.
      (4) Put the sterile gown on the patient.
      (5) Fold the sterile stretcher sheet up and over the patient.
      (6) Take the patient to the newly prepared room and transfer him into the sterile bed.
      (7) Make the patient comfortable.
   b. If a clean environment is sufficient:
      (1) Repeat steps 1 to 7. However, use clean rather than sterile linen.
7. Wash your hands (as you do after caring for any patient), leave the patient area, and remove barrier clothing (not germ carrying so no special removal technique required).

PROTECTING THE PATIENT IN THE REVERSE ISOLATION UNIT

This patient is extremely susceptible to illness and must be cared for by healthy nursing personnel. Practice good health measures (eat a balanced diet, get plenty of sleep, avoid worry, etc.) and stay healthy so that you can care for the patient without increasing his danger of infection. If you do get sick (cold, sore throat, or skin infection), tell the nurse immediately. She will recognize the danger you present with your high bacterial count, and she will send you off the ward to the personnel physician for treatment. Your illness will disrupt the patient care program on the ward, and it will necessitate a revision and a doubling-up of assignments. This increased work load may exhaust your co-workers and make them more susceptible to illness, or it may so overburden them that they take dangerous shortcuts in the patient's care. Try to avoid illness and maintain good health both for your own comfort and for the patient's safety.

Wear barrier clothing (sterile or clean) to block the flow of bacteria from you to the patient each time that you enter his room. Wash your hands thoroughly (and wear sterile gloves if the patient is in a sterile environment) before touching the patient or any of the equipment used in his care.

Use clean equipment (or sterile if indicated) each time that you care for the patient. This means that disposable personal hygiene equipment (bath basins, etc.) must be discarded after each use or that reusable equipment must be autoclaved. Give the patient clean drinking utensils each day.

Keep the patient's room clean and free of clutter. Remove used equipment promptly. Cover all solutions (bacteria from the air grow in these).

Nursing care plan

The nurse will give you a nursing care plan for this patient. Follow it carefully. It will tell you how to minimize your trips into the patient's room by planning them around his needs and by meeting many of these needs on each trip. In this way, you can accomplish the maximum with each visit and cut down on the number of your visits. Then, too, you will cut down on the patient's exposure to your bacteria.

Protect the patient from his own bacteria too. Give him mouth care frequently.

Instruct him to change his position often and to exercise his lungs by hourly deep breathing exercises. Check his vital signs carefully and notify the nurse promptly if fever develops. Temperature elevations indicate that life-threatening infection has begun.

SUMMARY

The patient with a decreased white blood cell count (leukopenia) is so susceptible to infection that he must be protected even from healthy staff members. He is placed in a clean or sterile environment, and the staff caring for him must wear barrier clothing (clothing to block the movement of bacteria out of the staff and into the patient).

Leukopenia (decreased white blood cell count) may be a symptom of a disease or it may be the result of a treatment that the hospital is giving the patient. The safety of any hospital treatment that lowers the patient's resistance to infection depends on the ability of the nursing staff to protect the patient from contact with bacteria. The success of most organ transplant surgery depends on this type of nursing care.

DISCUSSION QUESTIONS

1 Visit the operating room and observe the germ-free atmosphere of a surgical procedure. Why are caps, gowns, masks, and gloves worn by the healthy surgeons?
2 Why is the skin prepared with an antiseptic before a blood specimen is taken or a spinal tap is done?
3 Why should you wash your hands thoroughly between patients?
4 When is it safe to enter the room of the patient in reverse isolation without wearing barrier clothing?
5 Why are sterile sheets used on the beds of burn patients?
6 Why should the patient's room be labeled "reverse isolation"?

VOCABULARY

bacteria in the healthy person Bacteria normally living in the body and on the skin. Body defenses destroy these bacteria, thus controlling their numbers and preventing illness. Lowering *of body defenses permits the bacteria to grow in sufficient numbers to produce illness.*

cancer Disorderly growth of useless cells that soon overpower and destroy those that do the body's work.

clean Free of disease-producing bacteria.

disposable Can be discarded after use.

leukemia Cancer of the white blood cells and the white blood cell producing glands.

perfusion Intra-arterial injection of a cancer-destroying drug. The arteries carry blood to the organs. Therefore an intra-arterial injection of a drug such as 5FU means an injection into the artery that carries blood to the diseased organ. It ensures delivery of the anticancer drug to the organ. Arteries have much more pressure than veins; therefore perfusions must be forced into the artery with pressure pumps. Gravity is sufficient to push intravenous fluids into the vein.

radiation The destructive rays given off by roentgen-ray, cobalt, etc. Radiation is used in the treatment of cancer (to destroy it) or in the prevention of rejection (by lowering white blood cell production).

rejection phenomena White blood cells destroy foreign (not belonging to that body) substance or material entering the body. They destroy bacteria and this is beneficial, but they also destroy organs or skin grafts transplanted into the body from some other person. This destruction or rejection of transplanted organs is, of course, undesirable.

reverse isolation Protecting the susceptible patient from the bacteria present in the body and on the skin of healthy persons.

sterile Free from all bacteria.

white blood cells (1) Blood cells that defend the body from foreign substances; (2) soldiers who destroy invading foreign substances in the body.

35/Caring for the patient who is unable to cope with the problems in living

STUDY QUESTIONS

1. What is emotional illness?
2. How does it differ from physical illness?
3. Can a physically ill patient become emotionally ill too? Why?
4. Why is the patient's family life explored as a part of the medical history taking?
5. What are the symptoms of mental illness?
6. Why do most of the emotionally ill patients wear their own clothes?
7. What is neurosis?
8. What is psychosis?
9. What is anxiety?
10. How does the nursing assistant help the emotionally ill patient to get well?
11. Why do patients commit suicide?
12. How can you protect the patient from arriving at the need to commit suicide?
13. Why do we behave as we do?
14. How do we protect ourselves from physical danger? Emotional danger?
15. Why do emotionally ill patients have their own patient government?

EMOTIONAL PROBLEMS IN PHYSICAL ILLNESS

In Chapter 4 you learned that the patient who comes to the hospital with a diseased body also comes with a worried mind—a mind filled with annoying thoughts that remind him of his responsibilities to his job and his family and of his helplessness in meeting them; a mind filled with the disturbing thoughts that tell him how serious, how painful, and how destructive his disease is and of the dangerous state that his life is now in. He searches his thoughts for a way to solve these problems. How can he care for his responsibilities and save his life? He finds no answers. He realizes that he has lost control over his life and that he is at the mercy of the hospital staff members. They decide for him—they tell him—they cure him, and he just lies there waiting, hoping, worrying, and depending on them. He watches and he listens as he waits for the hospital staff to cure him. He looks for clues in their behavior to prove that his fears about becoming helpless or of having continuous pain or even that he is approaching death are correct. He distorts each word, look, and action of the staff into a verification of his fears. Listen to the patients on your ward. Observe how each one believes that his disease is the worst case that the doctor ever saw. And it really is "worse" from the patient's point of view because it is the only case on your ward that seriously interferes with his living. The other patient's problems or pains do not disturb him at all. Why is it useless to tell the patient that you have other sick patients on the ward who require care and that you cannot spend a great deal of your time caring for him?

When or if the patient proves to himself that he will be a burden to his family or that he is going to die and the staff cannot help him, depression (fear of living) occurs and suicide (destroying the worthless life) results. (Observe the daily papers for many stories about incurable patients jumping out of hospital windows and committing suicide.) The patient who believes that his living is impossible or unbearable will end it.

Depression and suicide of the physically ill patient can be prevented if you make his life worthwhile. In the chapter on colostomy and ileostomy care you learned how to avoid the development of this feeling that life is worthless by helping the incontinent patient to achieve continence. In Chapter 41 you will learn how to avoid depression by helping the patient to live comfortably (free of pain) and enjoyably (with hospital staff members who are friends) for as long as he can. Nursing the patient, then, really is more than caring for his body. It is helping him learn how to live successfully with that body. The focus of patient care is teaching the patient how to live effectively with what he has left rather than permitting him to lie helpless and grieving for the body part or function that he has lost.

EMOTIONAL ILLNESS

The emotionally (mentally) ill patient comes to the hospital because he has difficulty living comfortably. This difficulty, however, is caused not by his painful body but by his worried mind.

This worried mind occurs when the patient fails to meet his emotional (feeling tones) needs for comfortable living. These needs are as follows:

1. *Feeling of self-worth:* awareness of being a valuable human being
2. *Feeling of self-determination:* awareness of the ability to control one's own life
3. *Feeling of belonging:* awareness of one's value in relationships with significant others
4. *Feeling of safety:* awareness of freedom from danger
5. *Feeling of success:* awareness of one's achievement, significance, and contribution

Emotional illness means then that the patient is unable to satisfy his emotional needs and is therefore living uncomfortably and ineffectively. It means, too, that the patient, in his attempt to protect himself from this discomfort in living, is using his behavior to withdraw from or to fight the life of trouble and emotional pain (anxiety) that he has.

Satisfaction of emotional needs

Emotional needs are met in and through our relationships with others. The degree to which we meet them depends on our ability to form and maintain the relationships.

Relationships (feelings of belonging) with others develop when the togetherness creates feelings of safety, comfort, acceptance, and self-worth for the persons involved in them. And they continue as long as they are valuable helping, sharing, trusting, and rewarding experiences.

Emotional health depends on our skill in building a life filled with the kind of relationships that permit us to be a friend and to have one, to respect others and so be respected, to protect the rights and property of others and so be safe ourselves, to trust and be trusted. These skills, like all others, have to be learned; and they are learned in the basic relationship of family living. Here the child receives and learns to give love, is respected and learns to respect, belongs and learns the joy of belonging, is trusted and learns the responsibility involved, and learns to achieve by the rewards and satisfactions that the success brings. Here the child is safe, comfortable, accepted, wanted, and loved; and he soon learns to recognize and associate these emotions with home and family. The good family, like the good nursing assistant who cares for the helpless, physically ill patient, meets all the emotional needs of the infant and small child; but the good family also teaches and demonstrates how emotional needs are met through their pattern of family living. As the child grows the family encourages him to relate to his peers (develop relationships outside the family) in the neighborhood and in the school, to develop boy-girl relationships, and finally to establish his own family. The good family teaches its members to be self-determining, effective adults; it does not remain a prop for them to lean on throughout life.

The emotionally ill patient does not have such a family. His parent-child relationships are painful either in that they demand more than he can give and he always feels inadequate and worthless, or in that they possess him completely, smothering him with help and keeping him dependent upon them. Love becomes trouble, home uncomfortable, and closeness (in a relationship) demanding and destructive. The emotionally ill person learns early in life that relationships show up his deficiencies, control his behavior, rob him of his right to do, threaten his safety, and so are to be avoided; or that they take care of his every need, are substitutes for the helping mother-father relationship, are essential to provide him with the necessities of life, and so are to be attained and maintained at any personal cost to him.

The emotionally ill patient learns, incorrectly then, that relationships are to be avoided if he is to avoid the pain that they cause, or that parent-type relationships are essential to his living because of his dependent, childlike, helpless state. On the one hand he is doomed to a life of aloneness and loneliness, and on the other to a life of helplessness and dependency.

Emotional illness, then, is not some strange disease that creeps up in the dark to attack and destroy the patient, but is, instead, one that the patient brings on himself by his ineffective living patterns. He learned the wrong pattern of living. He cannot meet his emotional needs satisfactorily by living the way that he does and so he develops an emotional illness.

The treatment approach—the staff and patient work together at living

Emotional illness differs quite markedly from physical illness in many respects. In physical illness the patient is suddenly attacked, through no fault of his own, with a disease. The doctor assumes all the responsibility for the cure of this disease, and he operates, treats, or medicates the patient who just needs to lie there passively in bed waiting for the recovery to occur. The emotional illness, on the other hand, takes a long time to develop. The patient learned, as a child, incorrect living patterns for coping with life's problems. The problems became more frequent and complicated as he approached adult life, and so his inability to solve them became ever more evident. Soon the patient was either hiding (staying at home, afraid to go out, withdrawing from the mainstream of life) or fighting (hitting the boss, beating his family, breaking the laws—acting out his anger and fear of life). The psychiatrist (unlike the medical or surgical physician) cannot assume all the responsibility for the cure. He can only assist the patient unlearn his old inadequate ways of solving life's problems and relearn new and more effective ones. The psychiatrist becomes a teacher in the curative process, and the patient must become an active, participating learner.

Signs and symptoms of emotional illness

Emotional illness is defined in terms of painful, uncomfortable, ineffective living; and its signs and symptoms are identified when the patient's living pattern is explored. When the doctor takes a history, this exploration will reveal that the patient's life is a friendless one filled with family problems and job difficulties. It may even reveal self-destructive behavior patterns such as alcoholism, narcotics addiction, prostitution, and suicide attempts. You will not see these living difficulties when you visit the patient on the ward. In fact, you may even have difficulty identifying the patient as ill when you see him walking about the ward wearing his own clothes. Remember that emotional illness shows up in living and that this patient was admitted to the psychiatric ward because the living there is simple and easy and the demands on him are very few (much like the paralyzed patient who cannot live at home but who can live in the hospital because you become his substitute arms and legs and make life possible for him). Remember, too, that you will need to observe his ward living to discover how his life-problem-solving behavior is incorrect. The doctor and nurse must know what this is before they can teach the patient to unlearn it.

The signs and symptoms of emotional illness are ineffective living behavior, that is, behavior that prevents a significant relationship from developing or one that destroys it early in its formation. Think for a few minutes about the people you know and avoid. What behavior are you avoiding? Think of the irritating behavior of your loved one. This occurs only on rare (provoked) occasions, but suppose that it was his usual way of operating. What would happen to your relationship? Why? How do you behave when your emotional comfort is destroyed by factors that block the satisfaction of your needs? How do you feel and what do you do when the boss tells you about your "stupid" mistakes? When the boss constantly follows you around giving one direction right after the other? When the boss takes you into her office and closes the door? When your evaluation record is poor? How do you discuss this poor evaluation record with your friend, with your loved ones at home? This extreme behavior is occasional on your part, but it is the standard way of operating for the emotionally ill.

The emotionally ill patient responds (as we do) by running away from or by standing and fighting anything that threatens him. Unlike us, however, the emotionally ill patient sees threatening situations even where none exist. His ward behavior will be therefore one of withdrawal, avoidance, escape, and aloneness; or one of controlling, demanding, bossing, teasing, complaining, and fighting. On the other hand, the patient accepts his worthlessness, his failures, and his guilt and is protecting himself by escaping from life. Suicide is a good possibility. On the other hand, the patient is fighting these feelings. He is trying to deny them by acting out (like an actor plays a part) his importance or worth. A fight usually ensues if you degrade the patient who is trying to prove his worth with directions such as "keep quiet," "sit down," or "behave yourself."

Types of emotional illness

Emotional illness consists of two basic illness categories, neurosis and psychosis.

Neurosis is an emotional illness characterized by anxiety. You have learned already that we have only two ways of protecting ourselves from danger—to run or to fight. Therefore when a danger threatens us, we feel afraid and run away or stand and fight. (Running across the street to avoid the car bearing down on us might be an example of this.) Anxiety differs from fear only in the fact that the danger (the threat to our well-being) exists only in our own mind. (Anxiety on bridges or in tunnels or in the boss's office might be an example of this.) The danger or threat exists for no one but the anxious person whose own ideas, thoughts, and feelings are creating it. Why the particular situation—heights, or tunnels, or authority—creates a threat to one's well-being can be found only in an intensive psychoanalytic exploration of that one's previous life experiences. But the causative factors in the situation can be identified, and they are usually found to be associated with a disturbing and emotionally destructive experience. Reminders of this experience evoke the original emotional threat and result in overwhelming anxiety (body readiness to fight or flee; see Chapter 14). The anxiety may be expressed in the following ways:

1. *Free-floating anxiety:* generally tense feeling. Jittery, pacing, worried patient. See Chapter 14 for signs and symptoms of anxiety.
2. *Psychosomatic complaints:* anxiety focuses on body parts and the patient complains of headache, backache, heart trouble, etc. Patient really believes that he has the disease he is complaining about and he suffers the same intense pain he would have if he did. *Conversional-hysteria* is the term used to describe the converting of this emotional fear to a physical illness. Amnesia, paralysis, etc. occur frequently in the neurotic patient with conversional hysteria.
3. *Phobias*:* Anxiety in the patient is attached to some external object, and the patient then develops a deadly fear of the object. Elevators, heights, tunnels, subways, etc. are some examples of the fearful objects in phobias.

Psychosis is an emotional illness characterized by withdrawal from the painful, threatening situations in this world into an unreal and imaginary one where life is more comfortable. The psychotic patient who is living in a dream world (one of unreality) sees, hears, and believes things that do not exist for us. Therefore psychosis is characterized by:

1. *Hallucinations:* seeing visions, hearing voices, receiving God-given messages, etc. (false sensory experiences).
2. *Delusions:* Believing he has supernatural powers, that he is God, or Napoleon, or that he has no stomach, or that people are trying to kill him, etc. (false beliefs).

Therapeutic environment

The treatment for the emotionally ill patient consists of teaching him how to use those new behavior patterns that satisfy his emotional needs more effectively. The patient is using his learned behavior to do this now but it is ineffective. His needs are not met, and he has emotional pain (anxiety). Behavior is a learned way of meeting a felt need. Rewards strengthen and fix behavior while punishment (no reward) weakens it and permits it to drop out of our action patterns.

The environment on the psychiatric ward must be a rewarding, comfortable, safe, and interesting one for the patients if they are to learn how to lose their anxieties, recognize their value as human beings, and be motivated to try and learn to live again. This treatment or learning environment is created by developing a good familylike atmosphere where the staff and patients live together, sharing the authority, sharing the responsibilities, helping each other, and enjoying the living. The patients learn how to do by doing. They cannot be passive bystanders and learn. They must participate in patient government meetings to learn how to control themselves, and they must learn to belong by belonging to the group. They must learn how to work and play by

---
*These expressions of anxiety protect the patient by keeping him away from the threatening situation.

participating in planned work therapy and recreational programs, and they must learn the value of success by achieving it. They must learn to respect themselves because you respect them and you expect it from them in return. They must learn that people are trustworthy and safe by having comfortable relationships with the staff. They must learn to solve problems and resolve differences in an easy, friendly way without the pain of rejection. The opportunities to do this are present in their group therapy, in their ward living, and in their patient government meetings. The therapeutic approach for the emotionally ill patient consists of a teaching plan to help him learn effective living behavior. It must be simple at first, but it must grow in complexity as the patient's living skill increases until it becomes the patient's plan for living his life in a comfortable and effective way.

This plan will include all the activities of normal living (sleeping, eating, grooming, bathing, working, relating) and will include the doing of all these in group living, but it will identify a method of modifying these activities to the level of the patient's ability. In some activities, he may get assistance (bathing, toileting, grooming). Others may be simplified (work to occupational therapy like painting pictures). In others he may participate only by observation (sitting in the group that sings or dances). As the patient's living skill increases, his activities will be broadened into self-care, hospital-based work-for-pay program, and dancing with partners he chooses as well as by participation in competitive games. When the patient's ward living becomes more oriented to normal life, he will be encouraged to look for a job or to resume his old one, to spend days or weekends at home or in finding a place to live, and to participate in out-of-the-hospital social activities. After each out-of-the-hospital trip, he will return to the ward and share his experiences with his ward family (the staff and patients). They will listen to these experiences and help to minimize his problems and troubles through their companionship, and in doing so they will give him the courage and motivation to keep on trying. When he demonstrates that he is living effectively, the patient will be discharged from the hospital.

Medication program

The nurse will give the patient tranquilizers (such as chlorpromazine, promazine, chlordiazepoxide hydrochloride, or diazepam) to reduce his anxiety (fear of living) and to calm and quiet him. Tranquilizers do not cure the patient. They only relax, ease tensions, and soothe. They prepare the patient to participate in the learning of how to live more comfortably that you will teach him in your therapeutic ward environment.

The job of the nursing assistant

You are the patient's friend. You are the friend who understands the overwhelming anxiety, the frightening aloneness, and the painful rejection of the emotionally ill. You are the friend who sees the patient's behavior as symptoms of his illness, symptoms of his ineffective coping with life, but symptoms that are the ineffective methods he uses to protect himself from the emotional pain of rejection (feeling of being a friendless outcast of society) or that he uses to cry out against rejection in asking for the help he needs to relieve his lonely state—symptoms that you can relieve or eliminate by your caring, helping relationship with the patient; a friend who loves (develops a relationship that helps the patient to achieve a full, rich, happy life) and demands nothing in return; a friend who accepts the patient, regardless of his pathologic behavior, and the responsibility for the development of the relationship; the responsibility for giving his understanding, his interest, his concern, his help, and, most of all, his caring presence to the patient; a friend who is always available to share the joys of living and to dilute the pain; a friend who listens and encourages the patient to express and explore his feelings and thus to learn how to understand and control them.

You teach the patient how to live more effectively by your example of living in the accepting, nondemanding, sharing relationship you establish with him. In it he learns the joy of living, the value of friendship, the way to trust, the thrill of accomplishment, the right to express his feelings, and the way to solve problems. You can teach this only if you remember that mental illness is caused by relationships that evoke emotional distress and if you avoid evoking this distress in your nursing assistant–patient relationship. You cannot draw the patient into this learning if you reinforce his feelings of failure by dominating, by avoiding, and by rejecting. You can do it only by loving the patient, by considering his wishes, and by sharing the responsibility for ward living with him. You teach this in your every contact with the patient and not just when you decide to try to do it. Keep the nurse and doctor aware of how effectively the patient is living on the ward. Do this by observing, reporting, and recording the following aspects of the patient's ward living:

1. How does the patient eat?
   a. Does he refuse to eat?
   b. Does he eat too much?
   c. Is he afraid to eat?
   d. Is he eating enough to live? Is he adequately nourished?
2. How does the patient look? What is his grooming like?
   a. Does he bathe, shave, and dress neatly?
   b. Does he avoid bathing, shaving, etc.?
   c. Is his hair combed?
   d. Is his clothing buttoned and neat?
   e. Is his appearance disheveled?
3. What is the patient's sleep pattern?
   a. Does he sleep at night?
   b. Does he sleep all day?
   c. Is he awake most of the night?
   d. Does he need help in getting out of bed in the morning? In going to bed at night?
4. What is the patient's work pattern like?
   a. What does he do at activities? Occupational therapy? Recreation? Day room?
   b. How do his bed and unit look?
   c. Does he assist with the ward and day room straightening up?
   d. What does he do when he is left alone?
5. How does the patient get along with people?
   a. How does he work or play with the nursing assistants?
   b. How does he get along with other patients? In the day room? In activities? In ward government meetings?
   c. How does he get along with the nurse? The doctor?
   d. What does the patient do with his unoccupied time?
   e. How does he get along in the evening recreation with patients? With volunteers?
6. How is the patient living within the authority of the ward?
   a. Does he go to bed on time?
   b. Does he get up easily?
   c. Does he go to assigned activities readily or does he need assistance?
   d. Does he accept ward rules and obey them?
   e. Does he complain about ward rules and does he find it hard to live by them?
7. What effect is the patient receiving from his medication?
   a. Is he more or less anxious, agitated, hyperactive?
   b. Is his silence, withdrawing, and

depression increasing or decreasing?
c. Are physical symptoms developing? Identify? (Drowsiness, confusions, blood pressure drops, ataxia, rigidity, drooling, skin rashes, etc.)

These observations and the problems identified in your conversation with him should be recorded in your daily nursing note on the patient. The professional team or the nurse will diagnose the patient's living problems and will select specific treatment approaches for their elimination. Use these approaches to develop the relationships with the patient that permit you to redirect his behavior. Reward and fix the behavior that is desirable.

The suicidal patient

Suicide will occur when the patient feels that his life is too painful to live (when he feels trapped by the problems of life and sees no way to escape). The physically ill patient may arrive at this decision when he realizes that his cancer is incurable and that each day becomes more unbearable with its ever-increasing pain. The emotionally ill patient will plan suicide when his feelings of helplessness and worthlessness are verified by the rejection of all the significant people in his world and he is doomed to aloneness.

Suicide can be prevented by recognizing the deepening depression (disinterest in life) in the patient and reversing it by instituting a plan of care to:
1. Make his life worthwhile.
2. Give him significant caring relationships.
3. Protect him. This includes:
   a. Enriching his life with interesting activities so that he has no time or need to plan suicide.
   b. Protecting the patient from having the time or the opportunity to commit suicide.

This plan might include assigning you to care for the patient on suicidal precautions. This means that you must work with the patient throughout your entire tour of duty. You must help him live comfortably and interestingly with your constant caring and protecting presence. Remember that if you forget to care for your patient, he will have the time to plan and the opportunity to commit suicide.

The overactive patient

The extremely active patient who is so anxious that he cannot sit still for a minute roams about the ward interfering in everyone's business and dominating the ward activity program. He bosses everyone and is ready for a fight at the slightest provocation.

This patient is compensating (making up) for his feeling of worthlessness by acting important. He has learned that the important people in his life act this way. Attempts to control (stop) this behavior will only force the patient to show his importance by further exaggerating it. Telling him to stop will only increase the acting out. The treatment plan for this patient will include an approach to:
1. Develop a staff-patient relationship that recognizes the patient's value and eliminates the need for him to act it out.
2. Direct his anxious behavior into activities that are acceptable.
3. Reward him for acceptable behavior.
4. Protect him from the rejection his hyperactive behavior evokes from the other patients.

Somatic therapies

Electric and insulin shock therapy may be given to selected patients to block and eventually eliminate their self-degrading thoughts and ideas. The procedure for these treatments can be found in your hospital nursing service manual. The value in these treatments can be increased or minimized by your relationship therapy with the patient. It can be increased if your relationship encourages participation and fosters self-worth; it can be minimized if your relationship dominates and enforces worthlessness.

SUMMARY

You are the patient's friend, and through the privilege of this friendship you have the opportunity to help him to learn how to live a fuller, richer, more satisfying life.

You teach the patient not with words but with actions. You create a nonthreatening, comfortable, motivating ward environment by your caring presence and accepting manner. And you live with the patient in this environment, sharing, helping, and participating in a family-type living experience.

DISCUSSION QUESTIONS

1 Why do emotionally ill patients have a great deal of stomach distress? (See Chapter 8.)
2 Why do emotionally ill patients have difficulty sleeping? (See Chapter 14.)
3 Why do emotionally ill patients have a great deal of constipation? (See Chapter 8.)
4 What are the physical signs of anxiety? (See Chapter 14.) Why do these physical signs occur?
5 Why do emotionally ill patients have poor relationships with their family?
6 What behavior might the patient present when he is planning suicide?
7 Think about the last time you were angry. What behavior did you use to express this anger? What caused the anger?
8 Observe the hyperactive patient. Discuss his living pattern with the nurse. Discover whether it is as full of successes as he claims or whether it is full of failures.
9 What is a therapeutic staff-patient relationship?
10 Why do you form relationships with the people you do?
11 How do you behave when you are trying to form a relationship with a co-worker, a boy friend, a girl friend, a friend?
12 What behavior must you present in order to draw a patient into a significant relationship?
13 What causes anxiety? Have you ever been anxious? What made it worse? What relieved it?
14 What can you do to develop a ward environment that reduces anxiety, lessens hyperactivity, and prevents suicide attempts?
15 What can you do if you recognize that your own feelings toward a patient are those of intense dislike?
16 Why must you recognize and understand your own feelings before you can be a good psychiatric nursing assistant?

VOCABULARY

adult Person well qualified to meet and solve the problems of living.
agitated Roused to a sense of danger. The patient moves excitedly about the ward searching for the danger and the way to escape it. Since the danger is internal (feelings), this behavior solves nothing and increases until the patient receives help in controlling it.
anxiety Feeling of uneasiness caused by a danger that exists only in the patient's mind.
control Regulate or rule the life of another.
cope Meet and master the problems of living successfully.
delusion False belief. Ideas that exist only in the unreal world of a psychotic patient.
dependence Relying on another person for the essentials of life.
depression A feeling that life is not worthwhile. Forerunner of feelings to escape by suicide.
fight or flight The only two ways to meet and resolve a real danger. However, when the danger is unreal (exists only in the mind) both of these problem-solving methods become worthless in meeting it. Then the patient needs help in understanding the reasons for his feelings and in learning how to control them.
free-floating anxiety General feeling of uneasiness and danger but the threatening situation cannot be identified. There is no escape.
grief Feeling of helplessness and suffering caused by a loss. This loss may be a body part (leg) or a significant relationship (loved one).
hallucination Seeing, hearing, feeling, tasting, or smelling something that does not exist in the real world but exists only to the patient having the hallucination. Sensory experience of the psychotic living in a dream world.
helpless Unable to live one's own life without the aid of others.
hyperactive Excited and active patient who is searching for a danger that he is prepared and anxious to fight. (Paces, interferes, questions, annoys.)
neurosis An emotional condition in which the patient's feelings (of imagined dangers) limit his ability to achieve a full, rich life.
occupational therapy Treatment by work activity

program. The patient learns and does jobs such as making wallets or painting pictures. In the mentally ill patient treatment program, it serves to recreate feelings of worth through accomplishments.

patterns of living Ways of meeting and solving life's problems.

phobia Accusing an object of threatening your safety when all the time the real threat is your own feelings (fear of height, etc.).

psychiatrist Doctor who treats emotionally ill patients.

psychoanalysis Treatment of emotional illness by helping the patient to explore his present ineffective living patterns and his past living experiences in order to discover and eliminate the causes of his present feelings and thoughts and ideas.

psychosis An emotional condition in which the patient escapes from painful living by fleeing into unreality (dream world). Delusions and hallucinations occur.

psychosomatic Physical illness caused by emotional feelings (tension headaches, etc.).

psychotherapy Treatment of the emotionally ill patient through a helping relationship that teaches him how to live more successfully.

relationship Joining together (because of common interest, concern, and respect) and working together to achieve a common goal.

self-destructive behavior Doing things to hurt one's self (suicide, alcoholism, narcotics addiction).

silence Failing to utter a word or give a sign (look or gesture) that one is aware of what is going on about him.

somatic Physical—concerning the body.

suicide Ending one's own life.

therapeutic environment Circumstances or settings that treat the patient (interesting, permissive, satisfying life experiences).

threat Danger to one's life or to one's feeling of well-being.

SOURCES OF ADDITIONAL INFORMATION

1 Film: Preface to life; may be obtained from Central Office, Film Library, Veterans Administration, Vermont Avenue and H St., Washington, D. C. 20025. *(Shows parental influence in a child's developing personality.)*

2 Film: Psychiatric nursing: the nurse-patient relationship; may be obtained from Smith, Kline & French Laboratories and from the ANA-NLN Film Service. *(Demonstrates therapeutic nurse-patient relationship in the care of the emotionally ill patient.)*

3 Film: Special universe of Walter Krolick; may be obtained from ANA-NLN Film Service. *(Illustrates that good physical care is only one small part of the care of the long-term tuberculosis patient.)*

4 Pamphlet: Let your light so shine; available from Hoffman-LaRoche, Inc., Nutley, N. J. *(Excellent discussion of therapeutic relationship therapy.)*

36/Caring for the preoperative patient

STUDY QUESTIONS

1 Why does the preoperative preparation of one patient take longer than that of another?
2 What is the purpose of the preoperative preparation?
3 How is the outside of the patient's body prepared for an operation?
4 Why is the operative site shaved?
5 How is the inside of the patient's body prepared for an operation?
6 Why does a patient receive nothing by mouth for the 12 hours preceding the operation?
7 Why are the patient's false teeth removed before the operation?
8 Why is fingernail polish removed preoperatively?
9 How can you reduce the patient's fear of an impending operation?
10 Why does the doctor have the patient sign an operative permit for the most extensive type of operation that could possibly be done for the patient's condition?
11 Why is the patient's head shaved on the morning of brain surgery?
12 What is the most common postoperative complication? How does the preoperative care prepare the patient so that this complication is avoided or prevented?
13 What does preoperative patient teaching consist of? Why is the patient taught these things?

The patient may be admitted to the hospital for an operation, or it may be decided that he needs an operation after he has undergone several days or weeks of intensive study in the hospital. In both instances, however, the patient both wants and dreads the operation at the same time. He hopes that the operation will relieve his pain and suffering, but he is afraid that it might leave him helpless. He prays that his illness is not cancer, but he is sure that the operation will reveal that it is. He wants the operation and he knows that he must have it in order to get well, but he thinks of all the dangers involved and he becomes frightened by the thought that he might die on the operating room table. He feels trapped. He sees no way out and he turns to you for help. He asks you many questions and he listens carefully to your answers. He wants you to eliminate his fear by convincing him that the operation will be successful and that he will be cured quickly and painlessly.

The preoperative patient also checks up on the efficiency of the hospital staff by critically observing the care that they give to the newly operated upon patients. He knows that he can expect from you only the same kind of nursing care that he sees you give to others. So he watches to see how tenderly you handle the postoperative patient's painful body. He notices, too, how promptly you answer the postoperative patient's requests and how quickly you meet his toilet needs. He notices how the postoperative patient winces or cries out in pain, and he observes the time that it takes a member of the staff to respond to this call for help. The preoperative patient may be assured by these observation that the staff members are efficient workers who will take good care of him and his fear will subside; on the other hand, he may become aware of the fact that the staff members are careless, thoughtless, inefficient workers who will not take good care of him, and then his fear will develop into panic.

The preoperative patient observes also that the newly operated upon patient returns to the unit all connected up to intravenous infusions and noisy electrical equipment. Again, the preoperative patient experiences fear as he wonders about the tubes and bottles and machines that he sees. He asks you many more questions. If you are too busy or too uninformed to answer these questions, the patient will seek answers from those patients who actually went through the experience of having an operation.

The postoperative patient who had his operation just a few days previously will be very glad to have the monotomy of hospital life relieved by a visitor who is such a willing listener. Therefore the postoperative patient will describe his operation, his pain, and his discomfort in frightening detail for the preoperative patient. It is a well-established fact that a patient believes that his pain, his discomfort, and his operation were the worst in the world and, indeed, this is true. They are the worst problems in the world for him. The brain, which has little to keep it busy while the patient's activities are so limited, focuses on the pain and discomfort and exaggerates and distorts them until they are truly unbearable. However, the preoperative patient does not know that the recently operated upon patient is giving distorted and exaggerated information. The preoperative patient accepts this information and is truly convinced that a difficult and painful time awaits him during and after the operation.

This sequence of events can be avoided if the preoperative patient is adequately and carefully prepared for the operation by the doctor, the nurse, and the nursing assistant. When you receive your daily patient care assignment, listen to it carefully. Listen carefully to the information about those patients who are being prepared for an operation. Ask the head nurse or team leader to explain:

1. What the patient has been told about his impending operation
2. What you are to teach the patient in order to prepare him for his operation
3. How you are to answer the patient's questions
4. What nursing care you are to give to the patient

Proceed to care for the patient in the way assigned to you by the nurse. Listen carefully to the patient's questions. Answer the ones that you can. Keep the doctor and nurse informed of the kind and number of questions the patient is asking. Refer the questions that you are unable to answer to the doctor or nurse. The patient might be too fearful to ask the doctor and nurse these questions, yet they might be the very ones that are causing him emotional distress and worry. Try to keep the patient in an area on the ward or floor where he will not be subjected to the frightening sights of unconscious, vomiting patients returning from the operating room.

If the patient wants to talk to another patient who had the same type of operation that he is going to have, refer this request to the nurse. She may be able to have a recovered hospital patient return to do this therapeutic visiting. The recovered patient will discuss the operation much more truthfully because he can describe how the operation relieved his pain and permitted him to resume comfortable living. He can also give a much more accurate description of the kind and duration of postoperative discomfort. A visit from a recovered patient is very good therapy for a preoperative patient, for it helps markedly to decrease his fear and worry concerning impending surgery.

AIM OF PREOPERATIVE CARE

The aim of patient care during the preoperative period is to get the patient's body and mind into the best possible condition before the operation in order to ensure the following:
1. That the patient's body will function effectively during the operation
2. That the patient's body will recover and heal quickly after the operation
3. That the patient's body will not develop any complications because of the operation
4. That the patient's mind will be able to accept the results of the operation and remain alert and interested in a quick recovery and a speedy return to community living insofar as possible

The preoperative period varies in length from a few hours to a few weeks. Its length depends on the following factors:
1. How long it takes the doctor to make the diagnosis
2. How long it takes to build up the patient's body to its best possible condition so that the operation can be performed safely
3. How safe it is to delay the operation until the patient's body is built up and until his mind is prepared to accept the body changes that will occur during surgery

If the patient has an inflamed appendix that is very near the rupturing state, he is quickly and briefly prepared for the operation and rushed to the operating room for an appendectomy. However, if another patient comes into the hospital with a chronic inflammation of the appendix, his preoperative preparation will be extended over a 24-hour period. The first patient needed emergency surgery to save his life, so only the very essential preoperative preparation was done. However, the second patient's life is not threatened by a rupturing appendix, and he therefore receives a much more adequate preoperative preparation. The first patient's postoperative course will be more painful, more uncomfortable, and more likely to permit complications because of the limited preoperative preparation. The extensive preoperation preparation of the second patient results in a postoperative course that is likely to involve less pain, less discomfort, and less chance for complications to occur.

Every aspect of the preoperative preparation is important and is done for a specific purpose. However, when the patient's life is in danger, emergency surgery is done after only the minimum essentials of preoperative care. Then the patient who has emergency surgery is more likely to have a stormy postoperative course that is filled with the danger of complications. However, the emergency surgery has probably saved the patient's life, and you and the nurse will have to give the patient the special nursing care required to avoid the complications that limited preoperative care made possible.

GETTING THE PATIENT'S BODY IN THE BEST POSSIBLE CONDITION FOR SURGERY

The physician will examine the patient's body carefully to determine how it needs to be prepared for the coming surgery. Included in this examination will be such studies as a blood count, blood typing, blood sugar determination, a urinalysis, and an x-ray film of the chest.

A blood count

The blood count consists mainly of a count of the red blood cells (RBC) and of the white blood cells (WBC). The red blood cell count, which is normally about 4½ million, will tell the doctor whether or not the patient has a sufficient amount of blood. The white blood cell count, which is normally about 7,000 to 9,000, tells the doctor how many "soldiers" are in the blood to fight disease or infection. The white blood cell count also helps the doctor to diagnose the patient's illness, since it tells whether or not the patient has germs (infection) in his body. An example of this might be as follows.

A patient comes into the hospital complaining of pain in the right lower quadrant of his abdomen. The doctor palpates (feels) the painful area. He believes that this pain might be the result of an inflamed or infected appendix, so he requests the laboratory to do a white blood cell count. The count reveals that the patient has 13,000 white blood cells. The doctor then knows that the patient has a germ-invaded body area and that his white blood cells are fighting the germs. He knows too that the pain is in the area of the appendix, and he therefore schedules the patient for immediate surgery. However, if the white blood cell report revealed a count of 8,000, the doctor would know that the patient did not have a germ-invaded body area and that he had no need for immediate surgery. In this case the doctor would probably observe the patient for a few days and do some additional diagnostic tests.

Blood typing

The blood type merely tells the doctor what type of blood the patient has. If the red blood cell count indicates that the patient has anemia (inadequate supply of blood) or if the doctor feels that the operation will be lengthy and will result in some blood loss, he will send a specimen of blood to the laboratory for typing. He will further instruct the laboratory to prepare several pints of blood that he can use to transfuse the patient.

The laboratory will prepare blood for a transfusion by selecting from the blood bank blood of the same type as that of the patient and then examining the donor's blood and the patient's blood to see if they mix together without clumping or clotting. This testing of blood to determine its suitability for transfusion is called cross matching.

If the patient has a low red blood cell count, the doctor will probably give him a transfusion prior to surgery. However, if the scheduled surgery is to be extensive, the doctor may just want the cross-matched blood available in case the patient needs it during the surgery.

Blood sugar determination

The blood sugar report tells the doctor whether or not the patient is producing enough insulin to convert his blood sugar into energy. The doctor will regulate and correct an excessively high blood sugar level by putting the patient on a diabetic diet and by giving him injections of insulin to help him convert his blood sugar into the energy that his body needs. It is significant to point out here that the diabetic patient is unable to store sugar in his body so he will need to receive an intravenous infusion of glucose, insulin, and water throughout the entire operation. Remember, too, that the diabetic patient is a poor healer.

The blood sugar concentration is normally about 80 to 120 mg. per ml. of blood.

Urinalysis

Examination of the urine tells the doctor about the condition of the patient's kidneys. The anesthetic, which is given to make the patient unconscious and senseless to pain during the operation, is quite irritating to the kidneys. Therefore the doctor requests a urinalysis preoperatively so that he can be sure that the patient's kidneys are in good condition. If the urinalysis reveals the presence of albumin, sugar, red blood cells, or pus, it may indicate to the doctor that the kidneys are having some difficulty and will need help before they can safely undergo the additional stress of the operation.

X-ray film of the chest

The chest x-ray film tells the doctor about the condition of the patient's lungs. Since many patients develop chest complications after surgery, the doctor will want to be sure that the patient's lungs are in good condition so that complications can be avoided. Such complications usually develop because of the following reasons:
1. A general anesthetic (one that makes the patient unconscious) irritates the lungs, and this irritation increases the secretions in the lungs.
2. A newly operated upon patient is painful and sore, and because of this he does not move about in the bed nor does he breathe deeply and cough and spit up the increased secretions. Therefore these secretions plug up the bronchi (air tubes from the windpipe to the lungs) or the alveoli (air sacs in the lungs), and thus a lung infection develops. An example of such an infection is pneumonia.
3. A patient who smokes has an irritated respiratory system and an increased amount of mucous secretions. After the operation the patient is too painful and sore to cough up these secretions, so he is very likely to develop a lung infection or plugged bronchi and alveoli.
4. A new operated upon patient may vomit before he awakens from the anesthesia. This vomitus may be pulled down into the lungs from the back of the throat by a breath. The aspirated vomitus (vomit in the lungs) quickly causes lung infections to develop.
5. An unconscious patient (patient under anesthesia) cannot swallow his own saliva. This saliva falls back into the throat and is pulled down into the lungs with a breath. Saliva in the lungs causes infections (such as pneumonia) and occupies air space. Air cannot get into the saliva-filled lungs, so the patient develops shortness of breath and cyanosis. The doctor will try to avoid postoperative lung infections as follows:

a. By being sure that the patient's lungs are free of infection preoperatively. A preoperative cold may develop into postoperative pneumonia.
b. By having the patient stop smoking preoperatively. This will permit the lung irritation to heal and the respiratory secretions to diminish.
c. By teaching the patient in the preoperative period how to breathe deeply, cough productively, and spit up the lung secretions so that he will be able to do these postoperatively.
d. By teaching the patient to use an intermittent position pressure breathing apparatus (Bennett or Bird) preoperatively. The doctor will be especially careful to order this preoperative teaching of the use of the breathing apparatus for those patients who are particularly prone to develop lung infections (those in whom surgery involves an incision in the chest or upper abdomen). The breathing apparatus forces the patient to breathe deeply. Sometimes medications such as tyloxapol or isoproterenol are used in the machine to dilate (widen) the breathing tubes or to liquefy the thick mucus plugs that are blocking the breathing tubes.

• • •

Other tests may be ordered if the doctor feels that they are necessary. An example of such additional tests is the electrocardiogram (EKG) that the doctor requests on any patient who has abnormal heart sounds or pulse beats. The electrocardiogram tells the doctor how the patient's heart is functioning and what kind of support it will need to withstand the stress and strain of the operation. If the removal of a diseased lung or kidney is planned, the doctor will request extensive tests on the functioning organ. The doctor requests these tests to be sure that the good lung or kidney will be able to support the patient's body in such a way as to enable him to go on living after the diseased organ is removed.

THE PATIENT'S FEAR

During the period of preoperative preparation, the patient is subjected to intensive study. The patient lies in bed waiting and waiting. Each day brings more apprehension and more tests. The doctor and nurse give him the results of these tests by saying, "Your lungs are in good condition" or "Your blood is just right." This frightens the patient even more. He may have come into the hospital because he had some rectal bleeding, and he will therefore not understand why they are examining his blood and lungs when his trouble concerns the rectum. He feels sure that all he needs is to have his hemorrhoids (piles) removed. However, the doctor studies the patient in such a way as to prepare him for a hemorrhoidectomy (removal of piles) or for an extensive resection (cutting out) of the rectum if the bleeding is revealed (during the operation) to be caused by cancer. Therefore the doctor cannot even give the patient the emotional comfort of saying that his problem is a simple one of hemorrhoids. Instead, he refers to the patient's forthcoming operation in terms of an exploratory (exploring and examining) procedure. This frightens the patient, too, and makes him feel that he has some serious illness.

It is important for you to know the doctors' and nurses' operative plan for the patient. And it is important for you to help the patient by increasing his faith and trust in the medical and nursing staff. Help the patient to see that his whole body is being put into good condition for the coming operation. Just as you have your car overhauled before you start on a long trip, the patient's body is conditioned before it is subjected to the stress and strain of an operative procedure.

Keep the doctor and nurse aware of the patient's fears, doubts, and problems. Encourage the patient to talk to his priest, minister, or rabbi. Many patients are fearful of dying. However, they may be hesitant about talking this over with their pastor or rabbi because they believe that they have done something bad or that they have strayed far away from the church. This feeling of being on bad terms with God increases their fear of dying. In a very easy manner you can acquaint your patient with the fact that most hospital patients want to see their pastor or rabbi preoperatively. Then you might offer to arrange such a meeting for the patient if he so wishes.

SPECIAL PREOPERATIVE PREPARATION

When the patient is scheduled for surgery on the small or large bowel, special preparations begin about 72 hours prior to surgery. These preparations include the following:
1. A special diet that is soft and bland (nonirritating)
2. Administration of a series of antibiotics to sterilize the bowel

When a patient is scheduled for an operation on a bone, special preparations begin 48 hours preoperatively. Preparations might include the following:
1. Sterile preparation of the operative site. Forty-eight hours before surgery, the operative site is shaved and scrubbed with soap and water, and then it is wrapped in sterile towels.
2. Twenty-four hours preoperatively step 1 is repeated.

3. The patient then goes to the operating room with the sterile towels in place.

When the patient is scheduled for an operation on the stomach, a Levin tube is inserted into the stomach early on the morning of the operation.

When the patient is scheduled for an operation on the rectum, bladder, or uterus, a catheter is inserted preoperatively.

PREOPERATIVE PREPARATION— THE DAY BEFORE SURGERY

The day prior to surgery, the operative area is shaved. Hair harbors germs. It is impossible to sterilize the hair on the body; therefore it must be shaved off.

While the skin is being shaved preoperatively, it is inspected closely for infections such as pimples and abscesses and for infected scratches or cuts. If any of these conditions are found, the operation will be delayed until the skin heals, unless, of course, it is an emergency procedure. During the operation the skin is cut. Germs that are present on the skin thus have a freeway into the body and to the kidneys, heart, liver, bowels, etc. Therefore operations must be delayed when skin infections are present.

The areas to be shaved in specific operation sites are as follows:
1. In preparation for an operation on the elbow, shave the joints above and below the elbow. Thus the entire arm, including the shoulder, axilla, and wrist, is shaved.
2. Prior to surgery on the shoulder, shave the shoulder, the armpit, and the arm, down to and over the elbow. Also shave the entire side of the chest (front and back) on the operative side.
3. For surgery on the wrist, shave the entire hand and the arm up to and over the elbow.
4. Prior to an operation on the abdomen, shave the body area from the nipple line down to and including the genitals.
5. Prior to chest surgery, shave the body area from the chin down to and including the genitals. Shave this area on the operative side from the midline of the body in the front to the midline of the body in the back.
6. In preparation for surgery on the rectum, shave the body area from the waist down (front and back) over and including the genitals.
7. Prior to brain surgery, shave the head as directed by the nurse. A special permit is required to shave the patient's head. The physician usually shaves the patient's head just prior to the operation. Then the hair is too short to cause an infection. Shaving the head 24 hours in advance of the operation would permit the hair to grow enough overnight to make infection too great a possibility.
8. To prepare for surgery on the eye, check with the nurse and follow her directions.
9. Preparation for surgery on the genitals is the same as that for operations on the rectum. Shave from the waist down (front and back), to and including the genitals.
10. For surgery on the back, shave from the hairline at the back of the neck down to and including the rectal area.

The rule to follow in shaving a patient's skin preoperatively is to shave an area large enough so that the operation can be extended if necessary and large enough so that the germ-carrying hair is far away from the operative site.

Shaving the patient is done as follows:
1. If a razor is used:
    a. Lather the skin well with warm soapy water.
    b. Shave the area with a fresh razor blade.

c. Use a good light and be sure to remove all the hair.
   d. Ask the nurse to inspect the area when you are through.
   e. Clean off the area well. Clean out the umbilicus. Remove all adhesive tape marks, etc.
2. If hair-removing cream is use:
   a. Follow the directions on the container of cream.
   b. Apply a generous supply of cream to the area from which the hair is to be removed. Wait as instructed on the directions.
   c. Scrape the cream off with a tongue blade, a compress, or a piece of gauze.

Remember to avoid cutting the patient when you shave him. The cut that you make in the skin today may become infected tomorrow, resulting in delay of the operation until the infection heals.

Shaving the head is usually accomplished in the following manner:
1. Cut off the long hair with a pair of scissors.
2. Clip off the remaining hair with clippers.
3. Shave the scalp with a razor blade held firmly in a large Kelly hemostat or with a straight razor.

Listen to the patient carefully as you shave him and keep the body covered. Expose only the body area that you are working on. Report to the nurse any conversation that indicates extreme fear or apprehension on the part of the patient.

The surgeon will see the patient on the day before surgery and will explain to him what is to be done, when it is to be done, and what he can expect postoperatively. Then he will ask the patient to sign an operative permit. On the permit the doctor has written the name of the operation planned. However, he describes this operation on the permit in terms of the most extensive one that might be necessary rather than the least extensive one that might be planned.

For example, a woman with a very small lump in her breast may be asked to sign an operative permit for a mastectomy (removal of the breast). Of course, the doctor explains that he will examine the lump carefully when it is removed and, if nothing further is needed, he will do nothing more than remove the lump. However, he will go on and remove the breast if his study of the lump reveals that this procedure is necessary to stop the progress of the disease.

Although signing an operative permit for the most extensive operation anticipated is disturbing to the patient, the surgeon must have this permit because he will be unable to awaken the patient on the operating room table to explain to her that the examination of the lump reveals that her breast must be removed. Unfortunately, the patient sees only that her breast might be removed, and thus her fear increases. She will tell you about it. Listen to her carefully and visit her often. Let her talk through her fears. Do not tell the patient that this is a routine way of getting a permit because the patient may very well undergo a mastectomy. Then, when she returns to the ward after the operation, she will remember your false explanation, and she may believe that she will not be able to trust you again.

The nurse will visit the patient often on the day before the operation and try to dispel her fears. The nurse will also explain to the patient about the recovery room and the activities that she will need to do there. The nurse will teach the patient activities such as coughing, spitting, and deep breathing. The nurse may even ask you to take the patient down to the recovery room so that she can meet the nurses there and see the patient care facilities. This technique usually helps the patient to see that she will be in good hands and that she will receive good care after the operation.

The nurse will also explain to the patient about her preoperative enema, about the order not to eat after midnight, and about the time of her scheduled trip to the operating room. Then the nurse will encourage the patient to deposit her money and valuables in the hospital safe until she is alert enough to safeguard them herself.

PREOPERATIVE PREPARATION OF THE PATIENT—THE NIGHT BEFORE THE OPERATION

Instruct the ambulatory patient to take a tub bath or a shower or, when these are not possible, a thorough sponge bath. Instruct the female patient to wash the umbilicus well and, if she is wearing fingernail polish, to remove it. Instruct the male patient to wash the umbilicus well and to shave his face.

The umbilicus must be cleaned thoroughly or it will harbor enough germs to infect an abdominal incision. Fingernail polish must be removed so that the patient's nails can be observed for cyanosis.

The nurse will then give the patient a sleeping pill (hypnotic), which is ordered by the doctor. He usually prescribes this pill to help the patient get a good night's sleep. This prevents the patient from staying awake all night, tossing and turning and worrying about the coming operation.

The nurse will direct you to remove the pitcher and glass from the patient's bedside stand at midnight and to hang a sign saying "nothing by mouth" on the bed. (Sometimes the sign merely states "NPO," which is the abbreviation for nothing by mouth [*nil per os*] in Latin.) The reason for this is to be sure that the patient's stomach is empty at the time of surgery. Then, if vomiting occurs during surgery, either from the anesthesia or from the surgeon's handling of the stomach, the patient will have nothing in the stomach to bring up. This prevents him from aspirating any of the stomach contents.

PREOPERATIVE PREPARATION OF THE PATIENT—THE MORNING OF SURGERY

Either the night before or in the early hours of the morning of surgery (about 5 or 6 A.M.), you will be directed to give the patient an enema. This may be a soapsuds, tap-water, or prepackaged enema, depending on which one the doctor ordered. The purpose of this enema is to empty the patient's bowel for the following reasons:
1. So that the patient will not have a full bowel and defecate on the operating room table during the surgery
2. So that the patient's bowel will be empty and thus less likely to be injured by handling during surgery
3. So that the patient's bowel will be empty and therefore small, thus allowing the surgeon more room in which to operate
4. So that the patient will not need to move about, sit up on a bedpan, and defecate in the early postoperative period when he is so sore and painful
5. So that the patient will have less chance of developing abdominal distension from gas in the early postoperative period (Gas may occur from the action of the bacteria in the bowel on the fecal material stored there; such distention is very likely to occur in those patients who receive narcotics for pain because narcotics slow down and sometimes stop the peristaltic movement of feces and gas through the bowel.)

When the patient is scheduled to have an operation on the rectum or the large bowel, he may be given enemas until the return flow is clear. This is done to thoroughly clean out the part of the body that is being operated on.

It is extremely important to get back all the enema fluid that you injected. If it does not return (and it may not if the patient is tense or upset), reinsert the rectal tube through the tight anal muscle and into the rectum and siphon the enema fluid back.

If no fluid returns through the enema tube, notify the nurse at once. There is a possibility that the bowel or the rectum has ruptured. After you give the patient the enema, reexplain to him the plan for the operative day, as follows:

1. Advise him that he is not to eat or drink anything.
2. Tell him he will not receive any breakfast.
3. Tell him the specific time that he is scheduled for the operating room.

After you have explained the plan for the day, ask the patient (if he is ambulatory) to get up and brush his teeth and bathe. (If he is a bed patient, bring him the facilities and let him do these activities in bed.) Ask the patient to return to bed when he is finished.

Take the patient's vital signs carefully. Report abnormal temperature, pulse, respiration, or blood pressure readings to the nurse at once. Observe the patient carefully while you are taking his vital signs. Look for signs of respiratory infections (such as coughing or sneezing) and for signs of extreme fear (rapid pulse, increased perspiration, incessant talking, etc.). Report the presence of such signs to the nurse immediately, for the signs may be sufficient reason for calling the doctor. The doctor may even cancel the operation because of the patient's respiratory infection or extreme fear.

The patient will be permitted to rest in bed until time to get ready to go to the operating room. When this time comes, the nurse will instruct you as follows:

1. Put the operating room suit on the patient. This suit may consist of a cap (to cover the patient's hair), a short hospital gown, and a pair of leggings.
2. If the patient has false teeth, glass eyes, artificial limbs, or any other artificial and removable part, it must be removed.
   a. False teeth, including removable bridges, are removed because they may slip or be pulled down by a breath into the patient's windpipe, where they will obstruct his breathing during surgery while he is under anesthesia.
   b. Glass eyes, wigs, and artificial limbs are removed because they may fall and be lost or broken during surgery.
3. Offer the patient a bedpan or urinal and encourage him to void. This prevents him from voiding on the table while he is unconscious. It also empties the bladder, making it small and therefore getting it out of the way of the surgeon.
4. Remove the patient's jewelry (watch, rings, etc.).
5. Remove the patient's cigarettes and matches. This prevents the patient who is drowsy after preoperative medication from lighting a cigarette and falling asleep while he is smoking and thus risking setting himself and the hospital on fire. Instruct the patient that he is not to smoke from this time on until the operation is over.

The nurse will then give the patient the preoperative medication. This usually consists of a narcotic to dull the patient's brain, a hypnotic to help the patient sleep, and an anticholinergic drug to dry up the juices (saliva) in the patient's mouth. These drugs dull the patient's brain and make him sleepy so that he will be able to take the anesthetic easily. The anticholinergic drug (usually atropine) decreases the flow of saliva, thereby decreasing the possibility of the patient's aspirating saliva during the operation. After the nurse gives these drugs, she will instruct the patient to remain in bed and she will pull the crib sides up into position on the bed. She does this to prevent the drowsy preoperative patient from rolling out of bed.

You can help the patient obtain the full effects of these drugs by pulling down the shades in his room and by keeping his area of the hospital unit calm and quiet.

When the operating room attendant arrives on the floor to get the patient, accompany him to the patient's room. Check the patient's name tag to be sure that this is the patient the attendant came after. Then assist the patient onto the stretcher. Work calmly and quietly. Remember that the patient's brain is dulled with drugs so that he will take the anesthetic quickly. Do not make jokes or carry on senseless conversation. Answer the patient's questions quietly and simply. He will not be able to understand long, complicated conversation in his drowsy state. It will only tend to confuse him. However, it is necessary for you to do the following:

1. Check again to determine whether the patient needs to void. Do not ask him if he wants to; give him a urinal or bedpan and ask him to try and urinate.
2. Recheck to be sure that the patient's false teeth have been removed.
3. Check the name tag again to make certain that this is the patient the operating room attendant came for.
4. Check to see that all fingernail polish has been removed.

Fasten the stretcher straps over the patient and take him to the nurse's desk. The nurse will give the operating room attendant the patient's chart after she checks it again to be sure of the following:

1. That the operation permit is on the chart
2. That the reports of blood and urine examinations are on the chart
3. That the priest has seen the Catholic patient
4. That the result of the morning temperature, pulse, and respiration count is charted
5. That the preoperative medication is charted

The nurse will then check the patient's name tag, the patient's mouth, and the patient's need to void, after which the patient is ready to proceed to the operating room.

GETTING READY TO RECEIVE THE PATIENT AFTER THE OPERATION

Clean the patient's area as soon as he leaves it. Remake the bed with fresh linen and bring into the room all the equipment that you will need to care for the patient in the postoperative period. The patient usually goes to the recovery room until his vital signs become stable (stay the same) and then is returned to his unit. The nurse will explain to you what kind of an operation the patient is having and what kind of equipment you will need to care for him afterward.

While you are cleaning up the patient's room, be sure to safeguard his possessions. If he has false teeth, put them in a denture cup with cold water in it and then place them in his bedside stand. Give any jewelry or money that you find in the room to the nurse for safekeeping.

If the patient's family arrives, direct them to the visitors' lounge to wait for the patient. Do not forget about them. They are worried and upset, so visit them frequently and give them any information you can. Direct them to eating facilities at mealtimes. Treat them as you would want them to treat you if you were the one waiting for a member of your family to return from surgery.

SUMMARY

The preoperative period may vary from a few hours to a few weeks, depending on the length of time necessary to prepare the patient's mind and body for the stress and strain of the operation. The aim of treatment in this period is to get the patient in such good condition that he will recover quickly from the effects of the operation without any serious complications.

In emergency situations in which preoperative preparation is not possible because immediate surgery is needed to save the patient's life, the postoperative period is more difficult and complications are more likely to occur.

Just as the patient's body is prepared by cleaning it inside and out, the patient's mind is prepared by filling it with assurance that the doctor and the members of the nursing staff are skilled and will use this skill to take good care of him. This assurance is not given with idle promises but with actual demonstrations, that is, by giving good care to other patients.

DISCUSSION QUESTIONS

1. How do you care for the patient's false teeth while he is in the operating room? Have you ever lost any false teeth? If so, how could you have avoided this serious loss?
2. How do you safeguard the patient's money and valuables?
3. What is your hospital policy regarding a woman's wearing her wedding ring to the operating room? What is the purpose of this policy?
4. Do you put the preoperative patient near the postoperative patient in the ward? Why?
5. When do you give preoperative enemas to patients?
6. Why are crib sides pulled up into position after the patient receives his preoperative medication?
7. Why are postoperative patients usually very thirsty?
8. Do you have signs for the patient's bed stating "nothing by mouth"?
9. How do you help to eliminate the preoperative patient's fear?
10. How is fingernail polish removed? Why is it removed?
11. Would you notify the doctor if the preoperative patient's 8 A.M. temperature was 101° F.? Why?

VOCABULARY

anesthetic Drug that makes the patient senseless to pain.
aspiration Sucking of foodstuff, vomitus, or saliva into the lungs with the breath.
blood count Count of the red and white blood cells in the circulating blood.
blood typing Determining the kind of blood. There are four types that may be identified as 1, 2, 3, and 4, or A, B, AB, and O.
chronic Referring to a condition occurring over a long period of time and characterized by flare-ups that subside only to occur again.
cross-matched blood Blood of a patient that has been tested for its ability to get along well with the blood of a donor. This cross matching is done prior to a transfusion.
electrocardiogram (EKG) Electric heart tracing.
inflamed Invaded by germs.
Levin tube One type of stomach tube.
operating room Hospital area where operations are performed.
panic Trapped feeling that occurs when life is threatened and escape is blocked.
postoperative After surgery.
preoperative Before surgery.
red blood cells (RBC) Blood cells that carry oxygen to and carbon dioxide away from the body cells.
transfusion Injection of blood into the veins.
white blood cells (WBC) Blood cells that kill and engulf the bacteria that invade the body.

SOURCES OF ADDITIONAL INFORMATION

1. Film: Basic care of patients. Part VIII: Preoperative care; may be obtained from The Director, Armed Forces Institute of Pathology, Walter Reed Army Medical Center, 6825 16th St., N. W., Washington, D. C. 20025.
2. Film: Preoperative care; may be obtained from Director, Medical Film Library, United States Naval Medical School, National Naval Medical Center, Bethesda, Md. 20014.
3. Filmstrip and record: Preoperative and postoperative care; may be obtained from Trainex Corp., P. O. Box 116, Garden Grove, Calif. 92642.

37/Caring for the postoperative patient

STUDY QUESTIONS

1. What is the purpose of postoperative care?
2. What information do you need to have about the patient before you know what postoperative care to give him?
3. Why are postoperative patients put in a recovery room immediately after surgery?
4. What equipment is needed to care for the newly operated upon patient who has just been placed in the recovery room?
5. What special equipment would you add to the recovery room unit if the patient returning from the operating room had throat surgery?
6. Why is it necessary to take the patient's vital signs every 15 minutes when he comes to the recovery room?
7. How do you suction a patient?
8. Why do you suction a patient?
9. How is a binder applied?
10. What is the significance of an elevated temperature in a postoperative patient?
11. What is the significance of a falling blood pressure and a rising pulse rate in a postoperative patient?
12. Why are elastic bandages applied to a patient's legs postoperatively?
13. How do you cough a patient?
14. Why would the doctor order a patient to be coughed?
15. How does the drug that relieves the patient's pain endanger his recovery?
16. What nursing care should you give to the patient to prevent a pain-relieving drug from causing complications that could endanger his recovery?

Postoperative care is concerned with doing for the patient those activities of living that he is unable to do for himself, and doing these activities until the patient regains the physical and emotional ability to do them for himself. Postoperative care differs from patient to patient and depends on the following:

1. The kind of anesthesia the patient had
2. The kind of operation done on the patient
3. The condition of the patient's body

The surgeon who operated on the patient knows all about his condition, his operation, and his anesthesia. The surgeon knows too what activities of living the patient will not be able to do for himself and the consequences of neglecting these living activities. The surgeon will prescribe the patient care activities that you will need to do. These activities will include both those that help the patient get well and those that keep the patient from developing complications because of his inability to carry out his living activities effectively.

PREPARING THE UNIT FOR THE POSTOPERATIVE PATIENT

After the operation is completed, the patient is usually placed in a recovery room area, and he remains there until his condition indicates that he can be safely cared for in his room or on the ward. The recovery room area is usually located very near the operating room so that the surgeon or the anesthesiologist is immediately available if needed to give the patient emergency care. Nursing care in the recovery room is geared to helping the patient with the following activities of living:

1. Keeping him breathing
2. Identifying life-threatening situations and getting him help quickly
3. Preventing complications

The preceding purposes of the recovery room care tell you immediately that the patient's unit in the recovery room is well equipped to take care of any patient need. You can expect emergencies to occur in such a unit, and you must be prepared for them. In fact, emergency patient care needs are really not emergencies in the recovery room but are, instead, the expected needs of the newly operated on patient. Such an approach to patient care keeps the recovery room staff on the alert for situations that threaten the patient's life and ensure that the members of the staff are well equipped to reverse them.

To prepare the recovery room unit adequately for the patient, you must know what kind of an anesthetic he had, what kind of an operation was performed, and what condition his body is in. The first two items of information can be obtained from the operating room schedule. The third item of information concerning the condition of the patient's body may be obtained from the nurse who is circulating at the operation or from the anesthesiologist who brings the patient to the recovery room. Since you receive the information about the operation and the anesthesia early in the morning, you can set up the unit at this time. However, if the circulating nurse calls the recovery room and reports that the patient had a cardiac arrest on the operating room table (heart stoppage), you may need to add that additional equipment to the unit that is required to monitor the patient's heartbeat.

The patient who is being operated on is rendered senseless to pain by a general, a spinal, or a local anesthetic. These three types of anesthetics may be described as follows:

1. A *general anesthetic* depresses brain activity and makes the patient unconscious. When the patient is receiving this type of anesthetic and when he is recovering from it, he goes through a phase of restlessness and excitement.

2. A *spinal anesthetic* paralyzes the patient's body by blocking the nerves in the spinal cord. Therefore that part of the body that is blocked by the anesthetic cannot send nerve messages to nor receive nerve messages from the brain. Usually, the area of paralysis and lack of feeling extends from the umbilicus down to and including the legs and feet.

3. A *local anesthetic* acts much like the spinal anesthetic but differs from it in that it is used to paralyze and numb a much smaller area of the body. This is the kind of anesthetic you receive to numb (block sensation) one small area in your jaw and face when you are having a tooth pulled.

Therefore when you see listed on the operating room schedule the type of anesthesia that the patient is to receive, you will thereby receive information as to what his postoperative condition will be. For example, the patient who receives a general anesthetic will return to the recovery room in the following state:

1. He will be unconscious.
2. He will be unable to swallow his own saliva.
3. He will be unable to move.
4. He will be unable to control his tongue, and it will fall back in his throat and block his breathing.
5. He will be unable to drink fluids.
6. He will be unable to tell you about the condition of his body.
7. He will be unable to call for help.

The patient who receives a spinal anesthetic will return to the recovery room in the following state:

1. He will be conscious.
2. He will be paralyzed from the waist down. Sometimes, however, the level of paralysis is higher than this. Then the patient may have some breathing difficulty.
3. He will be unable to move the lower half of his body.
4. He will be able to swallow his own saliva and control his tongue.
5. He will be able to call for help.
6. He will be unable to feel the lower half of his body and so he will be unaware of its condition.

The patient who receives a local anesthetic will have such a minor interruption in body functioning that he will return directly to his room or area in the ward. However, the exception to this rule is the patient who has brain surgery under a local anesthetic. This patient will be taken to the recovery room in an unconscious state because of the interference in his brain functioning and not because of the action of the anesthesia.

Knowing the foregoing facts, you can prepare the recovery room unit for the patient in the following way:
1. Make the recovery room bed in such a way that the members of the operating room staff can lift the unconscious or paralyzed patient over into the bed easily. This is done by making the bed in the following manner:
    a. Clean the recovery room bed thoroughly.
    b. Make the bottom of the bed in the usual way.
    c. Place two rubber sheets on the bed—a large rubber sheet on the area of the bed that supports the operated upon part of the patient's body and a small one on the area at the head of the bed.
    d. Cover these rubber sheets with linen sheets. Fold the sheet that covers the large rubber sheet in half and the one that covers the small rubber sheet in quarters. Tuck the linen sheets under the mattress at the sides of the bed.
    e. Put the top covers on the bed in the usual way except for tucking them in. Instead, fold back the covers at the bottom to make a cuff like that at the head of the bed.
    f. Fold up the top covers at the sides of the bed into an 8-inch cuff.
    g. Stand the pillow on top of the mattress against the bed frame at the head of the bed.
    h. Label the bed with the patient's name.
    i. Attach a clipboard to the foot of the bed containing the necessary patient care records (temperature, pulse, and respiration sheet, blood pressure sheet, and intake and output sheet).
2. Attach side rails to the bed.
3. Attach an intravenous pole and an arm board to the bed.
4. Take the bed to the operating room.

When the operation is completed, the operating room staff will bring the bed into the room, flip back the top bed covers, lift the patient into the bed, flip the covers back over him, and tuck them in place. Then they will pull the side rails up into position, hook the container holding the patient's intravenous solution onto the pole attached to the bed, and take the patient to the recovery room. The side rails will prevent the unconscious or paralyzed patient from rolling out of bed, and the pole will support the intravenous solution while the patient is being transported from the operating room to the recovery room.

After you take the patient's bed to the operating room, but before the patient comes to the recovery room, set up the rest of the unit to receive him. This is done in the following way:
1. Set up the nasal oxygen equipment, which includes an oxygen supply, a nasal catheter, a supply of lubricant, and a roll of adhesive tape.

2. Set up the suction equipment, which includes a suction machine, a whistle-tip suction catheter, a container of antiseptic solution, and a container of cold water.
3. Set up the equipment to take the vital signs, including a thermometer, a blood pressure apparatus, and a stethoscope.
4. Set up the following patient care equipment in the patient's bedside stand:
   a. Emesis basin
   b. Supply of tissues
   c. Mouthwash cup, straws, and a supply of 2-inch-square or 4-inch-square compresses
   d. Tourniquets—alcohol sponges, etc. (for starting blood or giving intravenous injections)
   e. Safety pins
   f. Lubricant
   g. Tape
   h. Tongue depressors
5. Pin a paper bag on the patient's bedside stand. Then add any special patient care equipment as indicated by the scheduled operation. Such equipment is indicated as follows:
   a. Operation on the mouth or throat—tracheotomy set
   b. Operating on the gastrointestinal system (stomach, bowel, etc.)—(1) an intermittent suction setup (Gomco or wall) and (2) a Levin tube irrigating tray
   c. Operation on the heart or lungs—(1) underwater chest drainage setup, rack for transporting the underwater seal chest drainage bottles (2) a second suction setup (3) two hemostatic clamps, and (4) tape and pins to attach the tubing to the side of the bed
   d. Operation on the bladder—(1) a urine drainage tube, (2) a collecting bag or bottle, and (3) a catheter irrigating tray
   e. Operation on the brain—(1) a urine drainage tube and a collecting bag or bottle, (2) a catheter irrigating tray, and (3) a tracheotomy set
   f. Operation on the rectum—(1) an intermittent suction setup, (2) a Levin tube irrigating tray, (3) a urine drainage tube and a collection bottle, and (4) a catheter irrigating tray

RECEIVING THE PATIENT IN THE RECOVERY ROOM

The anesthesiologist will accompany the patient to the recovery room and will safeguard his life by keeping his airway open and free of saliva so that he can breathe adequately. As soon as you see the patient coming, help the anesthesiologist push the bed into the recovery room and place it in the unit that you prepared for the patient. The nurse will immediately come to admit the newly operated upon patient. Then she and the anesthesiologist will listen to the patient's breathing and they will correct any interference with normal breathing. Their actions might be as follows:

1. When *snoring* indicates that the patient's airway is blocked because his limp tongue is falling back in his throat, the nurse and the anesthesiologist will lift up the tongue by lifting up on the angle of the patient's jaw, and then they will slip an artificial airway into the patient's mouth to keep the tongue up in position. Since the tongue is attached to the jaw, lifting up on the angles of the patient's jaw also lifts up the tongue. The airway that they insert is a curved rubber or plastic tube that fits over the tongue and holds it up in place, thereby preventing it from falling back into the throat and blocking the windpipe.

2. When *gurgling* indicates that the patient's saliva is being pulled down into the lung with each breath, the nurse and the anesthesiologist will suction this saliva out of the patient's throat. They may also turn

the patient onto his side so that the back of his throat will be higher than his mouth. This position will cause the saliva to flow out of the mouth by the pull of gravity.

Then the nurse and the anesthesiologist will check the adequacy of the patient's respirations. Since the patient may have lost some blood during the operation, he may show signs of oxygen want. Remember that the blood carries oxygen to the tissues of the body. Therefore if the patient experienced some blood loss in surgery, he may have less blood in his body to carry the oxygen around. The patient with this difficulty will show the following signs of oxygen want:

1. Shortness of breath (dyspnea)
2. Rapid shallow respirations
3. Cyanosis of the fingernail beds and lips

The nurse and the anesthesiologist will assist the patient in meeting his oxygen needs by inserting a catheter into his nose and by connecting this catheter to a supply of oxygen.

When the patient is breathing adequately, the anesthesiologist will stand by and wait until the nurse checks the physical condition of the patient. The nurse does this by taking the patient's pulse, respirations, and blood pressure.

The nurse will report her findings to the anesthesiologist. If these signs have changed markedly from what they were before the patient left the operating room, the nurse and the anesthesiologist will check the patient carefully to determine the reason for the change. If the signs are unchanged, the anesthesiologist will report the following to the nurse:

1. The type of anesthesia the patient received
2. The extensiveness of the operation
3. The amount of intravenous fluids and blood the patient received in the operating room
4. The difficulties the patient experienced during the operation
5. The special care or observation the patient's condition warrants

After the anesthesiologist has given the nurse the necessary information, he will return to the operating room and the nurse will continue to care for the patient as follows:

1. She will take the patient's vital signs every 15 minutes.
2. She will chart these vital signs on the temperature, pulse, and respiration sheet attached to the clipboard at the foot of the patient's bed.
3. She will inspect the operative site for bleeding every 15 minutes when she takes the vital signs.
4. She will connect all tubes to drainage tubing.
5. She will observe whether the intravenous infusion is running adequately.

IMMEDIATE CARE OF THE PATIENT IN THE RECOVERY ROOM

The nurse will then check the chart to find out what nursing care the doctor prescribed for the patient. She will develop a schedule or plan for giving this care and outline the plan on his Kardex. The nurse will assign you to do those aspects of the patient's care that you know how to do. The nurse's instructions might include the following:

1. Take the patient's vital signs (pulse, respiration, and blood pressure) every 15 minutes and report immediately the following changes:
    a. Blood pressure that goes up or down 10 points
    b. Pulse rate that increases or decreases 10 points
    c. Respiratory rate that increases or decreases 5 points
2. Listen to the patient's breathing constantly and report immediately any sounds of difficulty such as snoring or gurgling.
3. Observe the operative site for bleeding and report immediately any

signs of blood on or around the dressings.
4. Observe the drainage bottles for (a) drainage and (b) blood in the drainage. Report any signs of bloody drainage or any failure of drainage to occur.
5. Observe the patient for pain and report it immediately, including in the report the kind of pain and its location.
6. Observe the patient's intravenous infusion or blood transfusion and report immediately if one of the following occurs:
   a. The fluid flow stops
   b. The needle site becomes swollen
   c. The patient develops any signs of a reaction such as chilliness or rash.
7. Observe the patient for nausea and vomiting. If vomiting occurs, you must turn the patient's head to the side immediately so that the vomitus will run out of his mouth and not be pulled down into his lungs with the next breath. Call the nurse. She will be able to clear the vomitus out of the patient's throat with the suction apparatus.
8. Protect the restless patient. Keep the side rails in place to prevent the patient from rolling out of bed. Notify the nurse immediately if the patient becomes extremely restless and tries to get out of bed or tries to pull off the dressings or pull out the tubes.
9. Watch the patient's color and report to the nurse immediately if the patient becomes cyanotic or extremely pale.
10. Watch the patient's skin and report immediately if the patient perspires excessively or if the patient's skin becomes cold.
11. Position the patient. The nurse will tell you what position the patient should be in and how often this position should be changed. She may tell you, too, what positions the patient should not be in. The positions to be avoided because they interfere with circulation in the legs are the following:
    a. Crossing the patient's legs
    b. Bending the patient's knees by elevating the lower part of the bed

The nurse may also assign you to make special observations in certain patients. These might be as follows:
1. Watch the patient with head surgery for signs of increasing intracranial pressure, such as the following:
   a. Restlessness
   b. Rising blood pressure
   c. Slowing pulse
   d. Slowing respiration
   e. Deepening stupor or coma
   f. Inequality of the pupils
2. Watch the patient with throat surgery for signs of breathing difficulty. Such signs include the following:
   a. Restlessness
   b. Increasing respiratory rate
   c. Shortness of breath
   d. Cyanosis
   e. Difficult or labored respirations
3. Watch the patient with chest surgery for signs of breathing difficulty and hemorrhage.
   a. The signs of breathing difficulty include:
      (1) Restlessness
      (2) Increasing respiratory rate
      (3) Shortness of breath
      (4) Cyanosis
   b. The signs of hemorrhage might include:
      (1) Restlessness
      (2) Falling blood pressure
      (3) Increasing respiratory rate
      (4) Increasing pulse rate
      (5) Cold, wet, pale skin (shock)
4. Watch the patient who has a cast on

a limb for interference with circulation of the blood in that limb. Signs of such interference might include the following:
  a. Coldness of the exposed fingers or toes
  b. Swelling of the exposed fingers or toes
  c. Numbness of the exposed fingers or toes
  d. Loss of movement in the exposed fingers or toes
  e. Feeling of burning or pain under the cast
  (The ends of the fingers or toes are always left out of a cast so that they they can be used to test circulation in the limb.)
5. Watch the patient with abdominal surgery for breathing difficulties or signs of hemorrhage as identified previously in item 3.
6. Watch the patient with blood vessel surgery for adequate circulation in the limb at those points beyond the operative site. Observation of circulation would include the following:
  a. Observing the radial pulse in the arm or pedal pulse in the foot for increasing strength or progressive weakness
  b. Observing the color and warmth in the operated limb as compared with the nonoperated limb (see signs of circulatory disturbance in item 4)

In the immediate postoperative period, from the end of the operation until the patient fully regains consciousness, the following life-threatening situations may occur:
1. The patient may choke on his tongue. The signs of this complication will be a snoring type of respiration with increasing cyanosis.
2. The patient may aspirate vomitus or saliva. The signs of such aspiration might be a gurgling type of respiration and cyanosis, or there may be no sign. However, after 48 hours the patient who has aspirated saliva or vomitus will develop many signs (atelectasis).
3. The patient may hemorrhage. He may do this without any blood being visible outside his body. Therefore external hemorrhage can be identified when you see the blood, but internal hemorrhage is identified only by a falling blood pressure, a rising pulse and respiration rate, and an increasing restlessness in the patient. However, the patient with intracranial hemorrhage has increased intracranial pressure brought on by the hemorrhage and has the following symptoms:
  a. Rising blood pressure
  b. Falling pulse rate
  c. Decreasing respiratory rate
  d. Increasing restlessness
4. The patient may suffer a heart attack either from the stress and strain of the operation or from the severe loss of blood associated with it. The signs of a heart attack include an increasing pulse rate and a decreasing pulse volume. The pulse may even become irregular and feel as though it is "skipping" beats.

NURSING CARE OF THE POSTOPERATIVE PATIENT AFTER HE REGAINS CONSCIOUSNESS

After the patient regains consciousness, the nursing care outlined previously will be continued. Even though the danger of the patient's choking on his own saliva has decreased, the danger of his aspirating fluid into his lungs still remains because the patient is in too much pain and is to sore to breathe deeply and cough up the secretions in his lungs. Therefore the need for suctioning the unconscious patient's saliva is replaced with the need to have the conscious patient move about in bed, breathe deeply, and cough up the secretions in his lungs.

The patient will need to be encouraged to move his legs each hour. This leg movement is necessary to keep the blood moving and to prevent blood clots from forming. Sometimes the doctor will try to prevent blood clots from forming by wrapping the patient's legs in elastic bandages from his toes to well over his knees. These elastic bandages cause the superficial veins in the legs to collapse and thus prevent blood from pooling there and clotting.

Even though the patient is receiving continuous intravenous fluids, he may be unable to urinate. The bladder muscles may have been injured by manipulation during the operation and may be as sore and as weak as the patient's abdominal muscles. Therefore the bladder may fill up with urine, making the patient quite uncomfortable, but he may be unable to void.

Observe the patient's postoperative output closely. Offer the patient a bedpan or urinal and encourage him to try to urinate. If he is uncomfortable but unable to void, use all the methods described previously (Chapter 32) to help him do so. If he is still unable to void, notify the nurse.

After the patient regains consciousness, he will complain of thirst. The nurse will tell you when he may have fluids by mouth. Until they are permitted, you can make the patient comfortable and relieve his thirst by the following measures:
1. Brush his teeth and rinse out his mouth every 2 to 4 hours.
2. Wipe his mouth and lips with 2-inch-square compresses moistened with cool water.

The patient may also complain of pain from the operation and irritation from the Levin tube in his nose. Report the patient's complaints of pain to the nurse, who will give him a pain-dulling or brain-depressing narcotic. This narcotic will relieve the patient's pain, but it will also slow down his breathing, slow down his moving, and slow down the peristalsis in the intestines. Therefore the narcotic relieves the pain, but it increases the patient's chances of aspirating saliva, developing blood clots in the veins in the legs, and having abdominal distention.

It is important for you to try and keep the patient comfortable so that he will need narcotics only when the operative pain becomes severe. Turn the patient frequently. Rub his back often. Position him comfortably. Keep his mouth moistened and clean. Visit him frequently and try to dispel his fears. Check on him often. Watch his vital signs closely. Encourage him to breathe deeply and move his legs hourly.

The Levin tube in the patient's nose is irritating and annoying. It increases the flow of juices in the nose and throat and increases the patient's need to swallow. Each swallow tugs on the tube and increases its irritation. Furthermore, the tube blocks the patient's nose and makes it necessary for him to breathe through his mouth. This mouth breathing dries the tongue and throat and increases the need for you to give good and frequent mouth care.

During the first 48 hours after the patient regains consciousness, you will know how the patient is progresssing by observing his vital signs. Therefore it is essential that the patient's temperature, pulse, respiration, and blood pressure be taken frequently and charted accurately. Abnormal findings should be reported to the doctor immediately. Complications (life-threatening situations) that may occur in this postoperative period include the following:
1. Congestion in the lungs from aspirated saliva or vomitus or from the lack of movement of the lungs
2. Aspiration of saliva
3. Hemorrhage
4. Retention of urine
5. Dehydration from insufficient fluids
6. Electrolyte imbalances from vomiting or electrolyte loss in tube drainage

7. Sore mouth
8. Abdominal distention

The signs and symptoms of the complications that may occur during the 48-hour period after the patient regains consciousness are as follows:

1. Lung congestion:
   a. Elevated temperature and increase in pulse and respiratory rate
   b. Shortness of breath
   c. Chest pain
   d. Cyanosis
2. Aspiration of saliva: same signs and symptoms as those indicating lung congestion (see item 1)
3. Hemorrhage:
   a. Falling blood pressure
   b. Increasing pulse rate
   c. Increasing respiratory rate
   d. Cold, pale, wet skin (shock)
   e. Restlessness and weakness
4. Retention of urine:
   a. Inability to pass urine
5. Dehydration:
   a. Concentrated (dark) urine
   b. Dry mouth
   c. Coated tongue
   d. Skin that has lost its elasticity (pinch does not disappear quickly)
   e. Elevation in temperature and increase in pulse and respiratory rates
   f. Restlessness and confusion
6. Electrolyte imbalance:
   a. Generalized weakness
   b. Vague aches and pains in the muscles
   c. Irritability, restlessness, confusion, and, at times, psychotic episodes
   d. Decreased pulse rate
   e. Rising temperature
7. Sore mouth: same signs as those indicating dehydration (see item 5)
8. Abdominal distention:
   a. Enlarged, swollen abdomen with skin over it becoming stretched, taut, and shiny
   b. Abdominal discomfort and pain
   c. Hiccoughing or nausea and/or vomiting
   d. Shortness of breath

During this period, the first 48 hours after the patient regains consciousness, he may receive oral fluids or he may receive all fluid intake intravenously. The method by which fluids are given depends on the operation that was done. If the patient had an operation on the gastrointestinal tract, he will probably receive nothing by mouth for 3 to 5 days. However, if the operation involved another system of the body, he may be started on oral fluids as soon as the nausea and vomiting from the anesthesia subside. However, if the patient's vomiting recurs, the oral fluids will be stopped immediately. Only the doctor knows the patient's condition. Therefore, only the doctor can determine when to start the patient on oral feedings.

The important thing for you to do is to carry out the patient care activities exactly as directed by the nurse. Then, the doctor will know from your accurate charting of intake and output and your careful measuring and charting of all drainage exactly what the patient's fluid and electrolyte needs are. Thus the doctor can give the patient the medical care that he needs to prevent complications and to achieve an early recovery.

POSTOPERATIVE NURSING CARE AFTER 48 HOURS

Forty-eight hours postoperatively the patient may be ordered out of bed for 15 minutes each morning and each evening. The doctor orders this out-of-bed treatment in order to increase the patient's physical movement and thus prevent clot formation in the legs and congestion in the lungs. The patient will still be quite sick and sore, even though he is allowed out of bed. He may still be receiving nothing by mouth and may be getting out of bed with the intravenous tubing attached to his arm. Therefore your nursing care during

this period will consist of the following:
1. Bathing the patient in bed
2. Assisting the patient out of bed twice a day for 15 minutes
3. Charting intake and output accurately
4. Encouraging the patient to breathe deeply, cough, and move his legs frequently
5. Taking the vital signs at least every 4 hours and reporting abnormal findings promptly
6. Providing the patient with an opportunity for interesting recreational activities
7. Observing the patient for signs of complications

Complications that may arise during the period after the first 48 hours are the following:
1. Congestion in the lungs, indicated by coughing, shortness of breath, cyanosis, chest pain, and elevated temperature
2. Persistent nausea and vomiting
3. Difficulty in voiding
4. Dehydration
5. Electrolyte imbalance
6. Abdominal distention
7. Dry, sore mouth
8. Pain in a body area other than the operative area with associated temperature elevation
   a. Pain in the calf of the leg—usually indicates thrombophlebitis (*thrombo*, clot; *phlebitis*, vein), or formation of a blood clot in the veins of the leg
   b. Pain in the left side of the chest that radiates down the left arm—usually indicates a heart attack
   c. Indigestion—usually indicates a heart attack
9. Evisceration, or reopening of the wound due to dissolving of the stitches before the wound is adequately healed; indicated by an increased amount of pink drainage on the dressings on or after the eighth postoperative day or the patient's complaint of a queer sensation in the operative site as though "something let go"

Complications can be prevented in this phase of the postoperative period if you recognize the fact that the patient is still very ill and needs your care and if you continue to give this care even when the patient is allowed out of bed. By being aware of the patient's condition, you will give him the care that he needs to keep on living effectively and you will make the observations that will identify a complication in this living.

One very common error nursing assistants make is to assume that every patient who is allowed out of bed is cured. When this happens, the newly operated on patient is required to care for himself long before he is able. This usually results in the patient's either doing so much that he falls or faints with weakness or doing so little that he lies in bed and develops a lung congestion such as pneumonia.

CLUES TO DIFFICULTY IN THE POSTOPERATIVE PERIOD

The vital signs keep you informed of the patient's condition. Therefore they should be taken every 15 minutes in the immediate postoperative period until they become stable. Then, they should be taken hourly on the operative day, and after this they should be taken at least every 4 hours.

The temperature shows whether the patient's body has been invaded by germs. This vital sign is the least significant sign in the immediate postoperative period, and it is therefore usually taken every 4 hours, even when the pulse, respirations, and blood pressure are taken every 15 minutes. However this is not true in those patients who have brain operations. In such patients, elevation of temperature indicates some interference with the heat-regulating mechanism of the brain. Therefore in the postoperative patient who has had brain surgery, the temperature is also taken every 15 minutes.

An elevated temperature during the postoperative period usually indicates the following:
1. First 72 hours postoperatively—infection in the lungs
2. Three to five days postoperatively—infection in the bladder
3. Five to eight days postoperatively—infection in the wound
4. Eight to ten days postoperatively—infection in the legs

The pulse and blood pressure indicate the condition of the heart, the blood vessels, and the blood, including the presence of blood loss or hemorrhage and excessive heart strain or heart failure. Therefore these signs are of special significance in helping you to observe the patient's progress throughout the postoperative period.

The respiration or breathing rate indicates the condition of the patient's lungs. The lungs are affected by the following conditions:
1. Decreased air space due to saliva or vomitus filling the lungs
2. Infections in the lungs that occur when the patient has too much pain to breathe deeply
3. Insufficient blood supply coming to the lungs to pick up oxygen for the body

Because of the foregoing effects, the respiratory rate will increase with hemorrhage and with lung infection or congestion. Respiratory infections are the most common postoperative complication. Therefore the respiratory rate is a significant vital sign to help you determine the patient's condition.

SUCTIONING THE THROAT OF THE POSTOPERATIVE PATIENT

The equipment that you need to suction saliva or vomitus out of the patient's throat includes the following:
1. Suction apparatus; either a wall suction apparatus or an electrically powered suction machine
2. Whistle-tip catheter and a T connector
3. Towel-covered suction tray containing:
   a. Small basin of benzalkonium chloride solution (1 to 750 dilution)
   b. Small basin of cold water
   c. Supply of tongue blades

Collect the equipment and set it up in the patient's room as follows:
1. Plug the wall suction apparatus into the wall suction outlet or plug the electrically powered apparatus into an electrical outlet.
2. Set up the suction tray on the patient's bedside stand.
3. Put the whistle-tip catheter into the benzalkonium chloride solution.
   a. Only one whistle-tip catheter and one basin of benzalkonium chloride solution needed for suctioning one orifice (the nose *or* the throat)
   b. Two basins of benzalkonium chloride solution and two whistle-tip catheters needed for suctioning two orifices (both the nose *and* the mouth)
   c. Label the catheter basins "nasal catheter in benzalkonium chloride" and/or "oral catheter in benzalkonium chloride"

Suction the patient's throat when he vomits or when you hear that his breathing is becoming moist and gurgling. Suction him in the following way:
1. Remove the catheter from the benzalkonium chloride solution and connect it to the suction apparatus.
2. Turn on the suction machine.
3. Dip the catheter into the basin of water and *rinse it thoroughly.*
4. Measure on the catheter the distance from the tip of the patient's nose to his ear. Add 2 inches to this measurement.
5. Insert the catheter into the patient's

nose for the distance that you measured off.

6. Permit the catheter to suction the saliva and mucus out of the patient's throat. Rotate the catheter to get out all of the secretions. Activate the suctioning by closing off the open end of the T connector with the tip of your finger.
7. Suction the patient's throat for approximately 15 seconds.
8. Release your finger to stop the suctioning. Remove the catheter from the patient's nose. Rinse it out.
9. Reinsert the catheter in the patient's nose and suction again if necessary. Suction until the respirations are again noiseless.
10. Turn off the suction apparatus. Disconnect the catheter and replace it in the benzalkonium chloride solution.
11. Make the patient comfortable.
12. Position the patient in a side-lying position with the back of the neck higher than the mouth so that the saliva will drain out of the mouth rather than down into his throat.
13. Return frequently to check the patient's respirations and to suction him.

Suctioning is continued for only 15 seconds at a time. Then it is stopped and the catheter is rinsed out. There are two reasons for this:

1. Discontinuing suctioning permits the patient to breathe.
2. Rinsing the catheter cleans out the thick mucus.

The mouth is suctioned in much the same way as just described, except that the procedure is a little more difficult for the following reasons:

1. The tongue gets in the way of the catheter.
2. The patient may clamp down on his teeth and prevent the entry of the catheter.
3. The patient may bite off the catheter.

Therefore when you are suctioning the patient's mouth or throat and are inserting the catheter through the mouth, you will need to use a tongue blade to keep the tongue down and out of the way and to keep the patient's mouth open. The oral catheter is used only for suctioning through the mouth, and the nasal catheter is used only for suctioning through the nose. The reason for this is that the mouth is filled with germs—the insertion of the oral catheter into the nose would inject the germs from the mouth down into the patient's throat, from which they would soon be pulled down into the lungs with his next breath.

If the patient coughs while you are suctioning his throat or nose, do not stop. The cough will bring up the lung secretions into the throat where you will be able

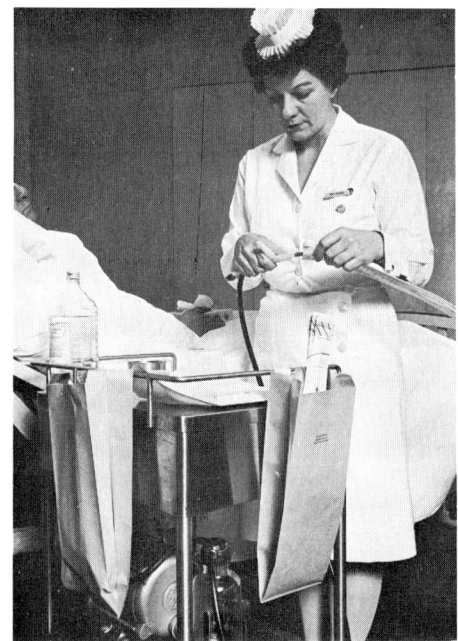

Fig. 37-1. The nurse is using sterile technique to connect the whistle-tip catheter to the suction source. Note the ample supply of sterile suctioning equipment.

to reach them with the catheter. Sometimes the doctor orders suctioning in a patient to stimulate this coughing and thus stimulate the removal of secretions from the lungs.

The patient with surgery on the air passages, the lungs, or the heart may be suctioned with sterile precautions. The additional equipment you will need to do this includes the following:

1. Sterile gloves
2. Supply of sterile catheters
3. Supply of sterile basins (for rinsing the catheter)
4. Supply of sterile rinsing solution
5. Container for used supplies

Use the technique described previously to suction the patient, but wear a glove and use a fresh sterile setup (catheter and basin) each time you do (Figs. 37-1 and 37-2).

GIVING THE PATIENT NASAL OXYGEN

The equipment that you will need to give the patient nasal oxygen is as follows:

1. Wall oxygen setup containing a humidifier or an oxygen setup on a tank, which contains a humidifier
2. Oxygen catheter
3. Piece of adhesive or Scotch tape
4. Lubricating agent
5. Tongue blades
6. "Oxygen in use" sign

Collect the equipment just listed and set it up in the patient's room as follows (Fig. 37-3):

1. Hang "oxygen in use" sign outside the patient's room.
2. Plug the wall oxygen setup into the wall oxygen outlet or attach the oxygen setup to the oxygen tank. (You will need a large wrench to attach the oxygen setup to a tank supply of oxygen.)
3. Unscrew the humidifier bottle from the oxygen apparatus and fill it with water up to the level indicated. (Use distilled water to prevent corrosion of the metal on the oxygen apparatus.)
4. Attach the catheter to the connector

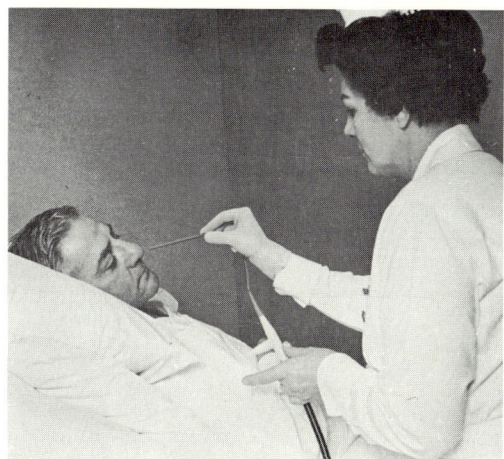

Fig. 37-2. The nurse is using sterile suctioning technique. Note that she inserts the nasal catheter with a glove-covered hand while she activates (nonsterile) the suction by closing off the open end of the T connector with an ungloved finger.

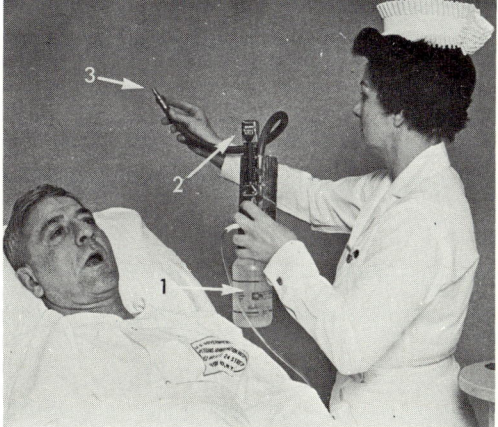

Fig. 37-3. The nurse is setting up the equipment to administer oxygen by way of a nasal catheter: **1**, oxygen humidifier, **2**, flow rate adjuster, and, **3**, connection to oxygen source (tank on wall).

on the tubing of the oxygen apparatus.
5. Start the flow of oxygen by turning on the oxygen supply valve on the wall outlet or on the tank. Adjust the flow of oxygen to that ordered by the doctor by turning the oxygen supply valve on the apparatus. The doctor usually orders an oxygen flow of 6 liters.
6. On the oxygen catheter, measure the distance from the tip of the patient's nose to his earlobe.
7. Lubricate the catheter with a water-soluble lubricating agent.
8. Insert the catheter into the patient's nose (Fig. 37-4) with the oxygen flowing. Insert it the measured-off distance (usually from 4 to 6 inches) (Fig. 37-5).
9. Attach the catheter to the tip of the patient's nose with a small strip of adhesive or Scotch tape.
10. Inspect the patient's throat. Use a tongue blade to hold down the tongue. If you can see the catheter at the back of the throat, the catheter is in too far. Pull it out a few inches until it cannot be seen in the throat.
11. Make the patient comfortable.
12. Return to the patient in 30 minutes and feel the stomach area (area in the middle of the body just below the ribs) with your entire hand. If the stomach area feels inflated (like a blown-up balloon), the nasal oxygen tube is inserted too far and the oxygen is going down into the patient's stomach instead of into his lungs. Remove the nasal tube and reinsert it as described previously.

You can easily understand the need for the humidifier bottle (bottle of water) and the reason the oxygen is bubbled through it before it is directed into the patient's throat if you take about six deep breaths through your mouth. Feel how dry your mouth is. You bypassed your nose with this mouth breathing and so your mouth has been dried out by the air.

When the patient receives nasal oxygen by catheter, the functions of the nose are bypassed as the oxygen is placed in the back of the throat. The oxygen dries the mucous membranes of the throat and makes the saliva thick and sticky. This drying can be avoided by wetting or humidifying the oxygen. You see now that one of the func-

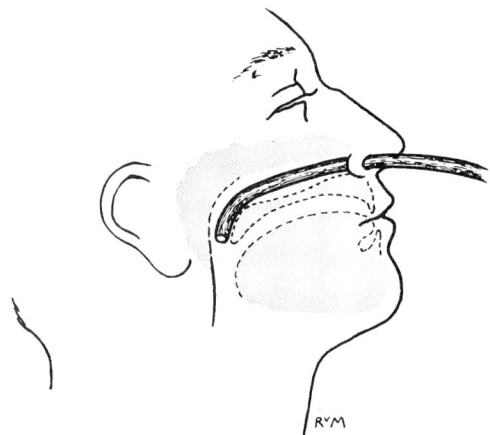

Fig. 37-4. The oxygen catheter in position.

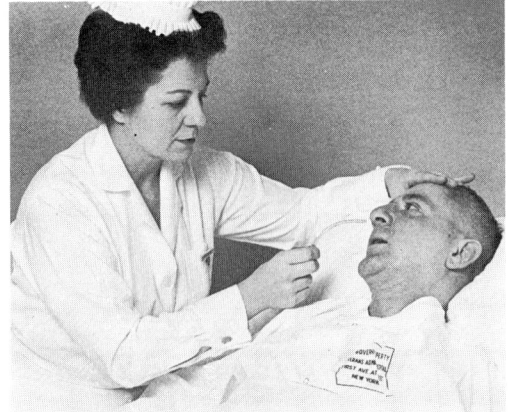

Fig. 37-5. The nurse is explaining and comforting the breathless patient while she inserts the nasal catheter to start the oxygen therapy.

tions of the nose is to moisten the air that you breathe.

Return to the patient frequently. Observe him carefully to determine whether or not cyanosis and dyspnea are decreasing. Report your findings to the nurse. Refill the humidifier bottle with water as needed. Change the patient's position every 2 hours. Remove the nasal catheter every 8 hours and reinsert a fresh one so that the holes in it do not become plugged with mucus.

A nasal cannula consists of a plastic base containing two 1-inch nasal projections and an elastic head strap. This nasal cannula can be used instead of a catheter to give the patient nasal oxygen. Administering oxygen through the nasal cannula instead of through the catheter has the following advantages:

1. Since the cannula nasal piece is short, the oxygen is introduced just inside the nose. This permits humidification of the oxygen by the patient's own nose.
2. Since the nasal cannula is short, there is no danger of directing the flow of oxygen into the patient's esophagus and thereby causing distention of the stomach (Fig. 37-6).

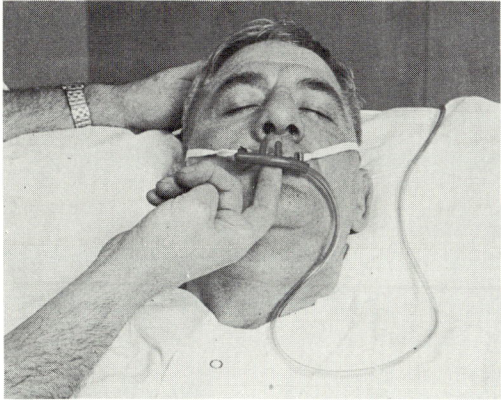

Fig. 37-6. Oxygen therapy via nasal cannula.

A disadvantage of administering oxygen to the patient by means of the cannula is that the mouth breather does not receive an adequate oxygen supply.

GIVING THE PATIENT DEEP-BREATHING AND COUGHING EXERCISES

Deep-breathing exercises that increase lung movements and assist in bringing up lung secretions can be done in the following way:

1. Position the patient so that there is the least possible limitation of chest movements by the bed. The most desirable position is a sitting position on the side of the bed. However, when this is not possible, a back-lying position with the patient's head elevated will be adequate.
2. Relieve the patient's discomfort and pain insofar as possible. Give him a urinal or bedpan if he needs it. Inform the nurse if the patient complains of pain.
3. Instruct the patient to breathe in deeply. Position one of his hands on his chest so that he can feel how deeply he is breathing.
4. Instruct the patient to exhale deeply.
5. Have the patient repeat this breathing in and out about ten times. He may feel silly just doing deep-breathing exercises, since he sees little or no purpose in them. A meaningful and interesting way to have the patient do these breathing exercises is to give him an inexpensive mouth organ and an instruction sheet and let him practice playing it.
6. Support the patient's operative area during breathing exercises if the muscular movement of the exercises increases his pain. This can be done by supporting and splinting the area with the palms of your two hands. This prevents movement in the operative area and avoids the pain that the movement causes.

Coughing exercises that help bring up lung secretions can be done in the following way:

1. Position the patient so that he has the least possible limitation of chest movement by the bed. The most desirable positions are as follows:
   a. Sitting on the side of the bed
   b. Sitting up in bed and leaning forward on an overbed table
2. Relieve the patient's pain or discomfort.
3. Support the patient's operative area by splinting it with your hands to prevent jerky muscle movements and pain.
4. Instruct the patient to exhale deeply.
5. Instruct the patient to breathe in deeply.
6. Instruct the patient to exhale with an explosive cough.
7. Instruct the patient to bring up loose secretions with this cough. Have him expectorate these secretions into a tissue.
8. Have the patient cough, by repeating this procedure, about six times.
9. Return the patient to a comfortable position in bed.
10. Return and cough the patient as frequently as ordered by the doctor (Fig. 37-7).

APPLYING ELASTIC BANDAGES TO THE PATIENT'S LEGS

If you are instructed by the nurse to bandage the patient's legs in order to prevent the formation of blood clots, collect the following equipment and take it to the patient's room:

1. Two 4-inch elastic bandages for each leg to be wrapped
2. Four bandage fasteners (or safety pins) for each leg
3. Firm pillow or box on which to elevate the leg (bed frame may be used)

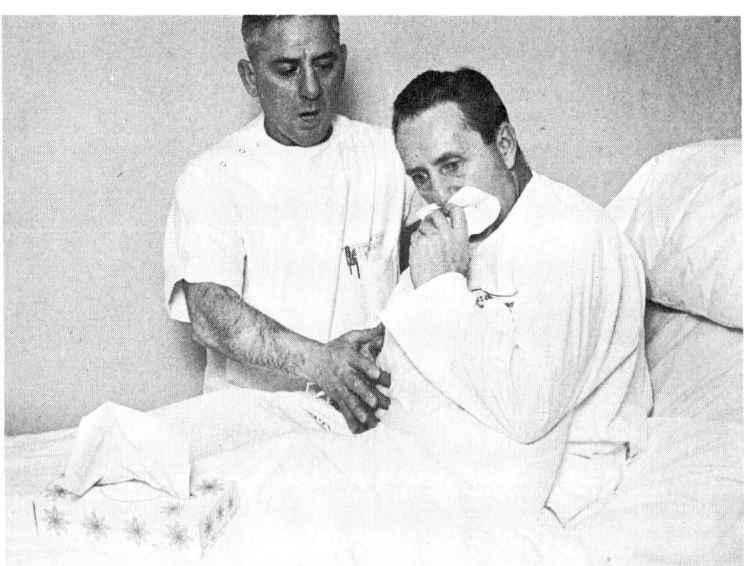

Fig. 37-7. The nursing assistant coughs the patient. Note: (1) the patient's chest is free of the bed, (2) the incisional area is supported with a pillow, and (3) the patient is coughing productively.

Caring for the postoperative patient   **367**

After all the necessary equipment has been brought to the patient's bedside, apply the bandage to the leg in the following way:

1. Elevate the leg on the pillow or box or on the frame of the bed.
2. Begin wrapping the leg just below the toes.
3. Wrap the bandage around the area of the foot just below the toes twice. This anchors the bandage.
4. Proceed to enclose the entire leg (to well above the knee) in the bandage. With each turn of the bandage, cover one third of the preceding turn. Hold the bandage firmly in your hand as you apply it, but do not pull it too tightly.
5. Fasten the bandage with clips or safety pins. Continue wrapping the leg with the second bandage.
6. Fasten the second bandage with clips or with a safety pin.
7. Wrap the second leg if you were directed to do so.
8. Return the patient to a comfortable position in bed.
9. Return in an hour and check the patient's leg for any signs that would indicate that the bandage is too tight. Such signs would include:
   a. Swelling of the exposed toes
   b. Coldness of the exposed toes
   c. Numbness of the exposed toes
10. Remove the bandage and rewrap the leg if signs occur indicating that the bandage is interfering with the circulation in the limb.
11. Remove the bandage daily and reapply it as just described. Be sure that you enclose the entire leg, including the heel, in the bandage (Fig. 37-8). If you do not, blood will pool in the unwrapped area and clots will form there. Clots will not form in the unwrapped toes because of

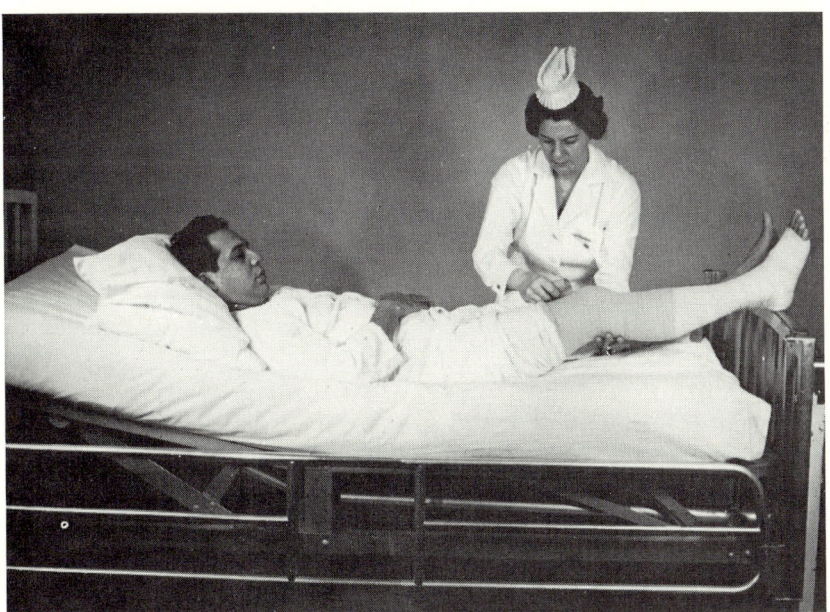

Fig. 37-8. The patient's leg is wrapped in two elastic bandages to prevent blood from pooling in the leg and forming clots.

the small blood supply in that area. However, the patient should be encouraged to wiggle his toes frequently.

APPLYING A BINDER TO THE PATIENT'S ABDOMEN

If you are instructed to apply a binder to support the patient's abdomen, collect the following equipment and take it to the patient's bedside:
1. Binder—Scultetus (many-tailed) or plain straight binder
2. Supply of safety pins—two if a Scultetus binder is used and six of a plain binder is used.

After the appropriate equipment has been brought to the patient's bedside, apply the binder as follows:
1. Expose that area of the patient's body to which the binder is to be applied by folding down the bed covers.
2. Turn the patient and put the binder under him just as you do when you put a fresh sheet on the bed under a patient.
3. Return the patient to a back-lying position, flat in bed over the binder.
4. Inspect the binder and be sure that it is positioned under the patient so that it will support the operative area but will not limit chest movements.
5. Apply the Scultetus binder as follows:
   a. Start wrapping it around the abdomen at the point that does not need the greatest support; in other words, start at the bottom of the binder for higher abdominal operations and at the top for lower abdominal operations.
   b. Bring one tail of the binder across the patient's abdomen and hold it in place by bringing a second tail, from the opposite side of the binder, over it.
   c. Cover two thirds of each tail on the binder with the next one, proceeding until you come to the last tail.
   d. Bring the last tail diagonally across the patient's abdomen (to hold all the tails in place) and fasten it there with a safety pin.
6. Apply the plain binder by pulling it firmly across the abdomen and pinning it in position.
7. Return the patient to a comfortable position in bed by replacing the top covers and by elevating the patient's head.
8. Return frequently to check the patient and see that he is comfortable and that the binder is not interfering with his breathing and chest movement.
9. Reapply the binder whenever it becomes displaced or uncomfortable.

CARING FOR THE PATIENT WITH DRAINAGE TUBES

If you are assigned the care of a patient with drainage tubes in place, collect the following equipment and take it to the patient's bedside:
1. Drainage bottle
2. Some connecting tubing
3. Tube irrigating tray

Connect the tube in the patient to the drainage bottle with the connecting tubing. Attach the drainage bottle to the bed with a holder or a hook. Set up the irrigating tray on the patient's bedside stand. This tray contains the following:
1. Basin of irrigating solution (usually saline)
2. Irrigating syringe
3. Emesis basin for the returning irrigating solution

The nurse will usually irrigate the patient's tubes. However, the principle of irrigation is much the same at that described for bladder irrigations (Chapter 32).

Your care of the patient with a tube in place will be to recognize that:
1. A tube is put into the patient to bring

something out. Therefore you will need to observe the drainage bottles to be sure that the tube is open and draining.
2. A kinked tube shuts off drainage. Therefore you will need to maintain the drainage tubing in a straight line from the bed to the drainage bottle (see Chaper 32).
3. A tube in the nose makes breathing through the nose difficult and forces the patient to become a mouth breather. Therefore you will need to:
   a. Give frequent mouth care
   b. Take the patient's temperature rectally
   c. Encourage the patient to breathe deeply to avoid lung complications
   d. Change the patient's position frequently
4. A tube drains material out of the patient's body. This drainage of material results in fluid and electrolyte loss, and the amount of material drained should be charted on the intake and output record.
5. If the patient hemorrhages, the tube may bring blood to the outside of the patient's body and into the drainage bottle. Therefore you will need to observe the kind and amount of drainage closely and report any bloody drainage to the nurse immediately. Excessive drainage or no drainage should be reported to the nurse immediately.
6. A tube in the throat irritates it and increases the flow of mucus. This mucus can be pulled down into the patient's lungs easily and may cause lung congestion. Therefore you will need to encourage coughing, spitting up secretions, moving about, etc. in the patient with a tube in place in order to prevent lung congestion from occurring.

The postoperative patient places his life in your hands. He will have an uneventful postoperative course and a speedy recovery if you take good care of him. On the other hand, dangerous complications may occur if you do not provide adequate care. Put yourself in the patient's place and take care of him in the same way that you would want him to care for you if your positions were reversed.

SUMMARY

Postoperative care consists essentially of doing the activities of living for a newly operated upon patient until he regains the physical and the emotional ability to do them for himself. Surgery and anesthesia interfere with the patient's ability to breathe, swallow, eat, move, and void. Therefore the members of the hospital staff must not only do these activities for the patient, but they must also teach and motivate the patient to do as many of them for himself as soon as he is able in order to prevent postoperative complications from occurring.

DISCUSSION QUESTIONS

1. Ask the nurse to suction a patient. Observe how she determines the distance to insert the suction catheter. How far does she insert it?
2. Why does a postoperative patient have difficulty breathing deeply or coughing up secretions?
3. Observe the intake and output records on your postoperative patients. How could they be improved?
4. How could you recognize that a postoperative complication, such as congestion in the lungs, is occurring in one of your patients?
5. Why are the fingers and toes left out of a cast or an elastic bandage?
6. Ask the nurse to supervise you as you suction a patient. How did you feel when the patient began to cough? Did you stop? Should you stop when a patient coughs while you suction him?
7. Where is the recovery room located in the hospital in which you work? Why is it located where it is?
8. What kind of operations were done on your patients? Why is it necessary for you to know about the patient's operation before you can safely care for him?
9. Which period is the most life-threatening one in the postoperative course? Why?

10 Who determines when the operated upon patient is to have oral liquids?
11 Why are postoperative patients thirsty? How can you relieve this thirst?

SOURCES OF ADDITIONAL INFORMATION

1 Film: Basic care of patients. Part IX: Postoperative care; may be obtained from Director, Armed Forces Institute of Pathology, Walter Reed Army Medical Center, 6825 16th St. N. W., Washington, D. C. 20025.
2 Film: Making a recovery bed; may be obtained from Director, Medical Film Library, United States Naval Medical School, National Naval Medical Center, Bethesda, Md. 20014.
3 Film: Postoperative care; may be obtained from Director, Medical Film Library, United States Naval Medical School, National Naval Medical Center, Bethesda, Md. 20014.
4 Pamphlet: Common medical terminology; may be obtained from Abbott Laboratories, North Chicago, Ill. 60064 (or ask your hospital pharmacist to get it for you).

38/Caring for the patient who is breathless

STUDY QUESTIONS

1. Why breathe?
2. What physical state gives the patient a feeling of breathlessness?
3. Why is the patient with pneumonia short of breath?
4. Why is the hemorrhaging patient short of breath?
5. Why is the patient with heart disease short of breath?
6. Why do you get breathless during strenuous exercise?
7. What makes us breathe?
8. Are all breathless patients given the same treatment?
9. Which breathless patients are treated with oxygen, with a tracheotomy, with artificial respiration? Why?
10. How do you care for a patient in order to "save his breath"?
11. How do you give artificial respiration?
12. What is the danger in oxygen therapy?
13. When do you suction a patient in a respirator?
14. How do you breathe for the respirator patient if the electricity fails?
15. What is an IPPB machine?
16. What is the difference between oxygen therapy and artificial respiration?

ESSENTIALS FOR CELL LIFE

The cells of the body live and work effectively only when they have an adequate oxygen supply and an efficient carbon dioxide removal system. This system is achieved by the following:

1. An adequate supply of air (inflow to and outflow from the lungs)
2. An effective exchange of oxygen and carbon dioxide between the air sacs (alveoli) in the lungs and the blood
3. An efficient transportation system that carries oxygen to the cells and carbon dioxide back from them to the lungs

Breathing (inspiration and expiration) is only one part of this system. It gets the air in and out of the lungs. The other two equally important parts are the lungs and the blood.

OXYGEN REQUIREMENTS

When the body is at rest (doing only the work of carrying on living), its oxygen need is quite small. The body meets this need by breathing about eighteen times per minute and by taking in about 350 ml. of air with each breath or about 6,300 ml.* per minute. The lung capacity (amount of air held without special exertion) is about 2,700 ml. Each expiration exchanges about one

---
*6,300 ml. is about equal to 6⅓ quarts; remember, 1,000 ml. = 1 quart.

seventh of the air in the lungs (350 ml.) and leaves behind approximately 2,350 ml.

The oxygen from the breathed-in air passes (diffuses like the odor of perfume diffuses through the air) through the air sacs in the lungs and goes into the blood. The blood picks it up and carries it to all the cells of the body.

The heart, when the body is at rest, pumps about 5,000 ml. (5 quarts) of blood around the body each minute. Each 1,000 ml. (quart) of blood carries about 50 ml. (less than 2 ounces) of oxygen, so that approximately 250 ml.* (½ pint) of oxygen is delivered to the cells of the body each minute by the 5,000 ml. (5 quarts) of circulating blood.

Activity increases the work of the cells, and it also increases the amount of oxygen that they need. Activity therefore increases the breathing rate, the pulse rate, and the oxygen–carbon dioxide exchange rate between the blood and the lungs. The cells of the extremely active adult (athlete) may require and receive as much as fifteen times 250 ml. (½ pint) of oxygen or 3,750 ml. (almost 4 quarts) per minute.

CONTROL OF BREATHING RATES

The breathing center in the brain (Chapter 22) is excited by increases in the carbon dioxide levels (waste material from the cells) in the blood and stimulates inspiration and expiration to occur. This breathing ventilates (brings in oxygen and gets rid of carbon dioxide) the blood and lowers the carbon dioxide level. The cells of the body are freed of the waste material (carbon dioxide) and the interference it causes in their functioning.

The breathing center in the brain is something of a carbon dioxide "stat," similar to a thermo(heat)stat, in that it regulates the amount of this gas in the bloodstream.

In some diseased conditions, like emphysema, the patient's ineffective breathing is unable to reduce his high level of carbon dioxide to that found normally in the blood. Although small increases in carbon dioxide blood levels do stimulate respirations, excess amounts depress them and throw the patient into coma and apnea (respiratory arrest) and death. As the patient's respirations decrease, his oxygen supply in the blood also decreases; and his body cells, deprived of oxygen, falter and then stop in their work of living. A second and emergency system for exciting respirations and maintaining life is activated in this emphysema patient by his oxygen need.

This emergency system consists of two special sets of cells that monitor the level of the oxygen supply in his body. These cells are located in the big blood vessel that carries oxygenated blood out of the heart (aorta) and in the one carrying oxygenated blood to the brain (carotid). These oxygen monitors get excited only when the blood oxygen level falls dangerously low, and they send an urgent demand for oxygen to the brain by way of a nerve. The breathing center is stimulated just in time, and the patient breathes. However, this patients feels dyspneic and breathes only when his cells scream for the oxygen that prevents their death rather than in the usual easy way triggered off by slight increases in carbon dioxide blood levels.

Remember that this second and emergency control of breathing is on the basis of oxygen want. It will be discussed in detail later. However, here it must be stressed that giving oxygen to this type of patient would eliminate the basis for stimulating his breathing center and would throw him into apnea (no breathing) and death. Oxygen cannot be given to the patient with emphysema unless it is accompanied by some method of artificial respiration (method of artificial breathing control).

---

*6,300 ml. of air taken in each minute. Air inspired contains 20% oxygen. Air expired contains 16% oxygen. Therefore, 4% (250 ml.) of the oxygen in the 6,300 ml. of air gets to the cells.

THE PATIENT WITH BREATHLESSNESS

Breathlessness occurs when the cells of the body need more oxygen than they are receiving. Conditions that interfere with an adequate oxygen delivery might be the following:

1. Conditions of the air passages:
   a. Obstruction to the inflow of air by a limp jaw and tongue, or a tumor, or an aspirated meal
   b. Obstruction to the outflow of air by a swelling and spasm in the bronchioles (small air tubes carrying air in and out of the air sacs) like that found in asthma
   c. Obstruction to the outflow of air by mucus plugs, or by swelling and infection in the bronchioles of emphysematous patients (patients whose lungs are blown up with old, retained air)
2. Conditions of the heart:
   a. Failure of the heart to pump the blood around the body effectively because of heart disease
3. Conditions of the blood:
   a. Insufficient supply of blood to carry the amount of oxygen that the body needs as in anemia or blood loss through hemorrhage
4. Conditions of the lungs:
   a. Inadequate lung area due to space-taking lung diseases such as pneumonia (air spaces fill with germs and fluid), atelectasis (collapse of the air sacs), pulmonary edema (blood stagnates in the heart because of left-sided heart failure; fluid seeps out of this blood and into the air sacs, thus filling them with fluid and decreasing the space for air), or silicosis (constant dust inhalation causes the lung tissue to become scarred and fixed and unable to move freely to bring in and give out the air)
5. Conditions of the brain:
   a. Failure of the respiratory center in the brain to work effectively because of pressure or tumors
6. Conditions of the muscles:
   a. Inability of the respiratory muscles to work because of muscle-wasting diseases such as amyotrophic lateral sclerosis
7. Diseases of the nerves:
   a. Inability of the nerves to carry the breathing message from the brain to the breathing muscles as in poliomyelitis, Guillian-Barré syndrome, or cervical (spinal cord) injuries

SIGNS AND SYMPTOMS OF OXYGEN NEED

Cyanosis

The flow of the blood through the small vessels gives the skin its color. Blood with a low oxygen content is dark blue, and it gives the skin the blue color that is called cyanosis. This cyanosis can be seen in the fingernail beds, the lips, the tip of the nose, and in the ear lobes. In a patient with a darkly colored skin, cyanosis is seen best in the mucous membranes of the mouth.

The anemic patient (decreased blood supply) looks pale even when the blood has a low oxygen content. This is because he has a decreased amount of blood circulating through the skin and so has little blood to get blue.

Dyspnea

Respirations are under the control of the voluntary and the involuntary nervous system. Dyspnea (a need or desire for air, air hunger) will occur with any condition that interferes with the oxygen supply to the cells, but it can also occur from abnormal thought patterns. Everyone who thinks about their breathing feels a little dyspneic and breathes more rapidly. Remember that in Chapter 22 you learned to count respirations with your fingers on the patient's pulse so that he would be unaware of your purposes and unlikely to change his breathing rate.

Sleeplessness

The patient with extreme dyspnea uses auxiliary muscles (those not normally used for breathing and those under the control of the will) to help him breathe. These are the muscles of the neck, shoulders, and upper arms. (Run up and down the stairs a few times. Observe your use of these auxiliary muscles to assist you breathe.) This extra breathing effort with the use of the auxiliary muscles uses more energy, requires conscious effort, and is very fatiguing.

When the dyspneic patient falls asleep, the auxiliary muscles of breathing (those under the conscious control of the will) stop helping his respiratory effort, and his breathing effectiveness decreases. Then, too, the bed splints his body and limits his chest movements and further impedes his breathing effectiveness. After only a short period of sleep, the dyspneic patient goes into oxygen want and wakes up frightened, breathless, and gasping for air.

Fear

The patient knows that his life continues as long as he breathes; therefore breathlessness frightens him, and he signals for help to prevent the death that he thinks is approaching. He is afraid to be alone, and he calls you constantly; or he may even come out of his room to find you. Fear increases the work of the cells. It makes them work harder to prepare the body to fight or flee the threatening danger, and so fear increases the cells' need for oxygen. It is a vicious cycle. Breathlessness causes fear. Fear increases the cells' oxygen need and so further increases the breathlessness.

Helplessness

Physical movement, whether it be work or play or just doing the activities of living, increases the cells' need for oxygen. The dyspneic patient (dyspneic at rest) can do nothing but lie motionless in bed in order to keep his oxygen need at the lowest possible level. In fact, he must use all his time and energy to breathe in enough air to maintain that level. He cannot even feed himself because that increases his activity and his oxygen need. Then, too, he needs the shoulder and arm muscles to help him bring in the life-supporting air much more than he needs food.

The dyspneic patient who is working hard at breathing will soon use up all his energy and become exhausted. Then his breathing effort will become ineffective and he will die.

Carbon dioxide intoxication

Carbon dioxide intoxication (poisoning) occurs when the lungs hold on to the air that they should expire. Then the blood not only fails to get rid of its carbon dioxide but it also fails to obtain fresh supplies of oxygen. Blood carbon dioxide levels increase and oxygen levels decrease. At first, the breathing center attempts to correct this situation by ventilating the body (increasing the breathing rate), but soon the brain, poisoned by the carbon dioxide and starved by the oxygen deficiency, falters and stops functioning altogether; the patient lapses into coma and death as his breathing rate slows and eventually stops (arrests).

FACTORS THAT INCREASE OXYGEN NEED AND SO ACCELERATE RESPIRATORY RATES

The cells of the body carry on the activities of living. Any factor that speeds up this living will, of course, increase all of the needs of the cells including their need for oxygen. These factors include the following:

1. Exercise (muscular movement) may increase the oxygen need of the cells up to fifteen times the amount required at rest.

2. Temperature elevations add to cell activity. A 1° temperature rise doubles or triples cellular activity and so doubles or triples oxygen need.
3. Emotional states function much the same as exercise in that they speed up cellular activity in order to prepare the body to fight or flee a danger. Therefore pain, fear, worry, etc. also intensify oxygen need.

The respiratory system

The respiratory system is a passageway that takes air from the outside of the body to the blood and then returns it to the outside. This system starts with the nose and ends with the thousands of tiny air sacs in the lung. It looks very much like a tree, beginning with one trunk planted in the earth and ending with the thousands of leaves that it exposes to the sun (Fig. 38-1).

Respiration, like all work in the body, is accomplished through muscle action. Inspiration occurs when the muscles surrounding the lungs contract (shorten) and pull away from them, thus enlarging the chest cavity and permitting the spongelike lungs to expand freely into the bigger space. During this expansion of the lungs, air is forced into them and inspiration occurs. Then the muscles relax and spring back (like a stretched elastic band returns to its original position), thus compressing (squeezing) the lungs into the smaller space and forcing the spongelike lungs to give up air, and expiration occurs (Fig. 22-1).

Respiration is accomplished by changing the size of the chest space. Situations that permit this to occur help breathing and those that hinder it limit breathing.

PROTECTIVE MECHANISMS IN THE RESPIRATORY SYSTEM

The respiratory system keeps the air passages open by preventing foreign material (anything but air) from getting into them and by clearing out anything that does happen to get in. You have already learned about the protective actions of the epiglottis and how it closes over the trachea (windpipe) during swallowing (Chapter 8). The other protective mechanisms are the following:

1. The *nose* warms, moistens, and filters (takes out dust particles) the air.
2. The mucus-coated, ciliated (hairlike projections) *lining of the air passages* (trachea and lungs) collects small particles (adhere to the fluid) and moves them up and out of the air

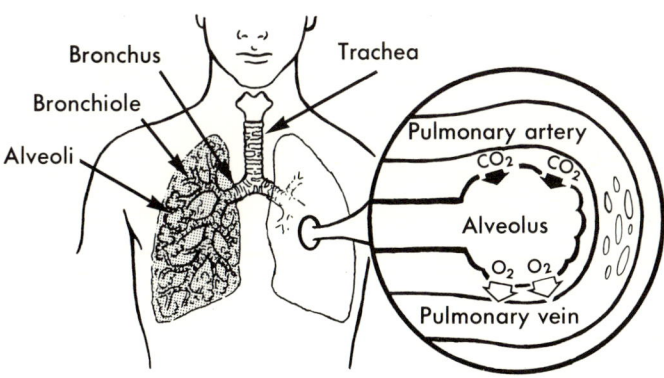

Fig. 38-1. Respiratory system. Note the CO_2—O_2 exchange between the alveolus and the blood.

passages (cilia sweep them up into the throat) (Fig. 38-1). (This material is then swallowed or expectorated.)
3. The *cough reflex* removes foreign material from the trachea or bronchi by sudden explosions of air outward. (This cough reflex is triggered off by the irritation of the sensitive trachea or bronchi with any foreign material.)
4. The *sneeze reflex* clears nasal passages of irritating foreign particles.

Remember that the unconscious patient loses the protective action of these mechanisms—you will have to take over and keep his air passages open and clean.

PREVENTION OF RESPIRATORY COMPLICATIONS

Respiratory complications occur when a foreign object gets into the air passages or when the mucus secretions are not swept up and out of the lungs.

The foreign objects most frequently sucked into the lungs with the air are saliva and food. The patient with swallowing difficulty is helped to aspirate this material by gravity when he is in a back-lying position. Prevent the aspiration, then, simply by avoiding this position. If it cannot be avoided, suction the patient frequently while he is in it. The patient with some swallowing difficulty should be fed very cautiously with the emergency suction apparatus standing by.

The mucus secretions are retained in the part of the lungs that is not working freely at breathing, the part that is splinted by the bed or the patient's muscles. You can prevent the pneumonia or atelectasis that complicates bed rest and surgery by changing the patient's position frequently and by encouraging him to cough and breathe deeply, thus using all his lung spaces.

The postoperative patient cannot be taught to cough and breathe because it hurts him to do so. This teaching must be done in the preoperative period.

Carbon dioxide inhalations (5% carbon dioxide and 95% oxygen) may be given through a mask to increase the rate and depth of the patient's slow, shallow breathing. These inhalations may be given three or four times a day for a period of 20 minutes. The nurse will give this treatment, but you must watch the patient closely (during this treatment) for signs of carbon dioxide intoxication, for example, slowing of the respirations, developing cyanosis, dulling of the consciousness, confusion, coma, and death. Remove the mask and get the nurse if you observe any of these symptoms developing.

CARING FOR THE DYSPNEIC PATIENT

The doctor will simplify the patient's living to the level that his respiratory system can support. This simplification may include the following medical directions:
1. Bed rest
2. Staff care (absolute bed rest)
3. Soft diet (little effort required to chew and digest it)
4. Stool softeners (soften and therefore decrease the energy required in defecation)
5. Bedside commode for defecation (utilize gravity and decrease effort required)
6. Tap water for drinking (ice water narrows blood vessels in the heart and decreases heart action)
7. Privacy (removes the patient from the excitement and the disturbances of the hospital)

The nurse will develop a plan of care that makes the patient's living as effortless as possible. In this plan she will direct you to do the activities of living for the patient.

You can make the patient's living easy by doing the following activities for him:
1. Reduce the patient's work at living:
   a. Keep the patient on absolute bed rest. Do all his care (Chapter 13).
2. Control pain and discomfort:

a. Report patient's complaints of pain to the nurse promptly.
b. Change the patient's position at 2-hour intervals.
c. Keep his personal articles close by. Prevent reaching, stretching, etc.
3. Eliminate emotional distress:
   a. Prevent feelings of helplessness and fear by your caring, comforting presence.
   b. Listen to the patient's problem and help him solve it, or report it to the nurse promptly so that she can do so.
   c. Avoid threatening experiences. Explain procedures before doing them. Work slowly and give the patient many rests. Do not hurry him.
   d. Protect the patient from disturbing situations. The nurse will discuss the patient's need for protection with his family. You will need to observe family visiting and its aftereffects on the patient and to report any signs of emotional distress indicating that the nurse's directions are not being carried out. Visiting may need to be stopped altogether if it distresses the patient.
4. Conserve the patient's energy:
   a. Assist him on and off the bedside commode.
   b. Answer his calls promptly or, better still, visit him frequently to determine his needs so that he does not need to call.
   c. Give him drinks that are neither hot nor cold.
   d. Follow the nurse's directions for bathing and positioning the patient. (These procedures may need to be modified or even eliminated if they use up the energy that the patient needs to breathe.)

You can make the patient's breathing easier by doing the following activities:
1. Place him in a semi-sitting (Fowler's) position. In this position gravity pulls the abdominal contents (bowels, stomach, etc.) away from the diaphragm (muscle at the bottom of the

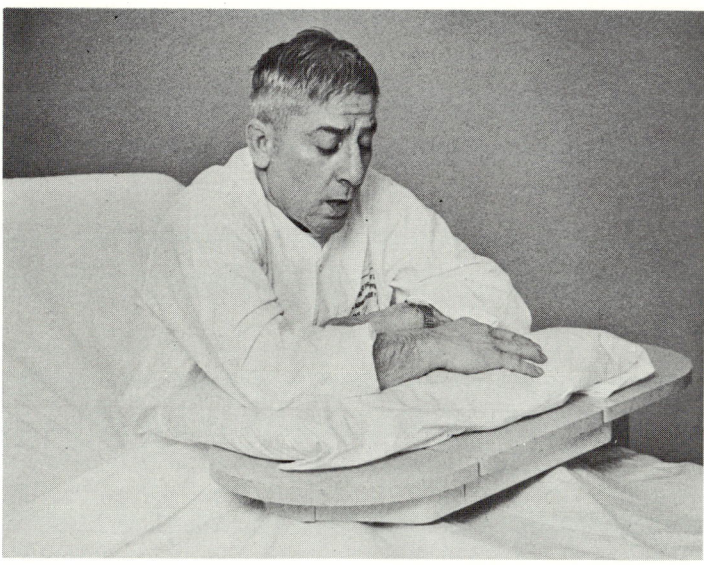

Fig. 38-2. The bed splint is removed from the chest of the breathless patient.

chest cavity) and permits it to move easily. This position also pulls fluid (pulmonary edema or infections such as pneumonia) to the bottom of the lung and frees the remaining lung space for breathing.
2. Free the patient's chest from the splinting effect of the bed. Place an overbed table in position in front of the patient and permit him to lean on it. Teach him to support himself with his arms (Fig. 38-2).
3. Change the patient's position frequently, if permitted. This rotates pressure-bearing and lung-splinting areas and helps to avoid not only decubitus ulcers but also the respiratory complications of bed rest. Protect weight-bearing buttocks areas with lamb's wool mats (absorb moisture and equalize pressure) or sponge rubber seats (equalizes pressure).
4. Avoid the use of powdery or pungent materials (like talcum and alcohol), which contaminate the patient's air, irritate his passageways, and increase his breathlessness.

TREATMENT FOR RESPIRATORY DISTRESS
From an obstruction of the airway

The patient with a blocked air passage will be cyanotic, gasping, and frightened. Send for help while you try to open the airway. Suction the airway. If unsuccessful, roll the patient over on his abdomen and position him across the bed. Slide him toward you and permit his upper body to hang over the side of the bed until his mouth is well below his chest. Cup (slap the chest with the hand held in the position of a cup) the chest vigorously. Cupping and gravity may loosen and dislodge the obstruction.

The professional staff (doctor and nurse) will do an emergency tracheotomy in the patient's room to bypass the obstruction if you are unsuccessful in removing it. Assist them as directed.

The unconscious patient in a back-lying position will obstruct his airway with his limp tongue. You can recognize this block by his struggling, snoring respirations.

Relieve it by placing the patient in a side-lying position and/or by putting an airway in his mouth over his tongue. The airway will keep his tongue up in his mouth (out of his throat) and his air passages open.

Remember that swelling in the throat will block the air passages too. Observe all your patients with infections, tumors, or surgery on the throat for adequate effortless breathing. Report any difficulty (effort required to breathe, dyspnea, or cyanosis) you observe to the nurse immediately. The doctor will need to do an emergency tracheotomy, so have the necessary equipment standing by and ready for use everytime you have a patient with throat conditions on your ward.

From oxygen need

The patient who is unable to meet his body's demand for oxygen because of lung disease, heart disease, or blood deficiency will get an oxygen-rich gas mixture* to breathe. Then each breath will deliver more oxygen to his lungs and to his blood.

The methods used to deliver this oxygen-rich gas can be a tent (40% oxygen), a nasal catheter or cannula (40% oxygen), a face tent (40% oxygen), or a mask (100% oxygen). The doctor will order the oxygen delivery method that the patient needs.

Oxygen therapy is relatively easy to start. However, it is a dangerous treatment because oxygen supports (encourages) combustion (burning) and blows a little spark into a huge fire. Eliminate this hazard by doing the following:
1. Prepare the patient:
   a. Explain that you are going to give him oxygen to help him breathe.
   b. Tell him that smoking is forbid-

---
*Air is 20% oxygen.

den. Remove his cigarettes and matches.
2. Prepare the room:
   a. Hang a "No smoking—oxygen in use" sign on the door *to* the room.
   b. Remove all spark-producing electrical equipment and all highly inflammable material (alcohol, grease, etc.)
   c. Place a fire extinguisher outside the door (Fig. 38-3).
3. Use the following additional precautions when an oxygen tent is used:
   a. Remove all wool and plastic material from the patient's bed. These things may ignite the oxygen-filled tent with a static electrical spark.
   b. Place a conductive (spreads the electricity throughout the sheet and so dissipates it) rubber sheet over the mattress and under the patient. Cover it with a bed sheet.
   c. Remove the bed linen and replace it with flame-resistant bed linen (less likely to ignite from a spark).
   d. Ground the tent (connect it to an object that takes the excess electricity off into the earth or into some other object that fails to carry it further but that is away from the treatment area).

Then deliver the oxygen to the patient:
1. Nasal oxygen by catheter or cannula (see Figs. 37-4 to 37-6)
2. Nasal oxygen by mask:
   a. Collect the equipment:
      (1) Oxygen supply
      (2) Flowmeter, tubing, and mask (humidifier not required—why?)
   b. Prepare the patient as outlined previously.
   c. Take equipment to the patient's bedside and initiate treatment as follows:

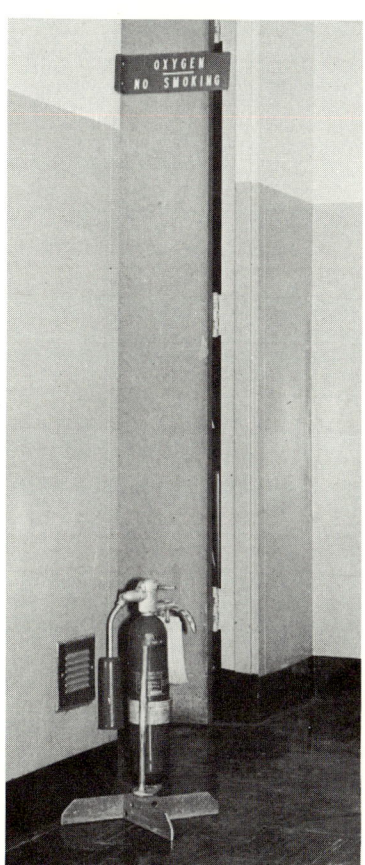

Fig. 38-3. Safety precautions during oxygen therapy.

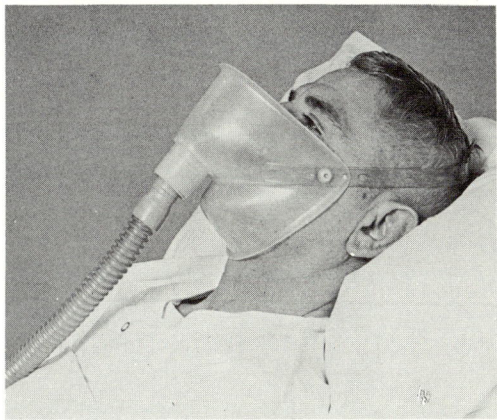

Fig. 38-4. The patient is receiving oxygen therapy with a face tent.

(1) Attach the flowmeter to the oxygen source.
(2) Turn on oxygen.
(3) Adjust flow to rate of 10 to 12 liters per minute.
(4) Permit patient to handle, explore, and apply his own mask. (Dyspneic patient is frightened by anything that covers his mouth and nose. Why?) Apply it for him if he can not. Mask must fit face snugly. Apply narrow part over the nose and position the wide part on the chin below the mouth.
(5) Fix the mask in position by fastening to strap (or straps) around patient's head.
(6) Readjust flow rate to that specified by the nurse (6 to 8 liters per minute).
(7) Sit with the patient until his apprehension decreases and his breathing resumes its usual pattern.
(8) Return and observe the patient frequently:
 (a) Check that the oxygen supply and the delivery rate to the patient are maintained. The bag should partially collapse on inspiration and fill during expiration. (Bag not filling may mean an exhausted oxygen source. This will suffocate the patient.)
 (b) Check for complications. Disadvantages of oxygen mask therapy are that the mask must be removed to suction the patient, that secretions or vomitus expelled into the mask will be aspirated with the next breath, and

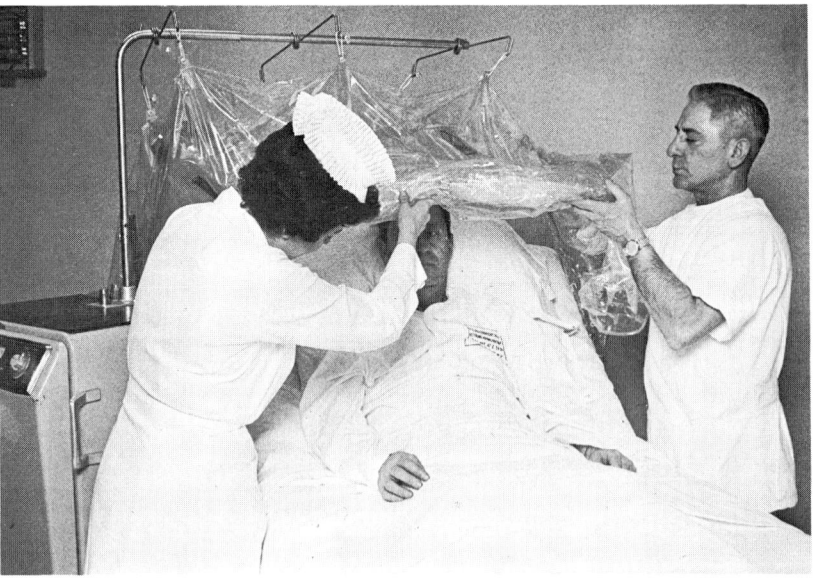

Fig. 38-5. The nursing assistant and his team leader position the oxygen tent canopy over the patient.

that a mask applied too tightly will irritate and blister the patient's face. If the patient needs frequent suctioning or starts to vomit, notify the nurse immediately. She may start another method of oxygen therapy.
3. Nasal oxygen by face tent:
   a. Apply in much the same way as the mask. The face tent is not as confining or as tight as the mask. Then, too, the patient's mouth and nose can be seen easily through the plasticlike face tent. However, the oxygen concentration delivered by this method is only 40% (Fig. 38-4).
4. Oxygen by tent:
   a. Collect the equipment:
      (1) Oxygen supply
      (2) Oxygen tent, connecting tubing, and flowmeter
   b. Visit the patient:
      (1) Explain that you are going to put him in an oxygen-filled environment to help him breathe.
      (2) Tell him of the need for no smoking. Remove all cigarettes and matches.
   c. Prepare the room (p. 379):
      (1) Remove inflammable material as described previously.
      (2) Prepare for the ever present possibility of fire.
   d. Take the equipment to the patient's bedside and start the treatment:
      (1) Connect the flowmeter to the oxygen source and turn on the oxygen full force (to flood) in order to fill the tent.
      (2) Plug tent electrical connection into wall outlet.
      (3) Turn on air conditioner (oxygen tent also contains an air

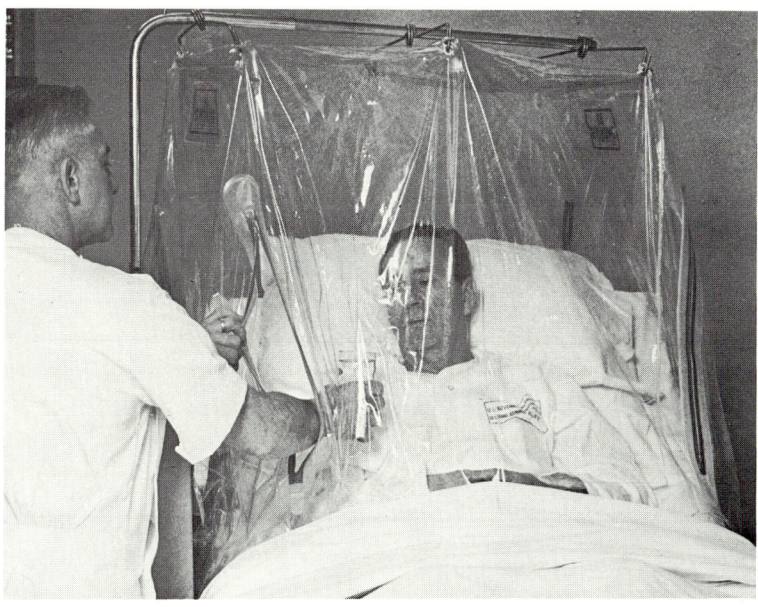

Fig. 38-6. The nursing assistant is giving the patient a drink of orange juice through the opened window in the oxygen tent. Note that the front part of the canopy is anchored in a folded sheet.

cooler to condition the air in the airtight tent).

(4) Set temperature control at 68° F. or at a temperature not more than 15° below that in the room.*

5. Lift the tent canopy over the patient and tuck it in at the top and sides of the bed (Fig. 38-5).
6. Fold a sheet in quarters widthwise and lay it over the patient's thighs.
7. Place front skirt of canopy in the sheet. Fold sheet up and over skirt. Then tuck the sheet in at both sides of the bed.
8. Readjust (after 15 minutes) oxygen flow rate to the one specified by the nurse (usually 10 to 12 liters per minute).
9. Stay with the patient until his apprehension ceases, his breathing returns to its usual rate, and he is comfortable.

The oxygen tent has zippered openings on both sides through which you can give the patient most of his care. Each time you open them, the oxygen concentration in the tent drops. It can be reestablished quickly by adjusting the flowmeter to flood for 1 minute. The nurse will help you plan the patient's care in such a way that opening the zippers and interfering with the oxygen therapy is kept at a minimum (Fig. 38-6). (How is the patient's temperature taken? Why?)

The tent that is used with a central oxygen source (piped in oxygen) has a safety valve that opens and draws in room air if the oxygen supply falls below 6 liters a minute. This not only makes the tent safe (prevents suffocation from a failing oxygen source or a turned-off supply when a fire occurs in a part of the hospital) but it also permits the tent to be used (without any oxygen supply) for cooling a patient (air conditioner). The tent that attaches to an oxygen tank may not have this safety valve. Monitor the oxygen supply carefully because this patient will suffocate if it runs out.

From retention of secretions or trapped air or both

The patient may receive postural drainage to rid the lungs of these secretions and/or intermittent positive pressure breathing to help him expel the trapped air.

The nurse may prepare the patient for postural drainage by giving him a drug like Isuprel (bronchodilator) or Mucomyst (mucus liquefier) to inhale through a nebulizer (device that breaks the liquid up into a mist that can be carried down to the alveoli [air sacs] with the air) for 15 or 20 minutes. Then she will tell you which lung areas are to be drained and how to position the patient to drain them.

Postural drainage requires you to put the patient in the position that creates a downhill path for the secretions from the lung area to the mouth. You can do this by instructing the patient to lie in a face-down position across the bed. Then assist him to

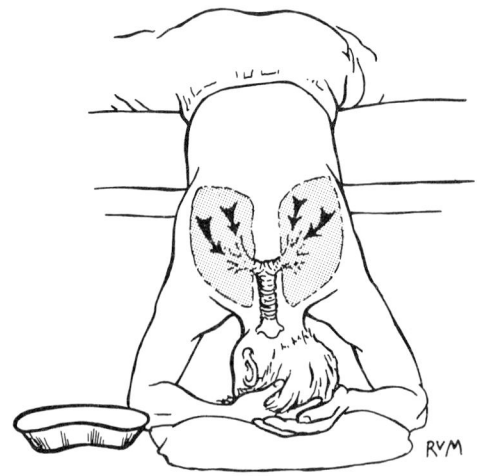

Fig. 38-7. Position for postural drainage.

---
*Air conditioner usually can handle only 15° of cooling.

slide forward, bringing his head and chest out of the bed. Instruct him to raise his arms over his head and place them on a low stool to support himself. Permit him to slide forward, supporting himself with his arms, until his chest is free of the bed and on a downhill path to the mouth (Fig. 38-7). Put an emesis basin near the patient's mouth. Instruct him to cough and breathe deeply. This position is effective in draining the lower and middle lobes of the lungs (Fig. 38-7). Have the patient roll to his right side (maintaining the same head-down position) to drain the left upper lobe, and to the left side to drain the right one. Have the patient maintain this head-down position for the time specified by the nurse (usually 20 to 30 minutes) or for as much of this time as he is able. Remain with the patient each time you do the postural drainage until he learns how to do it and is comfortable doing it. At first the patient will be afraid that he is falling, and he may even become lightheaded and dizzy. Discontinue the treatment if this occurs even if only 5 to 10 minutes have elapsed.

His tolerance and skill will increase, and soon he will be able to maintain the position for the specified time. The patient will expectorate some mucus during postural drainage and large amounts immediately after it. (Secretions are brought into the tracheobronchial tree with the drainage. These secretions then cause irritation and coughing, with emptying of the tracheobronchial tubes, for an hour or so after the treatment is over.)

The patient on IPPB therapy

The patient who receives intermittent positive pressure breathing (IPPB) therapy will probably be one who has a chronic chest disease and a higher than normal carbon dioxide blood level. His breathing may be stimulated by the oxygen want monitors in the aorta and carotid arteries rather than by the increased carbon dioxide levels in the blood and the need to reduce it (p. 372). Oxygen therapy may be avoided for this reason, and the intermittent positive pressure breathing may be given with compressed air.

The nurse will direct you to give the patient 15 or 20 minutes of therapy after she instills normal saline (wet the mucous membranes), Mucomyst (liquefy thick mucus plugs), or Isuprel (tracheobronchial dilator) into the nebulizer on the machine and sets the controls.

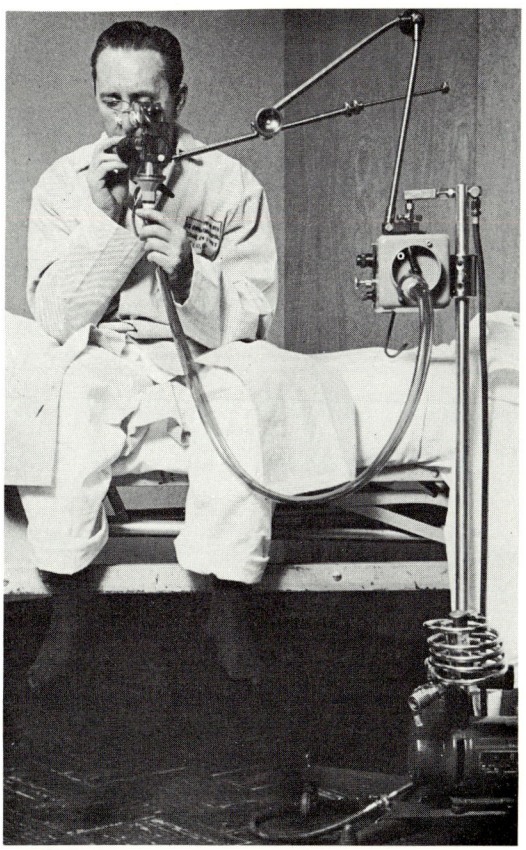

Fig. 38-8. The patient is receiving an intermittent positive pressure treatment with the use of the Bird respirator. Note that his chest is free of the bed and that his nose is closed with a clip. Oxygen from a wall source is being used for the treatment.

You can give the treatment in the following way:

1. Collect the equipment: IPPB machine (Bird and Bennett shown in Figs. 38-8 and 38-9), compressed air source (may be a motor attached to the machine, a tank or a wall supply), and a delivery system (may be a mouthpiece, mask, or tracheal adaptor).
2. Explain the procedure to the patient:
   a. Tell him to make a slight inspirator (breathing in) effort and that the machine will take over and inflate his lungs rapidly.
   b. Tell him that the machine will not help him exhale so he will have to do this for himself by using a gentle but forced expiratory (breathing out) effort.
   c. Ask the patient to place his hands on his upper abdomen (just below the rib cage) and to concentrate on moving this area (diaphragm) in and out. This type of breathing increases the size of the chest on inspiration and decreases it on expiration. The effective and forced expiration will help to rid the lungs of the retained air.
3. Place the patient in a sitting position on the side of the bed or the edge of the chair. Keep his chest free of supports and splinting.
4. Take the equipment to the patient's bedside.
5. Connect the IPPB machine to the gas source (wall source or tank).
6. Turn on the machine (Figs. 38-10 and 38-11).
7. Adjust the gas flow to the nebulizer until a fine mist is flowing (Bennett only, Bird has no separate control) through the open end of the delivery system (mask, mouthpiece, or tracheal attachment).

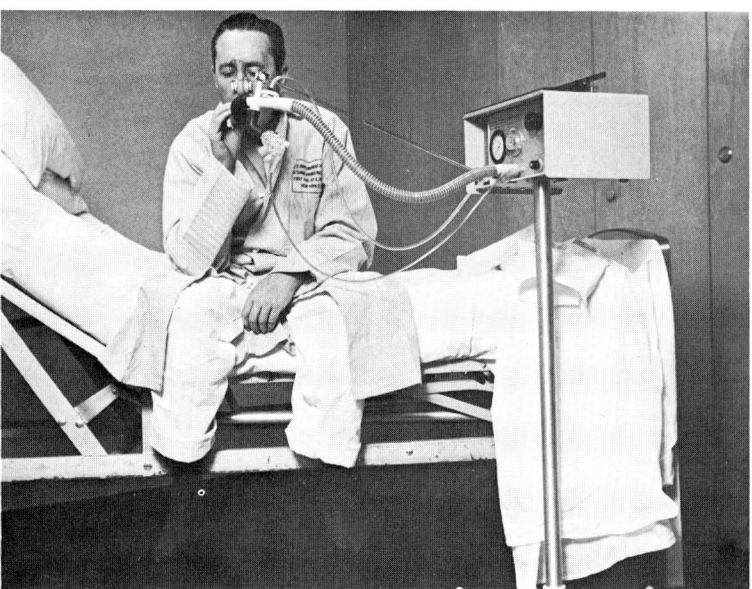

Fig. 38-9. The patient is receiving an intermittent positive pressure treatment with the use of the Bennett respirator. This machine contains its own air compressor and thus supplies its own source of air.

Caring for the patient who is breathless 385

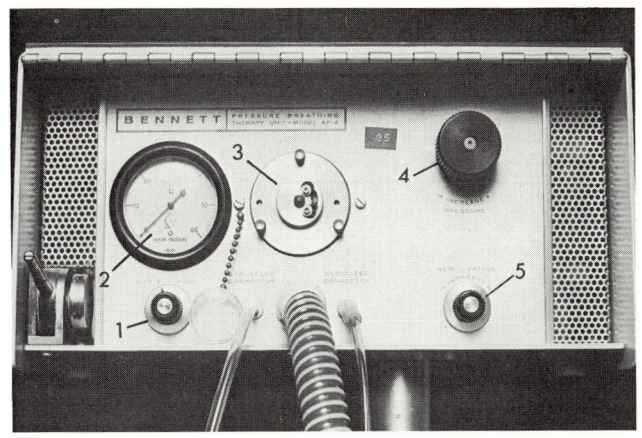

Fig. 38-10. Bennett IPPB unit: **1**, on-off switch, **2**, inspiratory pressure gauge, **3**, manual inspiratory control, **4**, pressure control, and **5**, nebulizer control.

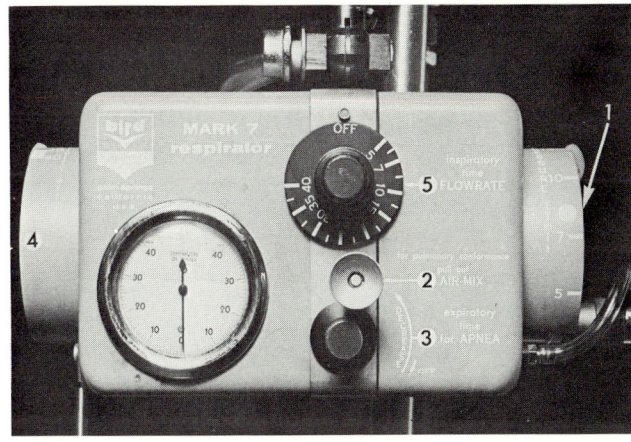

Fig. 38-11. Bird IPPB unit: **1**, inspiratory pressure control, **2**, air-mix control, **3**, automatic cycling control, **4**, sensitivity control, and **5**, flow rate control.

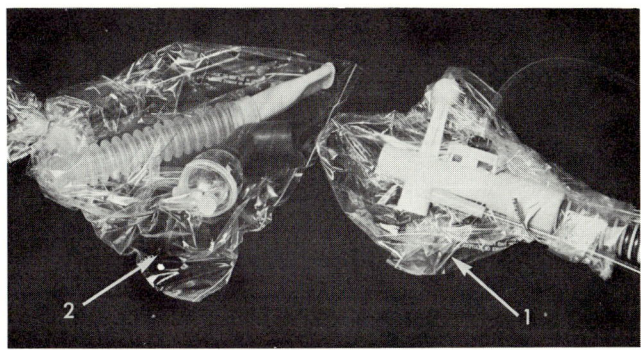

Fig. 38-12. Aftertreatment care of Bird IPPB unit: **1**, manifold is protected by enclosing it in a cellophane bag; **2**, nebulizer, mouthpiece, and connecting tubing are thoroughly washed, dried, and bagged.

386 The nursing assistant meets the needs of special patients in the hospital

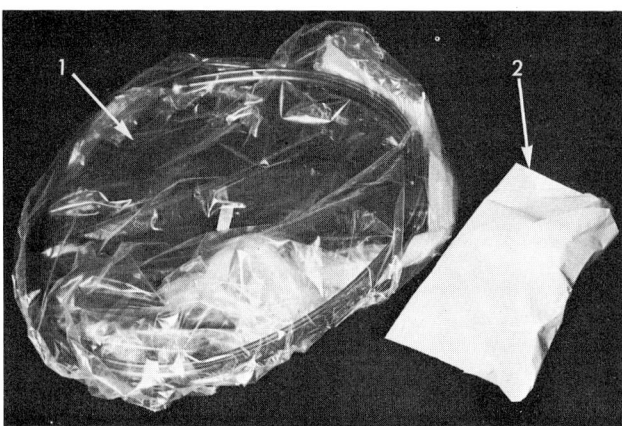

Fig. 38-13. Each day the complete tubing assembly (from machine to patient) is replaced with a sterile one: **1**, gas-sterilized assembly enclosed in a plastic bag; **2**, autoclaved manifold, connecting tubing, and mouthpiece.

8. Attach the mouthpiece, or mask, or tracheal adaptor to the patient.
9. Instruct the patient to breathe with a slight inspiratory effort to start the machine and with a gentle but forced expiration.
10. Encourage the patient to continue the treatment for the time specified by the nurse (usually 20 minutes) and until the medication is completely nebulized.
11. Discontinue the treatment by removing the mouthpiece, mask, or tracheal adaptor and by turning off the machine.
12. Disconnect the nebulizer from the IPPB apparatus. Wash the nebulizer and mouthpiece, mask, or tracheal adaptor thoroughly in warm, soapy water. Rinse and dry. Enclose in a clean plastic bag and retain it at the patient's bedside in readiness for the next treatment (Fig. 38-12).
13. Obtain a fresh setup (manifold tubing and patient attachment) (which has been gas sterilized and aired for 24 hours) for the patient each day (Fig. 38-13).

After the treatment is completed, the opened tracheobronchial tubes will drain and the patient will expectorate much thick mucus. The air that was trapped behind plugged air sacs or retained because of poor expiratory effort will be expelled too; and the patient will feel better, will be much less dyspneic, and will probably sleep.

The patient on IPPB therapy has chronic chest infections. Therefore germs (such as *Klebsiella*) are exhaled with the air. These bacteria will settle in the patient attachment (mouthpiece, mask, etc.) and in the nebulizing fluid. Here they will grow and reproduce at a very rapid rate in the moisture. An uncleaned apparatus will force, during the next treatment, germs down deep into the lungs with the air. Pneumonia will occur in 2 to 3 days.

From patient's failure to breathe

The patient stops breathing because of a brain, muscle, or nerve disease. Breathing stops because of a brain that fails to send the breathing message or because of nerves that fail to carry it, or because of muscles that fail to function when they receive it.

Caring for the patient who is breathless 387

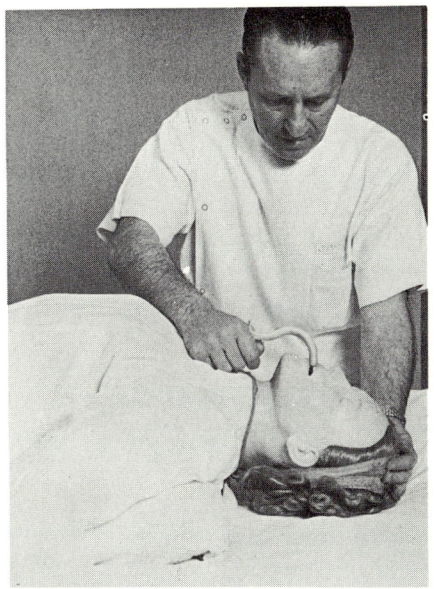

Fig. 38-14. The nursing assistant is preparing to administer artificial respiration by inserting an airway into the mouth of a manikin.

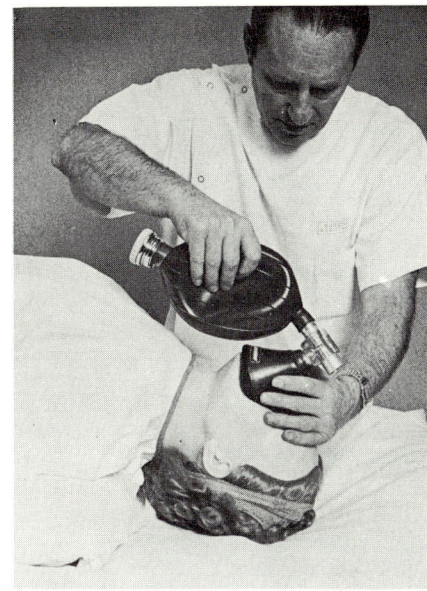

Fig. 38-15. The nursing assistant is giving artificial respiration with a Draeger resuscitator. Note the hyperextension of the head.

Apnea or respiratory arrest (stoppage) occurs quickly and quietly. You must expect apnea to occur in the patient with brain injuries or tumors, and in the one with a steadily worsening muscular weakness or paralysis on both sides of his body—and you must watch for it. Observe the patient frequently and check his respirations. Notify the nurse as soon as you discover any slowing of the breathing rate.

Respiratory arrest also occurs when the brain is so dulled by narcotics (drugs to relieve pain), or by hypnotics (drugs to produce sleep), or by carbon dioxide (waste material) that it becomes unaware of the body need for oxygen and is unable to function at activating breathing. Expect respiratory distress to occur in those patients receiving narcotics or hypnotics and in the ones with chronic lung disease such as emphysema (lungs blown up with trapped air). Count their respiratory rates frequently and report slowing to the nurse immediately. It is interesting to note here that the most usual cause of death in the person who attempts suicide with sleeping pills is respiratory arrest.

The patient who stops breathing needs help in getting the air into his lungs. He must get this help within 3 minutes or his cells (brain especially) will die from anoxia (no oxygen). Respiratory arrest is an emergency, and you must act quickly. Discover it as soon as it happens (because you suspect it may happen and you watch the patient closely) and start to breathe for the patient immediately (Figs. 38-14 to 38-16). (See Chapter 40 for technique of mouth-to-mouth resuscitation technique of reclaiming a patient from a condition resembling death.) Send for help or signal for it with the patient's communication system.

The professional staff (nurse and doctor) will arrive promptly and will take over the breathing for the patient. They may do this in any one of the following ways:

1. With a *Draeger respirator* (Fig. 38-

15), first an airway is inserted into the patient's mouth to keep his tongue up and out of the throat (Fig. 38-14). Then the mask is applied snugly over the patient's mouth and nose, and the bag (attached to the mask) is squeezed (about sixteen times a minute) to force air into his lungs.

2. With an *IPPB machine* (Figs. 38-17 and 38-18) (Bennett or Bird), the airway is again inserted. Then the IPPB machine is connected to an air or oxygen supply.

If an air compressor is included as part of the unit, it must be connected to an electrical outlet and turned on. The machine controls are set on automatic (machine controls set to inflate the lungs without any inspiratory effort from the patient) (Fig. 38-11, automatic cycling control no. 3) or prepared for manual operation (Fig. 38-17). The gauges (pressure, sensitivity, and flow) are set (Fig. 38-11), and the machine is attached to the patient by placing the mask snugly over his mouth and nose. Remember that you will need to continue the mouth-to-mouth breathing for the patient while these preparations are going on and until the machine takes over (Fig. 38-18).

3. With a *tank respirator* (Drinker), the carefully checked and known to be operating tank respirator with preset controls (positive and negative pressure and breathing rate) is connected to the electrical outlet and turned on. The airway is again inserted. The respirator is opened and the stretcher pulled out (Fig. 38-19). The patient is placed on the stretcher with the

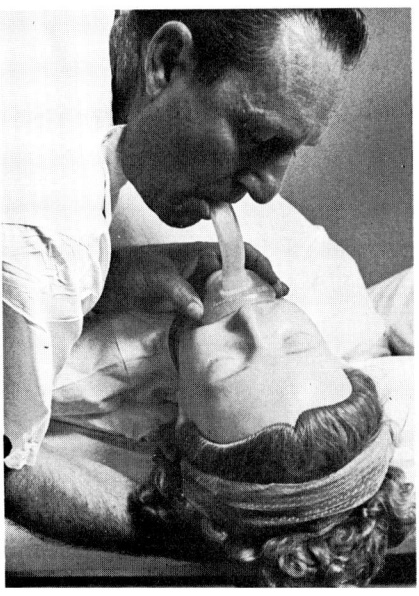

Fig. 38-16. The nursing assistant is artificially respirating the patient with a Rescussi-tube and his expired air. Note the hyperextension of the head and the tight seal around the lips. (The nose [air leak] pinch was eliminated only to present a visualization of the technique.)

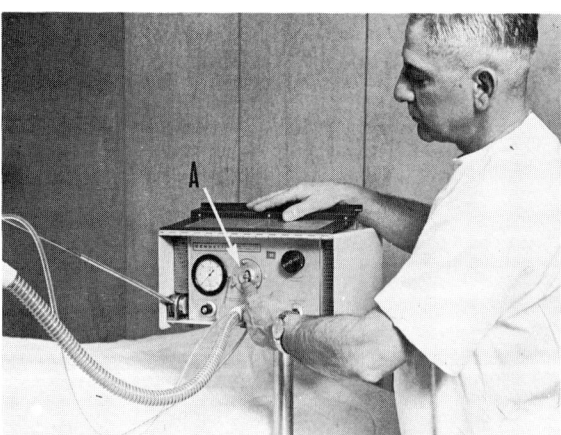

Fig. 38-17. Artificial respiration is given with the Bennett IPPB machine. Note that inspiration is initiated by moving the drum pin, **A**, upward.

Caring for the patient who is breathless 389

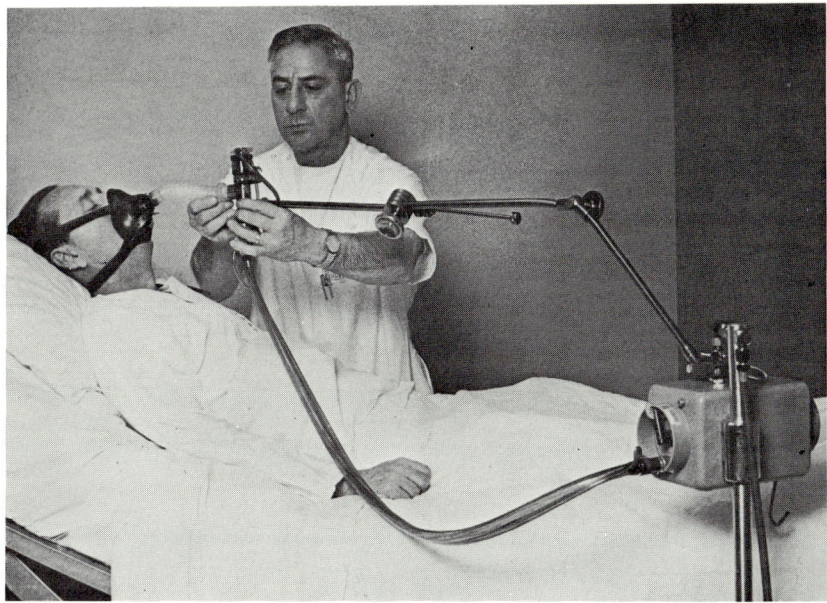

Fig. 38-18. The patient is being respirated (breathed) by the Bird respirator. The nursing assistant is checking to be sure that the nebulizer contains the prescribed medication. The machine is set on automatic cycling.

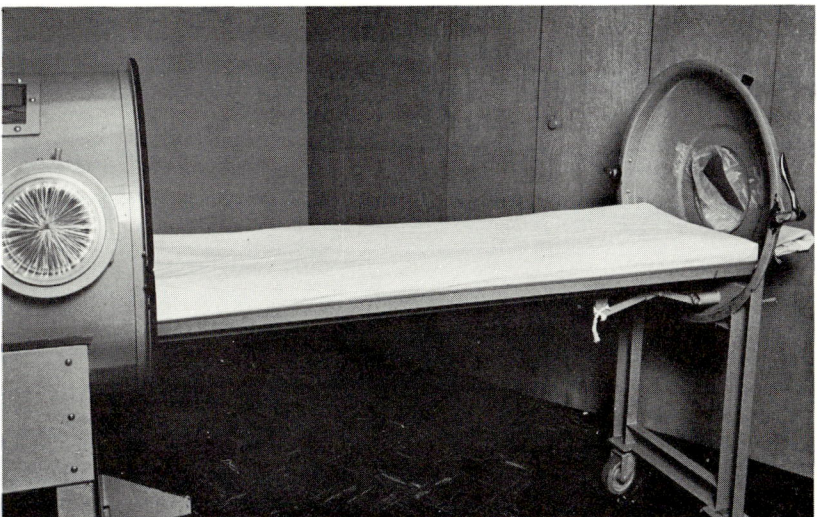

Fig. 38-19. The Drinker respirator is opened and the stretcher is pulled out. The respirator is positioned to receive a patient by placing it at right angles to the bed with the head of the stretcher at the foot of the bed (same positioning as for the Foster frame; see Figs. 12-4 and 12-5).

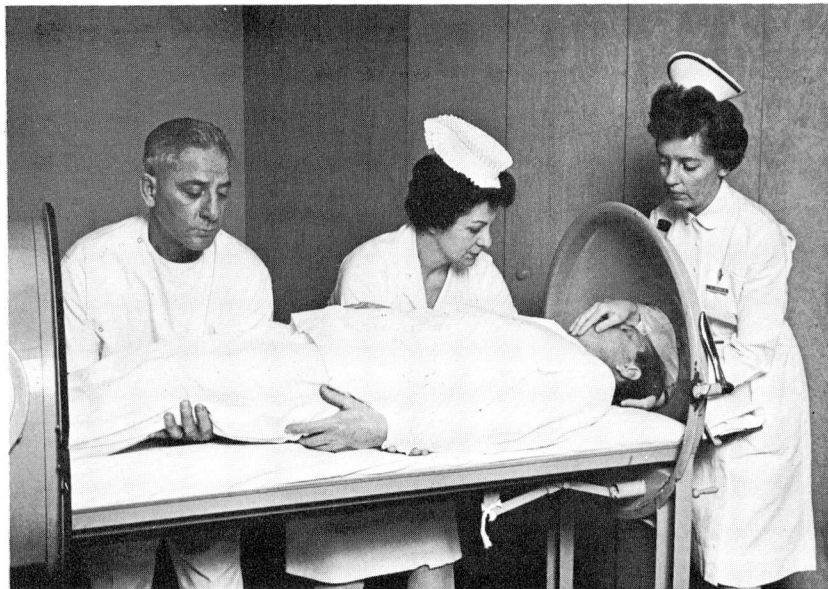

Fig. 38-20. The patient is lifted up and his head is guided through the Drinker respirator lid opening. Note that the nurse at the top of the respirator: (1) flexes the head (to obtain smallest diameter), (2) protects the face, and (3) carries the head through the lid opening.

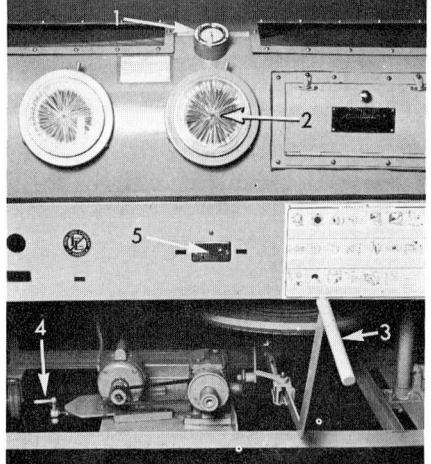

Fig. 38-21. Drinker respirator: **1**, pressure gauge (left side negative, right side positive); **2**, porthole for delivery of patient care; **3**, bellows manual operation handle; **4**, respiratory rate adjuster; and **5**, on-off switch.

"three-man carry" (Figs. 12-4 and 12-5). Then he is lifted up by two staff members while the third guides his head through the opening in the door (lid) of the tank (Fig. 38-20). The door is then closed, and the respirator collar is tightened around the patient's neck (to make the respirator airtight). The patient's inspirations are watched, and the pressure (positive and negative) and respiratory rate controls are manipulated until the desired rate and depth of breathing are achieved for the patient (Fig. 38-21). (Usually gauge settings are pressures of –10 to –20, and 0 to +5, with a respiratory rate of 15.)

These respiratory aids breathe for the patient in the following way:

1. The bag resuscitator or the IPPB machine. Air is forced through the mask and into the lungs during the positive pressure or squeezing phase. Then this phase stops and the stretched breathing muscles relax and spring

back to their normal position, thus crowding the lungs into the smaller chest spaces and forcing them to give up air.

2. The tank respirator. This machine has both a positive and negative phase. During the negative pressure phase, the pressure on the chest and abdomen is even less than that of the normal air pressure in the atmosphere. This causes the chest to expand and the lung space to increase. The air in the atmosphere (which is then under greater pressure than that in the lungs) flows toward the least pressure, that is, into the lungs (much like the air in a punctured tire flows out to the area of lesser pressure in the atmosphere). The lungs inspire. During the positive pressure phase, the pressure on the chest and abdomen increases to normal or above normal air pressure. The chest and abdomen spring back to their original position and crowd the lungs. The lungs must expire in order to fit into this smaller space and so exhalation occurs.

The patient who is unable to breathe for himself and is receiving artificial respiration by any one of these methods will be cared for by the nurse. You help her give this care and you must do it calmly, quietly, and skillfully. Remember that fear, worry, and movement increase oxygen need. Give the patient constant and skillful care. Prevent the occurrence of any disturbing emotional states. Avoid the use of any unnecessary or excessive movements in giving the care.

The patient who cannot breathe usually cannot swallow, and suctioning is an important part of his care. Unswallowed saliva in the throat will be pushed down into the lungs with the next inflow of air if it is not removed quickly. Of course, this patient cannot be fed. Artificial respiration by mask interferes with the care of the patient. The mask has to be removed to suction (and breathing stops), or the suctioning must be eliminated (and saliva is drawn into the lungs). Because of these facts, the mask-type resuscitator is usually replaced by IPPB machine to tracheal resuscitation or by the tank respirator as soon as possible.

The purpose of artificial respiration is to get lifesaving air into the lungs, and nothing should interfere with this process. Suction the patient on expiration only. The tank respirator has windows guarded by airtight diaphragms that you can open to insert your arms and care for the patient. Open these only during the positive pressure or expiratory phase. Do nothing to interfere with inspirations:

1. Remember that this lifesaving treatment depends on getting air and oxygen in. Do nothing to interfere with this phase of breathing. Feed the patient, teach him to talk, suction, etc. only during the expiratory or breathing-out phase.

2. In some instances, such as those in which the patient has weak or paralyzed breathing muscles only and little or no brain and nerve involvement, the patient may be able to swallow.

The patient receiving artificial respiration will die if the machine fails. Be prepared for electrical failures and a manual takeover (Fig. 38-21).

SUMMARY

All the cells of the body need oxygen to live. This need is met, and the patient breathes easily and effortlessly when:
1. There is an adequate outflow and inflow of air.
2. There is an effective oxygen–carbon dioxide exchange between the lungs and the blood.
3. There is an efficient oxygen delivery and carbon dioxide removal system maintained by the blood.

The patient has difficulty meeting this body need and is dyspneic when:

1. Conditions in the air passages block the inflow and outflow of air.
2. Conditions in the lungs occupy the air spaces and so decrease the amount of oxygen given to the blood and the amount of carbon dioxide taken back from it.
3. Conditions in the heart and blood cause the circulation to fail.

The amount of oxygen that the cells need depends on the amount of work they are doing. They work hard when the body is active—carrying on physical activity or fighting an infection—so oxygen need and breathing rates increase with physical exertion, with temperature elevation, and with strong emotional states. They do little work when the body is at rest—oxygen needs and breathing rates decrease with inactivity, hypothermia, and emotional peace. You can help the dyspneic patient breathe easier by taking all the physical and emotional exertion out of his living.

The treatment of the dyspneic patient depends on the cause of his breathlessness and may include oxygen therapy, positive pressure breathing therapy, or artificial respiration. The correct treatment will decrease breathlessness, but the incorrect one may result in the patient's death.

Life continues for only 3 minutes when respirations stop. Know how to give artificial respiration and start it immediately when the patient suddenly and unexpectedly ceases to breathe.

DISCUSSION QUESTIONS

1 Run up an down the steps two or three times. Observe what happens to your breathing rate. Why did this happen?
2 Check the method of supplying oxygen in your hospital. What precautions are taken to prevent fire? To put out the fire if it occurs?
3 What is the emergency plan of action for a fire in your hospital?
4 Check your ward emergency equipment. What equipment do you have to give emergency artificial respiration? Can you use it effectively? Demonstrate.
5 Observe the patients on your ward who have breathing problems. Ask the nurse why these problems occur. How can you help these patients breathe easier?
6 Do you have a cardiac and respiratory arrest team? How are they called? What is your job in helping them at the emergency?
7 Observe the nurse giving an intermittent positive pressure breathing treatment. Why must this equipment be cleaned after each treatment? How is it cleaned?
8 How can the preoperative patient be prepared for surgery so that respiratory complications do not occur in the postoperative period?
9 What equipment is required to do an emergency tracheotomy? Where do you get it?
10 What is a nebulizer? Why is it used?
11 Why do dyspneic patients wake up frequently at night?
12 Can you operate the Drinker respirator manually? How long do you think you could keep this up?
13 Does your hospital have an emergency electrical supply system? Where is it? Do you have access to it?

VOCABULARY

air sacs Tiny balloonlike structures at the end of the air tubes in the lungs. Around the balloonlike part is a blood vessel, and here internal respiration occurs. The oxygen passes through the sac wall and into the blood, and carbon dioxide passes from the blood into the sac.

airway Way for air to get into the lungs. An artificial airway is one that holds the limp tongue up in the mouth and out of the throat, thereby unblocking the air passages and making a way for the air to get into the lungs.

alveoli Medical term for air sacs.

amyotrophic Lateral sclerosis. A neurologic disease that steadily worsens from muscular weakness into muscular paralysis and death. Affects all the muscles including those of breathing.

anemia Not enough blood, deficiency of blood.

aorta The large artery taking oxygen-rich blood from the heart to the body. This artery subdivides into all the arteries in the body.

apnea No breathing (*a*, without; *pnea*, breathing).

aspirated meal Food that belongs in the stomach but is now in the lung.

asthma Spasm (muscle cramp) with narrowing in the inflow-outflow tubes of the lung (bronchi or bronchioles). Mucus is trapped behind the narrowed tube and fills up the air spaces.

atelectasis Collapsed and airless lung, or part of a lung caused by a plugged bronchiole (air intake and outflow tube). Usually the plug is one of mucus or food that has been sucked into the lung with the breath.

auxiliary muscles of breathing Shoulder, arm, and neck muscles that help breathing during emergency body needs.

Bennett A machine that forces air into the patient's lungs until a preset pressure is reached.

Bird A machine similar to the Bennett.

breathing center Area in the brain that sends the message to the breathing muscles to contract, thus causing inspiration to occur.

breathlessness Feeling that you cannot get your breath.

bronchi Large inflow-outflow tube from the trachea into the lungs. Subdivides and subdivides into smaller tubes called bronchioles.

bronchioles Small inflow-outflow tubes connecting the air sacs with the large bronchi.

carbon dioxide Waste product of living exhaled during expiration.

carbon dioxide "stat" Breathing center in the brain that regulates the blood level of carbon dioxide by stimulating breathing when it is high and slowing breathing when it is low.

carotid The first artery that comes off the aorta and takes oxygen-rich blood to the head.

central oxygen source Oxygen transported from a storage area to the patient's room through a system of pipes. Oxygen is obtained for the patient by merely hooking into the system.

cervical cord injuries Damage to the neck section of the spinal cord.

cilia Hairlike structures that sweep foreign material and secretions up and out of the air passages.

coma Not knowing or answering to body needs or to the environment. Deep, unwakeable sleeplike state.

complications Undesirable and preventable results of illness.

cyanosis Bluish skin color caused by oxygen want.

diaphragm Thick muscle of breathing below the lungs. It separates the chest from the abdominal cavity.

diffuse The movement of one gas into and throughout another (odor of perfume diffuses through the air of a room).

emphysema Lung disease where air is unable to flow out freely and becomes trapped in the lungs.

epiglottis Fingerlike protective structure that blocks off the trachea during swallowing.

expiration Breathing out.

Fowler's position Sitting up position in bed.

gas sterilized All bacteria are killed by a gas (usually ethylene oxide). Material that has been gas-sterilized must be aired (usually 24 hours) until the pungent fumes are dissipated.

inhalations Treatment associated with breathing in.

inspiration Breathing in.

intoxication Poisoning.

monitor Checker.

mucus plugs Thick, heavy mucus, usually because excess amounts are produced or because it is retained too long) that blocks off the inflow or the outflow (or both) of air. These plugs usually form in the smaller air tubes like the bronchi and bronchioles.

mucus-coated Covered with the normal secretion of the lining of the air passages.

nebulizer Device that breaks up a liquid into the small particles (mist), which can be carried down into the air sacs with the air.

nose clip Device to close off the nose and make an airtight connection between an IPPB machine and the lungs.

oxygen Colorless, odorless, tasteless gas that is essential for life. Air contains 20% oxygen.

oxygen therapy Treating a patient in oxygen want (cyanotic) by giving him a richer-than-air oxygen mixture to breathe.

pneumonia Germs invade and irritate the lungs and cause the air sacs to fill with fluid.

poliomyelitis Virus infection of the nervous system causing paralysis. This infection may paralyze a part or the entire body including the breathing muscles.

postural drainage Removing the retained secretions from the lungs by putting the patient in an upside down position so that there is a downhill path for them from the lungs to the mouth.

silicosis Lung condition caused by irritation of dust particles and resulting in a destruction of the air sacs by thickening and scarring.

spasm Sudden, severe muscle contraction (shortening) or cramp.

tracheal adaptor Device that connects a tracheotomy tube to a treatment system.

tracheobronchial tree Series of air inflow/outflow tubes from the throat to the blood.

SOURCES OF ADDITIONAL INFORMATION

1 Film: Anatomy and physiology: The respiratory system; may be obtained from the Audiovisual Support Center of the Army area in which you reside. (*Describes the anatomy and physiology of the respiratory system and illustrates in detail the exchange of oxygen for carbon dioxide in both internal and external respiration.*)

2 Film: Bronchitis and bronchiectasis; may be obtained from Pfizer Laboratories, 267 West 25th St., New York, N. Y. 10001. (*Illustrates diagnos-*

tic procedures and management regimes for these two diseases. Illustration of postural drainage excellent.)
3. Film: Introduction to prolonged artificial ventilation; may be obtained from the Audiovisual Support Center of the Army area in which you reside. *(Teaches the Army corpsman the principles of safe mechanical ventilation, safe tracheotomy care, and transportation of the apneic patient.)*
4. Film: Oxygen therapy—theory and practice; may be obtained from the Audiovisual Support Center of the Army area in which you reside. *(Describes symptoms of hypoxia and the treatment of it with oxygen.)*
5. Film: Prescription for life; may be obtained from your local heart association. *(Presents expired air ventilation and cardiac massage in emergency treatment of cardiac arrest. This film is particularly valuable as it shows actual emergency treatment being given. It pinpoints the errors and makes suggestions on how to avoid such errors.)*
6. Filmstrip and record: (a) Oxygen administration, (b) Cardiopulmonary resuscitation, (c) Congestive heart failure, and (d) Myocardial infarction; available from Trainex Corp., P. O. Box 116, Garden Grove, Calif. 92642.
7. Pamphlets available from your local tuberculosis association:
    a. Asthma and you
    b. Asthma, the facts
    c. Air pollution, the facts
    d. Bronchiectasis, the facts
    e. Chronic bronchitis, the facts
    f. Chronic cough, the facts
    g. Dust disease, the facts
    h. Emphysema, the facts
    i. Hay fever, the facts
    j. Pneumonia, the facts
    k. Pleurisy, the facts
    l. Shortness of breath, the facts
    m. TB, the facts
8. Slides with discussion guide: Emergency measures in cardiopulmonary resuscitation; may be obtained from your local heart association. *(Slides and discussion guide on expired air ventilation [mouth-to-mouth breathing] and use of the bag and mask in artificial ventilation.)*

39/Care of the aged person with problems in living

STUDY QUESTIONS

1. What is a nursing home?
2. What kind of people go to a nursing home?
3. Why do people go to a nursing home?
4. How does a nursing home differ from a hospital?
5. What are the diseases of the aged person?
6. How does the sick aged person differ from the sick young adult?
7. What is the job of the nursing assistant in a nursing home?
8. What is a living care plan?
9. What do you call the aged resident in a nursing home?
10. What makes the nursing home depressing?
11. What makes the nursing home comfortable and interesting?

THE NURSING HOME

At birth, the infant is helpless and depends on his parents for his every living need. They love and care for him, and soon he grows into a self-sufficient adult who can then leave his home and start a family of his own. As the infant grows and develops into a self-reliant married man, his parents grow old and deteriorate into feeble, infirm, and lonely people.

The stress and strain of living has exhausted the mind and body of these aged parents, and now they have difficulty taking care of themselves. Walking becomes difficult, and climbing steps is impossible. Falls occur frequently. Then, too, their worn minds have trouble taking in and holding onto the facts of daily living so their memory fails. Life-threatening situations result when they do not remember to turn off the gas, or to take heart-strengthening pills, or to get the right bus home from the store. Life becomes frightening and complicated and they need help, the kind of living help that a family situation gives in a home. Unfortunately, however, these aged parents do not have a family to give it. They cannot depend on married children, who are now parents themselves and so are overburdened with their own family responsibilities, but they can get it in a nursing home. A nursing home then is a loving, caring foster family for the adult who needs help in living.

THE NURSING HOME RESIDENT

The nursing home resident is a person who needs help in carrying on the activities of living, and not one who needs hospitalization. Therefore the focus in the nursing home is on helping the resident (not the patient) live as comfortably and as enjoyably as he can with the foster family's (the nursing home staff) loving and caring help.

Every good family is interested in helping its members live a happy and worthwhile life, and the foster family (nursing home) is too. Happiness is achieved, you remember from Chapter 37, when the person feels safe and worthwhile. These feelings develop in a person when he controls and directs his own productive life. They are replaced with feelings of fear and helplessness when life is controlled and useless. You can help the nursing home resident live this happy life then by assisting him to live the life that he wants to live. You can discover what this life is by just recognizing that each resident is an individual with special interests, abilities, needs, likes, and dislikes, and then by finding out what these things are for each person in the home. Now you and the nurse can study this information and from it create the living plan that the resident needs. This plan will not only identify the living assistance that you are to give, but it will also develop a schedule of interesting activities to make this life worthwhile.

THE LIVING NEEDS OF THE NURSING HOME RESIDENT

The wearing out process of aging is easily seen on the outside of the body in the graying hair, decaying teeth, sagging skin, bald head, and failing vision of the aged person. The effect on the inside is just as obvious when you observe the decline in living ability and the increasing number of living problems that develop. The muscles of the body, including those of the heart and bowels, weaken and tire just as easily as those of the eyes. Walking is exhausting, steps are difficult to climb, and sitting becomes very desirable. Breathlessness occurs with every exertion, and constipation is a constant source of worry. Why?

The bones, like the teeth, change too. They become brittle and fragile, and they fracture from only the slightest amount of injury. The weak body muscles and the failing vision create the ingredients for taking a misstep and a fall, and thus for providing the injury that then shatters the so easily broken bones.

The arteries narrow and harden as fat masses form in them. Blood is unable to circulate freely and easily through these half-plugged vessels so the heart must pump harder and harder—but even with this increased effort, it accomplishes less and less. The circulation is poor. The blood-starved body is always cold, and the fingernails and toenails (which are at the very ends of the body) become thick and horny. The blood-starved brain functions poorly, and it has difficulty taking in and holding onto the daily happenings of life. Recent events are not stored in the memory and are lost. Then the past becomes the present as the brain dwells on the facts of the long-gone times that are stored there.

The glands dry up too, and bodily secretions decrease. Sexual interest declines, and marital relationship becomes one of helping the partner live. Digestive ability is impaired or damaged, and frequent attacks of indigestion occur from food intolerances or allergies. The mouth dries, and mouth wetting, lip smacking habits develop.

Retirement on social security benefits makes life financially secure for the aging person who is unable to continue working, but it also forces upon him a life of idleness,* idleness that usually tells him he is no longer needed, or useful, or valuable in

---

*It is interesting to note that most retirees who are being given years of idle time also get a watch for a gift. Why? Is this to tell them that their time of living is running out, or is it to remind them that they will have time on their hands from now on in their idle life?

this world. He may fight this feeling of rejection by proving his value, and he usually does this by becoming the authoritative, directing, bossy parent and the loving, giving, and spoiling grandparent. These two roles irritate his children and make them angry. Soon the children avoid this overbearing, aged parent and he becomes rejected by them too. Idleness and loneliness almost smother him. When he does have a visitor, he talks and talks about the significant and valuable past when he was important, and this irritates his listener who has no interest in the world of yesteryear.

Death robs this aged person of his friends and even of his wife, and soon he is living in a world of unfriendly strangers. Depression occurs if and when he realizes that nothing remains for him but death.

The nursing home resident, then, is usually a person with such a worn-out body and mind that he is unable to take care of himself, and a person who has no family able and willing to take care of him.

THE DISEASES OF THE AGED

The same diseases that attack the young person may attack the aged person. Therefore the diseases of the aged are not new diseases but are really the same ones that we have been talking about all through this book. The only differences are that the aged person with a worn-out body and mind has less resistance to disease and less ability to fight it, so he is susceptible to frequent attacks of serious life-threatening illness. When he does get sick, the aged person is likely to develop complications. The already overworking heart is likely to fail with the additional stress. The blood-starved skin breaks down into decubitus ulcers with only a very short period of bed rest and its pressure. The poorly working brain mixes up day and night and home and hospital. The aged person gets out of bed in the middle of the night to go to the bathroom as soon as he receives the message that his bladder is full. Unfortunately, hospital beds are higher than those at home so he usually falls and breaks a bone.

Then, too, his tired, worn muscles work less effectively in bed and his constipation worsens, his breathing is more difficult, and his muscles weaken still further. Fecal impactions, pneumonia, and helplessness develop in only a few days of bed rest.

The sick older person rarely has only one disease; he usually has three or four. He may have an acute attack of intestinal obstruction, but he usually has chronic heart disease (hypertensive cardiovascular disease), chronic lung disease (emphysema), and chronic bone disease (arthritis) too. The stress and strain on the body by the acute intestinal obstruction further increase the work load on all his body parts (organs) and worsen their chronic diseased condition. This acute attack of illness, because of this fact, may cause the patient to have a stroke (bursted blood vessel in the brain), or to go into heart failure, or to develop breathlessness and severe bone and joint pain. You must observe each nursing home resident carefully and identify the early clues of illness. Report these to the nurse promptly, and she will get treatment started immediately.

A more effective approach, however, is to be aware of the resident's susceptibility to illness and accidents and to develop a protective plan of care to prevent them from occurring. This plan might include the following:

1. You stay healthy. Do not bring in colds or infections to the aged residents. Stay off duty when you are ill.
2. Recognize clues of minor illness and take the resident to the health maintenance clinic for prompt treatment.
3. Keep the environment safe. Mop up spilled water. Keep wheelchairs, etc. out of the resident's path. Be available when the residents awaken and after meals for toileting activities.
4. Give the residents low beds and protect them from falling out by supply-

ing side rails. Answer resident signals promptly. The aged resident with weak bladder and bowel muscles cannot wait for toileting, so he will attempt to get over the side rails and go to the bathroom.

5. Provide proper equipment for manicures and pedicures. Cut nails after tub baths when they are soft. Do not cut thick horny nails that are attached to the skin of the toe or finger. Refer these residents to the nurse. She will schedule them for an appointment with the podiatrist. Remember that the poor circulation in the feet will prevent the healing of any cut toe and may result in an amputation.
6. Protect the resident from falls or burns during tub bathing.
7. Avoid rearranging the resident's furniture. Keep things in the same place. This will protect the forgetful resident with poor eyesight from falls and injuries.
8. Keep the resident's eyeglasses, false teeth, and canes accessible.
9. Make nursing home life worth living. Be a caring, helping, loving family member. Create interesting activities like discussion groups, newspaper reading groups, work groups, etc. Busy work like cutting out paper dolls is ridiculous and forces the resident into childhood feelings and disgrace. Make the work activities worthwhile and valuable. Let the resident help with family life. Let the plumber fix, the clerk clerk, the mechanic repair, and the artist or teacher conduct work groups. Recognize the aged resident as the significant person that he is and permit him to retain his own identity and self-worth. Address him by his name. Avoid calling him "Pop," "Grandpop," "Dearie," etc., or by any other such personal terms that make him feel like a poor, dependent relative.
10. Plan out-of-the-nursing home trips for residents so that they can continue their interests in living. Accompany them only when they need your assistance.
11. Encourage family feelings to develop. Celebrate birthdays, anniversaries, holidays.
12. Help the resident to live and do not force illness upon him. Pattern the nursing home life after the normal living pattern. Develop day work programs and evening recreational ones. Plan the activities in these programs with the residents. Permit them to select and carry out the activities.

An interesting example of a loving caring foster family that reinforces living is found in the Mary Manning Walsh Nursing Home in New York City. Here the resident is assisted in his personal hygiene as needed, dressed in his own clothes, and permitted to live his own life. This life includes living with his spouse (if he has one), eating in the dining room (if he is able), buying evening snacks in the coffee shops or a drink in the bar, and conducting bazaars, shows, etc. It also includes and encourages out-of-the-home activity or family visiting trips. This home does not restrict life. It makes life possible and livable.

CARING FOR THE NURSING HOME RESIDENT

The nurse receives the new resident and identifies his living ability. Then she develops a nursing home care plan that simplifies the resident's living to the level of his ability. This is accomplished quite easily in some residents by merely providing them with the facilities for living (home, meals, etc.) while in others it is more difficult and requires the actual giving of assistance in the living. The most significant aspect of the plan is, however, that it must permit the resident to control and direct his own life. He retains the control and he lives his life successfully in the home with the staff's help. He cannot be pushed into a plan of routine physical management (bathing, feeding, etc.) that a controlling staff develops for their own convenience because this loss of control of one's own life forces the residents into a role of passiveness, helplessness, dependency, and depression.

The nurse's identification of the new resident's level of living ability and of the kind of living help he needs includes the following:
1. The resident's usual pattern of living, which includes the following: Explore family patterns, occupational contributions, interests, hobbies, abilities, social relationships, etc. Explore, too, previous life problems that disrupted the resident's living pattern and determine how effectively he coped with these. From this coping pattern, identify potential problems in adjustment to the nursing home in relation to personality patterns and to work and recreational patterns, which may occur out of the resident's way of living.
2. The resident is able to do the following living activities for himself and likes to do them in the way described. Explore eating, toileting, walking, bathing, talking, sleeping. Explore hour of arising in the morning and of going to sleep at night.
3. The resident cannot do the following living activities and needs the help specified. Identify these needs in relation to activities in item 2.
4. The resident has these special living problems. Explore the presence of chronic illnesses, medication therapy, constipation, urinary frequency, need to go to the toilet at night, allergies, food discrepancies, incontinence, etc.
5. The resident has the following emotional problems. Identify feelings of rejection, depression, and grief and describe situations that caused them. Identify confusion, disorientation, forgetfulness, etc., and describe the kind of protective supervision needed.

The nurse will validate this evaluation of the resident by observing his living carefully for several days and also by interviewing his family. Then she will be ready to develop a *living care plan*. You and the resident will participate in the development of this plan. It will include the following:
1. A work activity program for the resident's day. This will be a program of significant, worthwhile, productive activities. The aged resident is not interested in playing or carrying out useless but time-consuming activities such as cutting out paper dolls or waving flags.
2. A recreational activity program for the resident's evenings, Sundays, and holidays. This should evolve from his religious affiliations, his life interests, and his hobbies.
3. A plan for meeting the resident's living needs. This may include a way of preparing the facilities for the resident to do or for assisting him to bathe, dress, eat, toilet, ambulate, etc.
4. A health maintenance program.* This may include the development of schedules that remind the resident to take his daily medications and to make his weekly dispensary visits for physical and emotional evaluations.
5. A plan for visiting (receiving visitors in the home or visiting outside the home). This will include a way of assisting the resident to prepare for visitors in the home or for visiting outside of the home on Sundays and holidays.

---

*One such scheme is to place the daily pill allotment in paper cups and to staple these cups to the dates on the calendar.

PROBLEMS OF THE NURSING HOME ASSISTANT

You may have difficulty caring for aged nursing home residents because of your own fear and dread of getting old and dying. The residents with their sagging skin, gray hair, and feeble gait may activate your anxiety about aging and make you tense, short-tempered, and bossy. This behavior will incite the aged resident to rebel against you, and he will become either a demanding, uncooperative person, or a passive, dependent, and helpless one.

Evaluate you own effectiveness in carrying out the living care plan for each resident. Identify your failures and your successes, and discuss these with your nurse. Identify why you failed in some instances and why you succeeded in others. Remember that behavior is the mere acting out of feelings. Find out if your behavior irritates and identify what feeling it is expressing. Learn how to deal effectively with those threatening situations that are evoking the feelings and thus learn how to control them. All behavior has meaning, and the nurse can help you discover the meaning in your actions and the methods of changing them so that you can become a more successful nursing home assistant.

SPECIAL PROBLEMS IN THE CARE OF AGED RESIDENTS

The nursing home resident (especially the new one in the strange surroundings of the nursing home) may become confused at night. This is due to the fact that his brain functions poorly; he forgets recent events and may get the past mixed up with the present. This confusion can be minimized by keeping the surroundings familiar. One way of doing this is to keep lights on at night. (Remember how easily you distort and confuse objects in the dark when you awaken at night.)

The resident who lost his wife and his home has little left, but the little that he has soon becomes the objects of over-exaggerated value and significance. He owns the room, the wheelchair, the bathroom at certain hours, and the seat in the dining room; and he becomes furious if someone else takes them or even asks him to change them. It seems as though you destroy his very safety if you touch his possessions, and indeed you do. Change is disturbing and confusing because of his forgetfulness, and stability is comforting and secure.

The lonely nursing home resident lives with his memories, his photographs, and his few prized possessions, and he needs the privacy that permits him to display and enjoy them. He loves his room and spends all his unoccupied time in it just remembering—remembering and reliving the wonderful past when he was young and strong and life was beautiful. He needs time with his memories, but excessive periods of idleness, with all the emotional pain and boredom it creates, must be avoided. This idleness will force the resident to live in the past. Soon the past and the present will be fused into one, and the resident will develop that confusion so common in the aged person who merely exists in a dull, worthless world and who is anxiously awaiting the relief that death brings.

Change confuses and distresses the aged person with a memory loss. He rejects even the slightest disruption in routine. He knows the old way, and he has trouble remembering and rearranging his entire living pattern to adjust to new ones. He avoids the new and the errors he knows he will make by simply refusing to accept it.

The resident loves company, and he talks for hours on end about his past life. It seems as though a visitor gives him the opportunity to dream aloud about his glorious past or to prove his worth by telling of his past accomplishments in his family or his occupation. You may be surprised to hear this resident discuss fishing trips on Lake Erie of 50 years ago with great detail—yet he cannot remember what his fluid intake was at breakfast or what the instructions were that you gave him about not smoking in bed just 30 minutes ago. Remember that his brain cannot retain recent events so give simple instructions, repeat them often, and write them down whenever possible.

The aged nursing home resident has trouble taking in, understanding, and holding onto your conversation. His brain, like the rest of his body, acts slowly. Your usual conversation speed comes through to him like the garbled talk on a record played too fast. He does not understand what you said, so he figures out what it could have been and acts on this. Of course, his behavior is usually contrary to your directions, and you call the resident confused. Be aware of the resident's slowed down body and slowed down mind, and give him time— time to hear, time to understand, time to answer, as well as time to walk, time to eat, time to dress. Talk slowly (about half your usual speed). Give directions simply. Wait for answers. Check on the resident's understanding. Observe how quickly the confused patient becomes able to function correctly when your talk and your actions slow down to his speed level.

The aged person's appetite is poor, and his chewing is difficult because of his dentures. Food allergies and digestive disturbances are common. Malnourishment may occur unless you supervise mealtimes to be sure that the resident eats an adequate diet. Check on why certain foods are uneaten. Notify the dietitian of chewing problems or food dislikes. Modify the diet according to the resident's needs or wishes.

The resident's world narrows as his infirmity increases, and soon it becomes only a concern for his living needs. Each day he talks about his bowels, his sleeplessness, his pains, his loneliness, and his maltreatment by others (residents, staff, and family). It seems that his every word is a complaint, a criticism, and a rejection. The resident's family, already quite guilt-ridden by their rejection and placement of the family member in the nursing home, listen to these complaints and attempt to relieve their own guilt feelings by assuming the responsibility for reporting these deficiencies in care to the nursing home administrator. This complaining resident and his reporting family annoy and irritate you. You love the resident and you give him excellent care, but still they complain and report. You feel that it is impossible to please them, and you would like to stay away from the resident to keep out of trouble. You try this but things only get worse. Discuss this resident and his family with the nurse. She will help you understand that the resident's behavior is caused by his own anger at his fast-approaching helplessness and dependency and not by what you do. She will help you plan a way of caring for this resident that will minimize his emotional pain and will increase his interest in living, and she will include the family in making and carrying out this plan. She will help them understand the basis for the resident's behavior too, and she will show them how to prevent its occurrence by putting some fun and value in the life that the resident is living.

The resident's physical and emotional state deteriorates and his helplessness increases with each passing month. Eventually, some worn-out body part fails and the resident dies with a stroke, with heart failure, or with pneumonia. You begin to wonder about the value of your work in the nursing home. It seems as though the residents die no matter what you do or how much care you give them. Your living care plan does not reverse the problems of aging. You wonder if all the hard work, the careful planning, and the living activity programs are worthwhile when all the residents die anyway. You can overcome this feeling of helplessness and recognize the value in your care by focusing on the resident's daily living rather than on his eventual death. Identify the comforts and pleasures that the resident has in the life you help him live, and constantly seek ways of increasing them. The important aspect in life is not how long it lasts but how it is lived.

As the resident becomes increasingly more feeble and infirm, you will have to take over more and more of his care. You have already learned how to do this. Some of the particular problems he may present and the way they can be cared for are as follows:

1. Inability to move—see Chapters 12 and 13.
2. Inability to care for himself—see Chapters 8, 9, 10, 11, and 14.
3. Inability to control his bladder or bowels—see Chapter 11.
4. Inability to enjoy the life he is living (demanding, uncooperative, complaining resident)—see Chapter 37.
5. Inability to continue living—see Chapter 41.
6. Inability to live safely—see Chapter 40.

Identify these living problems in the resident and review the appropriate chapters to learn how to help him meet these living needs successfully.

SUMMARY

Aging wears out the mind and the body and brings on living problems. The aged person may receive a family type of helpfulness in living with the foster family of the nursing home staff.

The nursing home resident differs from the hospital patient in that he needs a living care plan rather than a nursing care plan. Therefore the focus of your care for the resident is identifying how he wants to live the life he has left and helping him to live it.

The aged person with a worn-out body and a worn-out mind has little resistance to illness and little ability to fight it when it does attack. Therefore a significant part of your care is protective supervision to prevent life-threatening illnesses or injuries.

The nursing home resident is usually discharged only by death. This fact can be depressing to staff members who focus on cure rather than on the real basis of care, which is making the life that the resident lives interesting, comfortable, and productive. The length of life matters not—the living that one does with it is all-important.

DISCUSSION QUESTIONS

1 What evidences of the wearing-out process of aging can you see in your residents?
2 What living help do you give the residents?
3 How much fun do the residents in your nursing home have?
4 What opportunities for valuable, productive work do your residents have?
5 How do the residents feel when one of their members dies? Why?
6 How sick does a resident get when he is attacked by a cold or by virus germs?
7 How can you help an incontinent resident to achieve continence?
8 How many of your residents fall? Why do they fall? Develop a plan to eliminate these falls.
9 How common are bedsores in your nursing home? Why? Develop a plan to eliminate their occurrence.
10 How do you talk to nursing home residents? Why?
11 Review the film, "Mrs. Reynolds needs a nurse." Identify the change in Mrs. Reynolds' nursing care and its effect on her. What ideas does this give you about caring for your residents?

VOCABULARY

acting out Expressing one's feelings through behavior (screaming with rage, etc.).
acute attack Sudden critical bout of illness.
aged person Person whose body and mind shows evidence of wearing out and so a lessening of their living ability.
allergy One person gets sick from food, drink, dust, etc. that does not bother others. (One man's drink may be another man's poison.)
appetite Interest in and desire for food.
arthritis Bone and joint disease.
authoritative Bossy.
complications Undesirable and avoidable worsening of a condition or situation.

confuse Failing to understand and so to respond correctly to the environment.
constipation The bowels hold the feces rather than expel it.
deficiency Shortage.
dependency Relying on another for the essential needs of life. Incomplete in one's self.
depression Sick of life.
deteriorate Decrease in efficiency.
family A group of related people living together and helping each other obtain the best life possible.
fat masses Deposits of fat that form in and plug up the arteries.
food intolerances Food that makes one person sick but does not bother another; allergies.
foster family A group of unrelated people who take over the function of the real family.
fractures Broken bones.
guilt Feeling of blame.
hypertensive cardiovascular disease Disease of narrowed blood vessels, enlarged overworked heart, and high blood pressure.
indigestion Food intolerance that causes stomach distress.
infirmity Feebleness.
intestinal obstruction Blocked bowels; feces cannot be expelled even with cathartics, enemas, etc.
living care plan Plan of meeting the physical and emotional needs for a happy life.
malnourishment Inadequate food intake for effective body functioning.
maltreatment Treatment that worsens the patients condition.
Mary Manning Walsh Nursing home in New York City.
memory Past learnings and life events that are stored in the mind and that can be used to direct daily living. Memory loss involves a difficulty in using these facts to control and direct living.
narrow hardened arteries Arteries plugged with fat masses (arteriosclerosis).
nursing home A foster family like situation for the patient with decreased efficiency in living.
recreational activity program Interesting relaxing activities that an individual likes to do and that make his life worth living.
rejection Discarding, ignoring.
resident Foster nursing home family member.
resistance to disease Ability to avoid illness.
retirement To leave one's occupation or useful work because of age.
Social Security Law Provides for financial safety of the retired worker. Money is withheld from his pay during his working years and is paid to him in monthly payments after retirement.
stroke Paralysis of one side of the body resulting from a broken or plugged blood vessel in the brain.
susceptibility Easiness in getting something.
validate evaluations Prove the observations of the resident are correct.
work activity program Useful, productive activities to replace the ones given up in retirement.

SOURCES OF ADDITIONAL INFORMATION

1. Pamphlet: After a coronary; may be obtained from the Metropolitan Life Insurance Co., 1 Madison Ave., New York, N. Y. 10011.
2. Pamphlet: A guide for the diabetic; may be obtained by your pharmacist from the drug company, Eli Lilly & Co.
3. Film: Cerebral vascular disease: the challenge of management; may be obtained from your local heart association.
4. Film: Diagnosis danger; may be obtained from A.N.A.-N.L.N. Film Services, 2 Columbus Circle, New York, N. Y. 10019. *(Shows a survey of hospital hazards.)*
5. Film: Diary of Connie McGregor; may be obtained from the Public Health Service Audiovisual Facility, Atlanta, Ga. 30333. *(Shows rehabilitation of the aged and chronically ill at a chronic disease hospital.)*
6. Pamphlet: Facts about heart and blood vessel diseases; may be obtained from your local heart association.
7. Film: Mrs. Reynolds needs a nurse; may be obtained from A.N.A.-N.L.N. Film Service, 2 Columbus Circle, New York, N. Y. 10019. *(Shows how a nursing staff resolved the problems of caring for an aged patient with a fatal disease when they added love to their nursing care.)*
8. Book: Phibbs, Brendan: The human heart, ed. 2, St. Louis; 1971, The C. V. Mosby Co.
9. Pamphlet: Strokes (a guide for the family); may be obtained from your local heart association.
10. Pamphlet: The nurse's role in epilepsy; may be obtained from Ayerst Laboratories, 685 Third Ave., New York, N. Y. 10017.
11. Film: The proud years; may be obtained from the A.N.A.-N.L.N. Film Service, 2 Columbus Circle, New York, N. Y. 10019. *(Shows the management of disabled, aged patients in the Home for Aged and Infirm Hebrews in New York in such a way as to preserve and promote movement.)*
12. Pamphlet: You and diabetes; may be obtained by your pharmacist from The Upjohn Drug Co.

40/Meeting the first-aid needs of the patient

STUDY QUESTIONS

1. What is first aid?
2. Is it necessary to call the doctor when you come upon an emergency situation?
3. How is bleeding stopped?
4. When do you use a tourniquet?
5. When do you loosen a tourniquet after you once apply it?
6. How do you give mouth-to-mouth resuscitation?
7. How long do you continue giving mouth-to-mouth resuscitation?
8. What is the first aid for a patient who has fainted?
9. What is the first aid for a patient who is having a convulsion?
10. How can you prevent the patient from reaching the need to commit suicide?

First aid is the emergency action that you take to save the patient's life while you are waiting for the doctor to arrive. The doctor is the only person who has the knowledge and the ability and the legal right to diagnose the patient's illness and to prescribe treatment. However, you have the right and the responsibility to give first aid without the doctor's direction or presence when the patient's life is threatened. Therefore you give the patient first aid under the following circumstances:

1. If the doctor is not present and the patient's life is threatened because of hemorrhage, suffocation, or shock
2. If the patient is trying to kill himself

You remain with the patient who is in danger of losing his life and give him first aid, but you use the patient's signal system to call the nurse. If another nursing assistant or even a patient arrives on the scene, send him to call the nurse or the doctor immediately.

The doctor or the nurse will arrive at the scene of the emergency with the ward emergency tray (sometimes called the cardiac arrest tray). You will be relieved of your first-aid responsibilities and the doctor or nurse (whoever arrived) will take over. Do not leave the room. Stand by to assist in the care of the patient or to get the emergency equipment needed to give this care. Listen carefully for directions from the nurse. If you do not fully understand any directions that she gives you, repeat them to the nurse in a questioning way. You will save valuable time and perhaps also save the patient's life by doing or getting exactly what is needed. In an emergency, every minute counts and you cannot waste these precious minutes by getting the wrong equipment or doing the wrong thing. Then, too, the doctor and the nurse may be so preoccupied with saving the patient's life that they may say one thing when they mean another. Repeating the directions that you receive will make them focus on what was said and will give them a chance to correct any errors or to clarify any vagueness.

Sometimes the nurse may be the first one at the scene of an emergency, and she may use the patient's signal system to summon you. When you arrive in the room, the nurse will continue with the first aid and she will direct you to call the doctor and to bring the emergency tray to the room. Therefore you must know how to get the doctor in an emergency and you must know where the emergency ward equipment is located. Learn these two things today. You will have no time to learn them when a patient's life is at stake and when minutes may mean the difference between life and death.

GIVING THE BLEEDING PATIENT FIRST AID

The patient may bleed internally or externally. Internal bleeding can be identified only through close observation of the vital signs, whereas external bleeding can be easily seen by any observer who looks for it. Bleeding can be expected to occur in the following patients:
1. Patients who have been operated upon recently
2. Patients who have been admitted to the hospital with a history of bleeding
3. Patients who have had diagnostic studies made by inserting a blunt needle into the liver, kidney, or spleen, for example:
   a. Liver biopsy
   b. Kidney biopsy
   c. Spleen biopsy
4. Patients who have fallen out of bed

In most of the instances just mentioned, the patient may have internal bleeding. This can be recognized only by close observation of the vital signs.* However, external bleeding can occur after a fall or after an operation. Therefore all hospital patients who might bleed are observed closely by:
1. Close observation of the vital signs at frequent intervals
2. Close observation of the operative site or the injury site at frequent intervals

As soon as any signs of internal bleeding occur (rising pulse, falling blood pressure, restlessness, thirst, and cold, wet skin), the doctor is notified. Until the doctor arrives, the nurse may direct you to stay with the patient and to try to keep him calm and quiet. You can do this best by being calm and quiet yourself so that the patient gets the feeling that he is safe in your hands. This calming and quietening of the patient will slow down the heartbeat and decrease the amount of bleeding. Remember, fear speeds up the heartbeat. Therefore the frightened patient will really increase his own bleeding difficulty.

Unexpected bleeding may occur in the following instances:
1. In patients who fall and lacerate (cut) the scalp or the skin
2. In patients who attempt suicide by cutting the wrists or the throat

In patients with unexpected bleeding, the bleeding will be external and therefore visible. If the patient has a lacerated scalp, wrist, or throat, the bleeding will be profuse. You will have to take emergency ac-

---

*Internal bleeding in the brain gives rise to signs of intracranial pressure, which are slowing pulse, rising blood pressure, and slowing respirations.

tions to save the patient's life. These actions are the following:
1. Keep the patient lying down.
2. Apply pressure over the wound with a sterile dressing, a clean cloth, or even your bare hand.
3. Use the patient's signal bell to summon help.
4. Continue to apply pressure until the bleeding stops, or until you are relieved by the doctor or nurse.
5. Work quickly but quietly and calmly.

A tourniquet may be used to control bleeding in a limb if you are unable to stop the bleeding with hand pressure. However, a tourniquet shuts off all the blood supply below it, and its use may result in the patient's losing the limb. Therefore use a tourniquet only as a last resort. A good tourniquet to use in the hospital is the blood pressure apparatus. It is applied by wrapping it around the limb (in the usual way) above the bleeding area and by inflating it. Once a tourniquet is applied, leave it on for the doctor to remove.

Remain with the bleeding patient until you are relieved by the doctor or nurse. Never run to get equipment. Use what is available to control the bleeding. Stay calm and do not forget to summon the nurse.

GIVING THE SUFFOCATING PATIENT FIRST AID

The patient suffocates when he is unable to get air into his lungs. Air is necessary for talking. Speech is actually accomplished by vibrating the vocal cords with air from the lungs. Therefore the suffocating patient will be unable to talk and unable to call for help. This means that you must observe your patients closely for breathing difficulties and for obstruction of the respiratory passages (breathing tubes). You might expect these difficulties to occur in the following patients:
1. Patients who are unconscious
2. Patients who are paralyzed and therefore have difficulty swallowing
3. Patients with diseases or operations on the mouth or throat
4. Patients who have nose or mouth packs in place
5. Patients who have inflated tubes in place in the stomach (Linton) or in the esophagus (Blakemore)

In the patients just mentioned, the respiratory passages may become obstructed (blocked) by the patient's tongue, by saliva, by food, by swelling, or by a slipped pack or tube. You can discover the patient with breathing difficulty and prevent suffocation from occurring if you investigate every time you can hear a patient breathing. Remember, normal breathing is soundless. Therefore when breathing is audible, the patient is in trouble, and this trouble must be corrected. Snoring is not a sound of valuable sleep; it is a symptom of a blocked breathing tube. Therefore you will need to take the following steps:
1. *Stop* when you hear noisy breathing.
2. *Listen* to identify the trouble.
3. *Look* at the patient to see if you can correct the problem.
4. *Act* quickly to help the patient restore effective breathing.

The actions that might be taken to correct the patient's breathing difficulty include the following:
1. Place the unconscious patient in a side-lying position. When this is not possible, check with the nurse and she will insert an airway to keep the patient's tongue up and out of the back of his throat.
2. Suction saliva out of the throat. Then place the patient in a side-lying position so that gravity will cause the saliva to flow out of the mouth rather than down into the breathing tube.
3. Summon the nurse if steps 1 and 2 do not restore effective breathing.

You can also prevent suffocation from occurring if you anticipate it and are prepared to take the emergency actions to

avoid it. Some anticipated complications and the methods for avoiding or relieving them are as follows:
1. Expect the paralyzed patient with swallowing difficulty to choke. Avoid his choking by:
   a. Feeding him slowly
   b. Placing the food in the nonparalyzed side of the mouth
   c. Having the suction apparatus ready for use
   d. Using the suction apparatus quickly if food gets into the air passages
2. Expect the patient with mouth or throat problems to develop enough swelling to block off the respiratory passages. Avoid suffocation by:
   a. Having his call bell within reach so that he can summon aid
   b. Answering the patient's call bell immediately
   c. Alerting the entire ward staff to this potential emergency
   d. Having an emergency tracheotomy set on hand in the patient's room

Another type of breathing difficulty may occur in which the patient suddenly and unexpectedly stops breathing. This may be due to an allergic reaction to a drug like penicillin or morphine, or it may be due to prolonged suctioning, or it may have no apparent cause. The first aid that you must give this patient immediately is mouth-to-mouth resuscitation. Continue this procedure and signal or send a patient for the doctor and nurse. When the doctor arrives, he may diagnose the patient's condition as cardiac arrest (heart stoppage), and he may summon the hospital emergency team to give cardiac massage and to continue the artificial respiration.

You give artificial respiration by the technique of mouth-to-mouth resuscitation in the following way:
1. Clean out the patient's mouth with your fingers, which are covered with a piece of cloth (patient's towel). Usually there is vomitus in the mouth or throat of the patient with cardiac arrest.
   a. If suction is available, use this to clean saliva, vomitus, blood, etc. out of the mouth and throat.
2. Pull the patient's tongue forward with your fingers.
3. Remove the pillow fnom under the patient's head. If possible, place the pillow under his shoulders.
4. Tilt the patient's head back as far as you can until he is resting on the top rather than on the back of his head.
5. Lift the patient's jaw and hold it in a jutting-out position by one of the following methods:
   a. Grasp the lower teeth with your thumb and the chin with your fingers and pull it forward.
   b. Lift the jaw upward by applying pressure to the angles of the lower jaw (corners of the jawbone near the earlobe).
   The tilted head and the jutting out position of the lower jaw will lift the tongue out of the throat and make a passageway for the air to the lungs.
6. Maintain this patient position by keeping your one hand on the crown of the patient's head to push it down while you pull up on his chin with the other hand.
7. Take a deep breath and open your mouth wide.
8. Place your lips widely around the patient's mouth. Press them firmly against the patient's skin to make a tight seal.
9. Lean your cheek against the patient's nostrils to close them off and prevent air leakage through them.
10. Watch the patient's chest.
11. Blow air into the patient's mouth until you see his chest rise.

12. Remove your mouth and let the air in the patient's chest escape.
13. Take your next breath as you listen to the sound of the patient's breath escaping.
14. Reinflate the patient's lungs as soon as the air has been exhaled by repeating the foregoing steps.
15. Continue to inflate the patient's lungs at the rate of ten to twelve times per minute.
16. Continue giving mouth-to-mouth resuscitation until the doctor or nurse arrives and gives you further directions.

Signs of difficulty that may occur when you are giving the patient mouth-to-mouth resuscitation are as follows:

1. The chest does not rise. This might indicate that there is an air leak. Seal your lips firmly over the patient's mouth and press your cheek more firmly against his nostrils.
2. The air will not go into the chest, and you feel a resistance when you blow into his mouth. This might indicate that the patient's tongue is still blocking the throat. Lift up his chin and push the top of his head back farther to get a better head tilt and to bring the tongue out of the throat.
3. The patient's breathing is noisy or gurgling. This might indicate that his mouth and throat need to be cleaned again or that his head-tilt position needs to be improved.

Artificial respiration (mouth-to-mouth resuscitation method) is of no value when the respiratory passages are blocked. The purpose of artificial respiration is to get air into the patient's lungs. Therefore any block in the respiratory passages caused by the tongue, food, or saliva must be removed before artificial respiration can be effective. Once the respiratory passages are blocked and breathing stops, you will need to remove the obstruction with your fingers or with suction and then you will have to give the patient mouth-to-mouth resuscitation in order to restart the respiratory process.

In those instances in which the respiratory obstruction cannot be removed, for example, when the patient has a swelling in the throat, artificial respiration (mouth-to-mouth resuscitation) is of no value. In such instances, the doctor must make an opening into the patient's trachea (windpipe) below the obstruction so that the patient can get air into his lungs. This opening is called a tracheotomy.

Some other instances in which you may be required to give the patient emergency artificial respiration by the mouth-to-mouth method and the procedures for giving first aid are the following:

1. The patient hangs himself with a rope, which puts pressure around the neck and squeezes the trachea closed. The first aid for this patient is as follows:
   a. Lift up on the patient's feet to take the pressure off of his neck and call for help.
   b. Continue to support the patient's body by lifting up while your assistant cuts the rope.
   c. Slide the patient to the floor.
   d. Start mouth-to-mouth resuscitation as your assistant goes for the nurse and doctor.
2. The patient is suffocating and stops breathing because his lungs are filled with smoke from a hospital fire.
   a. Remove the patient from the fire area by using the blanket drag (Chapter 13).
   b. Start mouth-to-mouth resuscitation immediately when you are clear of the fire area.
3. The patient is suffocating because he has taken an overdose of sleeping pills in a suicide attempt and his breathing has stopped.
   a. Start mouth-to-mouth resuscitation immediately.
   b. Send for the doctor or nurse.
4. The patient is suffocating because his

breathing stopped during or after a convulsion.
  a. Start mouth-to-mouth resuscitation immediately.
  b. Send for the doctor or nurse.
5. The patient is suffocating because his breathing stopped during or after an electric shock treatment for mental illness.
  a. Start mouth-to-mouth resuscitation.
  b. Send for the doctor or nurse.

The patient must breathe to live. The brain will stop functioning effectively within 3 minutes if its oxygen supply is interrupted. Therefore you must know how to give artificial respiration by the mouth-to-mouth method, and you must be ready to give it immediately when a patient emergency, as just described, occurs.

GIVING FIRST AID TO THE PATIENT IN SHOCK

Shock occurs when the blood supply to the brain is not adequate. It may be caused by pain, hemorrhage, fear, or even a heart attack. The signs of shock are the following:
1. Falling blood pressure
2. Rising pulse
3. Weakness and restlessness that may develop into unconsciousness
4. Pale, cold, wet skin

The first aid for shock is to reestablish the blood supply to the head. Therefore you will need to proceed as follows:
1. Lay the patient down flat in bed and remove the pillow from under his head.
2. Elevate the patient's feet by placing pillows under them. Gravity will cause the blood to flow downhill to the patient's head.
3. Keep the patient warm and calm and quiet. Use extra blankets.
4. Send for the nurse and doctor.

If the patient in shock has a head or chest injury, the head is kept elevated on one pillow. This is done to avoid increased bleeding in the head or chest.

Shock is prevented by recognizing the signs of its onset early and notifying the doctor immediately. Therefore you may be directed to take the vital signs on those patients in whom shock is a possibility, for example:
1. Patients who have recently been operated on
2. Patients with severe injuries or burns
3. Patients who are bleeding
4. Patients with heart difficulties

GIVING THE FAINTING PATIENT FIRST AID

Fainting occurs because the blood supply to the brain has been interrupted temporarily. This interruption may be due to fear, to a disturbing experience, or to great physical stress. Therefore you might expect the patient to faint under the following circumstances:
1. If he is getting a painful treatment that lasts for more than a few minutes
2. If he is terribly frightened by an approaching treatment or operation
3. If he is receiving more than one enema
4. If he is getting out of bed for the first time after a long period of bed rest
5. If he is receiving drugs that lower his blood pressure

You might also expect a relative or friend of a patient to faint when told that his loved one has died.

Fainting occurs in the following manner:
1. The patient feels "funny." After fainting, he might describe this feeling as becoming "light-headed" and then breaking out in a cold sweat.
2. The patient usually tries to go somewhere or do something to get help, but he never accomplishes it because he loses consciousness a moment after he notices the strange feeling, and he falls to the floor.

To revive the patient who has fainted, give the following first aid:
1. Lay the patient down.
2. Lower the patient's head.

3. Elevate the patient's feet to increase the blood supply to his head.
4. Give the patient a smell of a stimulant such as aromatic spirits of ammonia.
5. Send for the nurse.

When the patient recovers, he will still feel his prefainting urgency for getting help, and he may try to jump up and run. Keep the patient lying down for a few minutes after he regains consciousness and until his pulse is strong and regular again. Then assist him into bed to wait for the doctor.

You can prevent fainting from occurring by observing the following rules of patient care:
1. Help the patients out of bed gradually when they get up the first time.
2. Give the patient his enema in bed and encourage the weak patient to remain in bed and expel the enema in the bedpan.
3. Watch the patient's pulse and skin carefully during every treatment. If the pulse weakens or the skin becomes cold and clammy, stop the treatment. Return the patient to a back-lying position in bed and summon the nurse.
4. Have a patient's relative or friend sit down before the doctor or nurse arrives to give him disturbing news.
5. Anticipate fainting and watch for signs of its onset.

GIVING THE SUICIDAL PATIENT FIRST AID

First aid for the patient who has attempted suicide by hanging himself or slashing his neck or wrists has been discussed previously. There are also specific first-aid measures for the patient who contemplates suicide by threatening to jump out of the window or by threatening to slash his wrists.

If you enter a patient's room and find him perched on the windowsill or in the process of getting ready to slash his wrists, remain calm and do not jump for the patient. Send any available person for the doctor or nurse. Walk into the patient's room quietly at your usual pace and ask the patient to give you the sharp instrument or to come back into bed. Do not become frightened. Show your concern for the patient. The only reason the patient wants to die is that he believes life is worthless, impossible, and unbearable and that relief is unobtainable. Show him by your manner that you really do want to help him.

If the patient threatens to act if you come closer, stay where you are and encourage the patient to talk about his trouble. Listen to his conversation carefully. Accept his discussion of his problems. Tell him you know how terrible he feels and how discouraging things might appear; then tell him that you and the doctor and the nurse will help him. Do not argue, disagree, or make idle promises. Convince the patient of your sincere desire to help him. If you do, he will stop and return to bed. Then help him. However, you may have a difficult time convincing the patient if he is one of the incurable patients whom members of the ward staff have condemned to aloneness by their withdrawal from him.

This situation is easier to avoid than to correct. Therefore be sure that your patients never receive the impression that you do not care about them. You can prevent them from getting this idea by really caring.

GIVING THE PATIENT FIRST AID WHEN HE FALLS

When a patient falls, let him lie on the floor and examine him carefully. Determine if emergency action is needed. Check to determine the following:
1. Whether the patient is bleeding
2. Whether the patient is breathing
3. Whether the patient has fainted or is in shock

4. Whether the patient is injured (Look for bumps, bruises, and unnatural positions of the limbs.)

If the patient can tell you, ask him how he feels. Check the body part that he tells you is painful. If you find no need for first aid and if the patient is not injured, get help and return him to bed. Notify the nurse of this incident.

If the patient is bleeding, has stopped breathing, or has fainted, give him the proper first aid. If the patient has painful areas on the body or lumps and bruises, or if his limbs are in an unnatural or unusual position, permit him to stay on the floor. Stay with him and signal for the nurse or send another patient for her. Do not move an injured patient. Let him remain on the floor until the doctor or nurse arrives.

GIVING THE PATIENT FIRST AID WHEN HE HAS A CONVULSION

Before the patient has a convulsion, he notices a strange sensation that warns him that something is about to happen. This sensation causes him to scream out. However, he is unable to help himself in any way because the convulsion occurs one split second after the sensation. However, this scream or aura (warning) does notify members of the ward staff that something is happening to the patient, and it does bring them to him quickly.

When members of the ward staff arrive, the convulsion may have just started, and the patient may be in the tonic or rigid state. If so, he will be lying in bed or on the floor with every muscle of his body as tense as possible. His jaws will be closed tightly, and his tongue will have fallen back into his throat. His breathing will be the noisy, snoring type of obstructed breathing. His back may be so arched that he is touching the floor only with the back of his head and his heels. First aid for the patient at this stage is carried out as follows:

1. Keep the patient on the floor or wherever he is lying. Move him only if he is in a dangerous position such as on top of steps, near a radiator, or near a window. Open any tight clothing around his neck.
2. Open his jaws by applying pressure with your fingers to his jaw muscle. Apply pressure in front of his ears and between his jaws.
3. Insert a prepared tongue blade between his teeth and on top of his tongue. This prevents him from biting his tongue and it keeps his tongue up in his mouth, thus preventing it from falling back into his throat to obstruct breathing.
4. Protect his head from injury by placing a pillow under it.

After a few seconds, the patient will go into the clonic or shaking part of the convulsion, during which stage all the muscles are activated and he shakes all over. He jerks his head, his body, his arms, and his legs.

First aid for the patient during the clonic stage is to keep the tongue blade in place and to protect the patient from injury. The pillow will protect his head, but you will need to guide the movements of his arms and legs to prevent them from being injured. Do not try to hold his body still. Do not attempt to stop the body movements. You cannot stop them, but you could break the patient's arm or leg by attempting to do so.

After the clonic stage, the patient will become limp as all his muscles relax. Even his breathing will stop for a few seconds and he will become quite cyanotic. First aid consists of remaining with the patient and keeping the tongue blade in place. However, if the patient fails to resume breathing in a few moments, start mouth-to-mouth resuscitation (artificial respiration) at once.

When the patient regains consciousness, he will be frightened and a little confused. He will be unable to remember anything about the convulsion or anything that happened just before it occurred. He will try to jump up quickly and he may fall, or he may even have another convulsion. Encourage him to remain in the lying-down position for a few minutes until his confusion clears. Then assist him back into bed and summon the nurse.

You cannot prevent the convulsion. However, you can prevent the patient from injuring himself or from choking during a convulsion as follows:

1. Prepare a tongue blade to insert into the patient's mouth and attach the tongue blade to the top of the bed. The tongue blade is prepared by wrapping a 4-inch-square compress over two (double) tongue blades and securing it there with several strips of adhesive tape.
2. If the patient is ambulatory, prepare a second tongue blade and carry it with you.
3. Assist the patient in any patient care activity (such as taking a tub bath) during which his life might be threatened if he had a convulsion.
4. Place side rails on the bed to prevent the patient from falling out of bed during a convulsion.
5. Respond quickly to the patient's pre-convulsive scream and insert the tongue blade in his mouth immediately to prevent him from choking.
6. Give the patient mouth-to-mouth resuscitation if his respirations do not resume in a few moments.

SUMMARY

When the patient is in danger of losing his life, take those emergency actions indicated to save it. Such actions are the first-aid measures to stop bleeding, to start breathing, and to restore the blood supply to the brain. Remain with the patient and give this first aid, but always summon the nurse and doctor by using the patient's signal system or by sending another patient for them.

DISCUSSION QUESTIONS

1 Do you know what to do when a patient's life is threatened? Assume that a patient is choking on some food that is caught in his trachea (windpipe). The nurse is giving the patient first aid and she has sent you to call the doctor and to get the ward emergency equipment. Discuss what you would do.
2 Where is your ward emergency equipment located?
3 How could you summon a doctor in an emergency?
4 Is there a cardiac arrest team in the hospital in which you work? How do you summon the team when a cardiac arrest occurs on your ward?
5 What kind of patient emergencies do you expect on your ward? What is the first aid for these emergencies?
6 Can you give mouth-to-mouth resuscitation? Ask the nurse to demonstrate the procedure for you.
7 Enroll in a first-aid course sponsored by your local Red Cross chapter.
8 What first-aid equipment is standing by for your patients right now?
9 What patient emergencies does the doctor or nurse expect to occur? How would you recognize these emergency situations?
10 Why do some patients have a tracheotomy when they stop breathing, whereas others are given mouth-to-mouth resuscitation?

SOURCES OF ADDITIONAL INFORMATION

1 Film: Introduction to respiratory and cardiac resuscitation; may be obtained from Director, Armed Forces Institute of Pathology, Walter Reed Army Medical Center, 6825 16th St. N.W., Washington, D. C. 20025.
2 Film: First aid, Parts 1 and 2; may be obtained from your local Red Cross chapter.
3 Film: Mouth-to-mouth resuscitation; may be obtained from your local Red Cross chapter.
4 Pamphlet: First aid; may be obtained from The Superintendent of Documents, United States Government Printing Office, Washington, D. C. 20025.
5 Pamphlet: Rescue breathing; may be obtained from your local Red Cross chapter or your State Civil Defense Commission.
6 Program recommendation—Cardiac arrest: (a) Hospital policy identification; (b) American Heart Association—Film: Prescription for life; and (c) Practice session on cardiac massage and mouth-to-mouth breathing. Use model Rescussi-Anne.

41/Caring for the dying patient

STUDY QUESTIONS

1. What are the two parts of the hospital patient care program?
2. Why might nursing assistants avoid the dying patient?
3. Why does a patient get "cranky"?
4. How does the patient learn that he is going to die?
5. How does the pastor or rabbi help the dying patient?
6. Why do incurable, dying patients talk so much about their past life?
7. How is the care of an unconscious dying patient similar to that of an unconscious postoperative patient?
8. How can you help the patient's family live through the experience of seeing a loved one die?
9. What information are you permitted to give the family about the patient's condition?
10. How can you safeguard the patient's false teeth?
11. How is a body prepared for the morgue?
12. When is the patient considered legally dead?

THE HOSPITAL PATIENT CARE PROGRAM

All patients who are admitted to a hospital cannot get well. Some of them will die. Therefore the hospital patient care program has two parts:

1. Helping the patient to get as well as he can and then returning him to comfortable living at home
2. Helping the patient live as comfortably as he can for as long as he can

Sometimes the members of the hospital staff forget their second function. They try to help the patient recover, but when a diagnosis of an incurable illness is established, when the patient has repeated relapses with a constant worsening of his condition, or when the patient fails to get well despite the staff's efforts, they withdraw their caring from him. They still perform the essential parts of the patient's physical care. They wash him and they feed him, but they do it in a routine, "what's-the-use" kind of way.

The members of the staff may believe that they are wasting their time when they give it to the hopelessly incurable patient who gets progressively worse each day. They feel helpless and even a little guilty. They want to make the patient well, but they are not able to do so. All the knowledge and ability they have is not enough to cure the patient. Therefore each time the patient complains of discomfort or pain, they become annoyed at their own helplessness and they try to overcome it by reassuring the patient with false information about his ability to recover. The staff members are well aware of these misrepresentations, and they feel guilty about them. This feeling of guilt is uncomfortable, so they try to avoid it by avoiding the patient and thus the need to tell lies. However, the patient soon realizes that his condition is worsening, and he becomes angry at the staff members who keep promising him a cure while he gets sicker.

The patient may then accuse the staff of using him as a guinea pig and of giving him the wrong care. "If the staff promises me a cure," the patient reasons, "why am I getting worse?" Then he starts to fight for the cure that is being kept from him by the hospital staff. He complains about the poor meals, the incompetent staff, and the lack of proper hospital treatment facilities. Such complaints annoy the staff. They believe that they are doing everything possible for the patient and that he is not only ungrateful but nasty and complaining.

Having a reason to criticize the patient makes the staff members feel better. They justify their avoidance of the patient by telling themselves that he is miserable and ought to be left alone. Then the patient is condemned to spending his last few days or weeks alone, frightened by his illness, angry because of the promised cure that is not forthcoming, and annoyed at the staff members, who he believes are cheating him. The ward staff members spend this time uncomfortably, too. They avoid the cranky patient who criticizes them constantly, and they try to pacify the disturbed visitors who are caught between the patient's misery and the staff's apparent disinterest.

However, when the members of the hospital staff fully accept their two functions by accepting the fact that some patients will not get well, they can avoid this pattern of withdrawing from the patient. Then they can devote their nursing activities to relieving the patient's discomfort and to helping him enjoy living as long as possible. These nursing activities involve giving the patient the emotional care that he needs and giving the patient the physical care that he needs.

EMOTIONAL CARE OF THE DYING PATIENT

When the patient came to the hospital, he came for a cure. However, as the days pass and his disease continues and even worsens, he begins to wonder if he can be cured. Soon this wondering changes to the frightening thought that he might die. Of course, the patient does not want to die, and he tries to push this idea out of his thoughts.

The patient questions every staff member who enters the room about his condition and about his chance of recovery. He listens to the answers carefully. The staff members' vague answers and his own steadily worsening condition soon make the patient realize that he is going to die. He becomes frightened and he fights for his life. He is afraid to be alone, so he strives constantly to get your attention, and when he gets it, he holds it as long as he can. He signals you through the communication system frequently, and when you come to his bedside, he asks for such insignificant things as raising his bed about an inch or lowering his window shade a very little. When you start to leave his room, the patient tries to hold you with his talk or with new demands for care. As soon as you leave, he signals for you again.

In this frightening stage of life when the patient is getting his thoughts in order so that he can die comfortably, he needs you more than ever. He needs you to relieve his terrible feeling of aloneness and he needs you to help him organize his thoughts. Visit the patient frequently at regularly scheduled times. Each time you leave him, tell him when you will return. Plan your patient care activities in such a way that you can spend about 10 to 20 minutes with the patient each morning and afternoon just listening to him.

When you visit him, encourage him to talk while you just listen. The patient does not want answers. He knows that you do not have the answer to the mystery of death. He simply needs someone to listen while he tries to solve the mystery for himself. Listen to his talk about his past life. Listen to his talk about the good things that he did and the errors that he made. Listen to him talk while he works through his feelings about death. At first he will be angry, but he will gradually learn to accept death as he realizes the full and rich life that he had. The pain and discomfort that he has in his present living will help him reach this acceptance.

The patient will need all the assistance that he can get to help him accept and prepare for death. Most of this assistance will come from his religious beliefs. Therefore notify his pastor or rabbi, and when the clergyman visits, leave him alone with the patient. After he leaves, visit the patient and permit him to talk while you listen. The pastor or rabbi probably discussed dying, and now the patient may want to think and talk about this for awhile. Try to be comfortable and relaxed. Do not change the subject. Permit the patient to think and talk through his fear of dying while you listen. Do not feel guilty because you cannot help him avoid death. Everyone must die. Your role is not to cure the incurable but to help the patient die comfortably and fearlessly, in the presence of hospital staff members who really care about him.

PHYSICAL CARE OF THE DYING PATIENT

The physical care that the patient needs you to do for him depends on how many of the activities of living he is unable to do for himself. Therefore you will need to observe him closely. As he becomes weaker and more helpless, you will need to do more and more of his living activities for him. Be alert to these changes in the patient and discuss them with the nurse. Ask her what these physical changes mean in terms of what changes you will need to make in your nursing care plan. Help the patient with a living activity when he has difficulty doing it and before he realizes that he is no longer able to do for himself. You will reassure the patient by doing this because he will be aware of the fact that you are taking care of him, and he will not develop a feeling of helplessness and dependency.

As the patient becomes weaker and more helpless, provide for all of his physical needs. Bathe him, turn him, feed him, toilet him, etc., but permit him to do those things for himself that he can. Help him to feel that he is taking part in his own care. If you bathe the patient, let him comb his own hair. If you feed the patient, let him hold his own bread. If you turn the patient, let him hold onto the crib sides and help to pull himself over.

When the patient lapses into unconsciousness, you will need to perform all his living activities for him. You will need to bathe him, turn him, suction him, etc. However, you will need to develop a plan for doing these activities for the patient at regularly scheduled times. The patient will not ask for anything nor will he complain about your care. He will not even thank you for making him feel better. However, if you fail to move the patient and change his position, he may develop decubitus ulcers and lung congestion. Then, too, he will still need to void and defecate, and if you do not plan to meet these needs, he will urinate and defecate in bed. The bed that is soiled with urine or feces is sure to lead to the development of decubitus ulcers. Your nursing care of the unconscious patient will need to include a plan for carrying out the following living activities:

1. Bathing the patient
2. Giving him mouth care
3. Giving him toilet care
4. Moving him every 2 hours.
5. Keeping his airway open by the following methods:
   a. Keeping secretions out of his air passages
   b. Keeping his tongue from blocking his air passages
6. Feeding him by tube or observing his intravenous infusions
7. Identifying changes in his condition by close observation of his vital signs
8. Recording his intake and output
9. Charting the care you give and the observations you make on his nursing record

All of the preceding activities have been described previously with the exception of the toilet care of the unconscious patient.

MEETING THE TOILET NEEDS OF THE UNCONSCIOUS PATIENT

The doctor and the nurse will discuss the patient's toilet needs and will develop a plan for meeting them. This plan will take into consideration the fact that the patient is no longer able to control his bowels and bladder. This means that he may have a problem with urinary and fecal incontinence or with urinary retention and fecal impaction.

The plan for meeting the patient's toilet needs will attempt to reestablish bladder and bowel control. Since this control cannot be attained by an unconscious patient, it must be attained by the nursing personnel. Therefore the nursing care plan for this patient will include a method for having the patient's bladder and bowels empty in toilet facilities provided by the nursing personnel at times also established by the nursing personnel.

The plan for meeting the patient's need to evacuate fecal material may be as follows:

1. Each morning at a specific time (same time each morning), the patient is given a rectal irrigation. This irrigation is given in the same way as an enema, and it is given with the patient in a back-lying position on the bedpan.
2. When the patient has no fecal discharge between rectal irrigations, the irrigation is given every other day instead of daily.
3. As an alternative to rectal irrigation, suppositories may be used. Each morning at a specific time (same time each morning), the patient is turned to a side-lying position and a suppository is inserted. Absorbent pads are placed on the bed under the patient's buttocks in such a way as to catch the bowel movement that will occur about 30 minutes after the insertion of the suppository.
4. Another alternative plan is to give the patient a Fleet enema each morning. The patient is placed in a back-lying position on the bedpan.

The doctor will decide which method of bowel control is best for the patient, and he will write specific orders on the chart for carrying it out. You and the nurse will then plan together in a team conference to determine the best way of carrying out these orders to establish bowel control for the patient and thus eliminate fecal impactions or fecal incontinence.

The key to establishing bowel control in the unconscious patient is the same as it is in the patient with a colostomy, and this key is habit training. Habit training is accomplished by doing the same thing in the same way at the same time and by getting the same response. Therefore you will need to give irrigation, enema, or suppository each day at the same time and in the same way if you hope to train the patient's bowel.

The plan for meeting the patient's need to void may be as follows:

1. The patient's voiding time is determined by having a nursing assistant

check the patient every 30 minutes and record whether or not he has voided. This is done for 2 days. (The patient's fluid intake is kept the same.)
2. The nursing assistant's observations are checked, and the times that the patient voided are noted.
3. A schedule is then developed for providing the patient with voiding facilities. This schedule is as follows:
   a. One-half hour before his voiding time, the male patient is positioned on his side and a urinal is put in position. Success or failure is charted.
   b. After 5 to 7 days, a successful schedule can be developed for the male patient.
   c. A similar schedule may be followed in the female patient, too; however, at the scheduled voiding times the unconscious female patient is positioned on a low bedpan (fracture bedpan), since the female urinal is ineffective.
4. Alternate methods include the application of an external urinary drain over the penis or the insertion of a catheter into the bladder.

Urinary control is much more difficult to attain than fecal control. Remember, too, that voiding occurs much more frequently than does defecating. A patient's elimination needs may be met adequately with one bowel movement a day, but ten or twelve urinations may be required. Therefore you can expect urinary control to be ten to twelve times more difficult to obtain than fecal control, and, indeed, it is.

A valuable urination facility can be obtained for both the male and the female patient by placing the patient in a bed with a two-piece mattress. A funnel with drainage tubing attached can then be positioned between the sections of the mattress and in the area of the patient's urethra.

When an external urinary drainage system is used in providing for the voiding needs of the male patient, the condom-type attachment to the penis must be removed daily. The penis and the condom-type attachment must be washed thoroughly and then dried and powdered. Then the apparatus can be reapplied to the penis (Fig. 32-1).

EMOTIONAL SUPPORT FOR THE PATIENT'S FAMILY

The members of the patient's family do not have physical pain and discomfort. They do not feel the steadily worsening condition of the patient, and they are therefore unable to accept his impending death. Then, too, the family members have difficulty understanding how they can go on living without their loved one and so they fight to hold onto his life. They are at the patient's bedside constantly. They question the hospital staff hourly hoping to get some information that the patient's condition is improving. Each time the patient sighs, or moves, or eats, or drinks, or eliminates waste, they take this to be a "good sign" and they run out to report it to the doctor or the nurse, asking, "Now don't you think he'll get well?"

Even when the patient lapses into unconsciousness, the members of the family stay at the bedside, and they hope and pray. They feel miserable and helpless. They want to help their loved one get well. They want to relieve his discomfort and his pain. They want to help him breathe easier, and they want to help him eat and drink so that he will regain his strength. You need to help this worried, frightened family, and you can do it in two ways:
1. By giving the patient good care
2. By being kind and considerate to the troubled family

When the members of the family see you visiting the patient frequently and giving him care, they know that the hospital staff cares about the patient and is doing everything possible to make him well. They do not resent your coming into the room and evicting them while you care for the patient. In fact, they welcome you. On the other hand, if you delay the patient's care until the family leaves, they will be disturbed. If they do not see you coming into the patient's room, they begin to believe that the hospital staff has stopped caring about their loved one and has condemned him to death. Then they seek out the doctor and the head nurse and complain about the patient's care. When you hear them complain, ask yourself, "How did I let them get the idea that no one cared for the patient?" As soon as you have the answer, schedule your patient care in such a way as to correct this impression.

Treat the members of the patient's family as you would like to be treated if your situations were reversed. Speak to them kindly and courteously each time they come or each time you enter the patient's room. Each time you ask them to leave the patient's bedside, explain to them that you are going to give the patient some nursing care. Tell them how long this care will take, and suggest some place that they might go to rest or eat. Refer the family's questions about the patient's condition to the nurse. You do not know enough about the patient to give this kind of information. If you say that the patient looks better, the family who is begging for proof that the patient will not die may take this to mean that the patient is better. They may leave the bedside and go home for a much-needed rest, only to be called a short time later and informed that their loved one is dead. Then they may be angry. You can avoid this kind of situation by asking the head nurse what kind of information you may give to the family members and then by giving them only this information.

Visit with a family member who remains at the bedside of an unconscious patient for a few minutes after you give the patient his care. Do not give him any information other than that which the nurse has instructed you to give, but do listen, and encourage him to talk by your listening. Permit him to talk about his life with the patient and about the patient's helplessness and misery now. This talking and your concerned listening will help the family member to learn to adjust to a life without his loved one, and eventually it will enable him to accept the patient's forthcoming death.

Be concerned about the family member at the patient's bedside. Make arrangements for his meals. If possible, serve him a tray at mealtimes. If this is not possible, direct him to eating facilities. Orient him to those ward facilities that he will need. Show him where the ward toilet facilities are, where the phone is located, and where he can rest in the visitors' lounge. At night, serve him a cup of coffee when you have one.

SAFEGUARDING THE UNCONSCIOUS PATIENT'S BELONGINGS

When the patient lapses into unconsciousness and is no longer able to use the personal belongings that he brought to the hospital, arrange to have these belongings safeguarded. This can be done by placing them in the hospital clothing room or safe or by making arrangements for the family to take them home.

However, any replacements for lost or removed body parts (such as false teeth, wigs, glass eyes, or artificial limbs) should remain with the unconscious patient. You will need to safeguard these prosthetic appliances carefully. If the patient recovers he will want them immediately; if he dies, the undertaker will want them.

Safeguard the patient's prostheses in the following way:

1. If the patient has false teeth, label a container with the patient's name, room number, and ward. Then fill the container with cold water and put the false teeth in it. Place the container with the teeth in the patient's bedside stand. Make a notation on the nurse's record on the patient's chart

that you have removed the patient's false teeth from his mouth and that you have placed them in a labeled container in his bedside stand. If the patient is moved to another room or ward, carefully check his bedside stand for any belongings and send them with him. Note on the nurse's record what belongings accompanied the patient in this move from ward to ward or room to room. Each morning when you give the patient mouth care, check to be sure that his false teeth are still in his bedside stand. Then put fresh water in the container.

2. Place such prostheses as wigs and glass eyes in a box. Label the box with what it contains and with the patient's name, room number, and ward. Put this box inside the patient's bedside stand for safekeeping. Record in the nurse's notes in the patient's chart what you did with these patient belongings. Transfer these belongings with the patient when he is moved.

3. Label artificial limbs as described previously for other prostheses. Store them in the patient's clothes closet or in the hospital clothing room. Record in the nurse's record in the patient's chart where they are stored.

CARE OF THE BODY AFTER THE PATIENT DIES

On your frequent visits to the patient's room, observe his breathing and check his pulse. Notify the nurse immediately if he stops breathing or if you are unable to feel his pulse. The nurse will then check the patient immediately. If the patient has stopped breathing or if his pulse cannot be felt, she will call the doctor. The patient is not legally dead until the doctor determines that he is. Therefore treatments such as oxygen, intravenous infusions, or blood transfusions are continued until the doctor listens to the patient's heart with a stethoscope and, finding no beat, pronounces the patient dead. Then the doctor records the date and time of death on the patient's chart.

When the family is present at the time that the patient dies, they will be asked to wait outside the room while the doctor examines the patient. After the patient is pronounced dead, all treatments are discontinued and the body is placed flat in bed in a back-lying position with one pillow under the head. The bedclothes are arranged neatly and the room is straightened. Then the doctor or the nurse will bring the family in to see the body. They may at first be overcome with grief. However, the neat, relaxed atmosphere of the room, together with the calm, quiet repose of their loved one, comforts them. They see death now as a comforting, relieving, resting state. They may make remarks about how quiet, how calm, how peaceful, how relieved and restful their loved one looks. This helps them to control their grief, and eventually they leave the hospital to return home and pick up the threads of their living.

The nurse will ask you to assist her to prepare the body for the morgue. You can do this in the following way:
1. Collect the necessary equipment, including the following:
    a. Morgue pack containing:
        (1) Three strips of 4-inch-wide muslin bandage
        (2) Cotton padding
        (3) Tongue blades
        (4) Three strips of 1-inch gauze bandage
        (5) Safety pins if the sheet that encloses the body is pinned
        (6) Four morgue tags
    b. Bath basin
    c. Tongue blades and 4-inch-square compresses
    d. Stretcher
    e. Linen hamper
    f. Adhesive tape
2. Take all the equipment (except the stretcher) to the patient's room.
3. Remove the spread from the bed and fold it over a chair. You can

use this spread later to cover the body when it is on the stretcher.
4. Remove the blankets from the bed and discard them in the linen hamper.
5. Keep the body covered with the top sheet.
6. Remove the gown or pajamas from the body and discard them in the linen hamper.
7. Fill the basin with bath water, and wash any part of the patient's body that is soiled with drainage. If there is none, eliminate this step.
8. Clean out the patient's mouth.
   a. Wrap a 4-inch-square compress around a tongue blade, moisten it with water, and swab out the patient's mouth.
   b. If the patient's mouth is clean, eliminate this step.
9. If the patient has false teeth, place them in his mouth.
10. If necessary, secure the patient's teeth in his mouth as follows:
    a. Place a 4-inch-wide muslin bandage around the patient's face and under his chin.
    b. Put cotton padding under the bandage at the chin and at the top of the head.
    c. Bring the ends of the muslin bandage over the padding and behind the patient's ears, and tie them securely but not too tightly at the top of the head. (Padding and wide bandage are used to prevent marking the body.)
    d. If the patient has no false teeth, roll up a towel and place it on top of the patient's chest and under the chin to keep his mouth closed.
11. Hold the patient's eyelids closed for a few seconds. They may stay closed. If they do not, do nothing further. If the patient has an artificial eye, the nurse will insert it.
12. Cross the patient's hands on his abdomen and keep them in this position by wrapping well-padded, 4-inch-wide muslin bandage around his wrists and tying it there.
13. Tie the patient's legs together at the ankles with well-padded, 4-inch-wide muslin bandage.
14. Remove bulky dressings and cover any drainage area on the body with a small dressing. Make the dressing drainageproof by covering it completely with adhesive tape.
15. Turn the body to a side-lying position.
16. Twist a tongue blade so that it splits in half lengthwise.
17. Use the split tongue blade to pack the patient's rectum with cotton padding.
18. Place a lifting sheet on the bed. This is a regular bed sheet folded in half lengthwise and placed on the bed in the area from the patient's head to and including the hips. It is placed on the bed in the same manner as any clean sheet is placed under a patient.
19. Place the morgue sheet (if one is used) on the bed. This is put on in the same way as any clean bed sheet is placed under a patient.
20. Roll the patient to the opposite side of the bed and pull the morgue sheet and lifting sheet through and under the patient's body.
21. Place the prepared morgue tags on the body.
    a. The tags contain the patient's name, age, religion, time and date of death, ward, and the doctor's name.
    b. Two tags are usually placed on the body. One is tied to the wrists and the other to the ankles.
22. Enclose the patient in the morgue sheet or hooded paper shroud as follows:

a. If the morgue sheet is used, fold down the top over the head, bring up the bottom over the feet, bring in the sides and pin them closed.
   b. Place the hooded paper shroud on the patient by slipping the hood over the patient's head and tying the shroud at the neck and the feet. Then cover the front of the patient's body with the shroud and tuck the sides of it around and under the body.
23. Place the third prepared morgue tag on the body. It is usually pinned to the sheet or tied to the paper shroud at the neck.
24. Get the stretcher. Ask the ward clerk to call for a special elevator (usually the freight elevator is used).
   a. Get the Davis roller also if one is available.
   b. Obtain additional assistance for lifting if a Davis roller is not available.
25. Return to the patient's room with the stretcher and the Davis roller or with the lifting assistants.
26. Position the stretcher alongside the bed.
27. Lift the body onto the stretcher by means of the Davis roller or by using the lifting sheet with the help of several assistants.
28. Cover the body with the bedspread.
29. Signal the members of the ward staff that you are ready to bring the body to the freight elevator so that they can clear the hall and close the doors on the patients' rooms.
30. Take the body to the elevator and then to the morgue, taking an assistant to the morgue with you if one is needed to help lift the body from the stretcher to the morgue box.
31. Place the fourth tag on the outside of the morgue box in the slot provided.
32. Return to the ward promptly with all the ward equipment. This includes the stretcher and the sheets.
33. Clean the deceased patient's room and prepare it for the next patient. This is done in the same way as any discharge unit is cleaned.
34. Clean your equipment and return it to its proper place.

• • •

The patients on the ward usually feel bad after a death occurs. It reminds them that they, too, might die. Therefore you will need to visit your patients frequently throughout the day to comfort them. However, do not discuss the dead patient.

SUMMARY

The incurable patient creates feelings of guilt and helplessness in staff members who believe that their only function is curing. However, when the members of the staff accept their second function of caring for the patient even when cure is not possible, they are able to redirect their nursing activities toward helping the patient live as comfortably as possible for as long as possible.

The dying patient will become progressively weaker and more helpless and may lapse into unconsciousness. The weak and helpless or unconscious dying patient is cared for in the same way and with the same devotion and tenderness as is the weak and helpless or unconscious postoperative patient.

Bladder and bowel control is possible in the unconscious patient. This control is lost by the patient, but it can be established by the nursing personnel. However, it takes a concerned and caring nursing staff to achieve such control.

Religious beliefs and his pastor or rabbi are the patient's greatest sources of help in assisting him accept and prepare for death. Therefore the hospital staff members should notify the patient's pastor or rabbi as soon as they know that the patient may die. Just as the doctor is a co-worker in helping the patient get well, the religious counselor is a co-worker in helping the patient prepare for death.

DISCUSSION QUESTIONS

1. How can you safeguard the false teeth of an unconscious and dying patient?
2. If a patient has false teeth, do you always remember to transfer them with him if he is moved to the intensive care unit because he is acutely ill?
3. If possible, determine the number of times false teeth have been lost on your ward and develop a plan to prevent these losses from occurring.
4. Observe the family of your next dying patient. Listen to their conversation. What do they talk about?
5. Do you avoid visitors or do you help them? How many of your patient's visitors do you know?
6. How do you help the family member who stays at the patient's bedside for hours and hours? Have you oriented this family member to the comfort facilities on your ward?
7. *Discuss:* The ward staff members believe that they have a cranky patient and they avoid him, but the patient feels that he has miserable nursing assistants who do not like him.
8. Why is cotton padding put under the muslin bandage that is placed around the patient's face and chin in postmortem care?
9. Do you have incurable patients on your ward who make you feel so helpless that you avoid them? Keep a record of your activities for one day. Notice which patients you visit the most.
10. How do you know when the unconscious patient's condition changes?
11. Are your unconscious patients incontinent? How could you reestablish bladder and bowel control?
12. Do you know when your unconscious patient had his last bowel movement? Do you care? If so, how could you know?
13. Do your unconscious patients have decubitus ulcers? What methods do you employ to prevent these ulcers from developing?
14. How do you suction an unconscious patient?
15. How do you know when to suction an unconscious patient?

VOCABULARY

absorbent pads Pads put on the bed under the incontinent patient's genital area to absorb and collect urinary and fecal drainage.

dying patient Patient whose disease worsens constantly despite medical care and who finally dies after days, weeks, or months of pain and suffering.

external urinary drainage apparatus Rubber cover for the penis that is connected to urinary drainage tubing. (It is used instead of a catheter, which goes inside the patient's body to his bladder.)

habit training Reestablishing bladder and bowel control by the use of some artificial means after control has been lost. For example, the patient may learn to defecate in response to a suppository.

incurable patient Patient who receives comfortable hospital living through medical and nursing actions to relieve his pain and distress but who cannot be cured.

morgue sheet Sheet put on the body after the patient dies.

unconscious patient Patient who is totally and completely unaware of his environment and who does not respond to anything in his surroundings.

SOURCES OF ADDITIONAL INFORMATION

1. Film: Mrs. Reynolds needs a nurse; may be obtained from the A.N.A.-N.L.N. Film Service, 2 Columbus Circle, New York, N. Y. 10019. *(Shows a frightened, dying patient and an annoyed staff.)*
2. Film: Long day's journey; may be obtained from the A.N.A.-N.L.N. Film Service, 2 Columbus Circle, New York, N. Y. 10019. *(Shows care of the chronically ill patient in the home.)*
3. Filmstrip and record: (a) Care of the dying patient and (b) Spiritual needs of the patient; available from Trainex Corp., P. O. Box 116, Garden Grove, Calif. 92642.

42/Meeting the patient's need for comfort and safety on an off-ward trip

STUDY QUESTIONS

1. Why are patients taken off the ward so many times?
2. Why are all of the patient's studies and treatments not done on the ward?
3. How many different diagnostic and treatment areas may there be in a hospital?
4. What is a generalized escort service?
5. What is a departmental escort service?
6. How is a patient prepared for an off-ward trip?
7. Is it necessary for the nursing personnel to stay with the patient when they take him on an off-ward trip?
8. Can the patient wear his false teeth during an off-ward trip?
9. Why must the patient wear a name tag on his wrist when he leaves the ward for a study or treatment?

Because of the highly specialized environment and the expensive equipment required for diagnostic studies and therapeutic techniques, today's modern hospital sets up specific areas for them. Therefore the hospital in which you work will have many of the following off-ward areas:

1. The x-ray (or radiology) department, in which diagnostic x-ray films are made
2. The x-ray therapy (or radiation) department, in which x-ray treatment is given for patients with cancer and other diseases
3. The electrocardiogram laboratory, in which heart studies (EKG's) are done
4. The laboratories in which specimens (for example, blood, sputum, feces, urine, body cells, and pus) are studied to help the physician make a diagnosis
5. The electroencephalogram laboratory, in which brain tracing studies (EEG's) are done
6. The esophagoscopy and gastroscopy laboratory, in which the esophagus and/or stomach can be examined
7. The cardiopulmonary laboratory, in which cardiac catheterizations and breathing effectiveness studies are done
8. The B.M.R. laboratory, in which

basal metabolism rates (studies of minimum oxygen requirements for living) are made
9. The laboratory (radioisotope laboratory), in which radioactive substances are used for diagnosis and/or treatment
10. The operating room, in which surgical procedures are performed
11. The physical therapy (P.T.) department, in which rehabilitation treatments are carried out
12. The psychology department, in which psychological testing and/or psychotherapy is done

Soon after the patient is admitted to the hospital, the doctor examines him thoroughly and then orders those studies necessary for him to diagnose the patient's illness and those treatments necessary to cure or relieve the disease or disorder. Perhaps none of your patients will go to all the hospital areas just outlined, but most of them will go to at least three or four of them. Some may go daily to some treatment areas, such as the physical therapy department, the psychology department, or the x-ray therapy department.

ESCORT SERVICE

Because of the need to take so many patients to off-ward areas, some hospitals have established an escort service. Late each afternoon the ward clerk sends the escort service a report of all those patients scheduled for off-ward appointments the next day. This report includes the following:
1. The time of the appointment
2. The place of the appointment
3. The name of the patient scheduled for the appointment
4. The way the patient is to go (for example, by wheelchair, stretcher, or bed)

Early each morning, about 1 hour before the time of the first appointment, the foreman in the escort service reports on duty and prepares an assignment for each of his workers. When the members of the escort service report on duty (about 30 minutes before the first scheduled appointment), they pick up their assignments and proceed to take the patients to their appointments at the designated times. Although they return the patients to the ward, they do not remain with them in the study area. Therefore they must find out what time the studies will be completed and return for the patients at that time.

Those patients who are acutely ill and in need of constant nursing care during an off-ward trip to a diagnostic area (such as the x-ray department) should be taken on such a trip by a member of the ward nursing staff and not by a member of the escort service.

Departmental escort service

Some hospital departments have a great deal of difficulty adhering to a planned appointment schedule because of the emergency work they are required to do. In order to avoid having the patients wait for long periods of time off the ward, these hospital departments may have their own escort service. Examples of departmental escort services are those run by the operating room or by the x-ray department.

PREPARING THE PATIENT FOR AN OFF-WARD TRIP

Whether you are a member of the ward nursing staff or a member of the escort service, you must prepare the patient adequately so that he will be safe and comfortable throughout an off-ward trip. In order to prepare the patient, we might think of ourselves and how we prepare for a trip away from home. The hospital ward or room is the patient's home while he is ill. Therefore you should prepare the patient in much the same way that you prepare yourself for a trip, keeping the following considerations in mind:
1. You never start on a trip to nowhere. You always know where you are going and

why you are going there. The patient, too, should know where he is going and why. Tell him where he is going. If he has a great deal of apprehension about the trip, perhaps the nurse or doctor has been too busy to explain its purpose to him. Do not brush aside the patient's questions. Ask the nurse or doctor to answer them for him. If you fail to do this, the patient may be so upset throughout the study that false results are obtained. Perhaps the patient may even be too frightened to go.

2. You prepare your body for a trip. Perhaps you take a bath, shave, comb your hair, and even put on clean clothing. The patient, too, should have his body prepared for the trip. Check to be sure that the patient's body is clean, that he is free of soiled dressings, that colostomy or ileostomy bags are empty, and that his clothing (pajamas or gown) is clean.

3. You prepare your bladder and bowels for a trip. Just before you leave the house, you make a last trip to the bathroom. You want to be sure that you will be free of toilet needs when you are in unfamiliar areas where toilet facilities may not be available. The patient, too, must be taken to the bathroom if he is ambulatory or be given a bedpan and/or urinal if he is a bed patient. He must be given adequate time to use these toilet facilities. As mentioned previously (Chapter 11), fear and worry make it difficult to void; therefore give the patient time. When he is finished, give him the equipment he needs to wash his hands well.

4. You take with you those things you will need to be comfortable, such as money, glasses, and cleansing tissue. The patient, too, should take with him what he needs to be comfortable. This would include his glasses, cleansing tissue, etc. Also, let him insert his false teeth (if he is not actually ill and if he is not going to the operating room or any area where he will be put to sleep during the study or treatment). Other items might include an emesis basin if the patient is nauseated or a cushion for him to sit on if he has hemorrhoids. Find out if the patient's chart or his x-ray films are to be taken with him. If so, be sure to take them with you.

5. You dress adequately for the occasion. In summer you might take a light sweater, whereas in winter you may wear a heavy overcoat. The patient, too, should be properly dressed. His body should be adequately covered with a gown (or pajamas) and a bathrobe if he is in a wheelchair, or by a gown and adequate top covering (sheets and blankets) if he is on a stretcher. He should be dressed in the correct hospital attire (gown or pajamas) to permit free exposure of that part of his body to be studied while it keeps the rest of his body covered decently and modestly.

6. You take all the necessary precautions for protection during your trip. You check that you have identification in your pocket, that you have your auto license, etc. You should also check that the patient is protected. Check that he has a name tag attached to his wrist. Ask the nurse or check the appointment sheet to see if the patient walks or goes by wheelchair or stretcher, and, if necessary, place him in the proper carrier. Determine the patient's awareness of his surroundings. If he does not seem to know where he is or what is happening to him, check with the nurse to see if she wants you to remain with the patient. If he is placed on a stretcher, be sure that the stretcher safety strap is fastened over his body so that he will not roll off as you go around sharp corners. If the patient is unconscious, if he has difficulty in breathing, if he is in great pain, or if he is receiving an intravenous infusion, ask the nurse for specific directions about caring for him during the off-ward trip. Ask her, too, what she wants you to do if his condition suddenly gets worse.

7. You go on your trip at the right time. You start out in ample time to reach the movies, the store, the church, or the place

where you work. Occasionally you might be late, but this is rare. When you are late, you feel apologetic. The patient, too, should arrive for his appointment on time. The staff members of the various diagnostic and therapeutic services in the hospital are busy and have spent much time and effort preparing the appointment schedule. If the patient is late, his study may very well be cancelled for that day. This would be upsetting to the patient and would delay his entire treatment program. Each morning, as you receive your patient care assignment from the head nurse or team leader, find out what appointments have been scheduled for your patients for that day. Then plan your patient care around the appointment schedule. Care for the patient with the earliest appointment first. Have him ready in a wheelchair or stretcher when the escort employee comes to the ward. If you are taking the patient, leave the unit in sufficient time to get to the appointment at the designated hour. Remember to ask the technician when the patient will be ready to return to the unit and be sure to return for him at that time. Minutes spent waiting in a strange, drafty corridor will seem like hours to the patient.

RETURNING THE PATIENT TO THE WARD

Return the patient to the ward promptly and help him get comfortable. This may mean assisting him back into bed (if he is a bed patient) or into a comfortable chair (if he is an out-of-bed patient). Every off-ward experience is frightening for the patient because it is a trip to the unknown; therefore let him tell you about his experiences. Think how you might make this same kind of experience less frightening and more comfortable for the next patient who is scheduled for such a trip.

SUMMARY

Prepare the patient for an off-ward trip to a diagnostic or therapeutic area in much the same way as you prepare yourself for a trip. This preparation would include the following:

1. Tell the patient where he is going and why (check with the nurse for an explanation as to why).
2. Be sure that the patient is clean.
3. Give the patient an opportunity to void and defecate.
4. Take with him those things he needs to be comfortable (cleansing tissue, emesis basin, glasses, etc.) and those things the doctor needs (chart, x-ray films).
5. Dress the patient adequately for the appointment.
6. Keep the patient safe by having him adequately identified with his wrist band and safely stabilized on the stretcher to prevent him from falling off.
7. Get him to the appointment on time and return him to the ward as soon as he is finished.

Although the patient may resist giving up his false teeth, he must do so when he goes to the operating room or to any diagnostic or treatment area where he will be put to sleep. If in doubt, check with the nurse before you let the patient leave the ward wearing his false teeth.

DISCUSSION QUESTIONS

1. Does your hospital have an escort service? If so, what is your job in getting the patient ready for a member of this service? If not, who takes the patients to their appointments?
2. How many of your patients have an off-ward trip to a diagnostic or therapeutic area tomorrow? Where are they going?
3. How do the appointments scheduled for your patients affect the way you will carry out your patient care assignment?
4. Do the patients like to go to the x-ray department? What do they say about their experiences there when they return?
5. Why must you be sure that the patient is properly identified by a wristband when he goes to an off-ward area for study or treatment?
6. How effectively could the patient relax during a basal metabolic rate (B.M.R.) test if he had to void?

7 Why are the patient's studies not done on the ward? Would this not save the hospital time and money?

VOCABULARY

basal metabolism test A breathing test done to determine the patient's minimum requirements for oxygen when he is at complete rest. This test gives some indication of how much energy the patient is using in living.

cancer A tumor that grows rapidly and may spread quickly to other areas throughout the body. It destroys the body cells in the area in which it is growing. The patient has symptoms related to the body area destroyed by the cancer, as well as the symptoms of pressure caused by the tumor and the pain from irritated nerve endings.

cardiac catheterization Passing a tube through a vein in the arm and into the heart to withdraw blood from the heart for laboratory examination.

cardiopulmonary laboratory Laboratory in which cardiac (heart) and pulmonary (lung) studies are done.

catheterization Passing a tube into a body cavity to withdraw fluids.

diagnostic Refers to any test, study, sign, or examination that helps the doctor establish the nature of the patient's illness.

electrocardiography Study of the electrical impulses produced by the heart (*cardio*, heart; *graphy*, study).

electroencephalography Study of the electrical impulses produced by the brain (*encephalo*, brain; *gram*, study).

esophagoscopy Passing an instrument into the esophagus to permit the doctor to inspect it carefully for disease.

gastroscopy Passing an instrument into the stomach to permit the doctor to inspect it (look at it through the instrument) to determine whether it is diseased.

physical therapy Treatment of disease by heat, light, water, and massage.

psychology The branch of science that studies the mind in an attempt to understand and interpret the basis for behavior.

psychotherapy Method of treating the patient with mental illness. It is conducted by a psychiatrist or a psychologist who helps the patient understand the reasons for his present abnormal behavior and who then helps him learn how to change his behavior to a more comfortable and less stressful pattern.

radiations Rays of energy.

radioactivity The emission, by certain substances, of rays that can penetrate solid matter. These rays can kill living cells if the exposure to them is beyond the permissible range.

radioisotope Substance that possesses radioactivity. These substances are used in carefully determined dosages to treat patients with cancer. However, they are also used for diagnostic purposes (for example, in the diagnosis of thyroid disease or goiter).

radiology The branch of medical science that uses x-ray for diagnostic or therapeutic purposes.

rehabilitation Treatment program to help the patient regain his ability to live effectively, consisting of such training as helping the amputee to learn how to use his artificial leg in order to walk or helping the patient who is recovering from a heart attack to learn how to tolerate the activities of living again.

therapeutic Refers to anything that lessens the patient's discomfort or aids in curing his disease.

unconsciousness Condition in which body functions under the control of the will are no longer operating. The patient does not know what is going on about him, and he does not react to his environment. He is unable to understand or to meet any of his own body needs.

x-ray film Photograph of the inside of the body taken through the tissues of the body.

SOURCE OF ADDITIONAL INFORMATION

1 Film: The patient is a person; may be obtained from American Hospital Association, Film Library, 840 North Lake Shore Drive, Chicago, Ill. 60611. *(Emphasizes the importance of regarding each patient as a person with individual needs.)*

43/Assisting the patient to get ready to go home

STUDY QUESTIONS

1. What are some clues that the patient is getting better?
2. Why do some patients want to go home, whereas others behave as though they would like to remain in the hospital?
3. Why is the "ward pet" more penalized than helped?
4. How can a patient's pattern of living be changed?
5. How can the patient learn a new pattern of living?
6. What kind of patients does the ward nurse refer to the visiting nurse?
7. How is the patient's unit cleaned after he is discharged?
8. Why is bar soap used to clean a unit?
9. Why are harsh disinfectants dangerous?
10. Why is the unit cleaned after a patient is discharged?

THE CURED PATIENT WHO IS READY TO GO HOME

As the patient loses his pain and discomfort and regains his feeling of well-being, he begins to think of his job and his family responsibilities. Each morning he questions the members of the staff about when he can go home. He explains how his wife needs him, how the children miss him, how his boss is unable to hold his job much longer, or even perhaps how his bowling team is losing the trophy because he is not participating. Each day he becomes more and more anxious to get out of the hospital.

When the day of discharge finally comes, the patient gets up early, dresses hurriedly, and waits impatiently for his family to arrive. He is so anxious to get home that he usually overexerts himself and is completely exhausted by the time his family arrives.

You can help the patient avoid overexertion by visiting him early in the morning and making a plan for getting him ready for discharge. Find out what time he expects his family. Then tell him to rest in bed until you return (and state the time of your return) to help him dress. Explain to him that this is a big day. His body, which has been resting and healing, is going to resume the entire load of normal living. Explain that his body will not be able to resume this load immediately. Just as his weakened, stiff legs have difficulty supporting the weight of his body after a long train or auto trip, so his weakened recovered body will have difficulty carrying the weight of normal living after his illness. Explain how the morning rest will conserve his strength for dressing and going home later.

Return at the designated time and help the patient get dressed. He will be excited and in a hurry, so your manner must be a calm, quiet, efficient one that soothes him and conserves his energy. As you help him dress, check to be sure that he knows when to return to the doctor, that he has his prescriptions, and that he understands any treatment he is to continue at home. Ask the nurse to discuss his posthospital care with him again if you feel that he does not understand it.

Pack his belongings in a suitcase. Check his bedside stand carefully to be sure that he has everything.

Ask the nurse how the patient is to be taken to the hospital entrance. Have the wheelchair in readiness if one is to be used.

When the family comes, assist the patient with his coat and hat, help him into a wheelchair (if necessary), take his suitcase, and escort the patient and his family to the unit desk. The clerk or the nurse will check with the business office and will tell you where the patient goes next. Escort the patient and his family to these hospital areas (usually the business office) and then take him to the hospital entrance. Assist the patient into his car or help the family get a cab and assist him into this. Return to the unit (with the wheelchair if one was used).*

---

*Do not take a tip from the patient even though he is extremely grateful for your care and offers you one. Hospital care is very costly, and the patient has probably just paid a bill much bigger than he can really afford. Then, too, the bill he paid includes all the payment for your care. You will be getting some of that money on payday in your salary.

THE PATIENT WHO IS GOING HOME WITH A PROBLEM

Some patients do not go home able to resume the normal pattern of living. Although the disease has been treated, cured, or arrested (stopped), the effects of it may remain. The patient's body may be changed in a way that makes it necessary for him to relearn some activity of living. Some examples of such a situation might be as follows:

1. The patient who had a stroke received treatments and medication that lowered his blood pressure, but his paralyzed arm and leg remain. He must relearn how to move, eat, and care for his toilet needs with one arm and one leg.
2. The patient's cancer of the rectum is removed, but now he has a colostomy through which the bowels move.
3. The patient's ulcer has been removed, but now he has only one third of his stomach remaining. He must eat five small meals a day instead of the usual three.
4. The patient's heart has been slowed down and strengthened. However, he is unable to do the hard work he once did and so he must change his occupation.
5. The patient's diabetes has been brought under control. However, he must take insulin injections and stay on a low-carbohydrate diet the rest of his life.

This patient's signs and symptoms of illness decrease, but he usually does not develop a great interest in going home. Instead, he usually develops the feeling that only the hospital personnel know how to help him, and he becomes more and more afraid to leave the hospital and go home. He may even manufacture symptoms in order to stay in the hospital, or he may become the "ward pet" so that he is kept there.

You must recognize the fact that any patient whose body is changed has a problem learning to live again. You must also recognize that the patient will be unable to learn a new way of living if it is not taught to him. As long as the hospital does this activity of living for him, he needs the hospital.

As the head nurse or team leader gives you an assignment, listen to it carefully. When she assigns you to help the patient with his care, help him; do not do it for him. The kind of patient care activities that the patient must learn to do for himself include the following:
1. Testing his urine for sugar and acetone
2. Controlling his colostomy through irrigations
3. Changing his colostomy or ileostomy bag
4. Taking his own digitalis (medicine to slow and strengthen the heart) and checking his own pulse
5. Taking his own reserpine (medicine to reduce blood pressure) and checking his own blood pressure
6. Planning and preparing his own diabetic diet
7. Planning and preparing his own postgastrectomy diet
8. Learning esophageal speech (talking with swallowed air—burps)
9. Suctioning his own tracheotomy

When you do for the patient what he must learn to do for himself, you are only making him more aware of the fact that he cannot leave the hospital. Remember that the patient does not take you home with him. Take the time and effort to help him relearn how to manage and control his changed body. When the patient has learned to care for his needs he begins to think of his job and his family responsibilities and he is ready to go home.

The nurse knows that the patient's living at home will be a little more difficult than it was in the hospital. Therefore she will send a referral to the visiting nurse and ask her to visit the patient at home to help him with his living activities there.

On the day of discharge, you assist the patient who is going home with a problem in exactly the same way as you help the cured patient. However, the nurse will probably explain, demonstrate, and give written directions to the family about the patient's care.

CLEANING THE UNIT AFTER THE PATIENT'S DISCHARGE

After the patient leaves the hospital, the unit must be thoroughly cleaned and prepared for the new patient. You can do this as follows:
1. Set up the following cleaning material on a movable table:
    a. Basin
    b. Bar of soap
    c. Two or three large-sized cleaning cloths
    d. Brush
    e. Can of metal polish
    f. Can of porcelain cleaner
2. Take the table of cleaning equipment and a linen hamper to the room or unit to be cleaned.
3. Strip the bed of all linen (including the wool blanket) and discard it in the linen hamper.
4. Remove the patient's glass and pitcher and place it on the lower shelf of the movable table.
5. Discard the patient's towel, hospital gown, and hospital robe into the linen hamper.
6. Move the linen hamper outside the room.
7. Open the window in the room or the window in the ward near the bed.
8. Fill the basin with warm water.
9. Wash the chair with a wet soap-filled cloth. Rinse the cloth and wipe the chair to remove the soap. Dry the chair.
10. Wipe the pillow with a dampened cloth.

11. Place the damp-dusted pillow on the freshly cleaned chair.
12. Wash, rinse, and dry the plastic-covered mattress. (If the mattress is not plastic covered, damp dust it thoroughly with the brush.)
13. Turn the mattress sideways on the bed to expose one half of the springs (Fig. 43-1).
14. Dip the brush in the water and damp dust the bed springs.
15. Wash, rinse, and dry the bed frame on the exposed half of the bed.
16. Flip the mattress that was turned sideways so that the cleaned top of the mattress is now resting on the cleaned bed springs. The other (uncleaned) half of the bed is now exposed.
17. Dip the brush in the water and damp dust this half of the springs.
18. Wash, rinse, and dry the bed frames on the second half of the bed.
19. Straighten the mattress on the bed.
20. Wash, rinse, and dry the second half (uppermost part) of the plastic-covered mattress or damp dust the uncovered mattress.
21. Wash, rinse, and dry the bedside stand, inside and outside.
22. Polish the bedside tabletop with metal polish.
23. Wash, rinse, and dry the overbed table or any other equipment in the room.
24. Scour the sink.
25. Wash, rinse, and dry the bed lamp and the call bell or communication system.
26. Take the table of cleaning equipment to the utility room and return with clean linen to make the bed.
27. Make the unoccupied bed for the next patient.
28. Return to the utility room and wash the cleaning basin thoroughly, scour and autoclave it (when possible), and then return it to its proper place.
29. Return the used pitcher and glass to the ward kitchen for cleaning or autoclave it for 20 minutes at 250° F.
30. Clean the work table and return it to its proper place.

Remember that a bar of soap is used in the cleaning procedure. If liquid soap is used, two basins of water must also be

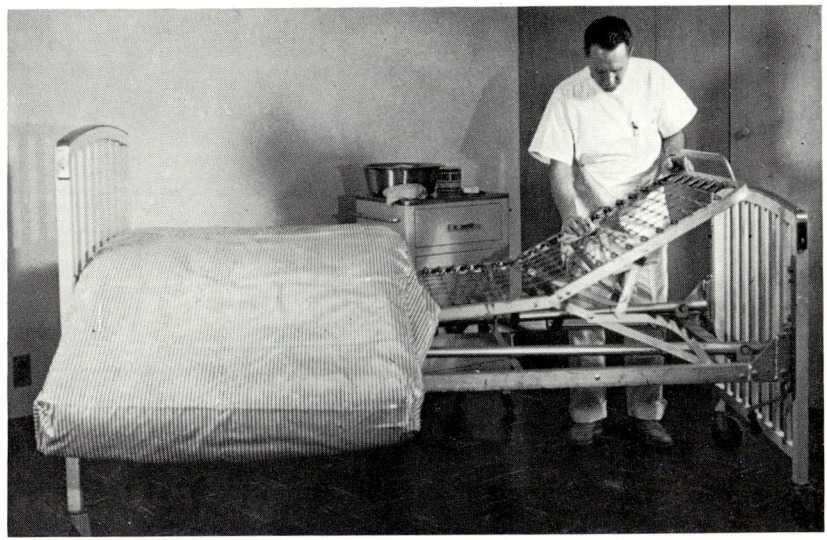

Fig. 43-1. Cleaning the patient's unit after he has been discharged.

used. One basin is filled with soapy water and used for washing, and the second basin is filled with clean water and is used for rinsing.

It is unnecessary to pour harsh disinfecting solutions into the water when you clean the patient's unit. Washing it well with soapy water, using a firm washing movement (friction), rinsing it thoroughly, and then drying it well will clean it adequately. Harsh disinfecting solutions will only irritate and excoriate your hands. Remember, we use our hands to care for the patient, and we clean them sufficiently by washing them with friction, soap, and water; therefore cleaning the bed with friction, soap, and water will suffice, too.

The method of cleaning a unit after the patient in isolation is discharged or taken out of isolation was already discussed. (See Chapter 33.)

Why the discharged patient's unit is cleaned

Every patient who comes to the hospital is sick. However, each patient has a different type of illness. Germs are present in body discharges such as sputum, feces, urine, nasal secretions, and pus. Therefore any hospital equipment that comes in contact with these secretions must be cleaned thoroughly before it can be safely used for another patient. The bed—the place where the patient eats, sleeps, takes care of toileting, and receives his treatments—has been in constant contact with body secretions. Therefore if it is not cleaned properly between patients, the bed may be covered with enough germs to infect the next patient and cause additional disease.

SUMMARY

The patient's bed—the place where he lives in the hospital—is in constant contact with body secretions and may be contaminated by germs. Therefore the bed must be washed thoroughly so that these germs will be removed after the patient is discharged and before the bed can be safely used for the next patient.

Bar soap and water together with firm washing movement (friction) are sufficient for ordinary cleaning. The hands you use for your personal care are cleaned adequately with soap, water, and friction to make it perfectly safe for you to use them to assist you in eating. Harsh disinfectants are not only unnecessary but are dangerous in that they dry and crack the skin on the hands.

The patient wants to go home when he is well if he is able to continue living in his usual way. If his body is changed so that his pattern of living must change, the patient will be afraid to go home until he knows how to carry out his new living easily and comfortably.

DISCUSSION QUESTIONS

1 Which patients assigned to you have a changed body that will necessitate their learning a new pattern of living?
2 How are you helping the patients referred to in question 1 learn the new pattern of living?
3 Discuss with the nurse those patients who must learn a new pattern of living and find out what more you can do to help them.
4 Carefully observe the patients assigned to you. Which ones are afraid to go home? Why?
5 Discuss with the nurse the patients referred to in question 4 and develop a plan for helping them to overcome their fear of going home.
6 How are your patient care units cleaned after a patient is discharged? Is this cleaning procedure adequate? Ask your nurse to send a culture from a cleaned mattress to the laboratory to find out if there are any disease-producing bacteria still present there.
7 If you use disinfectants, determine if they are necessary by performing the following experiment: Wash a bed with soap and take a culture from it. Then wash the bed with the disinfectant you usually use and take a culture from it. What are the differences in these cultures?
8 Should you accept a tip from a patient? Explain your answer.
9 Observe the patient's family. How anxious do they appear to be to take the patient home when his body is changed. Discuss with the nurse the ways you could help these visitors to understand and accept the patient with a changed body.

VOCABULARY

disinfectant Chemical that kills germs.
esophageal speech Speech produced by utilizing burps (swallowed air). The patient's voice box has been removed and he has a tracheotomy.
germicidal Germ-killing.
tracheotomy Opening made in the trachea (windpipe) to help the patient breathe.
visiting nurse Nurse who visits the patient in his home and gives him care. The patient pays for this care if he is able to do so.

SOURCES OF ADDITIONAL INFORMATION

1 Film: Almost a miracle; may be obtained from Public Health Service Audiovisual Facility, Chamblee, Ga. 30005; Attention: Film Distribution. *(Tells about the Visiting Nurse Service and shows how she cares for patients and their families.)*
2 Film: Basic care of patients, Part 1. Cleaning the patient's unit and making an unoccupied bed; may be obtained from United States Army (direct your request to Commanding General, Attention: Surgeon, of the Army area in which you reside).
3 Film: Nursing care: the diabetic patient; may be obtained from: Director, Medical Film Library, United States Naval Medical School, National Naval Medical Center, Bethesda, Md. 20014. *(Explains diabetes. Illustrates, for the hospital corpsman, the care of the diabetic patient, including urine testing, and teaching self-care.)*

Index

A

Abbreviations, 174
Abdominal distention, signs of, 359
Abdominoperineal resection, 228
Absolute bed rest, 108
Admission
　to hospital, 17-18
　to ward, 131-141
　　acquainting patient with facilities in, 134
　　initial interview in, 133-134
　　initial observations in, 132-135
　　recording information on patient chart in, 134-135
Adrenocortical hormones, effect on blood pressure, 187
Aged person; *see also* Nursing home resident
　care of, 395-403
　diseases of, 397-398
Alertness, 194
Alternating pressure mattress, 105
Ambulatory patient, safety of, 157
Amino acids, body use of, 41
Analgesics, effect on levels of consciousness, 196
Anesthesia
　general
　　effect on levels of consciousness, 196
　　state of patient returning from surgery with, 352
　local, 352
　spinal, 352-353
Anticholinergic drugs, in preoperative care, 348-349
Anxiety
　alleviation of, 16
　and blood pressure, 187
　and bowel movements, 219
　as characteristic of neurosis, 332-333
　and colostomy irrigation, 237
　and defecation, 81-82
　and digestive system, 44
　free-floating, 333
　in preoperative care, 344
　and pulse, 179
　as sign of oxygen need, 374

Aquamatic K-Pad, 264
Aramine, 188-189
Arteriosclerosis, 187
Artificial respiration, 387-391
Asepto syringe barrel, 45
Axilla, washing, 70

B

Ball-and-socket joint, normal movement of, 66
Barbiturates, 196
Bath
　alcohol sponge, 275-277
　cold sponge, 277
　complete bed, 67-74
　　body care in, 69-73
　　finishing, 70-73
　　mouth care in, 67-69
　ice-water sponge, 278-279
　medicated, 265-266
　　oatmeal, 266
　　saline, 266
　　starch, 265-266
　　sulfur, 266
　observations of patient's body during, 78
　out-of-bed, 74-78
　　on bath stretcher, 77
　　in bathroom, 74-75
　　shower, 76-77
　　time for, 78
　　in tub, 75-76
　partial bed, 74
　reasons for, 65-66
　sitz, 264-265
Bathroom privileges, for patient needing bed rest, 108
Bed
　with alternating pressure mattress, 105
　with alternating pressure pad, 32
　assisting patient out of and into chair, 109-115
　assisting patient out of and onto stretcher, 115-118
　with board under mattress, 32
　as body splint, 92-93
　Circ-O-lectric, 102-105

Bed—cont'd
　complications of lying in, 93-94
　with cradle, 32
　high-low, 32
　individualization of, 27
　patient who may get out of, 107
　positions of, 37-38
　positions of patient in, 96-102
　　face-lying, 97-98
　　side-lying, 96-97
　postoperative, 32
Bed rest, 108-109
　absolute, 108
　and ambulatory or out of bed ad lib, 109
　with bathroom privileges, 108
　dangling with, 108-109
　doctor's orders in, 108-109
　and out of bed
　　in chair for 30 minutes, 109
　　no weight bearing on right (left) leg, 109
　　on stretcher, 109
　　to use bedside commode, 108
　　walking, 109
Bed trapeze, 114
Bedmaking, 28-37
　aseptic precautions in, 36
　basic, 28
　　modifications of, 28, 32
　need for smoothness, 34, 36
　organization of, 36-37
Bedpan, assisting patient with, 82-84
Bedside commode, 84
Bile, role of, 46
Bisacodyl, 224
Bladder
　approach to in catheterization, 288
　exercises, 299
　reasons for problem in control of, 88-89
　training, 87
Bland diet, 44-45
Bleeding
　first aid for, 405-406
　internal, signs of, 405
Blood count, in preoperative care, 341-342
Blood pressure, 189-193
　conditions that affect, 187-188
　effect of adrenocortical hormones on, 187
　effects of high and low, 188-189
　equipment, 192
　normal, 187
　reporting of abnormal, 165
　taking, 186-193
Blood sugar, determination of, in preoperative care, 342
Blood supply, increased in infection, 260
Blood typing, in preoperative care, 342
Body functions, nervous control of, 81
Body heat, 167-168
Body needs; see Needs of body
Bowels
　control, of, reasons for problem in, 87-88
　retraining, 64
　training, 81

Breathing
　control of rate of, 372
　signs of difficulty in, 356
Breathlessness
　caring for patient with, 371-394
　reasons for, 373
Bromides, 196

C

Calcium, body use of, 41
Calorie, 55
Carbon dioxide intoxication, as sign of oxygen need, 374
Care, 4-5
　after-meal, 52
　before-meal, 52
　plan of, 136-139
　planning conference of, 9
　team, 9-14
Carotid artery, and taking pulse, 176
Cathartic, 222
Catheter, irrigating, 295-299
Catheterization; see also Urinary drain, internal
　dangers in, 293-295
　of female patient, 293
　as last resort, 295
　of male patient, 288-292
　reasons for, 287
　tray for Foley, 288
Cell
　use of food in, 41
　use of oxygen in, 41
Century tub, 76
Chest, x-ray film of, in preoperative care, 343
Chills, 272
Chlorpromazine hydrochloride, in treatment of shivering, 280
Circ-O-lectric bed, 102-105
Circulation, signs of interference in, 357
Circulatory system, 40
Codeine, 196
Colectomy, 249
Colostomy, 226-247
　irrigation of
　　patient assistance in, 243
　　procedure for, 234-242
　　purpose of, 234
　permanent, reasons for, 227-229
　reasons for, 227-228
　role of nursing assistant in, 246
　temporary
　　double-barreled, 228
　　reasons for, 227
　types of, significance in patient care of, 229-231
Colostomy bag
　disposable
　　applying, 233-234
　　emptying, 234
　permanent, care of, 245-246
Coma, 195
Communicable disease(s)
　caring for patient with, 303-323
　facts about common, 308

Communicable disease(s)—cont'd
  immunity from
    acquired, 306-307
    natural, 307
    skin in, 307
  nature of, 305
  prevention of spread of, 305
    handwashing in, 315-316
    protective techniques in, 307-309
    wearing protective clothing in, 310-311, 314-315
  protection of nursing assistant from, 306-307
Compresses, effect of cold, 281-282
Consciousness, levels of, 194-195
  charting, 197
  effect of drugs on, 196-197
  meanings of, 195
  observing, 195-197
  reporting abnormal, 165
Constipation, 50
  as result of bed immobilization, 93
  use of suppository in, 224
Convalescing patient, 143-146
Conversional-hysteria, 333
Convulsions, first aid for, 411-412
Culture
  feces, method of obtaining specimen for, 207
  urine, voided specimen for, 206-207
Cyanosis, 93, 373
Cyclopropane, 196

D

Dangling, and bed rest, 108-109
Davis roller, 117-118
Death, care of body after, 419-421
Decontamination
  of isolation unit, 320-321
  of items used in patient care in isolation unit, 321
Decubitus ulcers, 92, 94
  methods of prevention, 118-119
  in patient confined to bed, 92
Defecation, 49, 80-84
  assisting patient with lack of muscle control in, 84
  bedpan in, 82-84
  bedside commode in, 84
  effects of anxiety on, 81-82
  facilities for, 81-82
  reasons for problems with, 87-88
  suppository to stimulate, 224
Dehydration, 63, 359; see also Fluids, loss of
Delusions, as characteristic of psychosis, 333
Demerol, 196
Depression, 330
Diabetes, treatment for, 47
Diarrhea, 50
Diastole, 187
Diet
  bland, 44-45
  individualization of, 41
  low-fat, high-carbohydrate, high-protein, 47
  milk and cream, 44
  smooth food, 44-45

Diet card, 51
Digestion, 41
Digestive system, 40
  functions of, 41
    significance of, in feeding patient, 50-52
  influence of anxiety on, 44
  parts of, 42-50
    esophagus, 43
    functions of, 42-50
    large intestine, 49-50
    mouth, teeth, and tongue, 42
    small intestine, 45-49
    stomach, 43-45
    throat, 42-43
Digitalis, 59
Discharge of patient
  assisting in, 428-433
  cleaning of unit after, 430-432
  who is cured, 428-429
  who is going home with a problem, 429-430
Diuril, 59
Dorsalis pedis artery, and taking pulse, 176
Draeger respirator, in artificial respiration, 387-388
Drainage, postural, 382-383
Drainage tubes, postoperative care of patient with, 368-369
Drinker tank respirator, in artificial respiration, 388-390
Drinking water, 62
Dulcolax, 224
Duodenostomy, 48
Dying patient
  caring for, 413-422
  emotional care of, 414-415
  emotional support for family of, 417-418
  physical care of, 415-416
Dyspnea
  care of patient with, 376-378
  as sign of oxygen need, 373-374

E

Edema, 58-59, 92
Electric shock therapy, 336-337
Electrocardiogram, in preoperative care, 343-344
Electrolyte imbalance, signs of, 359
Electrolytes, 85
Embolus, 93
Emergencies, moving patient in, 120-121
Emotional health, care of, 142-146, 330-331
Emotional illness, 330-337
  caring for patient with, 329-338
  medication program in, 334
  role of nursing assistant in, 334-336
  signs and symptoms of, 332
  somatic therapies in, 336-337
  therapeutic environment in, 333-334
  treatment approach to, 331
  types of, 332-333
Enema
  administration of, 209-225
  barium, 222
  cleansing, expelled in 5 minutes, 209-211
    before proctoscopic or sigmoidoscopic examination, 222-223

Enema—cont'd
  cleansing, expelled in 5 minutes—cont'd
    giving prepackaged, 219-220
    procedure for, 213-219, 221-222
    reasons for failure of patient to expel, 218-219
  doctor's orders in, 212-224
  Fleet, 210
  order for in patient who is not eating, 223
  patient position for, 213
  prepackaged units, 210
  reasons for, 210-211
  retention, 209, 211-212
    administration of, 220-221
    medicated, 221
    never expelled, 212
    oil, 211, 212
    for period of time up to 4 hours, 211-212
    starch, 211, 212
  temperature of, 213
  types of, 209-212
  until clear, 210-211
Enterostomatist, 258
Escort service, 421
Esophagus, as part of digestive system, 43
Ether, 196, 212
Examination
  pelvic, assisting physician with, 136
  rectal, assisting physician with, 136-137
Exercises, 73-74
  bladder, 299
  deep-breathing and coughing in postoperative care, 365-366
  effect on pulse rate of, 179
  encouraging patient to do, 105

F

Fainting, first aid for, 409-410
Falling; see also Injuries to patient, falling
  first aid for, 410-411
Fatty acids, body use of, 41
Feeding
  gastrostomy, 45
  intravenous, 53, 55
  Levin tube, 52-55
  of unconscious patient, 52-55
Fever, 168-169, 271-272; see also Temperature, elevated
  effect on pulse rate, 179
  as sign of injury or infection, 261
Fire, patient evacuation procedures in, 120-121
First aid, 404-412
  for bleeding patient, 405-406
  circumstances calling for immediate, 404
  for convulsions, 411-412
  for fainting, 409-410
  mouth-to-mouth resuscitation in, 407-408
  for patient who falls, 410-411
  for shock, 409
  for suffocation, 406-409
  for suicidal patient, 410
Fleet enema, 210
Fluids
  amount needed by body, 58

Fluids—cont'd
  body requirements for, 58; see also Water
  extra, 62
  limiting intake of, 58-59
  loss of
    signs of extreme, 63
    sources of, 58
  recording input and output of, reasons for, 62-63
Foley catheterization tray, 288
Food
  body requirements for, 40-41
  use of in cell, 41
Foster frame, 98, 102

G

Gas, in intestine, 223
Gastrostomy, 45
Gastrostomy feeding, 45, 46
General anesthetics, effect on levels of consciousness, 196
General hospitals, 3
Genitalia, washing, 70
Germs, 305-306
  culture of, 202-203
  types of, 203
Glucose, body use of, 41
Glycerin, 224
Glycerol, body use of, 41

H

Hallucinations, as characteristic of psychosis, 333
Heat
  amount applied to body, 261-263
  application of
    Aquamatic K-Pad in, 264
    care of patient receiving, 263
    dangerous situations in, 273-274
    hot-water bottle in, 263
    for infection, 260-270
    lamp in, 263, 268
  excess, effect on body of, 272-273
Helplessness, as sign of oxygen need, 374
Hemiplegia
  assisting patient out of bed with, 110-111
  complication of feeding in, 42
Hemorrhage
  effect of, on blood pressure, 188
  effect of, on pulse rate, 179
  signs of, 356, 359
Heroin, 196
Home Health Aides, 5
Hospital
  and extended care facility, 3-5
  living in, helping patient adjust to, 135-136
  movement of patient about, 21-22
  ownership of, 3
  patient care in, 4-5
  patient care program of, and dying patient, 413-414
  patient's home in, 20-23
    changes of, 21
    needs in determining conditions of, 21
  programs of, 3-4

Hospital—cont'd
  purposes of, 3
  reasons patient comes to, 142-143
  responsibility of, 4
  types of, 3
Hot-water bottle
  giving patient, 264
  proper temperature for, 263
  times to use, 268
Hydrodiuril, 59
Hypertension, 188
Hypertrophy, 188
Hypnotics, 126-127, 196
Hypotension, 188
Hypothermia-hyperthermia machine, 279-281

I

Ice cap, application of, 279
Identification, needs for, 22
Ileostomy, 48
  caring for patient with, 248-254
  explanation of, 249-250
  reasons for, 248-249
  "wet"
    caring for patient with, 254-259
    explanation of, 256-257
    reasons for, 254-255
Ileostomy bag
  permanent, applying of, 252-254
  temporary, applying of, 251-252
Illness, emotional aspects of, 15
Immunity
  acquired, 306-307
  function of body secretions, in, 307
  function of skin in, 307
  natural, 307
Infection
  care of entire body in presence of, 269
  caring for patient with, role of nursing assistant in, 261
  elevating limb in presence of, 268-269
  heat in treatment of, 260-270
  signs of, 261
Injuries to patient
  falling, 147, 149-150
  signs of, 261
  wrong medication in, 147-149
Insulin, role of, 46-47
Insulin shock therapy, 336-337
Intensive care unit, 21
Intermittent positive pressure breathing therapy, 383-386
Intestinal system, 41
Intestines, gas in, 223
Intracranial pressure, signs of, 356
Intravenous feedings, 53, 55
Intravenous infusions
  determination of proper needle placement in, 189
  observations in, 189
Involuntary nervous system
  functions of, 81
  and sleep, 122-123
  and urination, 86

Isolation
  caring for patient in, 316-320
    giving fresh ice water in, 317
    giving a treatment in, 317-318
    off-ward trips in, 318-319
    removing bedpan or urinal in, 316-317
    serving patient's tray in, 316
    taking temperature, pulse, and respiration in, 319-320
  loneliness in, 304
  nursing care plan in, 327
  patient in, 303-304
    getting ready to care for, 311-314
  reverse; *see* Reverse isolation
Isolation unit, 309-310
  decontamination of, 320-321
  patient leaves, 320
Isuprel, 382, 383

J

Jaundice, 47
Jejunostomy, 48
Joints
  ball-and-socket, 66
  sliding, 66

K

Kardex, 12

L

Large intestine, as part of digestive system, 49-50
Laryngectomy, 45
Levin tube feedings, 52-55
Levophed, 188-189
Lift
  mechanical, 113-114
  one-man, in emergencies, 120-121
  three-man, 119-120
  two-man, 111-113
Loneliness, as problem in isolation, 304
Low-fat, high-carbohydrate, high-protein diet, 47
LSD, 196
Lung complications, after surgery, 343
Lung congestion, signs of, 359

M

Mechanical lift, 113-114
Medicated bath; *see* Bath, medicated
Meperidine hydrochloride, 196
Milk and cream diet, 44
Morphine, 196
Mouth care
  in bed bath, 67-69
  frequency of, 69
Mouth, teeth, and tongue, as part of digestive system, 42
Mouth-to-mouth resuscitation, 407-408
Movement
  body's need for, 91-92
  exercises for, encouraging patient to do, 105
  meeting patient's need for, 94-102
  normal body, 66-67
Moving of patient
  assisting out of bed into chair in, 109-115

Moving of patient—cont'd
  assisting out of bed onto stretcher in, 115-118
  with breathing difficulty, 117-118
  with Davis roller, 117-118
  getting out of bed in, 107-121
  mechanical lift in, 113-114
  one-man carry for emergencies in, 120-121
  quick, of helpless patient, 119-120
  three-man carry in, 119-120
  two-man lift in, 111-113
  use of bed trapeze in, 114
Mucomyst, 382, 383

N

Nasal oxygen, administering in postoperative care, 363-365
Needs of body
  movement; see Movement, body's need for
  in presence of infection, 260-261
  urination and defecation, 80-90
  water; see Fluids; Water
Needs of patient, 18-19
  cleanliness and movement, 65-79
  for cleanliness, difficulty in, 161
  comfortable bed as, 27-39
  emotional, 15-16
  feeling of dignity, signs of difficulty in, 161
  food, 40-56, 160
  freedom from discomfort as, signs of difficulty in, 161
  in getting out of bed, 107-121
  identifying, recording, and reporting, 159-164
  mental and emotional, 19
  movement, 91-106, 160-161
  nursing assistant meeting particular, 129-300
  oxygen, 371-372
    factors that increase, 374-375
    signs and symptoms of, 373-374
  physical, 18-19
  sleep, 122-127, 161-162
  water, 57-64, 160
Neomycin, in enema, 212
Nervous system
  involuntary
    functions of, 81
    and sleep, 122-123
  voluntary
    functions of, 81
    and sleep, 122-123
Neurosis, 332-333; see also Emotional illness
Night rounds, observations in, 162
Nonanalgesics, effects on levels of consciousness, 196
Nurse, duties of, 6-7
Nursing assistant, duties of, 6-8
  assisting doctor in, 7-8
  care of patient's hospital home in, 7
  meeting patient's basic daily needs in, 25-127
  patient care in, 7
  training program for, 10-11
Nursing care team, 9-10
  operation of, 13
  role of leader in, 11-13
Nursing home, 395

Nursing home assistant, problems of, 400
Nursing home resident, 396; see also Aged person
  caring for, 398-399
  living needs of, 396-397
  special problems in care of, 400-402

O

Observation of patient, 159
  clues to report in, 160-163
    method of reporting, 162-163
  reporting of abnormal vital signs in, 165-166
Off-ward trip
  care of patient in, 423-427
  escort service and, 424
  preparing patient for, 424-426
  returning patient after, 426
One-man lift, in emergencies, 120-121
Operation, preparing to receive patient after, 349
Osteoporosis, 93
Ostomy bag, applying temporary, 242-243
Ostomy, care of patient with, 258
Overactive patient, 336
Oxygen therapy, 378-382
Oxygen, use of in cell, 41; see also Needs of patient, oxygen

P

Packs
  cool wet
    applying, 277-278
    using fan with, 278
  ice water sponge, 278-279
Paraldehyde, 196, 212
Patient
  admission of; see Admission
  convalescing, 143-146
  dying; see Dying patient
  emotional health of, 142-146, 330-331
  moving of; see Moving of patient
  needs of; see Needs of patient
  observation of; see Observation of patient
  as person, 17-19
  safety of; see Safety of patient
  special, meeting needs of, 301-433
Pelvic examination, assisting physician with, 136
Pentothal sodium, 196
Peristalsis, 48
Phobia, as characteristic of neurosis, 333
Physician's examination, 136-138
Planning conference, 9, 11
Positions
  face-lying, 97-98
  side-lying, 96-97
  Trendelenburg, 188
Posterior tibial artery, and taking pulse, 177
Postoperative care, 351-370
  administering nasal oxygen in, 363-365
  applying binder to abdomen in, 368
  applying elastic bandages in, 366-368
  clues to difficulty in, 360-361
  deep-breathing and coughing exercises in, 365-366
  after 48 hours, 359-360

Postoperative care—cont'd
  of patient after regaining consciousness, 357-359
  preparing recovery room in, 351-354
  suctioning throat in, 361-363
Postural drainage, 382-383
Preoperative care, 339-350
  aim of, 341
  anxiety in, 344
  day before surgery, 345-347
  morning of surgery, 347-349
  night before operation, 347
  preparation of patient's body in, 341-344
    blood count in, 341-342
    blood typing in, 342
    electrocardiogram in, 343-344
    urinalysis in, 342-343
    x-ray film of chest in, 343
  shaving hair in, 345-346
  signing operative permit in, 346
  special, 344-345
  variation in length of, 341
Proctoscopic examination, cleansing enema before, 222-223
Promethazine hydrochloride, in treatment for shivering, 280
Psychosis, 333
Psychosomatic complaints, as characteristic of neurosis, 333
Pulse
  charting, 198-200
  correct time for taking, 177-178
  definition of, 176
  elevated rate, as sign of injury or infection, 261
  factors affecting rate of, 179
  normal rate of, 179-180
  places for counting, 176-177
  reporting of abnormal, 165
  rhythm and volume of, observations of, 178-179
  taking, 176-180
Pulse graph, 199-200

R

Radial artery, and taking pulse, 176
Recovery room, 21
  immediate care of patient in, 355-357
  nursing care in, 352
  receiving patient in, 354-355
Rectal bladder
  caring for patient with, 257
  and colostomy, 256
  explanation of, 255-256
  reasons for, 254-255
Rectal examination, assisting physician with, 136-137
Respiration
  charting, 198-200
  control of, 182-183
  counting, 181-185
  definition, 181
  normal, 183
  process of, 181-182
  rate of
    conditions that decrease, 194

Respiration—cont'd
  rate of—cont'd
    conditions that increase, 183-184
    elevated, as sign of injury or infection, 166
Respiration graph, preparing, 199-200
Respiratory arrest, 386-391
Respiratory complications, prevention of, 376
Respiratory distress
  from obstruction of airway, 378
  from oxygen need, 378-382
  from patient's failure to breathe, 386-391
  from retention of secretions or trapped air, 382-383
  treatment for, 378-391
Respiratory system, 40, 375-376
Restlessness, 194-195
Restraining devices, 151-153
  arm and leg, 151-153
  chest harness as, 151
  complications in use of, 154
  safety belt as, 151
  safety net as, 151
Reverse isolation
  caring for patient in, 324-328
  problem of staff health in, 324-325
  reasons for, 323
  unit for, 325-326
    protecting patient in, 326-327

S

Safety of patient, 147-158
  ambulatory, 157
  in bed, 150-153
    arm and leg restraints in, 151-153
    chest harness in, 151
    safety belt in, 151
    safety net in, 151
  in chair, 154-157
    supportive measures in, 155-156
  during treatment, 153-154
  maintaining safe environment in, 147-158
  matching patient to prescribed treatment in, 147-149
  prevention of falling in off-ward areas, 157-158
Serum, 58
Shaving hair, 345-346
Shock, first aid for, 409
Shock position, 188
Sigmoidoscopic examination, cleansing enema before, 222-223
Sitz bath, 264-265
Sleep
  individualization of amounts needed, 124-125
  interruption of, reasons for, 123
  observations of, 126
  patient's need for, 122-127
  preparing patient for, 125-126
Sleeping pills, 126-127
Sleeplessness
  consequences of, 162
  as sign of oxygen need, 373
Sliding joint, normal movement of, 66
Small intestine, as part of digestive system, 45-49

Smears, 202
Smooth food diet, 44-45
Soaks
  arm, 266
  continuous warm wet, 266-268
  foot, 266
Social relationships, 330
Specialty hospitals, 3
Specimens
  biopsies, 204
  blood, 204
  collecting, 201-208
  as diagnostic measure, 201-202
  feces, 204
  identification of germs from, 202-203
  information obtained from, 203-205
  kinds of, 202
  obtained by needle aspiration, 202
  obtained by resection, 202
  spinal fluid, 204
  sputum, 204
  urine, 204
Stomach, as part of digestive system, 43-45
Stupor, 195
Suffocation, first aid for, 406-409
Suicide, 330
  attempted, first aid for, 410
  preventing, 336
Supportive devices for patient in chair, 156-157
Suppository, 224
Surgery, lung complications after, 343
Swallowing, 42
Systole, 187

T

Team assignment, 11
Temperature
  charting, 198-200
  definition of body, 167-168
  elevated
    in postoperative period, 361
    reducing, 274-279
    role of nursing assistant in reducing, 282
  how body reduces, 274
  how brain controls, 271
  methods of taking
    axillary, 170
    choice of, 170
    oral, 169-170
    rectal, 169-170
  normal body, 168
  reducing, 271-283
  reporting of, 169
    abnormal, 165
  slight elevation in, dangerous situations in, 273
  taking, 167-175
  very high or very low, verifying, 169
Temperature graph, 199-200
Temporal artery, and taking pulse, 176
Thermometer, 167
  oral, 169
  reading, 170-172
  rectal, 169-170

Thiopental sodium, 196
Thirst, 57
Three-man lift, 119-120
Throat
  as part of digestive system, 42-43
  suctioning of, in postoperative care, 361-363
Trendelenburg position, 188
Two-man lift, 111-113

U

Unconscious patient
  feeding of, 52-55
  meeting toilet needs of, 416-417
  safeguarding belongings of, 418-419
Uremia, 59
Ureterostomy
  caring for patient with, 254-259
  explanation of, 257
  reasons for, 254-255
Urinals, cleaning, 87
Urinalysis, in preoperative care, 342-343
Urinary control problem, patient with, 284-285
Urinary drain
  external
    applying, 285-287
    caring for patient with, 286-287
    reasons for, 285
  internal; see Catheterization
    reasons for, 287
  internal and external, 284-300
Urinary system, 40
  function and description of, 285
  output of, 59
Urination, 84-87
  facilities for, 85-86
  increased, care of patient with, 86-87
  patient with problems with, 88-89

V

Visiting Nurses Service, 5
Vital signs, 165-166
  changes in, as result of infection, 261
  charting, 198-200
Vitamins
  body use of, 41
  K, role of, 46
Voiding; see Urination
Voluntary nervous system
  functions of, 81
  and sleep, 122-123

W

Wakefulness, 123
Water
  body use of, 41
  drinking, 62
  patient needing increased intake and output of, 62-63
  recording intake and output of, 59-62
Weighing, 138
White blood cell count, normal, 261
Wrist labels, purpose of, 149
Wyamine, 188-189